PRECLINICAL SPEECH SCIENCE

Anatomy Physiology Acoustics Perception

Thomas J. Hixon, Ph.D
Gary Weismer, Ph.D
Jeannette D. Hoit, Ph.D

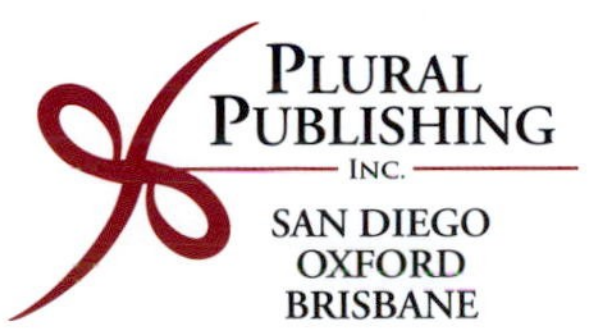

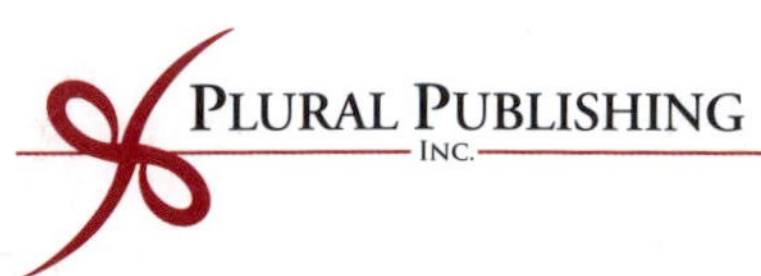

5521 Ruffin Road
San Diego, CA 92123

e-mail: info@pluralpublishing.com
Web site: http://www.pluralpublishing.com

49 Bath Street
Abingdon, Oxfordshire OX14 1EA
United Kingdom

Typeset in 10.5/13 Palatino by Flanagan's Publishing Services, Inc.
Second printing, April 2009. Printed in Hong Kong by Paramount Printing.

Library of Congress Cataloging-in-Publication Data:

Hixon, Thomas J., 1940-
Preclinical speech science : anatomy, physiology, acoustics, and perception / Thomas J. Hixon, Gary G. Weismer, and Jeannette D. Hoit.
p. ; cm.
Includes bibliographical references and index.
ISBN-13: 978-1-59756-182-2 (alk. paper)
ISBN-10: 1-59756-182-7 (alk. paper)
1. Speech--Physiological aspects. 2. Respiratory organs--Anatomy. 3. Respiration. 4. Speech perception. 5. Phonetics, Acoustic. I. Weismer, Gary. II. Hoit, Jeannette D. (Jeannette Dee), 1954- III. Title.
[DNLM: 1. Speech--physiology. 2. Respiratory System--anatomy & histology. 3. Speech Disorders. 4. Speech Perception. WV 501 H676p 2008]
QP306.H59 2008
612.7'8--dc22

2008007787

Contents

Acknowledgments

There are many people to thank for the book you see before you. Maury Aaseng created the artwork for the book. His images reflect his enormous talent and add a special dimension to the book. Sandy Doyle oversaw the production of the book from beginning to end. Her thoughtful thumbprint is on the text in many ways. Many colleagues and students made important contributions through their advice on content and their critiques on different sections. These include Julie Barkmeier-Kraemer, Sam Brown, Kate Bunton, Yun-Ching Chung, Susan Ellis Weismer, Harry Hollien, Kristen Kalend, Joel Kahane, Yunjung Kim, Dave Kuehn, Amy Lederle, Julie Liss, Robin Samlan, Sara Finch Schubert, and Brad Story. The University of Wisconsin-Madison provided GW with two sabbaticals that provided much needed release time to complete work on this text. Finally, the considerable guidance and encouragement of Angie Singh and Sadanand Singh during the long course of this project deserves special recognition.

1

Introduction

Welcome to *Preclinical Speech Science: Anatomy, Physiology, Acoustics, Perception*. Two preliminaries are offered here at the start. One is a discussion of the focus of the book. The other is a discussion of the domain of preclinical speech science.

FOCUS OF THE BOOK

Preclinical Speech Science: Anatomy, Physiology, Acoustics, Perception is designed as an introduction to the fundamentals of speech science (inclusive of voice science) that are important to aspiring clinicians and practicing clinicians. The text is suitable for courses that cover the anatomy and physiology of speech production and swallowing, and the acoustics and perception of speech. The material is user friendly to beginning students, yet integrative and translational for graduate students and practicing speech-language pathologists. Certain topics in the text are novel to the speech science and speech-language pathology literatures and suggest important new conceptualizations.

This book is an outgrowth of the three authors' many years of teaching experience with several thousand undergraduate and graduate students. The development of the book is the result of a sifting and winnowing of the broad range of facts, principles, and methods associated with its topics. The outcome is an integrated fabric that is a logical precursor for clinical study and practice. The age-old questions of "What should I study for the final examination?" and "Which parts of the material are most relevant to me clinically?" are answerable as "Everything in the book." Chapters in the book are infused with clinical scenarios, sidetracks of clinical and historical interest, considerations of the scientific bases of clinical protocols and methodologies, and discussions of clinical personnel involved in the evaluation and management of disorders of speech production, speech, and swallowing.

The illustrations are a key feature of this book. These are done by a single illustrator and provide a consistency that will appeal to students and instructors. These original illustrations, largely in full color, are supplemented by a small number of illustrations from other sources. The original illustrations were carefully chosen and drafted to convey only salient features, an approach in line with the written text. Occasional cartoons lighten the material, but carry educational messages.

DOMAIN OF PRECLINICAL SPEECH SCIENCE

The domain of preclinical speech science is portrayed in Figure 1–1. This domain encompasses speech production, speech acoustics, speech perception, and swallowing. Within this domain, consideration is given to levels of observation, subsystems of speech production and swallowing, and applications of data.

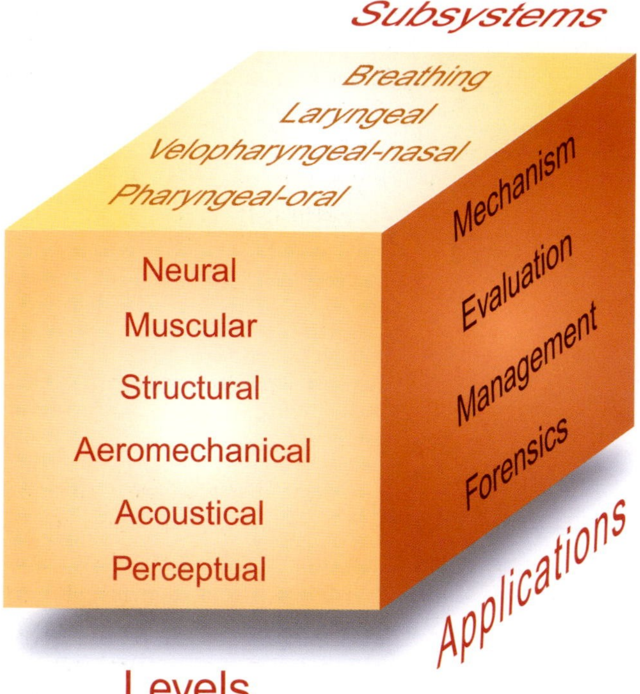

Figure 1–1. Domain of preclinical speech science.

Levels of Observation

Speech production and swallowing are processes. They result in acoustical products (more so for speech than swallowing) and perceptual experiences. These processes, products, and experiences involve different levels of observation. Six such levels are represented in Figure 1–1: (a) neural, (b) muscular, (c) structural, (d) aeromechanical, (e), acoustical, and (f) perceptual.

The *neural* level of observation encompasses nervous system events during speech production and swallowing. These include all events that qualify as motor planning and execution and all forms of afferent and sensory information that influence the ongoing control of speech production and swallowing. The neural level of observation pertains to the parts of the brain, spinal cord, and cranial and spinal nerves important to speech production and swallowing and to all underlying neural mechanisms, some voluntary and some automatic, some that involve awareness, and some that do not. Neural data are often derived from physical or metabolic imaging methods that reflect patterns of activation of different regions of the brain. Activation at the neural level can also be inferred from events associated with other (downstream) levels of observation.

The *muscular* level of observation is concerned with the influence of muscle forces on speech production and swallowing. Muscle forces are responsible for powering these two processes. Muscles are effectors that respond to control signals from the nervous system. The muscular events of speech production and swallowing are manifested in mechanical pulls and are often indexed at the periphery through the electrical activities associated with muscle contractions. Inferences about muscle activities are also made from measurements of the forces or movements generated by different parts of the speech production apparatus and swallowing apparatus. Nevertheless, there are ambiguities introduced when attempting to infer individual muscle activities from forces or movements, because forces and movements are usually accomplished by groups of muscles working together. Such inferences, if they can be made at all, require a detailed knowledge of anatomy and physiology.

The *structural* level of observation deals with movements of the speech production apparatus and swallowing apparatus. This level of observation is concerned with the displacements, velocities, and accelerations/decelerations of structures and how they are timed in relation to the movements of other structures. Certain structural observations can be made with the naked eye, whereas others are hidden from view or are too rapid to be followed with the naked eye and require the use of instrumental monitoring. To the person on the street, the structural level of observation is public evidence of speech production and swallowing. Speech reading (lip reading) has its roots at this level of observation.

The structural movements of speech production and swallowing give rise to an *aeromechanical* level of observation. It is at this level that air comes into play. Movements of structures impart energy to the air by compressing and decompressing it and causing it to flow from one region to another. The raw airstream generated in association with the aeromechanical level is modified by structures of the speech production apparatus and swallowing apparatus that lie along various passageways. The products of the aeromechanical level are complex, rapid, and nearly continuous changes in air pressures, airflows, and air volumes. These products are usually "invisible," especially for swallowing. However, those who speak and smoke at the same time or who speak in subfreezing temperatures often provide the observer with the opportunity to visualize certain aeromechanical events.

The *acoustical* level of observation is fully within the public domain. Although certain aspects of swallowing may be accompanied by sounds, primacy at this level pertains to the generation of speech sounds. The raw material of the acoustical level is the buzz-like, hiss-like, and pop-like sounds that result from the speaker's valving of the airstream in different ways and at different locations within the speech production apparatus. This raw material is filtered and conditioned by its passage through the apparatus and radiates from the mouth or nose, or both, in the form of nearly continuous changes in atmospheric pressure. The sound waves that are formed propagate spherically from the speaker and can be coded in terms of frequency, sound pressure level, and time. These sound waves are what constitute speech, an acoustical representation of language. The acoustical level is important in face-to-face communication and in the use of telephones, radios, televisions, and various forms of recording. It is this level that makes it possible for many listeners to be engaged simultaneously and makes it possible to communicate effectively around corners, through obstacles, in the dark, and over long distances.

The *perceptual* level of observation has somewhat different manifestations for speech production and swallowing. For speech production, it pertains primarily to auditory events. Kinesthesia (movement sensation), proprioception (position-in-space sensation), and touch-pressure sensation are important as bases for staying informed about ongoing speech production events, but the principal factor is audition (hearing sensation). Visual information is sometimes important as well, and experience and knowledge of the language is critical for extracting meaning from speech. In contrast, swallowing is highly dependent on kinesthesia, touch-pressure sensation, and even taste, with relatively little reliance on auditory or visual information. Cognitive processes contribute to various degrees at the perceptual level of observation for both speech production and swallowing.

The levels of observation portrayed in Figure 1–1 are not completely separate entities, but have important interactions. These interactions are not shown in the figure, but are discussed in subsequent chapters.

Subsystems of Speech Production and Swallowing

The speech production apparatus and the swallowing apparatus perform different activities. However, they share many structural and functional components and, although different in their control and movement, can be viewed along similar lines. It is convenient, for discussion purposes, to partition the speech production apparatus and swallowing apparatus into subsystems. Speech production subsystems may differ when chosen by a linguist versus a speech scientist versus a speech-language pathologist. And swallowing subsystems may differ when chosen by a swallowing scientist versus a gastroenterologist versus a speech-language pathologist. For the purposes of this book, four subsystems are used for speech production and swallowing. As illustrated in Figure 1–1, these include the (a) breathing apparatus, (b) laryngeal apparatus, (c) velopharyngeal-nasal apparatus, and (d) pharyngeal-oral apparatus. The role of each of these subsystems is considered in detail in subsequent chapters. The functional significance of each of the four subsystems differs between speech production and swallowing, but each subsystem is critically important to its respective behaviors and each manifests in clinical signs that can reveal abnormality.

The *breathing* apparatus is defined in the present context to include structures below the larynx within the neck and torso. These are, most importantly, the pulmonary apparatus (pulmonary airways and lungs) and chest wall apparatus (rib cage wall, diaphragm, abdominal wall, and abdominal content). The breathing apparatus provides the driving forces for speech production, while simultaneously serving the functions of ventilation and gas exchange.

During swallowing, the breathing apparatus engages in a period of apnea (breath holding) to protect the pulmonary airways and lungs from the intrusion of unwanted substances (food and liquid). The breathing apparatus is the largest of the subsystems and its role in speech production and swallowing is fundamentally important.

The *laryngeal* apparatus lies between the trachea (windpipe) and the pharynx (throat) and adjusts the coupling between the two. At times, the laryngeal airway is open to allow air to move in and out of the breathing apparatus, whereas at times it is adjusted to obstruct or constrict the airway. During speech production, obstructions and constrictions enable the generation of transient and sustained noises, respectively. Very rapid to and fro movements of the vocal folds within the larynx create voiced sounds and give the laryngeal apparatus its colloquial label "voice box." For swallowing, the laryngeal apparatus is active in closing the laryngeal airway to protect the pulmonary airways. Food and liquid are then able to pass over and around the larynx and into the esophagus on their way to the stomach.

The *velopharyngeal-nasal* apparatus is positioned between the pharyngeal and nasal cavities and adjusts the coupling between the two. The velopharyngeal-nasal airway is open when breathing through the nose. During speech production, the size of the velopharyngeal port varies, depending on the nature of the speech produced. For example, consonant sounds that require high oral air pressure are typically associated with airtight closure of the velopharyngeal port, whereas nasal consonants are associated with an open velopharyngeal port. Function of the velopharyngeal-nasal apparatus during swallowing is concerned mainly with keeping the velopharynx sealed airtight. This prevents the passage of food and liquid into the nasal cavities, while substances are moved backward and downward through the oropharynx.

The *pharyngeal-oral* apparatus comprises the pharynx, oral cavity, and oral vestibule. During running speech production, the apparatus is open during inspiration and makes different adjustments for consonant and vowel productions during expiration, including the generation of transient, voiceless, and voiced sounds and the filtering of those sounds. During swallowing, the pharyngeal-oral apparatus prepares food and liquid for propulsion through the apparatus in transit to the esophagus.

Applications of Data

There are many applications of data obtained about speech production and swallowing. These applications depend on who selects and defines the data and what the goals are for collecting and analyzing them. For the purposes of this book, applications of data are categorized into four areas: (a) mechanism, (b) evaluation, (c) management, and (d) forensics. These four are shown in Figure 1–1.

One application of data is the understanding of *mechanism*. This use provides the foundational bases for knowing how speech is produced and how swallowing is performed. Such foundational bases are important for their heuristic value in elucidating fundamental processes and working principles and for differentiating normal from abnormal.

Another application of data is its use in *evaluation*. This use is usually practical in nature and involves quantitative determinations of the status and functional capabilities of an individual's speech production, speech, and swallowing. Evaluation first enables a determination as to whether or not abnormality exists. If abnormality does exist, then appropriate evaluation may contribute to (a) making a diagnosis, (b) developing a rational, effective, and efficient management plan, (c) monitoring progress during the course of management, and (d) providing a reasonable prognosis as to the extent and speed of improvement to be expected. For example, a specific use of subsystems analysis in the evaluation of speech production is the determination of how individual subsystems contribute to deficits in speech intelligibility. Two individuals may have equivalent intelligibility problems as determined by formal tests, but have different subsystems "explanations" for their deficits. The careful evaluation of subsystems performance can point to which parts of the speech production apparatus may be particularly responsible for speech intelligibility deficits, and how those parts should be addressed in management to improve intelligibility. Evaluation relies on an understanding of what constitutes normal function.

A third application of data is *management*. Different interventions may be based on any of the six levels of observation and include any of the four subsystems of speech production and swallowing. Different management strategies may include adjusting individual variables or combinations of variables, staging the order of different interventions, and providing feedback about speech production and swallowing processes, products, and experiences. Management data provide information about outcome and whether or not interventions are effective, efficient, and long lasting. Management data can also be used to compare and contrast different interventions to arrive at optimal choices.

The remaining application of data is their use in *forensics*. This application is concerned with scientific facts and expert opinion as they relate to legal issues. The speech scientist and speech-language pathologist are sometimes called on to give legal depositions or to testify in courts of law in a variety of forensic contexts. Forensic uses of data may include issues pertaining to speaker identification, speaker status under the influence of drugs or alcohol, and speaker intent at deceit, among others. Forensic uses of data may also relate to personal injury claims or malpractice claims. These may involve speech production, speech, or swallowing alone, or in different combinations, and may include adversarial depositions and testimonies of other experts. Under such circumstances, the status and capabilities of the individuals claiming personal injury or malpractice may be considered from the perspective of underlying mechanism, evaluation, and management.

REVIEW

Preclinical Speech Science: Anatomy, Physiology, Acoustics, Perception is intended as an introduction to the fundamentals of speech science (inclusive of voice science) that are important to aspiring clinicians and practicing clinicians.

The text is suitable for different courses that cover anatomy and physiology of speech production and swallowing, and the acoustics and perception of speech.

The material in the text is strongly integrative and translational, applicable to both undergraduate and graduate students, and a source of continuing education and reference for practicing speech-language pathologists.

The domain of preclinical speech science encompasses different levels of observation, different subsystems of speech production and swallowing, and different applications of data.

Levels of observation include the neural, muscular, structural, aeromechanical, acoustical, and perceptual levels.

Subsystems of speech production and swallowing include the breathing apparatus, laryngeal apparatus, velopharyngeal-nasal apparatus, and pharyngeal-oral apparatus.

Applications of data include the understanding of mechanism, evaluation, management, and forensics.

Sidetracks

Throughout the book you'll find a series of sidetracks. These are short asides that relate to topics being discussed in the main text. Many of the sidetracks in the book are a bit less formal and a bit more lighthearted than the main text they complement. This is intended to enhance your reading enjoyment and to put some fun in your study of the material. We hope you enjoy reading these sidetracks as much as we enjoyed writing them.

2

Breathing and Speech Production

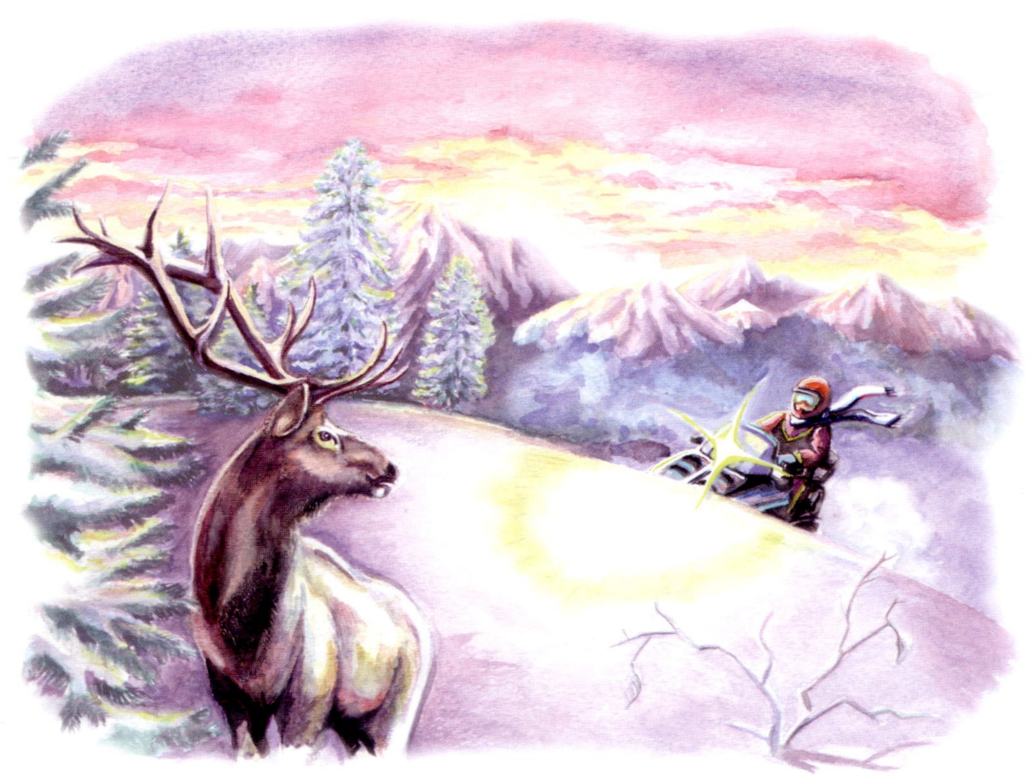

Scenario

The continental divide was in sight. It was near dusk and the peaks of the San Juan Mountains were pink with the last sun of December. This was a time of day she loved. She had just turned 20. He was 4 years old. He weighed 500 lbs, was massive through the shoulders, and respected. She weighed less than 100 lbs, was petite, and a college sophomore favorite of her classmates. His winter life was about survival and moving slowly. Hers was about thrills and a craving for speed.

When she crested the hill they met. The headlight of her snow machine momentarily shined on his eyes and his massive antlers. The impact was full on and it was over in a few seconds. She never managed to scream. His life was snapped and hers changed forever. She awoke to a new vibration and the sound of a voice on a radio. She was strapped down, her head, neck, and body braced. She heard talk of Durango and the activation of landing pad lights. She tried to move but could not. Her arms and legs had taken leave from her control. Her worst fears were confirmed in the emergency room. It was an unmercifully long night full of tears.

The morning's choice was Denver or Albuquerque, where a new mountain would have to be climbed, one higher than any she had ever seen or imagined. By midday a decision was made, with her family, and she again would hear the sound of a voice on a radio. This time it was in a fixed-wing air ambulance that was given clearance for takeoff on runway 9 with a straight-out departure. From then on she slept, with a flight nurse and her mother at her side. Denver came into sight below the front range of the Rocky Mountains. She was now on a leave of absence of indeterminate duration from her studies in veterinary science.

Six months passed and her abilities and disabilities were now known and part of her new life. Her spirit was returning and she had some optimism, some of it realistic and some of it not. She had a cervical spinal cord lesion (C6) and was quadriplegic, except for some movement in her arms and hands. She was thinking about getting a service dog to assist her with daily activities. A counselor from an agency visited with her and expressed some concern about whether or not she could control a dog because her voice was so soft. Her neurologist made a referral to a speech-language pathologist with a request to determine her potential to increase the power of her voice.

Auditory-perceptual examination revealed problems with reading aloud, extemporaneous speaking, and conversational speaking. Her speech was low in loudness, characterized by short breath groups (typically about 4 syllables each), and interspersed with relatively slow inspirations. Her speech phrasing was abnormal and her voice trailed off and became inaudible toward the ends of her expirations. She could not increase her loudness much, could not generate heavily stressed syllables, and could not increase the lengths of her speech expirations. She tired when speaking for more than a couple of minutes and needed to take frequent breaks while conversing to "catch her breath." Her conversational style was low keyed and gave the impression that she lacked energy. She reported that her breathing was uncomfortable when she spoke for too long and that it took a lot of effort to speak.

Physical examination revealed paralysis of the abdominal wall and severe paresis of the rib cage wall for both inspiration and expiration. Neck muscle function and diaphragm function were intact. During forced inspiration, the intercostal spaces were sucked inward and the upper rib cage wall moved inward (paradoxically). She required trunk support to maintain an upright body position. The abdominal wall was distended and the rib cage wall was positioned low. Forced expiration was weak, as was cough.

Her inspiratory capacity was 0.90 L and her expiratory reserve volume was 0.04 L. These values were 35% and 3% of their predicted values, respectively. Maximum inspiratory pressure was –28 cmH_2O and maximum expiratory pressure was 3 cmH_2O, as measured at the resting tidal end-expiratory level, 31% and 2% of their predicted values, respectively. She failed a screening of alveolar pressure for speech production (criterion 5 cmH_2O for 5 seconds). Impairment of inspiratory function was rated as moderate to severe and impairment of expiratory function was rated as severe to profound. Measurements on a breathing discomfort scale revealed moderate dyspnea in association with reading and mild dyspnea in association with conversational speaking.

Diagnostic interventions were tested and results were positive. With intervention, she could be made to inspire deeper and more forcefully and increase her loudness and phrase length. Certain intervention probes also reduced her dyspnea. A report was prepared for the neurologist with recommendations that included mechanical intervention and subsequent behavioral management.

Meanwhile, life continued as usual in the San Juan Mountains. It was now summer. The creeks were swollen, the meadows in color, and Lobo Lookout revealed the splendor of Wolf Creek Pass and the Weminuche Wilderness. She wondered about her chances of returning there.

INTRODUCTION

Speech breathing disorders are often encountered in clinical practice. It has been estimated that among individuals who present with speech disorders, 15% will have problems that are caused, at least in part, by one or more abnormalities of speech breathing. A speech breathing disorder may be the result of functional and/or organic causes and may present as a problem of breathing movement, gas exchange, breathing comfort, or any combination of these (Hixon & Hoit, 2005).

This chapter begins by considering the fundamentals of breathing, then turns to the consideration of breathing for normal speech production. This is followed by description of selected methods for the measurement of breathing. Next, general information about speech breathing disorders and the clinical professionals who work with them is considered as a bridge between the areas of basic science discussed in the chapter and their clinical application. The chapter ends with a review and the completion of its opening scenario.

FUNDAMENTALS OF BREATHING

The breathing apparatus is a mechanical air pump. This pump includes an energy source and passive components that couple this source to the air it moves. The present section considers the nature of this pump and how it functions. Topics discussed include the anatomical bases of breathing, forces and movements of breathing, adjustments of the breathing apparatus, output variables of breathing, neural control of breathing, and ventilation and gas exchange during tidal breathing. For the purposes of this chapter, the breathing apparatus is considered to include the pulmonary apparatus and chest wall (both defined below). Structures of the laryngeal apparatus, velopharyngeal-nasal apparatus, and pharyngeal-oral apparatus are covered in other chapters.

Anatomical Bases of Breathing

The breathing apparatus is located within the torso (body trunk). A skeleton of bone and cartilage forms a superstructure for the torso. This superstructure is depicted in Figure 2–1.

Skeletal Superstructure

At the back of the torso, 34 irregularly shaped vertebrae (bones) form the vertebral column or backbone. The uppermost 7 of these vertebrae are termed cervical (neck), the next lower 12 are called thoracic (chest), and the next three lower groups of 5 each are referred to as lumbar, sacral, and coccygeal (collectively, abdominal). The vertebral column constitutes a back centerpost for the torso.

The ribs comprise most of the upper skeletal superstructure. They are 12 flat, arch-shaped bones on each side of the body. The ribs slope downward from back to front along the sides of the torso, forming the rib cage and giving roundness to the superstructure. At the front, most of the ribs attach to bars of costal (rib) cartilage, which, in turn, attach to the sternum or breastbone. The sternum serves as a front centerpost for the rib cage. The typical rib cage includes upper pairs of ribs attached to the sternum by their own costal cartilages, lower pairs that share cartilages, and the lowest two pairs that float without front attachments.

The remainder of the upper skeletal superstructure is formed by the pectoral girdle (shoulder girdle). This structure is near the top of the rib cage. The front of the pectoral girdle is formed by the two clavicles (collar bones), each of which is a strut extending from the sternum over the first rib toward the side and back of the rib cage. At the back, the clavicles attach to two triangularly shaped plates, the scapulae (shoulder blades). The scapulae cover most of the upper back portion of the rib cage.

Coming to Terms

Terms can enlighten you or get you into verbal quagmires. Respiratory physiologists have gone out of their way to be precise in their use of terms. They've even held conventions to iron out their differences in language. It's a good idea to take a little extra time and care when reading the early sections of this chapter. Let the lexicon of the respiratory physiologist take firm root. Don't be tempted to skip over parts just because the words in the headings look familiar to you. You may be surprised to find that a term you thought you understood actually has an entirely different meaning to a respiratory physiologist.

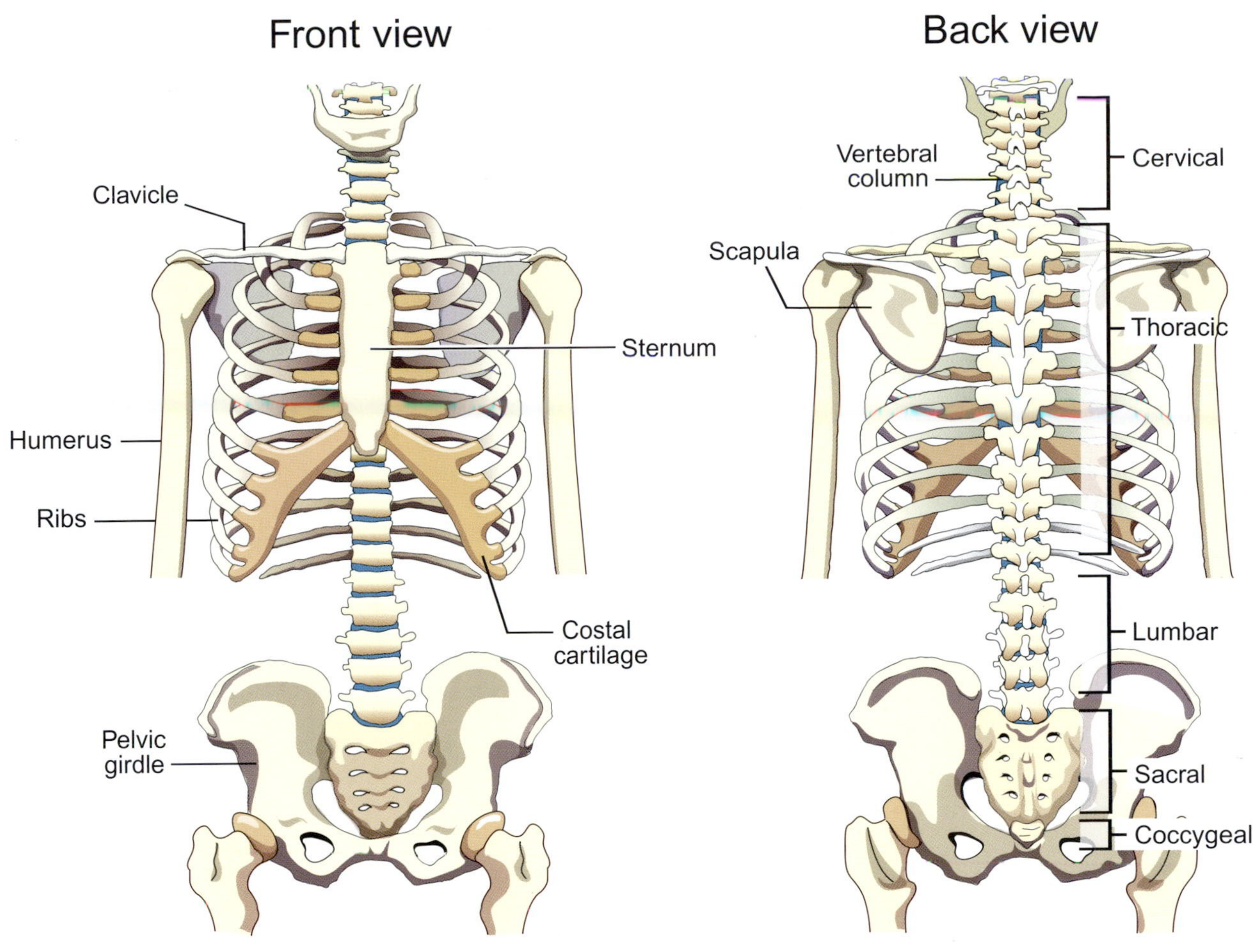

Figure 2–1. Skeletal superstructure of the torso.

Two large, irregularly shaped coxal (hip) bones are located in the lower skeletal superstructure. These two bones, together with the sacral and coccygeal vertebrae, form the pelvic girdle (bony pelvis). The pelvic girdle comprises the base, lower back, and sides of the lower skeletal superstructure.

Breathing Apparatus and Its Subdivisions

The breathing apparatus (breathing pump) and its subdivisions are depicted in Figure 2–2. The torso, which houses the apparatus, consists of upper and lower cavities that are partitioned by the diaphragm. The upper cavity, the thorax or chest, is almost totally filled with the heart and lungs, whereas the lower cavity, the abdomen or belly, contains much of the digestive system and other organs and glands. The structures of the breathing apparatus form two major subdivisions, the pulmonary apparatus and chest wall. These subdivisions are concentrically arranged, with the pulmonary apparatus being surrounded by the chest wall.

Pulmonary Apparatus. The pulmonary apparatus is the air containing, air conducting, and gas exchanging part of the breathing apparatus. Figure 2–3 portrays some of its salient features. The pulmonary apparatus provides oxygen to the cells of the body and removes carbon dioxide from them. The apparatus can itself be subdivided into two components, the pulmonary airways and lungs.

Pulmonary Airways. The pulmonary airways constitute a complex network of flexible tubes through which air can be moved to and from the lungs and between different parts of the lungs.

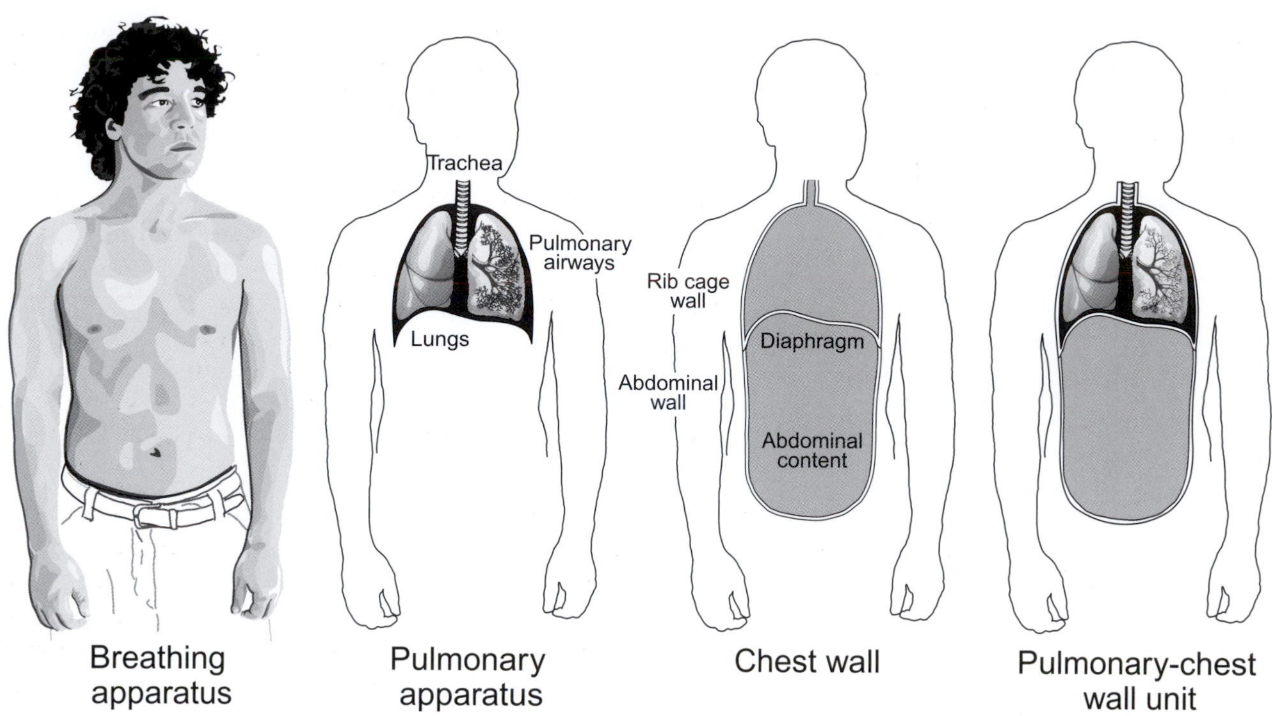

Figure 2–2. Breathing apparatus and its subdivisions. From *Evaluation and management of speech breathing disorders: Principles and methods* (p. 13), by T. Hixon and J. Hoit, 2005, Tucson, AZ: Redington Brown. Copyright 2005 by Thomas J. Hixon and Jeannette D. Hoit. Modified and reproduced with permission.

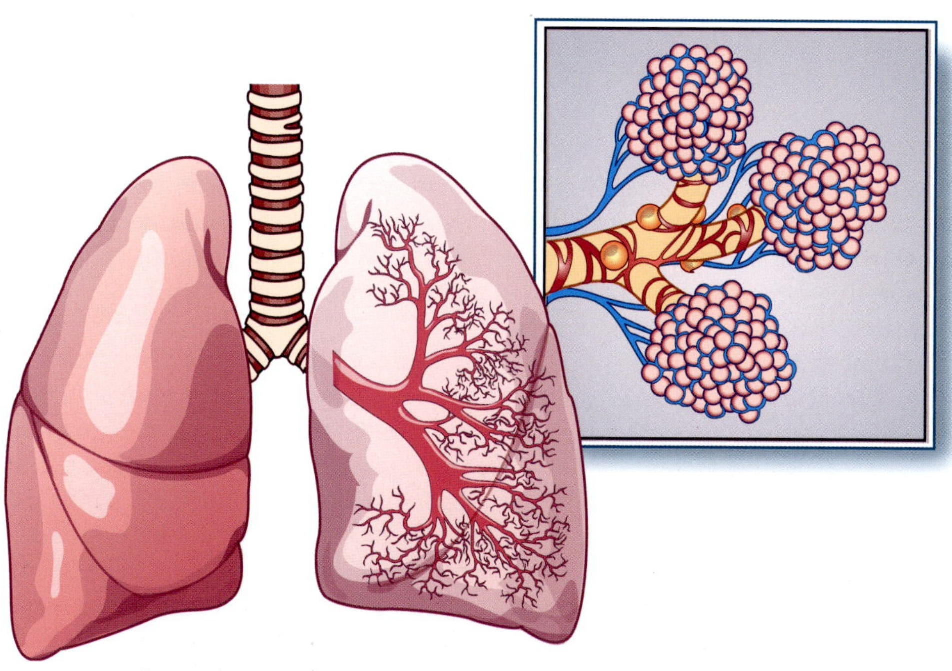

Figure 2–3. Salient features of the pulmonary apparatus.

These tubes are patterned like the branches of an inverted deciduous tree. The network is, in fact, commonly referred to as the pulmonary tree.

The trunk of the pulmonary tree (the top part) is the trachea or windpipe. The trachea is a tube attached to the bottom of the larynx (voice box). It runs down through the neck into the torso. The trachea is composed of a series of C-shaped cartilages whose open ends face toward the back where the structure is completed by a flexible wall shared with the esophagus (a muscular tube leading to the stomach). At its lower end, the trachea divides into two smaller tubes, one running to the left lung and one running to the right lung. These two tubes, called the main-stem bronchi, branch into what are called lobar bronchi, tubes that run to the five lobes of the lungs (two on the left and three on the right). The five lobar bronchi each branch and their offspring also each branch, and so on, through more than 20 generations. Each successive branching leads to smaller and less rigid structures within the pulmonary apparatus. These include, in succession, segmental bronchi, subsegmental bronchi, small bronchi, terminal bronchi, bronchioles, terminal bronchioles, respiratory bronchioles, alveolar ducts, alveolar sacs, and alveoli. The last, the alveoli, are extremely small cul de sacs filled with air. They number more than 300 million and are the sites where oxygen and carbon dioxide are exchanged.

Lungs. The lungs are the organs of breathing. They are a pair of cone-shaped structures that are porous and spongy. Each lung contains an abundance of resilient elastic fibers and behaves like a stretchable bag. The outer surfaces of the lungs are covered with a thin airtight membrane, the visceral pleura. A similar membrane, the parietal pleura, covers the inner surface of the chest wall where it contacts the lungs. Together these two membranes form a double-walled sac that encases the lungs. Both walls of this sac are covered with a thin layer of liquid, which lubricates them and enables them to move easily upon one another. The same layer of liquid links the visceral and parietal membranes together, in the manner that a film of water holds two glass plates together. Thus, the lungs and chest wall tend to move as a unit, such that where one goes the other follows.

Chest Wall. The chest wall encases the pulmonary apparatus. There are four parts to the chest wall—the rib cage wall, diaphragm, abdominal wall, and abdominal content.

Rib Cage Wall. The rib cage wall surrounds the lungs and is shaped like a barrel. Recall that the rib cage superstructure includes the thoracic segments of the vertebral column, the ribs, the costal cartilages, the sternum, and the pectoral girdle. The remainder of the rib cage wall is formed by muscular and nonmuscular tissues that fill the spaces between the ribs and cover their inner and outer surfaces.

Diaphragm. The diaphragm forms the convex floor of the thorax and the concave roof of the abdomen. The diaphragm separates the thorax and abdomen, and thus, gets its name—diaphragm meaning "the fence between." The diaphragm is dome-shaped and has the appearance of an inverted bowl. The left side of the structure is positioned slightly lower than the right. At its center, the diaphragm consists of a tough sheet of inelastic tissue, the central tendon. The remainder of the structure is formed by a sheet of muscle that rises as a broad rim from all around the lower portion of the inside of the rib cage and extends upward to the edges of the central tendon.

Abdominal Wall. The abdominal wall provides a casing for the lower half of the torso. This casing is shaped like an oblong tube and runs all the way around the torso. The lower portion of the skeletal superstructure of the torso forms the framework around which the abdominal wall is built. This includes a back centerpost of 15 vertebrae (lumbar, sacral, and coccygeal) that extends from near the bottom of the rib cage to the tailbone and pelvic girdle. Much of the abdominal wall consists of two broad sheets of connective tissue and several large muscles. The two sheets of connective tissue cover the front and back of the abdominal wall and are called the abdominal aponeurosis and lumbodorsal fascia, respectively. Muscles are located all around the abdominal wall—front, back, and flanks—and combine with the abdominal aponeurosis, lumbodorsal fascia, vertebral column, and pelvic girdle to form its encircling casing.

Abdominal Content. The abdominal content is everything in the abdominal cavity. This includes a wide array of structures, such as the stomach, intestines, and various other internal structures. This content is close to unit density (the density of water) and constitutes a relatively homogeneous mass. This mass is suspended from above by a suction force at the undersurface of the diaphragm and is held in place circumferentially and at its base by the casing of the abdominal wall. Together, the abdominal cavity and the abdominal content are the mechanical equivalent of an elastic bag filled with water.

Pulmonary Apparatus-Chest Wall Unit. The pulmonary apparatus and chest wall form a single functional unit that derives from the linkage effected by the pleural membranes. As shown in Figure 2–4, the resting positions of the pulmonary apparatus and chest wall in this intact unit are different from their individual resting positions when the two are separated. When the pulmonary apparatus is removed from the chest wall, its resting position is a collapsed state in which it contains very little air. In contrast, the resting position of the chest wall, with the pulmonary apparatus removed, is a more expanded state. With the pulmonary apparatus and chest wall held together by pleural linkage, the breathing apparatus assumes a resting position between these two separate positions such that the pulmonary apparatus is somewhat expanded and the chest wall is somewhat compressed. This resting position of the linked pulmonary apparatus-chest wall unit involves a mechanically neutral or balanced state in which the force of the pulmonary apparatus to collapse is opposed by an equal and opposite force of the chest wall to expand.

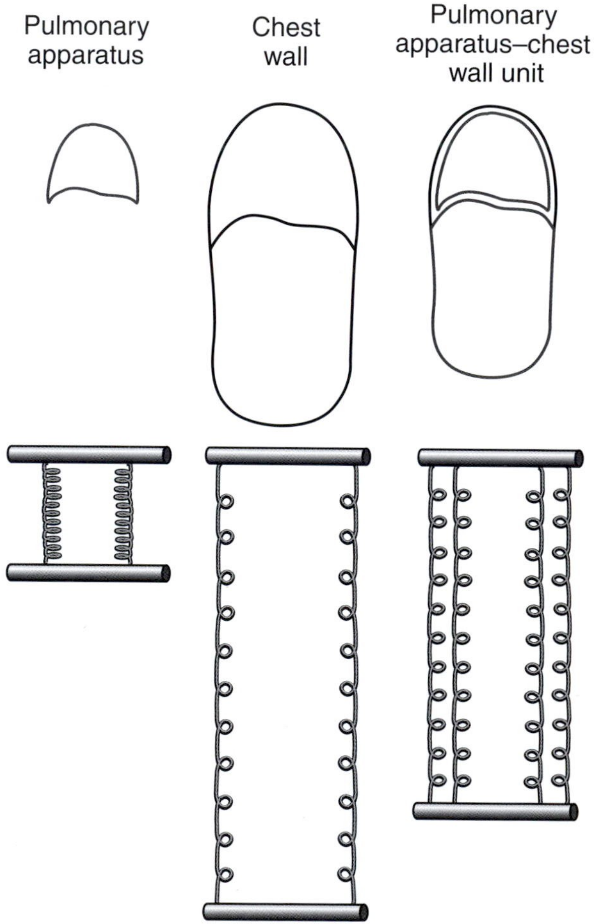

Figure 2–4. Unitary nature of the pulmonary apparatus and chest wall.

Forces and Movements of Breathing

Forces applied to and by different parts of the breathing apparatus result in movements. Such forces and movements constitute breathing at the mechanical level.

Forces of Breathing

Passive and active forces operate on the breathing apparatus. Passive force is inherent and always present. Active force, in contrast, is applied willfully and in accordance with ability.

Passive Force. The passive force of breathing comes from (a) the natural recoil of muscles, cartilages, ligaments, and lung tissue, (b) the surface tension of alveoli, and (c) the pull of gravity. These factors cause the breathing apparatus to behave like a coil spring, which, when stretched or compressed, tends to recoil toward its resting length.

The sign (inspiratory or expiratory) and magnitude of passive force depends on the amount of air in the breathing apparatus. When the apparatus contains more air than it does at its resting level, it recoils toward a smaller size (expires), like a stretched spring. The more air in the apparatus, the greater the recoil force. In contrast, when the apparatus contains less air than it does at its resting level, it recoils toward a larger size (inspires), like a compressed spring. The less air in the apparatus, the greater the recoil force. Thus, like a coil spring, the more the breathing apparatus is deformed from its resting level, whether in the inspiratory or expiratory direction, the greater the passive recoil force it generates.

Active Force. The active force of breathing comes from the actions of muscles of the chest wall. The sign (inspiratory or expiratory) and magnitude of this force depends on which muscles are active and in what patterns. Active force also depends on the amount of air in the breathing apparatus. The more air in the apparatus, the greater the active force that can be generated to expire, and the less air in the apparatus, the greater the active force that can be generated to inspire.

The roles of individual muscles in generating active force are described below for the rib cage wall, diaphragm, and abdominal wall. These descriptions assume that only the muscle under consideration is active and that it is shortening during contraction. It should be noted, however, that several factors might influence the contribution of an individual muscle, including the actions of other muscles, the mechanical status of different parts of the chest wall, and the breathing activity being performed.

Muscles of the Rib Cage Wall. The muscles of the rib cage wall are defined to include muscles of the neck and rib cage. These muscles are depicted in different views in Figure 2–5.

The ***sternocleidomastoid*** muscle is a broad, thick structure positioned on the front and side of the neck. It originates in two subdivisions, one at the top and front of the sternum and the other at the top of the sternal end of the clavicle. Fibers from these subdivisions pass upward and backward and insert into the bony skull behind the ear. When the head is fixed in position, contraction of the ***sternocleidomastoid*** muscle results in elevation of the sternum and clavicle. The force generated is transmitted to the ribs through their connections to the sternum and clavicle. Consequently, the ribs are also elevated.

The ***scalenus anterior***, ***scalenus medius***, and ***scalenus posterior*** muscles are three separate muscles that form a functional group. These are positioned on the side of the neck. The ***scalenus anterior*** muscle originates from the third through sixth cervical vertebrae and runs downward and toward the side to insert along the inner border of the top of the first rib. The ***scalenus medius*** muscle arises from the lower six cervical vertebrae and descends along the side of the vertebral column to insert into the first rib behind the point of insertion of the ***scalenus anterior*** muscle. And the ***scalenus posterior*** muscle originates

Rib Torque

Sounds like leftovers. Actually, it refers to rotational stress produced when one end of a rib is twisted out of line with the other. Some have suggested that when the ribs are elevated during resting tidal inspiration they're twisted outward (placed under positive torque) and store energy, which is then supposedly released during expiration. Not so. The ribs are actually twisted inward (are under negative torque) at the resting tidal end-expiratory level. The lungs are pulling inward on the rib cage wall at that level. The ribs untwist during resting tidal inspiration, but do not reach neutral (zero torque) in the upright body position until the 60 %VC (percent vital capacity) level is attained. Resting tidal inspiration involves only about a 10 %VC increase, from say, 40 to 50 %VC. Thus, rib torque actually opposes resting tidal expiration rather than assists it. The only thing leftover about rib torque in this context is the folklore.

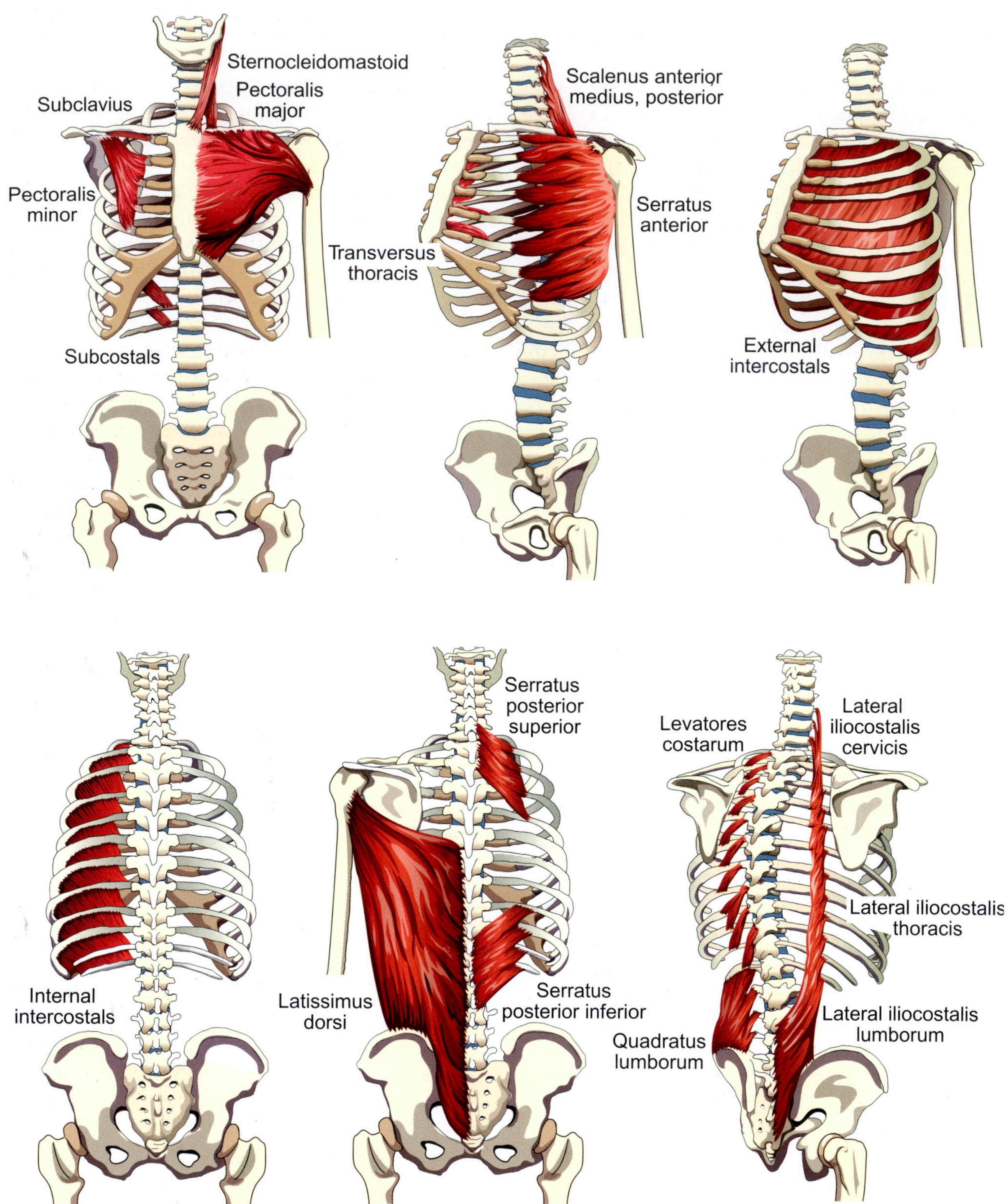

Figure 2–5. Muscles of the rib cage wall. From *Evaluation and management of speech breathing disorders: Principles and methods* (pp. 19–20), by T. Hixon and J. Hoit, 2005, Tucson, AZ: Redington Brown. Copyright 2005 by Thomas J. Hixon and Jeannette D. Hoit. Modified and reproduced with permission.

from the lower two or three cervical vertebrae and passes downward and toward the side to attach to the outer surface of the second rib. When the head is fixed in position, contraction of the ***scalenus anterior*** and/or ***scalenus medius*** muscles results in elevation of the first rib, whereas contraction of the ***scalenus posterior*** muscle results in elevation of the second rib.

The ***pectoralis major*** muscle is a broad, fan-shaped muscle positioned on the upper front wall of the rib cage. This muscle has a complex origin that includes the front surface of the upper costal cartilages, sternum, and inner half of the clavicle. Fibers run across the front of the rib cage wall and converge to insert into the humerus (the major bone of the upper arm). When the humerus is held in position, contraction of the ***pectoralis major*** muscle pulls the sternum and ribs upward.

The ***pectoralis minor*** muscle is a relatively large, thin muscle that lies underneath the ***pectoralis major*** muscle. Its fibers originate from the second through fifth ribs near their cartilages. From there, they extend upward and toward the side, where they insert into the front surface of the scapula. When the scapula is fixed in position, contraction of the ***pectoralis minor*** muscle elevates the second through fifth ribs.

The ***subclavius*** muscle is a small muscle that originates from the undersurface of the clavicle. It runs slightly downward and toward the midline, where it attaches at the junction of the first rib and its cartilage. When the clavicle is braced, contraction of the ***subclavius*** muscle elevates the first rib.

The ***serratus anterior*** muscle is a large muscle positioned on the side of the rib cage wall. It originates from the outer surfaces of the upper eight or nine ribs. Fibers pass backward around the side of the rib cage, where they converge and insert into the front of the scapula. When the scapula is fixed in position, contraction of the ***serratus anterior*** muscle results in elevation of the upper ribs.

The ***external intercostal*** muscles are 11 muscles that fill the outer portions of the rib interspaces. Each is a thin layer of muscle that runs between adjacent ribs. The fibers of the muscles are oriented forward and downward. Together, the 11 muscles form a large sheet of muscle that links the ribs to one another. This sheet of muscle is anchored from above to the first rib, the cervical vertebrae, and the base of the skull. When the muscle in any rib interspace contracts, it elevates the rib immediately below and, perhaps, other ribs below through their linkage to the sheet of muscle. The ***external intercostal*** muscles may activate individually in different rib interspaces or they may activate collectively. En masse activation causes the ribs to move upward as a unit. Muscle activation also stiffens the tissue-filled rib interspaces. This prevents them from being sucked inward and pushed outward as internal pressure is lowered and raised, respectively.

The ***internal intercostal*** muscles are 11 muscles that lie in the inner portions of the rib interspaces. They are located underneath the ***external intercostal*** muscles and extend from around the sides of the rib cage to the sternum. The ***internal intercostal*** muscles do not fill the rib interspaces at the back of the rib age. Fibers of the ***internal intercostal*** muscles run downward and backward and at a right angle to those of the ***external intercostal*** muscles. The ***internal intercostal*** muscles form a large sheet of muscle that links the ribs to one another and to the pelvic girdle through other muscles, especially those of the abdominal wall. When muscle in a rib interspace contracts, it pulls downward on the rib immediately above and, perhaps, on other ribs above through the linkage created by the muscle sheet. The ***internal intercostal*** muscles may activate individually in any rib interspace or they may activate collectively. For the latter, the ribs tend to move downward as a unit. Muscle contraction stiffens the tissue-filled rib interspaces and prevents them from being sucked inward and bulged outward during the lowering and raising of internal pressure, respectively.

The portion of the ***internal intercostal*** muscles that lies between the costal cartilages (the ***intercartilaginous internal intercostal*** muscles) is arranged such that the muscle tissue exerts an upward pull on the rib cage wall rather than the downward pull exerted by the portion of the muscle that lies between the bony ribs (the ***interosseous internal intercostal*** muscles). Thus, the ***internal intercostal*** muscles play a functional role in the intercartilaginous region that is similar to that played by their companion ***external intercostal*** muscles throughout the rib cage wall. Stated otherwise, the two layers of intercostal muscles (external and internal) function similarly toward the front of the rib cage, but dissimilarly at other locations.

The ***transversus thoracis*** muscle is a fan-shaped structure located on the inside, front wall of the rib cage. It originates at the midline on the inner surface of the lower sternum and fourth or fifth through seventh costal cartilages. From there, it fans out across the rib cage and inserts into the inner surface of the costal cartilages and bony ends of the second through sixth ribs. The upper fibers of the muscle run nearly vertically, whereas the intermediate and lower fibers course at other angles. When the ***transversus thoracis*** muscle contracts, it exerts a downward pull on the second through sixth ribs.

The ***latissimus dorsi*** muscle is a large muscle positioned on the back of the body. It has a complex origin from the lower six thoracic, lumbar, and sacral vertebrae, along with the back surfaces of the lower three or four ribs. Fibers run upward across the back of the lower torso at different angles to insert into the humerus. When the humerus is fixed in position, contraction of the fibers of the ***latissimus dorsi*** muscle that insert into the lower ribs will elevate them. Contraction of the muscle as a whole, in contrast, compresses the lower portion of the rib cage wall. Thus, the ***latissimus dorsi*** muscle is capable of generating active force of different signs (inspiratory and expiratory).

The ***serratus posterior superior*** muscle is located on the upper back portion of the rib cage wall. It is a thin muscle that originates from the back of the vertebral column. Points of origin include the seventh cervical and first three or four thoracic vertebrae. Fibers course downward across the back of the rib cage and insert into the second through fifth ribs. When the ***serratus posterior superior*** muscle contracts, it pulls upward on the second through fifth ribs.

The ***serratus posterior inferior*** muscle is a thin muscle positioned on the lower back portion of the rib cage wall. It arises from the lower two thoracic and upper two or three lumbar vertebrae and slants upward across the back of the rib cage where it inserts into the lower borders of the lower four ribs. Contraction of the ***serratus posterior inferior*** muscle results in a downward pull on the lower four ribs.

The ***lateral iliocostalis*** muscle group includes three muscles located on the back of the torso. These are positioned to the side of the vertebral column and extend between the cervical and lumbar regions. The ***lateral iliocostalis cervicis*** muscle originates from the outer surfaces of the third through sixth ribs and courses upward and toward the midline to insert into the fourth through sixth cervical vertebrae. The ***lateral iliocostalis thoracis*** muscle arises from the upper edges of the lower six ribs and courses upward to insert into the lower edges of the upper six ribs. And the ***lateral iliocostalis lumborum*** muscle originates from the lumbodorsal fascia, lumbar vertebrae, and back surface of the coxal bone. It courses upward and toward the side to insert into the lower edges of the lower six ribs. Contraction of the ***lateral iliocostalis cervicis*** muscle causes elevation of the third through sixth ribs, whereas contraction of the ***lateral iliocostalis lumborum*** muscle results in depression of the lower six ribs. Contraction of the ***lateral iliocostalis thoracis*** muscle stabilizes large segments of the back of the rib cage wall and makes them move in concert with either the rib elevation or depression caused by the cervical and lumbar elements of the muscle group, respectively.

The ***levatores costarum*** muscles are 12 small muscles positioned on the back of the rib cage wall. Their origin is from the seventh cervical and upper eleven thoracic vertebrae and they extend downward and slightly outward to insert into the back surface of the rib immediately below the vertebra of origin. When an individual muscle of the ***levatores costarum*** muscle group contracts, it elevates the ribs into which it inserts. When the muscle group contracts collectively, its action is similar to that effected by collective contraction of the ***external intercostal*** muscles (the ribs elevate as a unit).

The ***quadratus lumborum*** muscle is a flat, quadrilateral sheet of muscle located on the back of the torso. It arises from the top of the coxal bone and runs upward and toward the midline where it inserts into the first four lumbar vertebrae and lower border of the inner half of the lowest rib. When the ***quadratus lumborum*** muscle contracts, it pulls downward on the lowest rib.

The ***subcostal*** muscles comprise a group of thin muscles located on the inside back wall of the rib cage. They differ in number from person to person and are most often located and best developed in the lower portion of the rib cage wall. The ***subcostal*** muscles originate near the vertebral column on the inner surfaces of ribs and course upward and toward the side where they insert into the inner surfaces of ribs immediately above, or skip a rib or two and insert into higher ribs. When the ***subcostal*** muscles contract, they pull downward on the ribs into which they are inserted.

Muscle of the Diaphragm. The muscular features of the diaphragm are portrayed in Figure 2–6. The ***diaphragm*** muscle is a large, complex muscle that subdivides the torso into two compartments. Its origin is around the internal circumference of the lower rib cage. This includes the bottom of the sternum, the lower six ribs and their cartilages, and the first three or four lumbar vertebrae. From this internal rim, muscle fibers radiate upward to insert into the circumference of the central tendon, a broad sheet of inelastic tissue that forms the centermost portion of the diaphragm. When the ***diaphragm*** muscle contracts, it can effect two actions. As portrayed in Figure 2–7, one of these is to pull the central tendon downward and forward, thus enlarging the thorax vertically, whereas the other is to enlarge the thorax circumferentially through elevation of the lower six ribs. The actions of lowering the base of the thorax and expanding its circumference occur in patterns that depend on the relative stiffness of the rib cage wall and abdominal wall.

Muscles of the Abdominal Wall. The muscles of the abdominal wall are depicted in Figure 2–8. Different views are shown.

The ***rectus abdominis*** muscle is a ribbon-like structure located on the front of the lower rib cage wall and abdominal wall just off the midline. It arises from the upper, front edge of the coxal bone and runs upward vertically to insert into the outer surfaces of the fifth, sixth, and seventh costal cartilages and lower sternum. The ***rectus abdominis*** muscle is compartmentalized into four or five short segments by tendinous breaks. The entire muscle is encased in a fibrous sheath formed by the abdominal aponeurosis. The muscle and sheath form a centerpost along the front of the abdominal wall that is a continuation of the front centerpost formed by the sternum on the rib cage wall. When the ***rectus abdominis*** muscle contracts, it pulls the lower ribs and sternum downward and forces the front of the abdominal wall inward. The compartmentalized segments of the muscle are also capable of independent contraction.

The ***external oblique*** muscle is a broad structure located on the side and front of the lower rib cage wall and abdominal wall. It originates from the upper surface of the coxal bone and abdominal aponeurosis near the midline. Fibers course upward across the abdominal wall at various angles. The most prominent course is upward and toward the side, with insertions being on the outer surfaces and lower borders of the lower eight ribs. When the ***external oblique*** muscle contracts, it pulls the lower ribs downward and forces the front and side of the abdominal wall inward.

The ***internal oblique*** muscle is a large muscle positioned on the side and front of the lower rib cage wall and abdominal wall. It lies underneath the ***external oblique*** muscle. The ***internal oblique*** muscle originates from the upper surface of the coxal bone and lumbodorsal fascia. Its fibers fan out across the abdominal wall to insert into the abdominal aponeurosis and the lower borders of the costal cartilages of the lower three or four ribs. The fibers of the ***internal oblique*** muscle run at a right angle to those of the ***external oblique*** muscle. When the ***internal oblique*** muscle contracts, it pulls the lower ribs downward and forces the front and side of the abdominal wall inward. Thus, its functional potential is similar to that of the ***external oblique*** muscle.

The ***transversus abdominis*** muscle is a broad structure located on the front and side of the abdominal wall. It lies underneath the ***internal oblique*** muscle. The ***transversus abdominis*** muscle has a complex origin that includes the upper surface of the coxal bone, lumbodorsal fascia, and inner surfaces of the costal cartilages of ribs seven through twelve. Fibers of the muscle run horizontally around the abdominal wall and insert at the front into the abdominal aponeurosis. The paired left and right ***transversus abdominis*** muscles encircle the abdominal wall. When the ***transversus abdominis*** muscle contracts, it forces the front and side of the abdominal wall inward.

The four muscles just described are located on the front and sides of the abdominal wall and are routinely referred to as "the" abdominal muscles. However, the abdominal wall runs all the way around the torso and includes more than just its front and sides. Three other muscles traverse the abdominal wall at the back and are as much a part of the abdominal wall as the muscles just discussed.

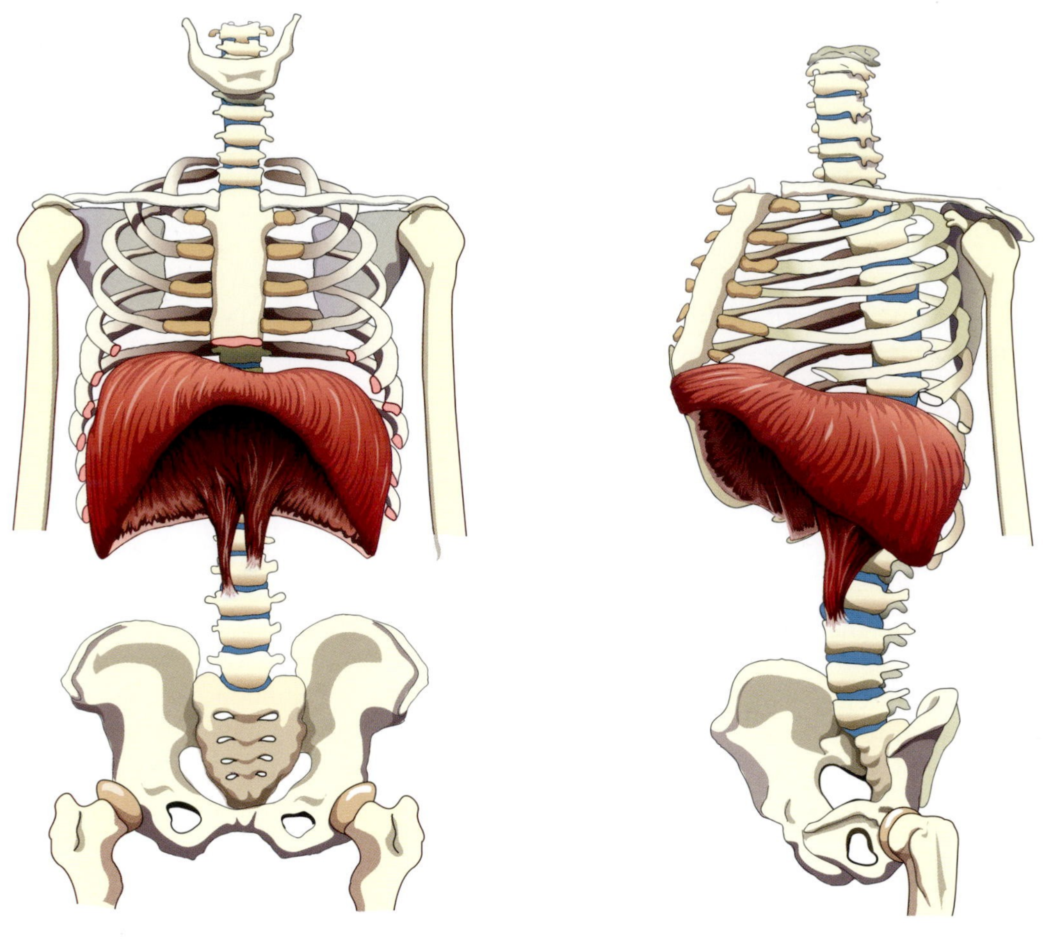

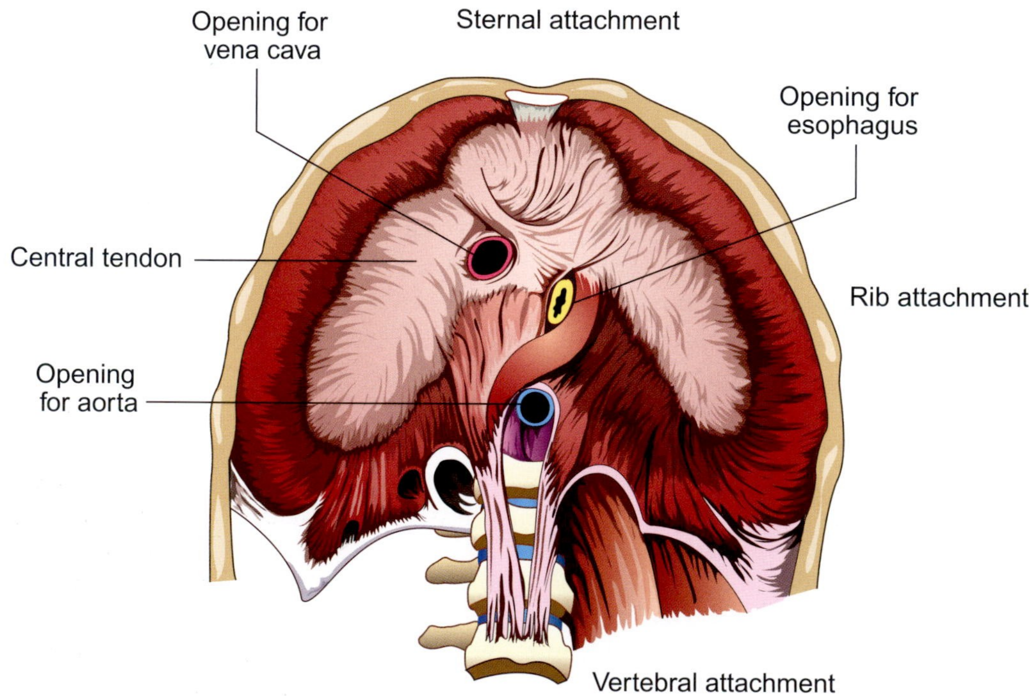

Figure 2–6. Muscle of the diaphragm. Upper panels from *Evaluation and management of speech breathing disorders: Principles and methods* (p. 25), by T. Hixon and J. Hoit, 2005, Tucson, AZ: Redington Brown. Copyright 2005 by Thomas J. Hixon and Jeannette D. Hoit. Modified and reproduced with permission.

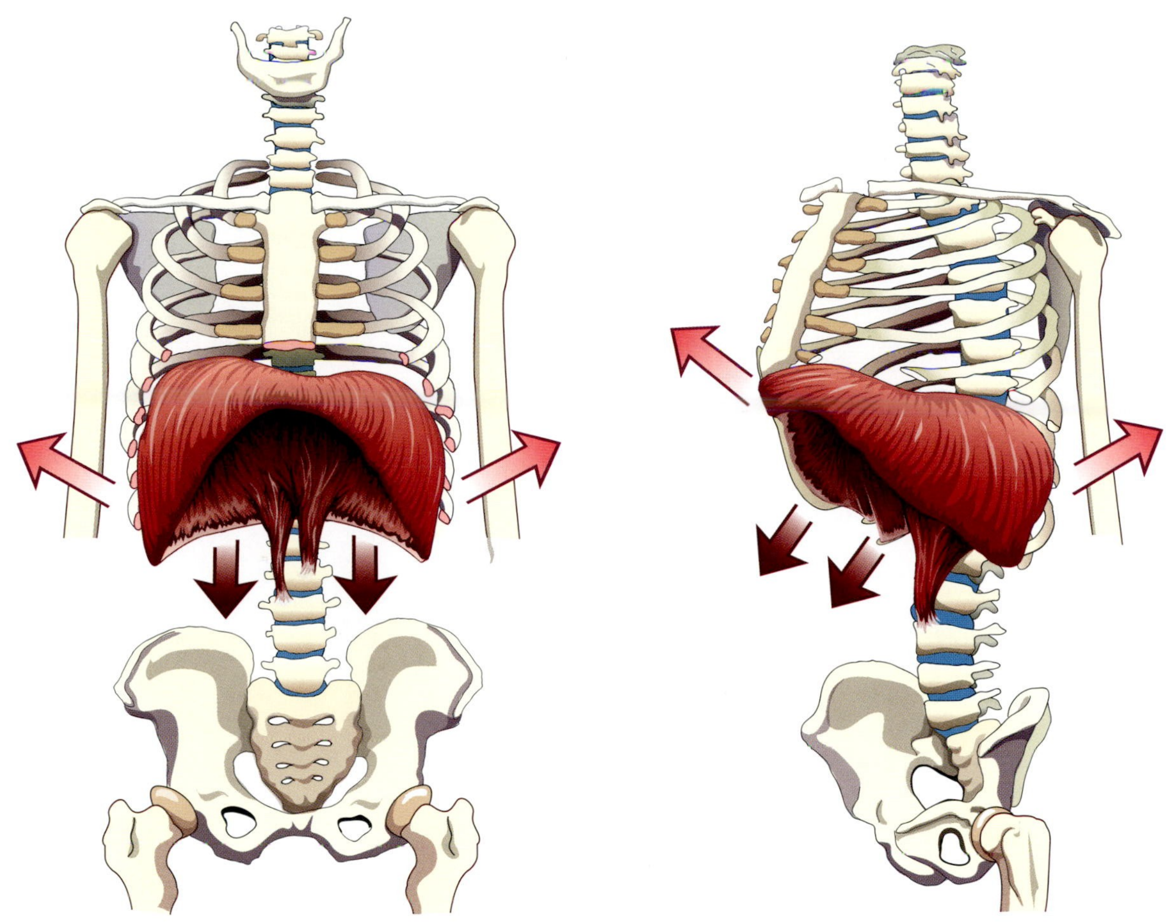

Figure 2–7. Actions of the diaphragm. Structural features from *Evaluation and management of speech breathing disorders: Principles and methods* (p. 25), by T. Hixon and J. Hoit, 2005, Tucson, AZ: Redington Brown. Copyright 2005 by Thomas J. Hixon and Jeannette D. Hoit. Modified and reproduced with permission.

These three muscles are described above in the context of the rib cage wall. They include the ***latissimus dorsi, lateral iliocostalis lumborum,*** and ***quadratus lumborum*** muscles. These muscles do not effect major displacements of the abdominal wall. Nevertheless, they can brace the abdominal wall at the back and alter its stiffness. Accordingly, they are important functional partners with the other four abdominal muscles.

Realization of Passive and Active Forces

Forces of breathing are realized in two ways. One is through pulls on structures and the other is through pressures developed at various locations. Pulling forces are distributed in a complex fashion. Fortunately, they are uniformly distributed at certain points where they manifest as pressures. The locations of the most important of these pressures are indicated in Figure 2–9.

Included among these pressures are alveolar pressure, pleural pressure, abdominal pressure, and transdiaphragmatic pressure. Alveolar pressure is the pressure inside the lungs. Pleural pressure is the pressure inside the thorax but outside the lungs (between the pleural membranes). Abdominal pressure is the pressure inside the abdominal cavity. And transdiaphragmatic pressure is the difference in pressure across the diaphragm (the difference between pleural pressure and abdominal pressure).

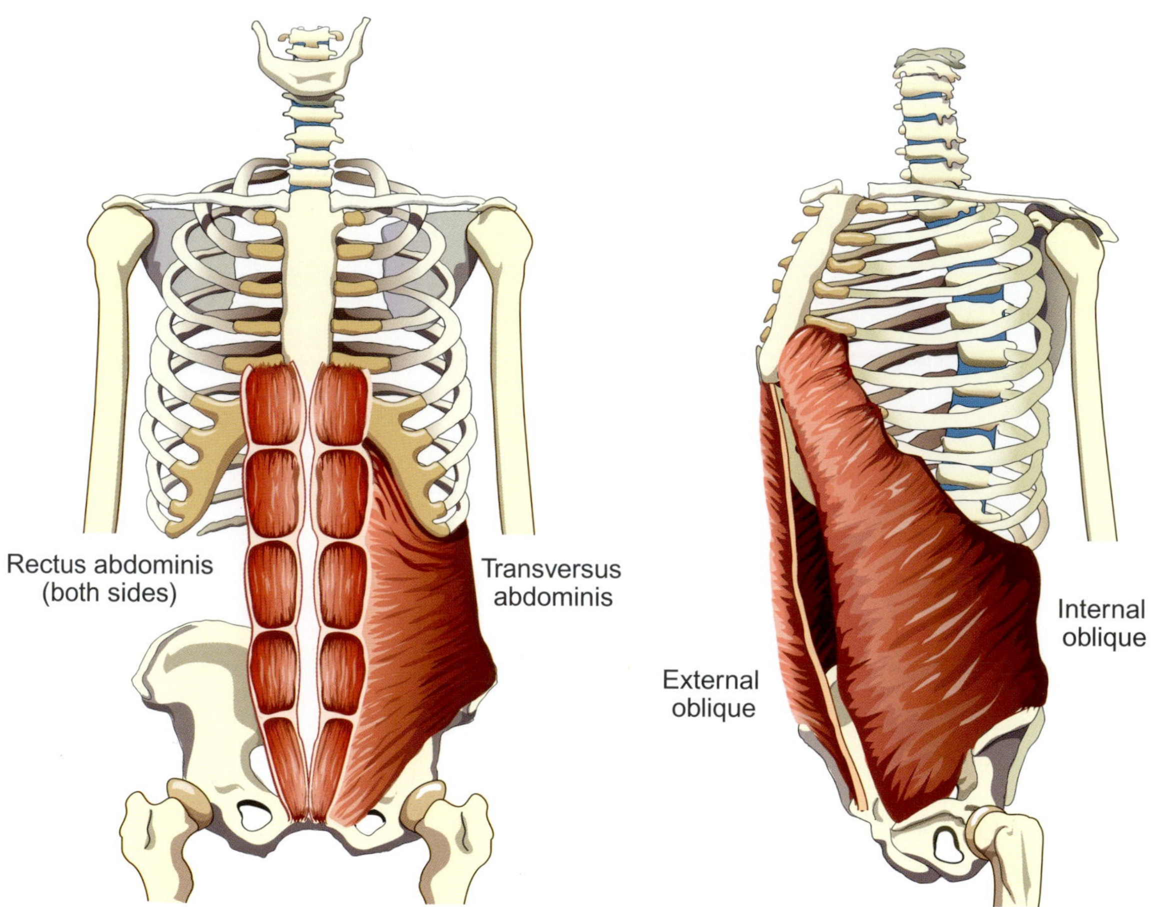

Figure 2–8. Muscles of the abdominal wall. From *Evaluation and management of speech breathing disorders: Principles and methods* (p. 26), by T. Hixon and J. Hoit, 2005, Tucson, AZ: Redington Brown. Copyright 2005 by Thomas J. Hixon and Jeannette D. Hoit. Modified and reproduced with permission.

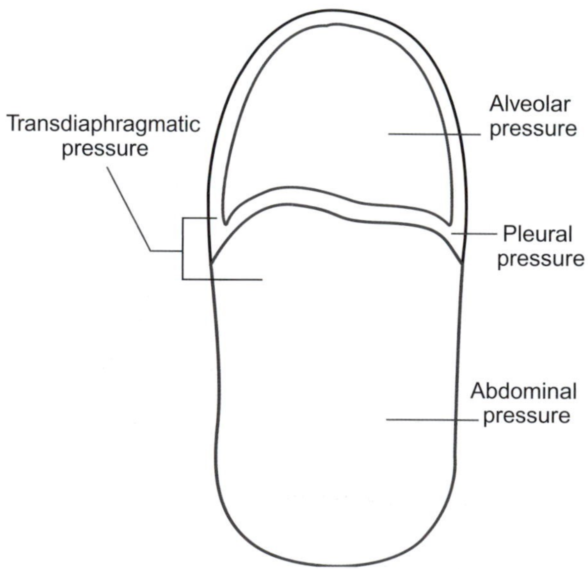

Figure 2–9. Pressures of the breathing apparatus.

Movements of Breathing

The movements of breathing occur in the rib cage wall, diaphragm, and abdominal wall. Movement potential is considered here apart from the forces responsible for it.

Movements of Rib Cage Wall. The rib cage wall is able to move because of two sets of joints, those between the ribs and sternum (costosternal joints) and those between the ribs and vertebral column (costovertebral joints). Actual movement differs somewhat from rib to rib, owing to differences in the lengths and shapes of individual ribs. Nevertheless, two forms of rib movement are typical and are illustrated in Figure 2–10.

One form of rib movement involves a vertical excursion of its front end. This excursion is either

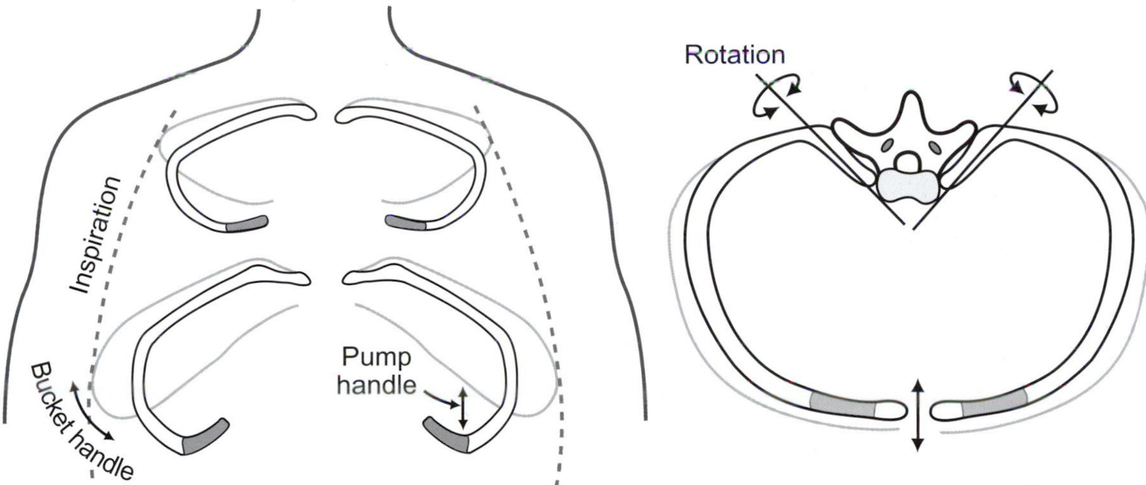

Figure 2-10. Movements of the ribs.

> **Not Doing What Comes Naturally**
>
> The initiation and execution of voluntary breathing movements comes "naturally" for most of us. But, for some individuals with maldeveloped or damaged brains, these may not be easy, or even possible, to do. Their problem is praxis or action. They have dyspraxia when they have difficulty with action, and apraxia when they are unable to carry out action at all. One of the most perplexing clients we ever encountered was a young man who showed difficulties with breathing actions following a traumatic brain injury. When he attempted to initiate voluntary inspirations or expirations on command, he often became frozen in position. Occasionally, his attempt resulted in movement in the opposite direction (he breathed in when trying to breathe out). He knew exactly what he wanted to do, but just couldn't do it. Imagine the depth of his frustration.

upward and forward or downward and backward and results in an increase or decrease, respectively, in the front-to-back diameter of the rib cage. Each rib rotates through the axis of its neck (at the back near the vertebral column) and the pattern of movement that results is akin to the raising and lowering of the handle on a water pump.

The other form of rib movement is vertical excursion along the side of the rib cage. This excursion involves a rotation of the rib around an axis extending between its two ends. The rotation is either upward and outward or downward and inward, the result being an increase or decrease, respectively, in the side-to-side diameter of the rib cage. Such movement is similar to the raising and lowering of the handle on a water bucket.

These two types of rib movement occur together and in phase. Thus, the circumference of the rib cage wall increases and decreases along with increases and decreases in its two diameters (front-to-back and side-to-side).

Movements of the Diaphragm. Movements of the diaphragm are hidden from view and must be inferred from movements of other structures of the chest wall. Such movements are manifested in changes in the radius of curvature of the diaphragm and depend on the relative fixation of the central tendon and lower ribs.

As depicted in Figure 2–11, the diaphragm can be made to flatten or become more highly domed. Flattening is brought about by descent of the central tendon and/or elevation of the lower ribs, and can range from slight to marked. When marked, the diaphragm assumes the shape of an inverted pie pan. Increased doming of the diaphragm results from elevation of the central tendon and/or descent of the lower ribs, and can also range from slight to marked. When marked, the diaphragm assumes the shape of a rounded bullet nose.

When the rib cage is fixed in position, the movement of the diaphragm is coextensive with the movement of the central tendon. In contrast, when the central tendon is fixed in position, the movement of the diaphragm is coextensive with the movement of the abdominal wall.

Movements of the Abdominal Wall. The configuration of the abdominal wall differs from person to person. Factors such as abdominal muscle tone and body type contribute to such differences. When standing or sitting erect, the lower abdominal wall is distended somewhat. This is because the pressure inside the abdomen is greater near the bottom than near the undersurface of the diaphragm and forces the lower abdominal wall outward. Two movements can change the configuration of the abdominal wall. These include moving the wall inward and outward.

Inward movement flattens the abdominal wall. Such flattening can range from slight to marked. When flattening is marked, the configuration of the wall is linear or may actually be curved inward slightly in someone who is exceptionally lean. More pronounced distension of the abdominal wall is accomplished by moving it outward. Outward movement increases the degree to which the wall is protruded. When such protrusion is marked, the configuration of the wall makes the torso appear much like a pear in side view.

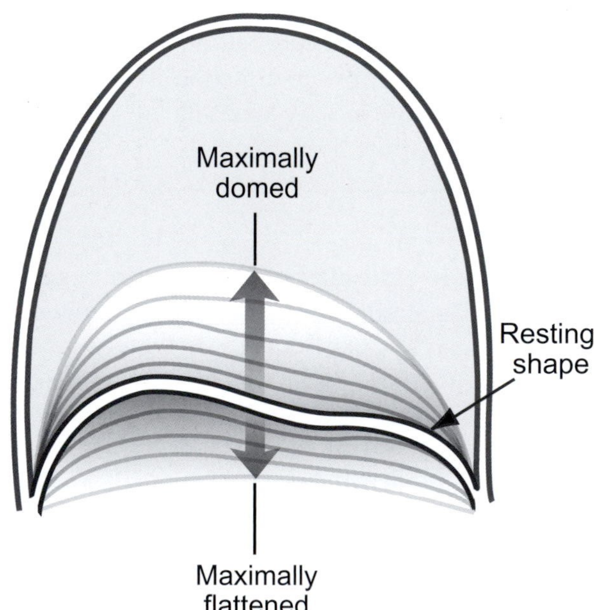

Figure 2-11. Movements of the diaphragm.

Relative Movements of the Rib Cage Wall, Diaphragm, and Abdominal Wall. Figure 2–12 illustrates that the movements of the rib cage wall, the diaphragm, and the abdominal wall can have different functional consequences. The reason is that the rib cage wall and diaphragm-abdominal wall are in contact with different proportions of the surface of the lungs.

The rib cage wall contacts about three fourths of the surface of the lungs. Thus, its movement has a major influence on alveolar pressure and the movement of air. Even a small movement of the rib cage wall can cause a significant pressure change or move a large amount of air into or out of the pulmonary apparatus.

In contrast, the diaphragm contacts only about one fourth of the surface of the lungs. This means that the diaphragm must go through a much greater excursion than the rib cage wall to accomplish the same alveolar pressure change or move the same amount of air into or out of the pulmonary apparatus.

The abdominal wall presents a similar situation. The abdominal wall and diaphragm are opposite surfaces of a very large chest wall part (the diaphragm-abdominal wall), with the abdominal content lying between them. Thus, the abdominal wall is indirectly in contact with the pulmonary apparatus by way of the diaphragm and has access to the same one fourth of the surface of the lungs as does the diaphragm. Like the diaphragm, then, the abdomi-

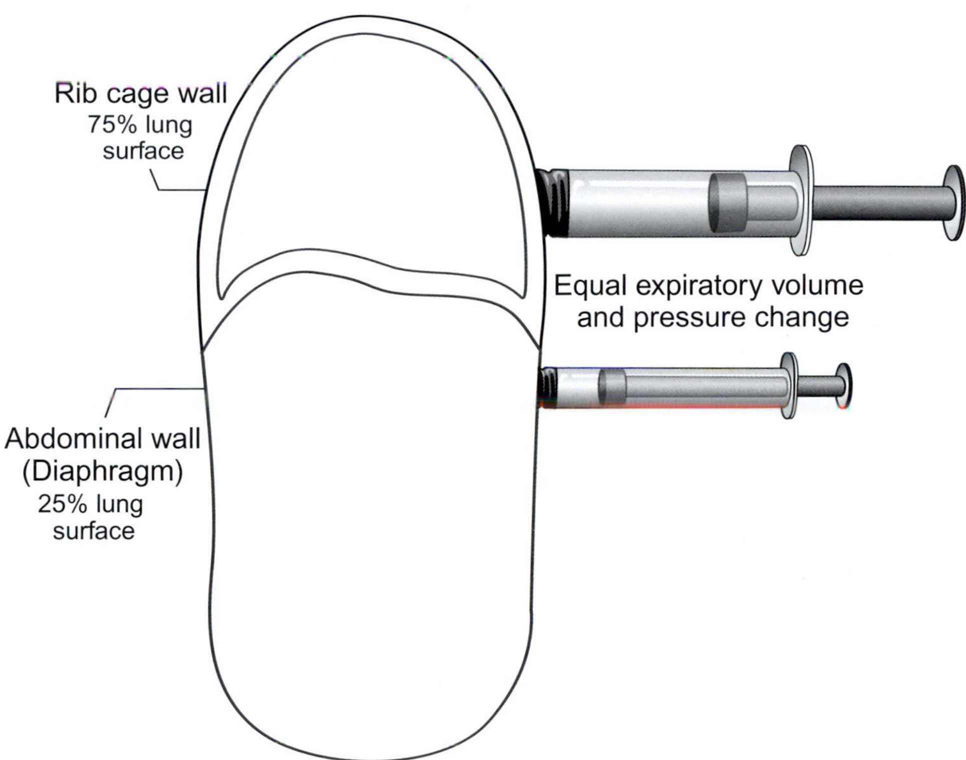

Figure 2–12. Relative movements of the rib cage wall, diaphragm, and abdominal wall.

nal wall must go through a much greater excursion than the rib cage wall to effect the same alveolar pressure change or move the same amount of air into or out of the pulmonary apparatus.

Adjustments of the Breathing Apparatus

The breathing apparatus can make many adjustments. Some of these are confined to the parts of the chest wall in which they occur. Others are the result of actions between and among different parts of the chest wall. Figure 2–13 summarizes the passive and active forces that can contribute to adjustments of the breathing apparatus. These are depicted for the pulmonary apparatus, chest wall, and the three components of the chest wall individually—rib cage wall, diaphragm, and abdominal wall. Negative and positive signs in the figure represent forces that tend to inspire and expire the breathing apparatus, respectively.

Pulmonary Apparatus

The pulmonary apparatus only participates passively in adjustments of the breathing apparatus. It recoils toward a smaller size at all times, like a stretched coil spring. Thus, it operates only in the expiratory direction.

Chest Wall

The chest wall can participate both passively and actively in adjustments of the breathing apparatus. It recoils inward at large chest wall sizes and outward at small chest wall sizes. Thus, it complements the recoil of the pulmonary apparatus at large chest wall sizes and opposes it at small chest wall sizes. Muscles of the chest wall can generate active force to either inspire or expire the breathing apparatus at any chest wall size. Muscles that inspire the apparatus are located in the rib cage wall and diaphragm, and muscles that expire the apparatus are located in the rib cage wall and abdominal wall. Active force

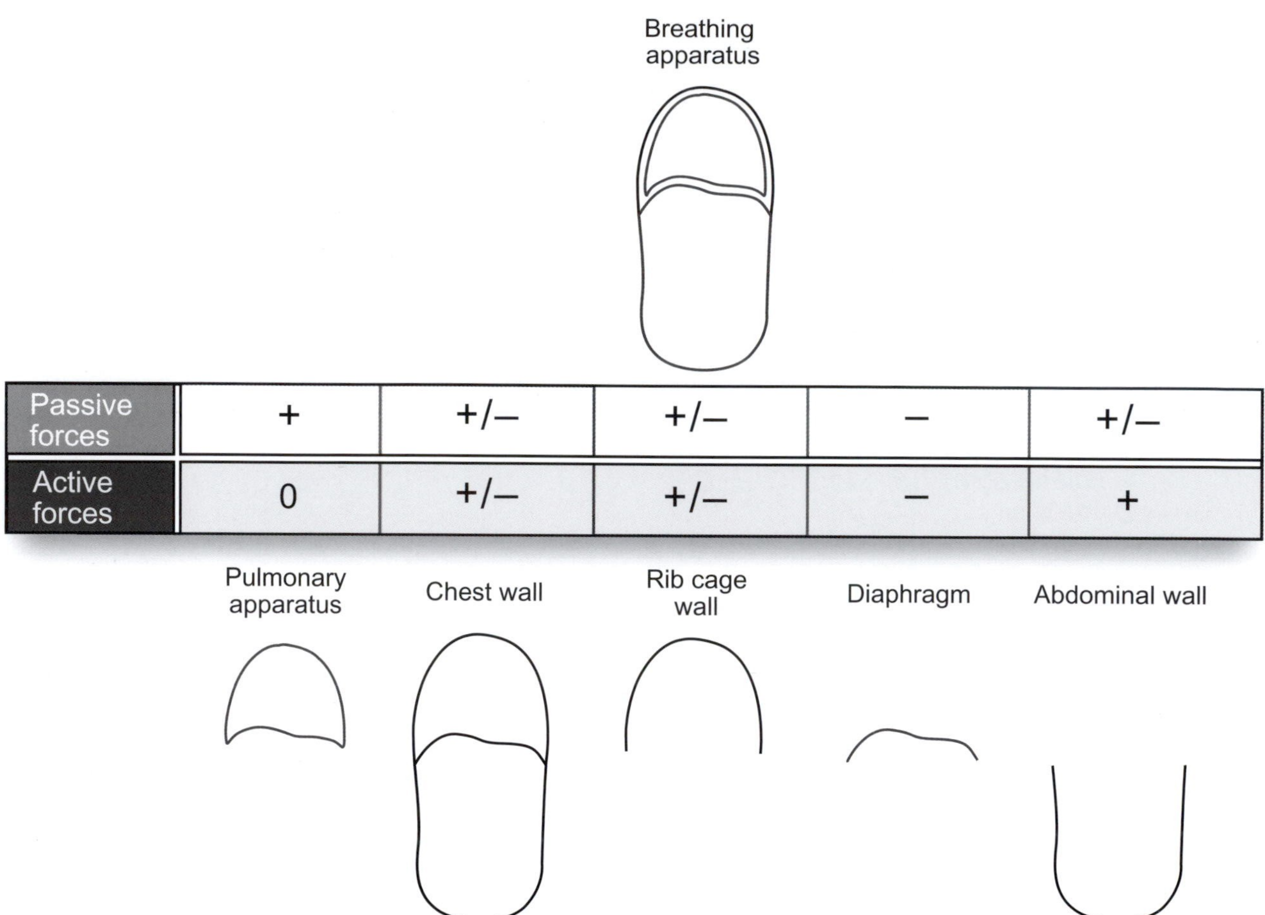

Figure 2–13. Passive and active forces of breathing. From *Evaluation and management of speech breathing disorders: Principles and methods* (p. 31), by T. Hixon and J. Hoit, 2005, Tucson, AZ: Redington Brown. Copyright 2005 by Thomas J. Hixon and Jeannette D. Hoit. Modified and reproduced with permission.

available to inspire the breathing apparatus is greater at small chest wall sizes, whereas active force available to expire the apparatus is greater at large chest wall sizes. This is because the inspiratory and expiratory muscles of the chest wall are on more favorable portions of their length-force characteristics at small and large chest wall sizes, respectively.

Rib Cage Wall. The rib cage wall can contribute both passively and actively to adjustments of the breathing apparatus. It recoils inward at large sizes and outward at small sizes (except in downright body positions). Thus, it complements the recoil of the pulmonary apparatus at large rib cage sizes and opposes it at small rib cage sizes. Muscles of the rib cage wall can generate active force in both the inspiratory and expiratory directions. Those responsible for inspiratory force are located in superficial layers of the rib cage wall and those responsible for expiratory force are located in deep layers of the wall. Active force available to inspire the breathing apparatus is greater at small rib cage wall sizes, whereas active force available to expire the apparatus is greater at large rib cage wall sizes. The force advantages at different sizes of the rib cage wall relate to more favorable length-force characteristics for the inspiratory and expiratory muscles at small and large rib cage wall sizes, respectively. The smallest muscles of the breathing apparatus are located in the rib cage wall and provide it with the capability for fast and precise action.

Diaphragm. The diaphragm is capable of contributing both passively and actively to adjustments of the breathing apparatus. When displaced footward and being less highly domed, as it is at large lung volumes, it develops no recoil. In contrast, when displaced headward and being more highly domed, as it is at small lung volumes, it recoils in the inspiratory direction. Inspiratory recoil is caused by passive stretch of the muscle fibers of the diaphragm brought about by forces acting across the structure. Thus, the diaphragm opposes the recoil of the pulmonary apparatus at small lung volumes. The diaphragm can generate active force in the inspiratory direction only. The more highly domed the configuration of the diaphragm, the more active force the structure is able to exert. This is because its muscle fibers are elongated and are on more favorable portions of their length-force characteristics.

Abdominal Wall. The abdominal wall can make both passive and active contributions to adjustments of the breathing apparatus. It recoils in the expiratory direction at large abdominal wall volumes and in the inspiratory direction at small abdominal wall volumes (except in downright body positions). Thus, it complements the recoil of the pulmonary apparatus at large abdominal wall volumes and opposes it at small abdominal wall volumes. The abdominal wall can only generate active force in the expiratory direction. Such active force can be greater at large abdominal wall volumes because the abdominal wall muscles are on more favorable portions of their length-force characteristics.

Pulmonary Apparatus-Chest Wall Unit

Mechanical arrangements between different parts of the pulmonary apparatus-chest wall unit condition how actions of the breathing apparatus are manifested. Such arrangements make it possible for one part of the breathing apparatus to cause adjustments in other parts of the apparatus, as illustrated in Figure 2–14 and discussed in the following examples.

Actions of the rib cage wall can cause adjustments in both the diaphragm and abdominal wall. For example, when the rib cage wall expands and the diaphragm and abdominal wall are quiescent, pleural pressure lowers and pulls the diaphragm headward and the abdominal wall inward. This action is akin to the way in which liquid is pulled upward in a drinking straw (hence the phrase "sucking it in" when referring to the consequence on the abdominal wall). In contrast, when the rib cage wall compresses, pleural pressure rises and pushes the diaphragm footward and the abdominal wall outward.

Actions of the diaphragm can cause adjustments in both the rib cage wall and abdominal wall. The nature of these adjustments will depend on the mechanical status of the rib cage wall and abdominal wall. For example, when the rib cage wall is fixed in position, movement of the diaphragm is resolved into footward displacement and abdominal wall distention. In contrast, when the abdominal wall is fixed in position, movement of the diaphragm is

Laundry Starch

The stiffness of the breathing apparatus changes across life. The term that pertains to this is compliance and it refers to the tendency to yield to an applied force. In the lexicon of the respiratory physiologist, compliance is quantified in terms of how much volume is displaced for the pressure applied. We are reminded of laundry starch when we think of this concept. You get a little more in the "fabric" of your breathing apparatus as time goes by. The compliance of the breathing apparatus of a newborn is relatively high and somewhat like that of a dishrag. In contrast, the compliance of the breathing apparatus of a senescent adult is relatively low and somewhat like that of a plastic garbage can lid. Thus, we start out life being relatively floppy and end up life being relatively stiff (no pun intended on the stiff part, honestly).

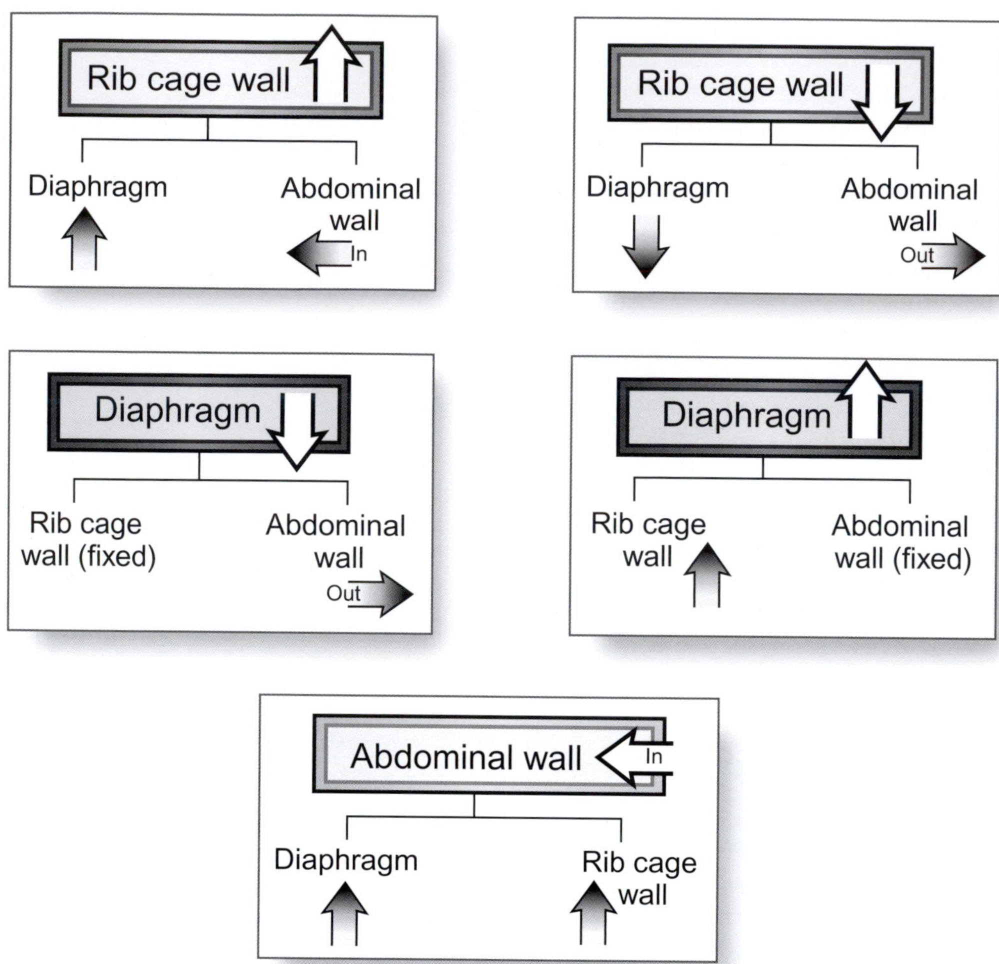

Figure 2–14. Influence of rib cage wall, diaphragm, and abdominal wall components on one another.

resolved into headward displacement of the rib cage wall. Usually, neither the rib cage wall nor abdominal wall is rigidly positioned, so that they move in accordance with their relative compliance (floppiness).

Actions of the abdominal wall can cause adjustments in both the rib cage wall and diaphragm. For example, when the muscles of the abdominal wall contract, they force the abdominal wall inward and raise abdominal pressure. This forces the lower rib cage wall outward and the diaphragm headward. The combination of these two effects causes a passive lifting of the rib cage wall, such that it moves higher and higher with more and more inward movement of the abdominal wall.

Actions of the breathing apparatus often seem deceptively simple and can be erroneously ascribed as being caused only by the parts of the apparatus in which they are observed. As noted above, however, the mechanical interplay between and among different parts of the breathing apparatus is significant and must be considered when trying to understand any adjustment of the breathing apparatus.

Output Variables of Breathing

The breathing apparatus controls a number of variables. Those that are important in the present context are volume, pressure, and shape.

Volume

Volume is defined as the size of a three-dimensional object or space. The volume of interest here is the volume of air inside the pulmonary apparatus. This volume is termed the lung volume and it reflects the size of the breathing apparatus. Lung volume is important because the behavior of the breathing apparatus depends on lung volume.

Movements of the breathing apparatus can cause a change in lung volume by moving air into or out of the pulmonary apparatus. Such volume change, termed volume displacement, can occur only if the larynx and upper airway are open.

The volume variable can be partitioned into what are called lung volumes and lung capacities. Volume is often displayed in a spirogram, a record of lung volume change over time obtained from a spirometer (a device that records volume displacement). A spirogram is shown in Figure 2–15.

There are four lung volumes. Each covers a portion of the lung volume range that is mutually exclusive of the others.

The *tidal volume* (TV) is the volume of air inspired or expired during the breathing cycle. When recorded in the resting individual, this volume is termed the resting tidal volume.

The *inspiratory reserve volume* (IRV) is the maximum volume of air that can be inspired from the tidal end-inspiratory level (the peak of the tidal volume cycle).

The *expiratory reserve volume* (ERV) is the maximum volume of air that can be expired from the tidal end-expiratory level (the trough of the tidal volume cycle).

The *residual volume* (RV) is the volume of air in the pulmonary apparatus at the end of a maximum expiration. This volume cannot be measured directly, because the pulmonary apparatus cannot be emptied voluntarily.

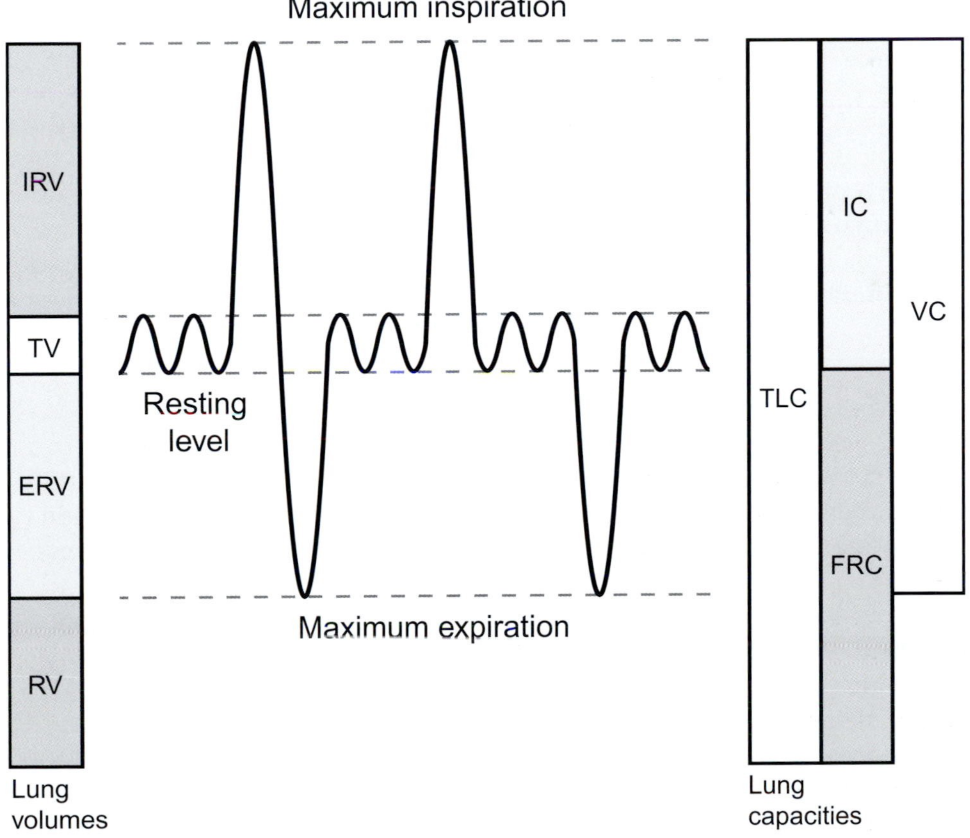

Figure 2–15. Lung volumes and lung capacities. From *Evaluation and management of speech breathing disorders: Principles and methods* (p. 36), by T. Hixon and J. Hoit, 2005, Tucson, AZ: Redington Brown. Copyright 2005 by Thomas J. Hixon and Jeannette D. Hoit. Modified and reproduced with permission.

There are four lung capacities. Each includes two or more of the lung volumes discussed above.

> The *inspiratory capacity* (IC) is the maximum volume of air that can be inspired from the resting tidal end-expiratory level. It is the sum of the tidal volume and the inspiratory reserve volume.
>
> The *vital capacity* (VC) is the maximum volume of air that can be expired following a maximum inspiration. It includes the inspiratory reserve volume, the tidal volume, and the expiratory reserve volume.
>
> The *functional residual capacity* (FRC) is the volume of air in the pulmonary apparatus at the resting tidal end-expiratory level. This capacity includes the expiratory reserve volume and the residual volume.
>
> The *total lung capacity* (TLC) is the volume of air in the pulmonary apparatus at the end of a maximum inspiration. It includes the inspiratory reserve volume, the tidal volume, the expiratory reserve volume, and the residual volume.

Figure 2–16 depicts the range of manipulable lung volumes (in percent vital capacity, %VC) in a different graphic format than that just considered for the spirogram. This display indicates the lung volumes used in a number of everyday breathing activities. The 40 %VC level represents the resting level of the breathing apparatus.

Pressure

Pressure is defined as a force distributed over a surface (pressure = force/area). The most important pressure for present purposes is the pressure inside the lungs. Recall that this pressure is termed the alveolar pressure. Alveolar pressure represents the sum of all the passive and active forces operating on the breathing apparatus.

Alveolar pressure is generated by the collision of air molecules within the lungs. When air molecules are more crowded, more collisions occur and pressure is higher. In contrast, when air molecules are less crowded, fewer collisions occur and alveolar pressure is lower. When the larynx and/or upper airway are closed, lung volume and alveolar pressure are inversely related. That is, a halving of volume causes a doubling of pressure, and a doubling of volume causes a halving of pressure (provided temperature remains constant).

One way to display alveolar pressure is in a volume-pressure diagram, such as that shown in Figure 2–17. The vertical axis of the diagram represents lung volume (in %VC) and the horizontal axis represents alveolar pressure (in centimeters of water, cmH_2O). The solid horizontal line represents the resting level of the breathing apparatus, shown to be 40 %VC in the diagram. The solid vertical line

Where Did That Come From?

We have seen many young children with cerebral palsy and breathing disorders. Many of these children, especially those who are quadriplegic and show major signs of spasticity, seem to have a governor on them. That is, they behave like there's a device that is limiting the degree to which they can willfully adjust the breathing apparatus. For example, when asked to perform an inspiratory capacity maneuver ("Take in all the air you can"), they may only be able to inspire to their resting tidal end-inspiratory level. Try it over and over again and the same thing happens. Then, out of the blue, the child shows you a gaping yawn of boredom and takes in an enormous breath. The breath may actually be several times the size the child could generate during voluntary inspiration. Now, you're faced with a dilemma. What do you record as the child's inspiratory capacity? Think about it, carefully.

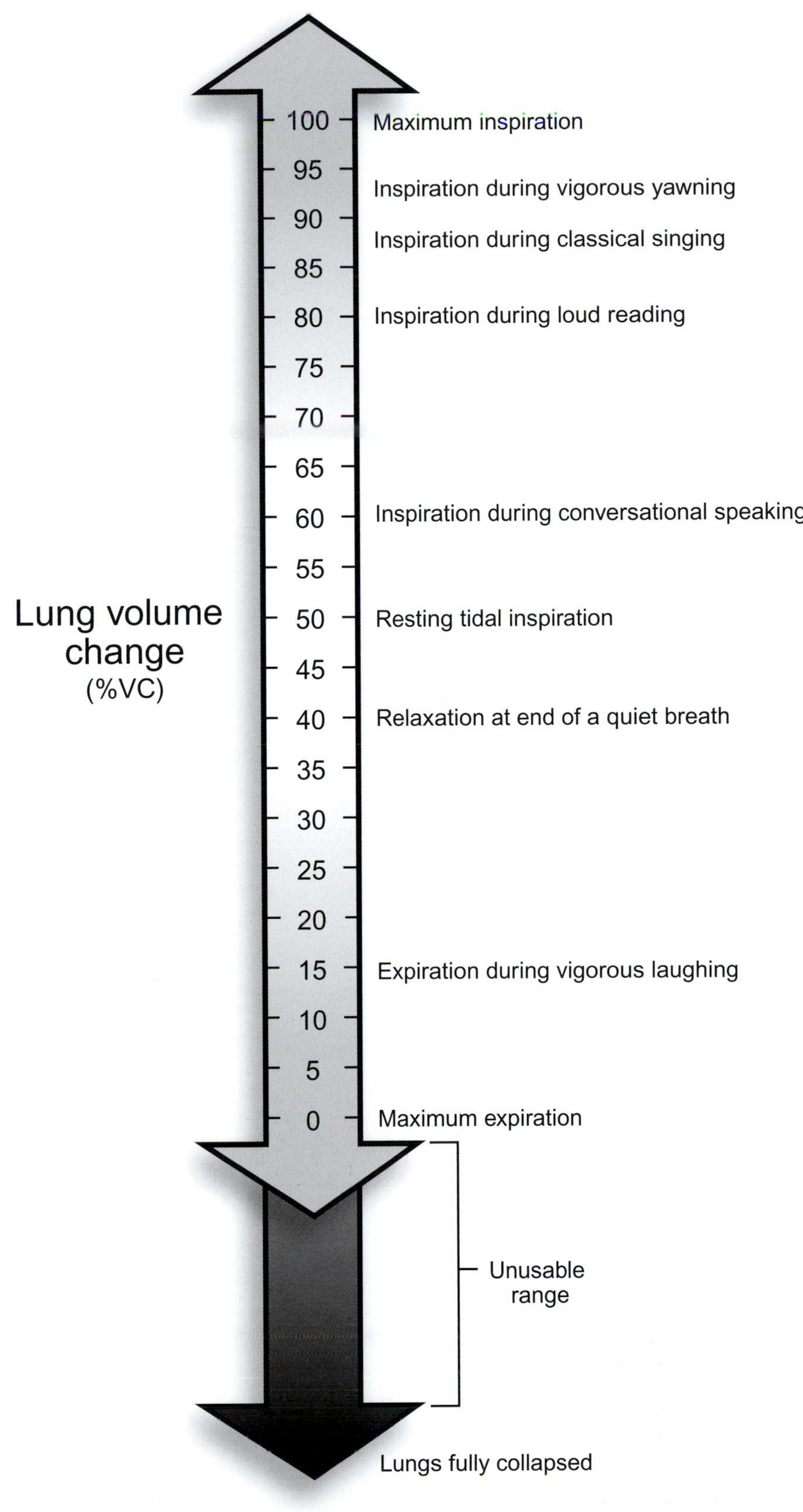

Figure 2–16. Lung volumes used in some everyday activities.

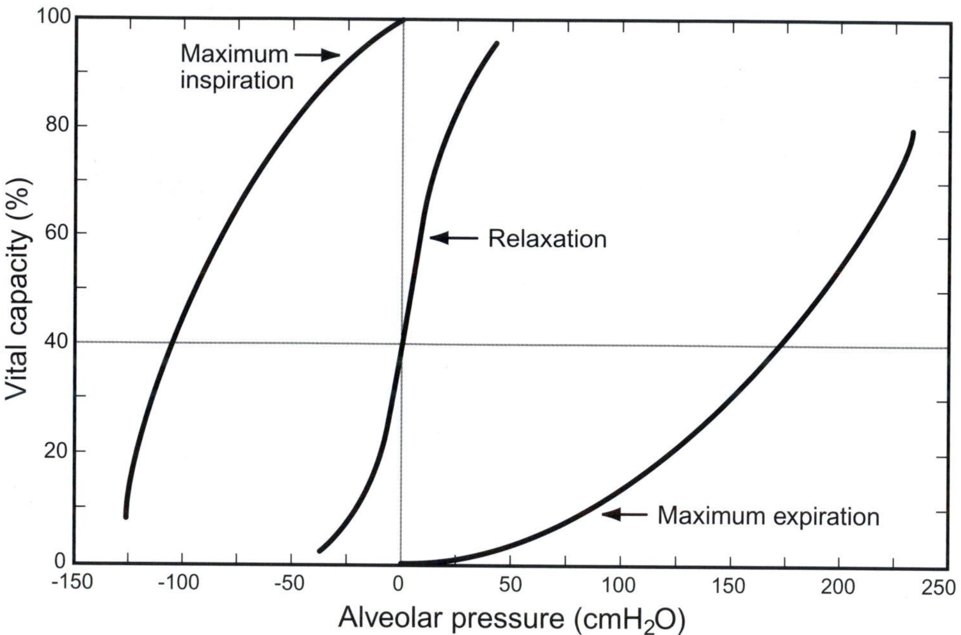

Figure 2-17. Volume-pressure diagram. From *Evaluation and management of speech breathing disorders: Principles and methods* (p. 38), by T. Hixon and J. Hoit, 2005, Tucson, AZ: Redington Brown. Copyright 2005 by Thomas J. Hixon and Jeannette D. Hoit. Modified and reproduced with permission.

Always Under Pressure

The zero pressure seen on breathing diagrams really doesn't mean zero. It actually represents atmospheric pressure, the pressure we are under all the time. Far from zero, atmospheric pressure has a magnitude of 1.01325×10^5 newtons per square meter (N/m^2). That's roughly 1000 centimeters of water (cmH_2O), a unit of pressure measurement often used by respiratory physiologists. When we blow our hardest, we might (on a good day) develop 225 cmH_2O of alveolar pressure. That's interesting. We blow as hard as we possibly can and we can only increase our alveolar pressure to about one fourth the magnitude of the pressure that is operating on us as we just sit there. Most of us probably aren't even aware that we have 1000 cmH_2O of pressure continuously trying to squash us. But, in fact, we're always under pressure.

represents atmospheric pressure (zero, by convention). Points to the left of this line represent pressures that are below atmospheric (negative, by convention) and points to the right of this line represent pressures that are above atmospheric (positive, by convention). The three curves represent volume-pressure relations during relaxation, maximum inspiration, and maximum expiration.

The relaxation pressure is the pressure produced entirely by the passive force of the breathing apparatus. As shown in Figure 2–17, the relaxation pressure varies with lung volume. Relaxation pressure is positive at lung volumes larger than the resting level of the breathing apparatus, and negative at lung volumes smaller than the resting level. The greatest positive relaxation pressure is generated at the largest lung volume, and the greatest negative relaxation pressure is generated at the smallest lung volume. In the midrange of the vital capacity, the relaxation pressure changes nearly in direct proportion to lung volume change, whereas at the extremes of the vital capacity, pressure changes more abruptly with volume change. This is because the breathing apparatus is stiffer at very large and very small lung volumes.

Departures from the relaxation pressure require active muscular effort. A net inspiratory muscular pressure is needed to generate pressure that is lower than the relaxation pressure (to the left of the volume-pressure relaxation curve) at the prevailing lung volume. In contrast, a net expiratory muscular pressure is needed to generate pressure that is higher than the relaxation pressure (to the right of the curve) at the prevailing lung volume. When net is specified, as it is here, it means that both inspiratory and expiratory muscular pressures may be operating simultaneously, but one or the other is predominating. When pressure is equal to the relaxation pressure, this may mean that all the muscles of the breathing apparatus are relaxed, or it may mean that equal inspiratory and expiratory muscular pressures are being exerted so that they cancel one another.

The maximum inspiratory pressure that can be generated by the breathing apparatus is represented by the leftmost curve in Figure 2–17. The maximum inspiratory pressure is greater at smaller lung volumes than larger lung volumes. This is because negative relaxation pressure is more forceful at smaller lung volumes, and because the inspiratory muscles are operating under more favorable length-force conditions at smaller lung volumes.

The maximum expiratory pressure that can be generated by the breathing apparatus is represented by the rightmost curve in Figure 2–17. The maximum expiratory pressure is greater at larger lung volumes than smaller lung volumes. This is because positive relaxation pressure is more forceful at larger lung volumes, and because the expiratory muscles are operating under more favorable length-force conditions at larger lung volumes.

Figure 2–18 shows the range of achievable alveolar pressures (in cmH_2O) in a different form of graphic display. Shown along the pressure scale is a list of activities and typical alveolar pressures associated with those activities.

Shape

Shape is the configuration of an object, independent of its size or volume. The shape of interest in the present context is the shape of the chest wall. More specifically, shape is the surface configuration of the rib cage wall and abdominal wall, the two parts of the chest wall that can be observed externally. Shape is important because it provides information about the prevailing mechanical advantages of different parts of the chest wall.

The rib cage wall and abdominal wall each usually behave with a single degree of freedom with respect to their movement. Thus, it is possible to characterize the shape of the chest wall when the relative sizes (which can be converted to volumes) of the rib cage wall and abdominal wall are monitored. One convention for illustrating shape is to display the relative sizes of the rib cage wall and abdominal wall against one another. This convention is portrayed in Figure 2–19, which displays rib cage wall anteroposterior (front-to-back) diameter (a measure of size) on the vertical axis, increasing upward, and abdominal wall anteroposterior diameter on the horizontal axis, increasing rightward.

The dashed line in Figure 2–19 represents the relaxation characteristic of the chest wall. This is the shape assumed by the chest wall at different lung volumes when the breathing muscles are completely relaxed. The circle at the top of the relaxation characteristic represents the total lung capacity, whereas the circle at the bottom of the characteristic represents the residual volume. The filled circle near the middle of the characteristic represents the resting level of the breathing apparatus. The circumscribed area in the diagram depicts the full range of shapes that the chest wall can assume. The range of shapes is smaller near the diameter extremes, where both the rib cage wall and abdominal wall are very large or very small. The range of shapes is greatest in the diameter midrange.

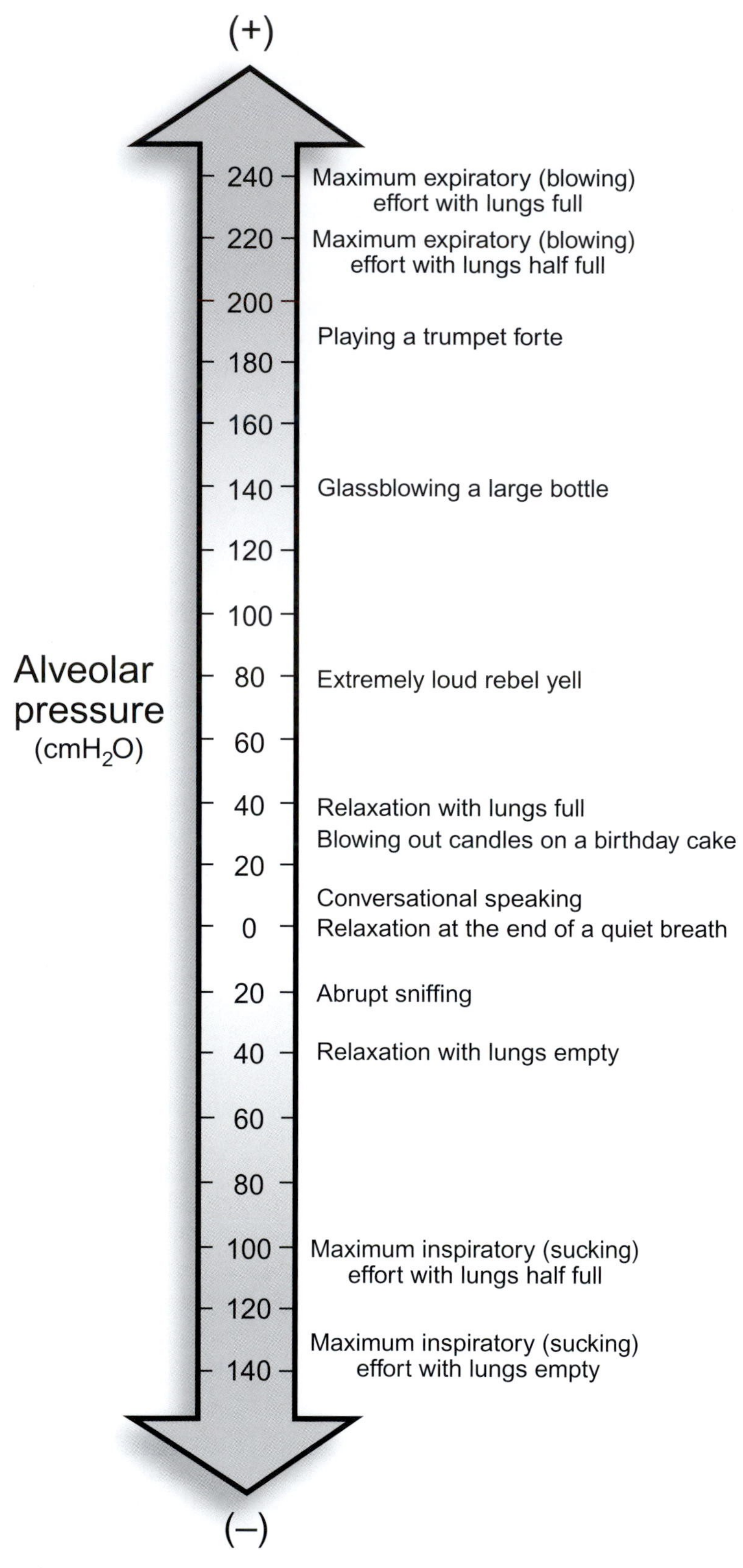

Figure 2–18. Alveolar pressures used for different activities.

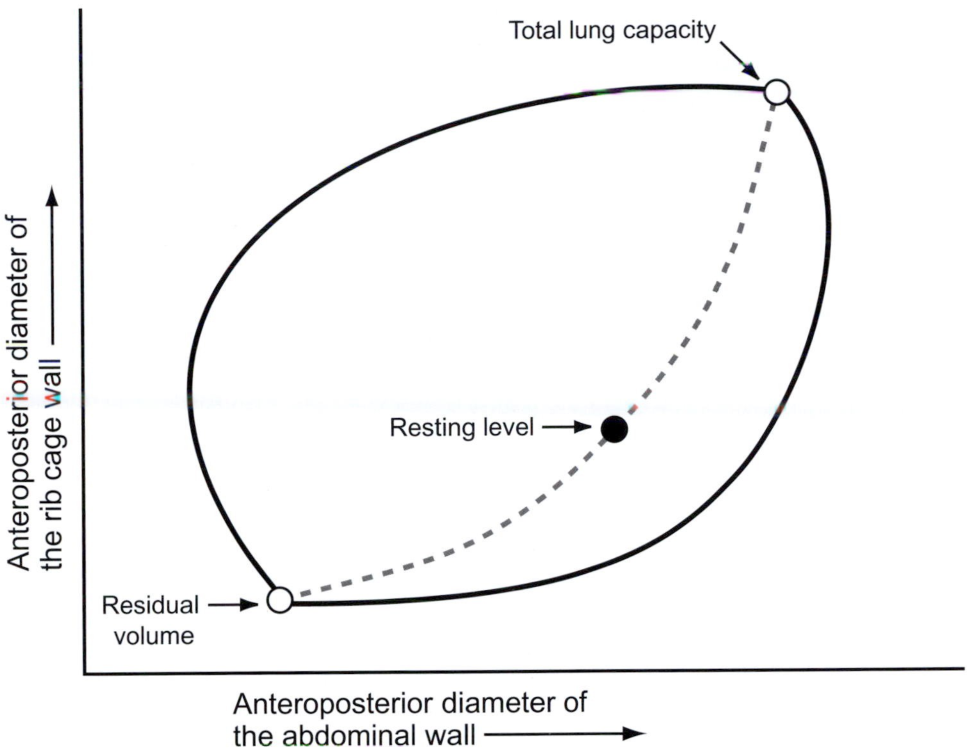

Figure 2–19. Relative diameter diagram. From *Evaluation and management of speech breathing disorders: Principles and methods* (p. 41), by T. Hixon and J. Hoit, 2005, Tucson, AZ: Redington Brown. Copyright 2005 by Thomas J. Hixon and Jeannette D. Hoit. Modified and reproduced with permission.

Each point in Figure 2–19 represents a unique combination of chest wall shapes and lung volumes that can be interpreted in relation to underlying muscular mechanism. Figure 2–20 illustrates how this can be done.

Points on the relaxation characteristic in Figure 2–20 represent either complete relaxation of the muscles of the chest wall or equal and opposite muscular forces that cancel one another. Points that are not on the relaxation characteristic can only be achieved using active muscular force. Points to the left of the relaxation characteristic can be achieved using (a) a net inspiratory rib cage wall force, (b) an expiratory abdominal wall force, (c) a net inspiratory rib cage wall force and an expiratory abdominal wall force, or (d) a net expiratory rib cage wall force and a greater expiratory abdominal wall force. Points to the right of the relaxation characteristic can be achieved using (a) a net expiratory rib cage wall force, or (b) a net expiratory rib cage wall force and a lesser expiratory abdominal wall force.

Figure 2–21 shows the range of achievable chest wall shapes (in relative terms) in a different form of graphic display. Shown along the scale in the figure is a list of events and conditions and the chest wall shapes associated with them.

Neural Control of Breathing

Breathing movements are controlled by the nervous system. This section describes the neural bases of breathing with focus on its substrates and their participation in the control of tidal breathing and special acts of breathing.

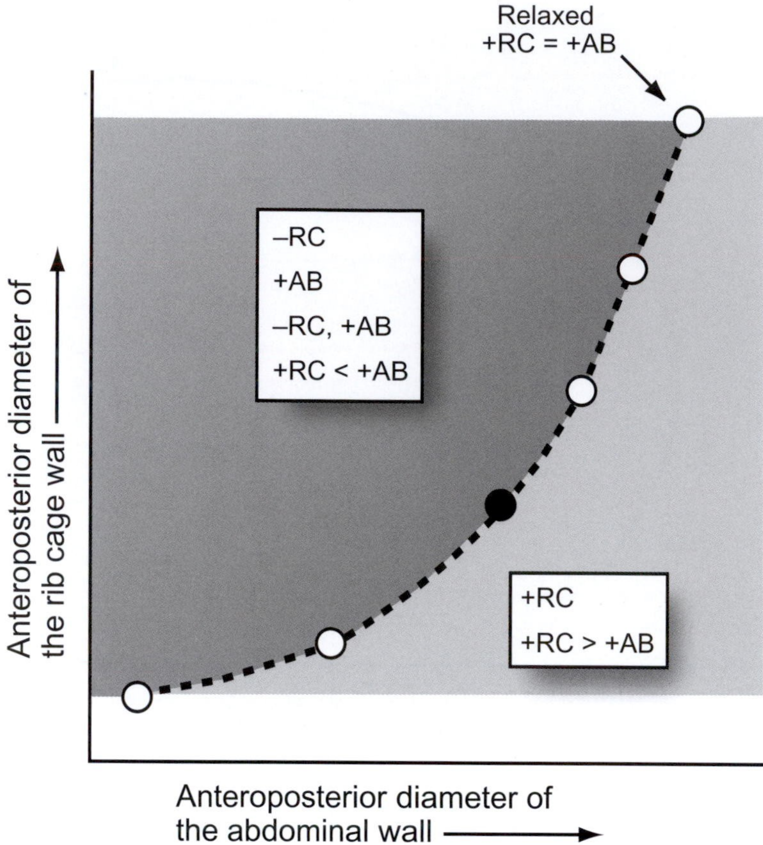

Figure 2–20. Interpretation of muscular mechanism from the relative diameter diagram.

Neural Substrates

Figure 2–22 depicts the structures of the nervous system that are important to the control of breathing. These structures are located in two major subdivisions of the nervous system, the central nervous system and the peripheral nervous system.

The central nervous system includes the brain and spinal cord. The former is a mass of neural tissue within the skull and the latter is a long appendage of the brain that extends downward through the vertebral column.

The peripheral nervous system connects the central nervous system with different parts of the breathing apparatus. These connections are effected through cranial and spinal nerves. Four cranial nerves are participants in the control of breathing. These include cranial nerves IX (glossopharyngeal), X (vagus), and XII (hypoglossal), which innervate muscles that dilate the larynx and upper airway during inspiration, and cranial nerve XI (accessory), which innervates the ***sternocleidomastoid*** muscle that elevates the sternum, clavicle, and rib cage.

Twenty-two spinal nerves contribute to the control of breathing. These are listed in Table 2–1 along with the muscles they innervate. As shown there, the spinal nerves relevant to breathing include the eight cervical (C) nerves, the twelve thoracic (T) nerves, and the first two lumbar (L) nerves. Successively lower spinal nerves generally provide motor nerve supply to successively lower regions of the breathing apparatus. An exception is the diaphragm, which derives its motor nerve supply from C3–C5, a collection of motor nerves designated as the phrenic nerve. Table 2–1 lists only the motor nerve supply to the muscles of the chest wall. The sensory nerve supply to the chest wall is generally similar in pattern to its motor nerve supply, a notable exception being that the sensory supply of the diaphragm is vested in the phrenic nerve and lower thoracic nerves.

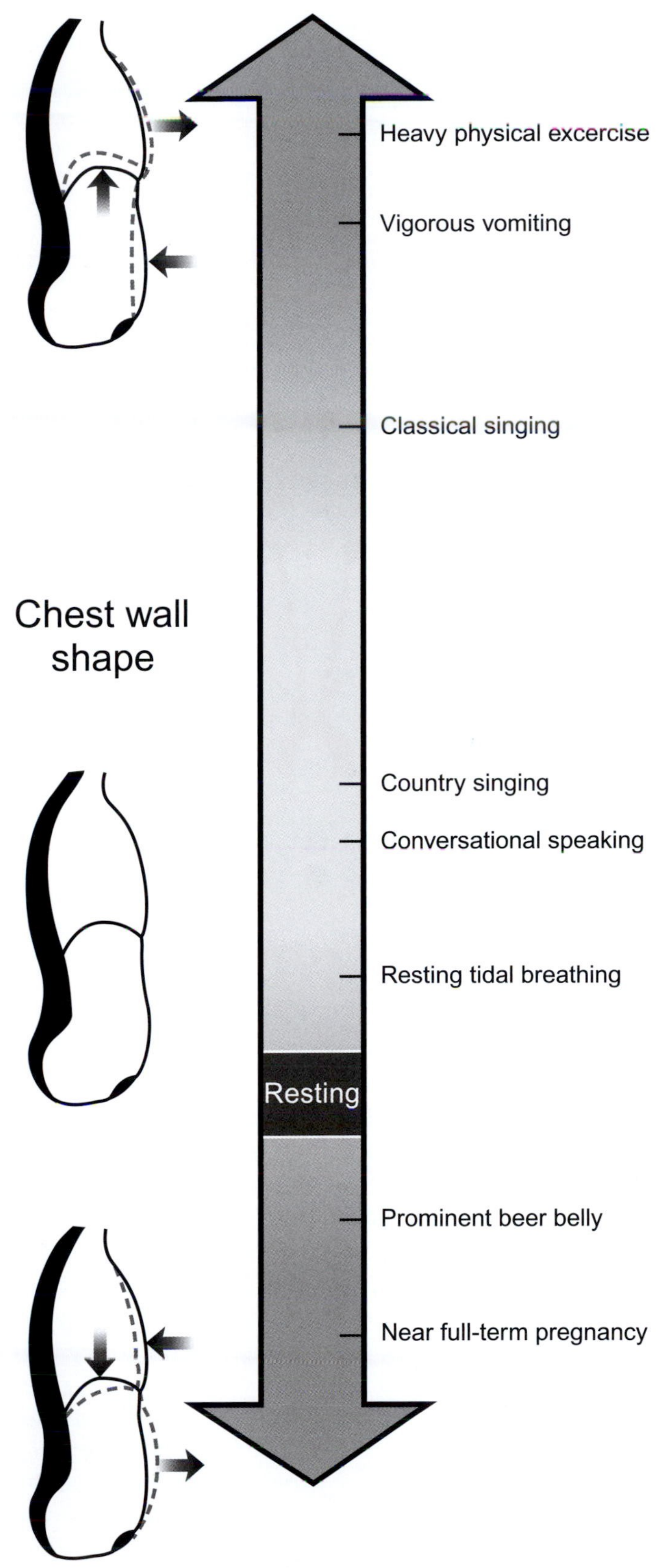

Figure 2–21. Chest wall shapes characteristic of different events and conditions.

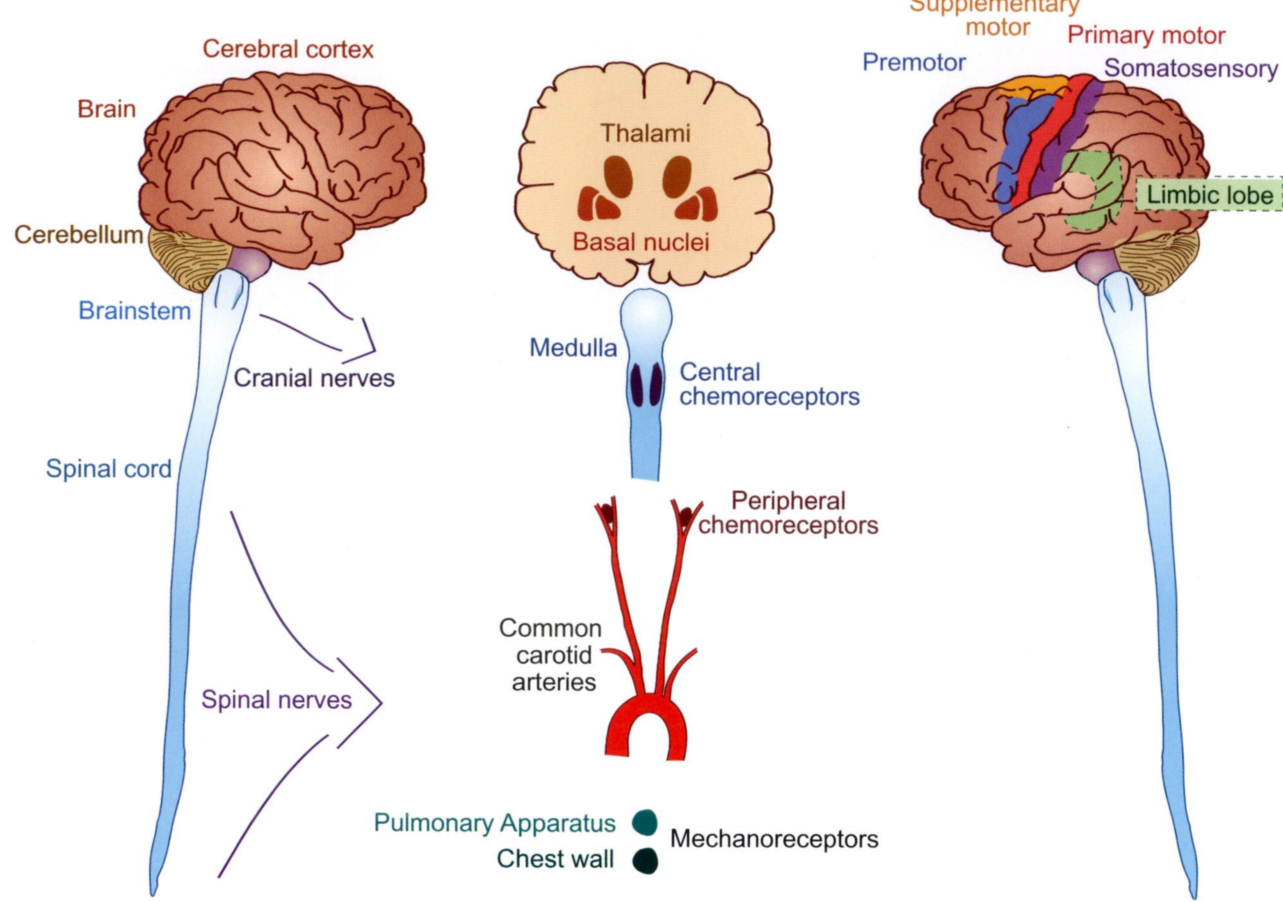

Figure 2-22. Adult nervous system. From *Evaluation and management of speech breathing disorders: Principles and methods* (p. 43), by T. Hixon and J. Hoit, 2005, Tucson, AZ: Redington Brown. Copyright 2005 by Thomas J. Hixon and Jeannette D. Hoit. Modified and reproduced with permission.

These neural substrates control a wide variety of breathing activities. Such activities can be associated with different states, including being awake, alert, aroused, asleep, conscious, or unconscious. Such activities can also be classified using different schemes that include terms such as automatic, metabolic, reflexive, learned, voluntary, behavioral, purposeful, or emotional. For present purposes, discussion of the control of breathing is organized around the simple dichotomy of tidal breathing and special acts of breathing.

Control of Tidal Breathing

Tidal breathing, the most common form of breathing, is sometimes called automatic breathing, metabolic breathing, or involuntary breathing. The control of tidal breathing is vested in the brainstem. Of special importance are structures located in the medulla, the region of the brainstem that is contiguous with the spinal cord. These structures include a network of neurons that are collectively designated as the lower brain center for breathing. The primary tasks of this lower brain center are to generate a rhythmic pattern of breathing and to regulate gas levels (oxygen and carbon dioxide) in arterial blood by adjusting ventilation (Feldman & McCrimmon, 1999; Lumb, 2000). The lower brain center can run breathing on its own automatically without input from higher brain centers and is often called the central pattern generator for breathing.

Signals from the brainstem travel via peripheral nerves to reach the muscles of the chest wall. For example, for inspiration, signals from the brainstem

Table 2-1. Summary of the Segmental Origins of the Motor Nerve Supply to the Muscles of the Chest Wall (C = cervical, T = thoracic, L = lumbar).

MUSCLE	SPINAL NERVE
RIB CAGE WALL	
Sternocleidomastoid	C1-C5
Scalenus group	C2-C8
Pectoralis major	C5-C8
Pectoralis minor	C5-C8
Subclavius	C5-C6
Serratus anterior	C5-C7, T2-T3
External intercostals	T1-T11
Internal intercostals	T1-T11
Transversus thoracis	T2-T6
Latissimus dorsi	C6-C8
Serratus posterior superior	T2-T3
Serratus posterior inferior	T9-T12
Lateral iliocostalis group	C4-T6, T1-T11, T7-L2
Levatores costarum	C8-T11
Quadratus lumborum	T12-L2
Subcostals	T1-T11
DIAPHRAGM	
Diaphragm	C3-C5
ABDOMINAL WALL	
Rectus abdominis	T7-T12
External oblique	T8-L1
Internal oblique	T8-L1
Transversus abdominis	T7-T12
Latissimus dorsi	C6-C8
Lateral iliocostalis lumborum	T7-L2
Quadratus lumborum	T12-L2

Source: Based on Dickson and Maue-Dickson (1982).

reach the ***diaphragm*** muscle via the phrenic nerve and cause its fibers to contract. Signals may also travel to the ***external intercostal*** muscles, causing them either to stiffen the rib cage wall (during resting tidal inspiration) or to assist the diaphragm as a supplemental prime mover (during more forceful tidal inspiration). Signals sent simultaneously to laryngeal and upper airway muscles increase the size of their associated airways to reduce the resistance to inspiratory airflow and stiffen the tissues that line them to reduce their chances of being sucked inward.

The breathing pattern generated by the brainstem is strongly conditioned by afferent (incoming) information from a variety of sources. Most of the time, this afferent information is received and processed unconsciously. Sometimes, however, afferent information is processed to a level of awareness (sensation) or to a level of meaning and association (perception). At such times, individuals may begin to consciously attend to their breathing and to develop breathing-related perceptions having to do with forces, movements, and feelings of breathing comfort, to give a few examples.

The most important afferent information comes from chemoreceptors and mechanoreceptors. Chemoreceptors are sensitive to chemical status and those most relevant to breathing are called central and peripheral chemoreceptors. Central chemoreceptors, which are located on the front and side surfaces of the medulla, respond primarily to changes in the amount of carbon dioxide in cerebral spinal fluid. Peripheral chemoreceptors are located in the carotid bodies at the bifurcation of the common carotid arteries, near the major blood supply to the brain. These are the primary oxygen receptors for the body, although they also respond to changes in the level of carbon dioxide and acidity-alkalinity balance in arterial blood. Central and peripheral chemoreceptors generally act synergistically to stimulate adjustments in breathing by providing moment-to-moment updates on the concentration of gas in the blood. Changes in the concentration of gas stimulate the brainstem to make appropriate adjustments in ventilation. For example, an increase in carbon dioxide or a decrease in oxygen stimulates the brainstem to send signals through the peripheral nerves to the chest wall muscles to increase ventilation.

Mechanoreceptors are sensitive to mechanical changes and those of special importance to the control of tidal breathing are located in the pulmonary apparatus and chest wall. Those in the pulmonary apparatus respond to stimuli such as the stretching of smooth muscles (such as occurs with an increase in lung volume), airway irritants (such as smoke, dust, chemicals, or cold air), and distortions of the alveolar wall (such as might occur when excess fluid surrounds the alveoli). Signals from these pulmonary mechanoreceptors reach the central nervous system by way of cranial nerve X. Mechanoreceptors in the chest wall respond to changes in muscle length (such as occur with changes in rib cage wall or abdominal wall volume) or changes in force (such as occur with changes in inspiratory or expiratory muscular efforts). Their afferent signals reach the central nervous system via spinal nerves.

Other afferent input can also influence tidal breathing (Shea, Walter, Pelley, Murphy, & Guz, 1987; Wyke, 1974). For example, afferent signals from mechanoreceptors located in the larynx or upper airway and signals from cranial nerves that transmit visual and auditory information (cranial nerves II and VIII, respectively) can affect breathing. Thus, tidal breathing can be altered by the presence of an irritant in the larynx or upper airway, by the images in an action-packed movie, or by rhythms of a musical concert.

Tidal breathing can also be influenced by internally generated activity from brain areas outside the brainstem (Mador & Tobin, 1991; Shea, 1996; Shea, Murphy, Hamilton, Benchetrit, & Guz, 1988; Western & Patrick, 1988). For example, cognitive activity (originating from cortical areas), such as that associated with the performance of mental arithmetic, can change tidal breathing. In fact, merely being consciously aware of breathing can change its pattern. Emotional influences (originating from limbic areas) can also have a profound influence on tidal breathing. Feelings of excitement, anger, or fear, for example, can be associated with hyperventilation, breath holding, or erratic breathing. Changes in tidal breathing can even be a primary sign (and feelings of breathlessness a primary symptom) of certain psychogenic disorders, such as anxiety disorder or panic disorder. These types of disorders have been so strongly linked to breathing that they are sometimes classified as hyperventilation disorders (Gardner, 1996).

Control of Special Acts of Breathing

Special acts of breathing can be defined as acts of breathing that are not effected for the primary purpose of maintaining homeostasis of arterial blood gases (Shea, 1996). They are controlled by higher brain centers that either override or bypass activity of the lower (brainstem) center for breathing. Special acts of breathing can be voluntary (highly conscious), such as breath holding or performing a guided breathing exercise. Or, they can be learned, well practiced, and require little conscious control of breathing—for example, breathing associated with glass blowing, wind instrument playing, singing, or speaking. Other special acts of breathing, such as laughing or crying, are driven primarily by emotions.

As with any voluntary motor act, a voluntary act of breathing requires a motor plan. Motor plans and the process of generating them are complex and only partially understood. What is known for sure is that many brain centers participate in the process, including subcortical structures (in particular the

Breathing as a Laughing Matter

Breathing plays a huge role in laughter. Much of laughter, especially the hearty type, goes on within the expiratory reserve volume. Laughter also involves large movements of the abdominal wall. This is probably the reason our folk language is riddled with statements like "I busted a gut laughing," "He kept me in stitches with his jokes," and "We laughed 'til our sides hurt." The neural mechanisms that underlie laughter are different from those that underlie speech breathing. This is illustrated dramatically in persons who can't move the abdominal wall on command or use it for speech production, but show vigorous movement of the wall during involuntary laughter. Thus, even if someone appears to be paralyzed, it's always wise to ask the question, "Paralyzed for what activity?"

basal nucleus, cerebellum, and thalamus) and cortical structures in the frontal and parietal lobes of the brain (in particular the primary motor cortex, premotor cortex, supplementary motor area, and somatosensory area). As a behavior becomes learned and less consciously guided, there is likely to be less reliance on cortical participation in the development of the motor plan. Commands from higher brain centers can be integrated at the brainstem level such that they override the central pattern generator for breathing. Commands can also be routed directly from the cortex to spinal nerves, bypassing the brainstem altogether (Corfield, Murphy, & Guz, 1998) and imposing cortical control over the breathing act.

Special acts of breathing that are associated with emotional expression are driven by the limbic system, a phylogenetically old part of the brain. The limbic system has a strong influence on the control of special acts of breathing such as crying and laughing. Crying and laughing can even override voluntary acts of breathing, indicating that limbic drive can prevail over cortical drive. Consider, for example, the situation of attempting to speak while sobbing.

It is common for the nervous system to manage multiple breathing-related drives simultaneously, and often these drives compete with one another. Voluntary breath holding is one example. Breath holding is controlled by the cerebral cortex and is a clear demonstration of the ability of the cortex to override the brainstem. Nevertheless, cortical control must eventually give way to brainstem control as danger signals from chemoreceptors make it impossible to continue to inhibit inspiration. Less dramatic examples of competing drives occur frequently and include situations such as attempting to speak while exercising, or playing a wind instrument while experiencing stage fright.

Ventilation and Gas Exchange During Tidal Breathing

Tidal breathing is the type of breathing engaged in most of the time. Its name comes from the ebb and flow of air that resembles the ebb and flow of an ocean tide. Tidal breathing is driven by the need to ventilate (to move air in and out of the pulmonary apparatus) for the purpose of gas exchange (to deliver oxygen, O_2, to the body and remove carbon dioxide, CO_2, from it).

Figure 2–23 depicts the process of gas exchange during tidal breathing. Air, which consists of approximately 21% oxygen, enters the alveoli during tidal breathing. Oxygen then leaves the alveoli and enters the bloodstream to travel to tissues throughout the body. Tissues absorb oxygen from the blood and return carbon dioxide (a byproduct of metabolism) to the blood. The carbon dioxide then travels through the bloodstream and eventually reaches the

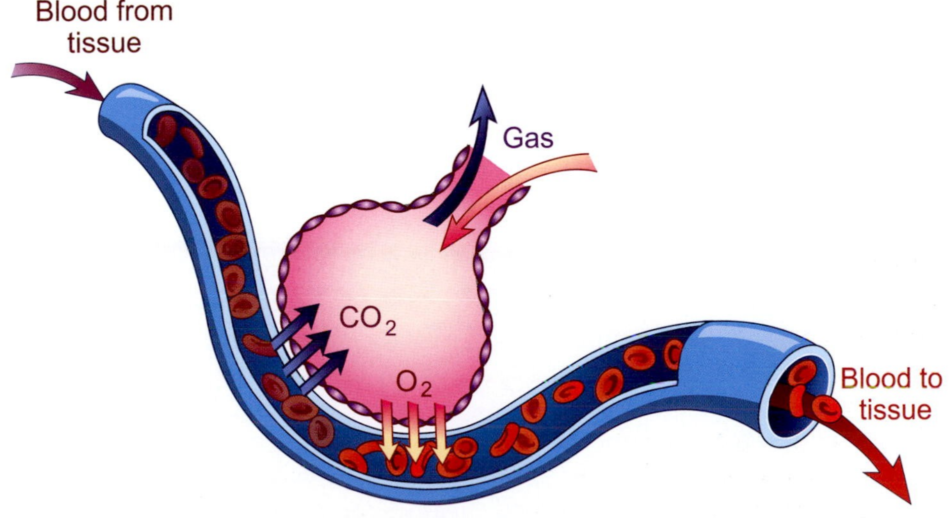

Figure 2–23. Process of gas exchange during tidal breathing.

alveoli where it is released. When metabolic demand increases, as with increased physical or mental activity, more oxygen is consumed and more carbon dioxide is produced.

Tidal breathing at rest is associated with a relatively regular inspiration-expiration pattern that begins and ends at the resting level of the breathing apparatus. This pattern is exemplified for lung volume (in liters, L), airflow (in liters per second, LPS), and alveolar pressure (in cmH_2O) in Figure 2–24. During inspiration, the chest wall expands, causing the lungs to expand and alveolar pressure to fall. This creates a pressure gradient, with the pressure inside the pulmonary apparatus being lower than that outside the apparatus. As a result, air flows into the pulmonary apparatus. When equilibration is reached (the pressure outside and inside the pulmonary apparatus are equal) inspiratory airflow ceases.

Expiratory airflow begins as the lungs compress and alveolar pressure rises. Such airflow continues until the resting level of the breathing apparatus is reached. These patterns of volume, airflow, and pressure change are generally the same across body positions, except that the absolute lung volume range differs with body position.

Resting tidal breathing is driven by a combination of passive and active forces. These are summarized graphically in Figure 2–25 for the upright and supine body positions. During inspiration, essentially all of the active force comes from the diaphragm. The diaphragm contracts and displaces the rib cage wall and abdominal wall outward. This is true for all body positions. In the upright body position, some rib cage wall muscles and abdominal wall muscles are also active during inspiration (Hixon, Goldman, & Mead, 1973; Loring & Mead, 1982). Rib cage wall muscle activity stiffens the rib cage wall to prevent it from being sucked inward when the diaphragm contracts. Abdominal wall muscle activity usually causes the abdominal wall to move inward. When the abdominal wall moves inward, the rib cage wall is lifted and the diaphragm is pushed headward. This stretches the fibers of the diaphragm so that they are placed on more favorable portions of their length-force characteristics for contraction. In the supine body position, the abdominal wall muscles are relaxed. This is because the abdominal wall is already pulled inward and the diaphragm is already pushed headward by the force of gravity.

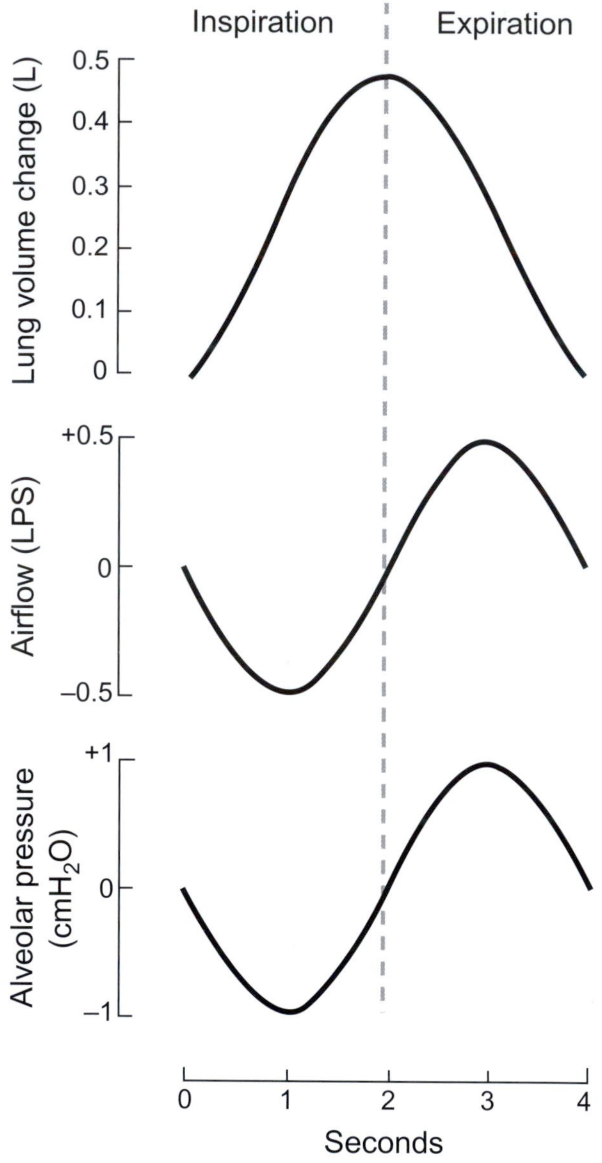

Figure 2–24. Pattern of resting tidal breathing.

During expiration, the relaxation pressure of the breathing apparatus moves the rib cage wall and abdominal wall inward. Thus, resting tidal expiration is primarily a passive event. Nevertheless, in the upright body position, the abdominal wall muscles remain active throughout the resting tidal breathing cycle.

Although resting tidal breathing shares general features across individuals, its specific details differ from person to person. In fact, each person has what

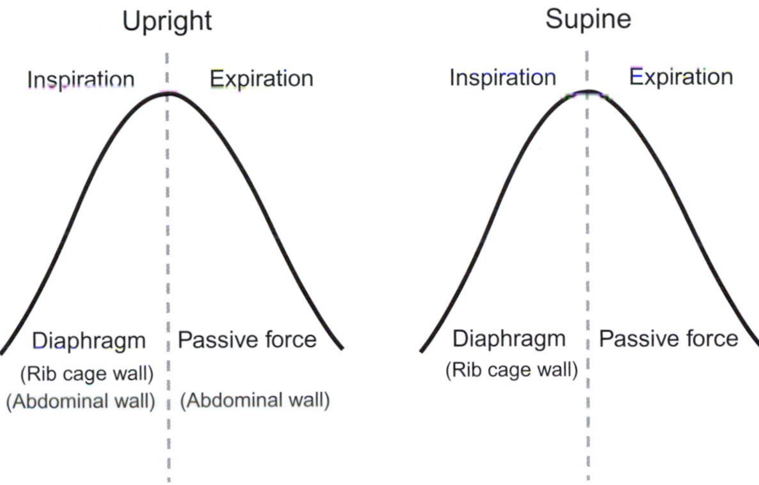

Figure 2–25. Passive and active forces of resting tidal breathing.

> **Ribbit, Ribbit**
>
> Ever watch a frog breathe? Did you notice how its cheeks moved? Frogs don't have a diaphragm to pull air into their lungs. They push the air in using their mouths like pistons. Frogs are positive pressure breathers. People are negative pressure breathers. A frog doesn't have the ability to emulate us (except, perhaps, Kermit) if its positive pressure pump fails. But, we have the ability to emulate the frog if our negative pressure pump fails, by doing what is called glossopharyngeal breathing. And what would you suppose is the common name for such breathing? Well, it's "frog breathing." In frog breathing, the tongue and throat are used to pump air into the lungs. Air is gulped in small portions (mouthfuls), each held in place by closing the larynx as a one-way valve. Frog breathing isn't difficult to learn and once mastered can be used to fill the lungs in a stepwise fashion all the way to the top.

might be thought of as a signature resting tidal breathing pattern that remains relatively unchanged over the years (Benchetrit et al., 1989; Dejours, 1996; Shea & Guz, 1992; Shea, Horner, Benchetrit, & Guz, 1990; Shea, Walter, Murphy, & Guz, 1987).

BREATHING AND SPEECH PRODUCTION

The breathing apparatus provides the driving forces that enable the generation of speech. Actions of the breathing apparatus during speech production contribute to the control of speech intensity (loudness), voice frequency (pitch), linguistic stress (emphasis), and the segmentation (division) of speech into units (syllables, words, phrases). At the same time the breathing apparatus performs these speech-related functions, it continues to serve its primary functions of ventilation and gas exchange.

This section describes two forms of speech breathing—extended steady utterances and running speech activities—as performed in the upright body position (standing or seated erect). Following these descriptions, consideration is given to speech breathing as it relates to other body positions, ventilation and gas exchange, drive to breathe, cognitive-linguistic factors, conversational interchange, body type, development, age, and sex.

Breathing in Extended Steady Utterances

Extended steady utterances are those that are produced throughout most of the vital capacity. An extended steady utterance begins after taking the deepest inspiration possible and continues until the air supply is depleted. Such an utterance might be a sustained vowel, a series of repeated syllables of equal stress, or a sung note. Extended steady utterances are considered here following the conceptualizations and elaborations of others (Hixon, 1973; Hixon & Hoit, 2005; Hixon, Mead, & Goldman, 1976; Weismer, 1985).

Figure 2–26 shows the volume, pressure, and shape events associated with a sustained vowel produced at a usual and steady loudness, pitch, and voice quality. As can be seen in the figure, lung volume decreases at a constant rate throughout the utterance. Alveolar pressure rises abruptly, remains steady throughout the utterance, and falls abruptly as the utterance ends. Rib cage wall volume and abdominal wall volume, which together reflect the shape of the chest wall, decrease at constant and similar rates.

Both relaxation pressure and muscular pressure contribute to extended steady utterance production. This is illustrated in Figure 2–27 for the same utterance depicted in Figure 2–26. In the top panel of Figure 2–27, alveolar pressure (in cmH_2O) is plotted on the horizontal axis, ranging from negative (inspiratory) to positive (expiratory). Lung volume (in %VC) is plotted on the vertical axis, with 40 %VC

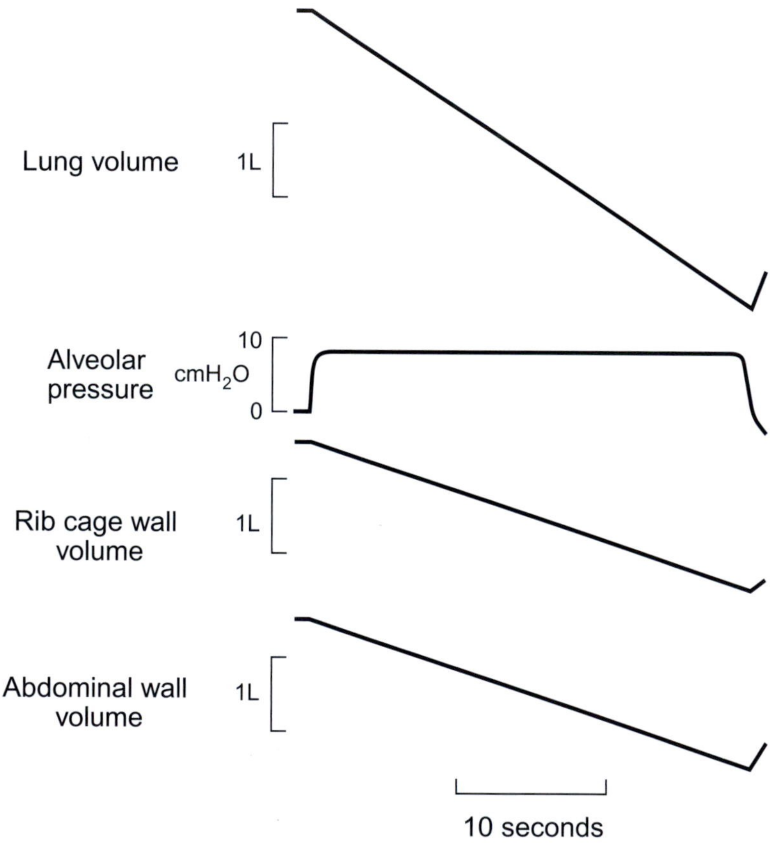

Figure 2–26. Volume, pressure, and shape events for an extended steady utterance produced in the upright body position. From *Evaluation and management of speech breathing disorders: Principles and methods* (p. 57), by T. Hixon and J. Hoit, 2005, Tucson, AZ: Redington Brown. Copyright 2005 by Thomas J. Hixon and Jeannette D. Hoit. Modified and reproduced with permission.

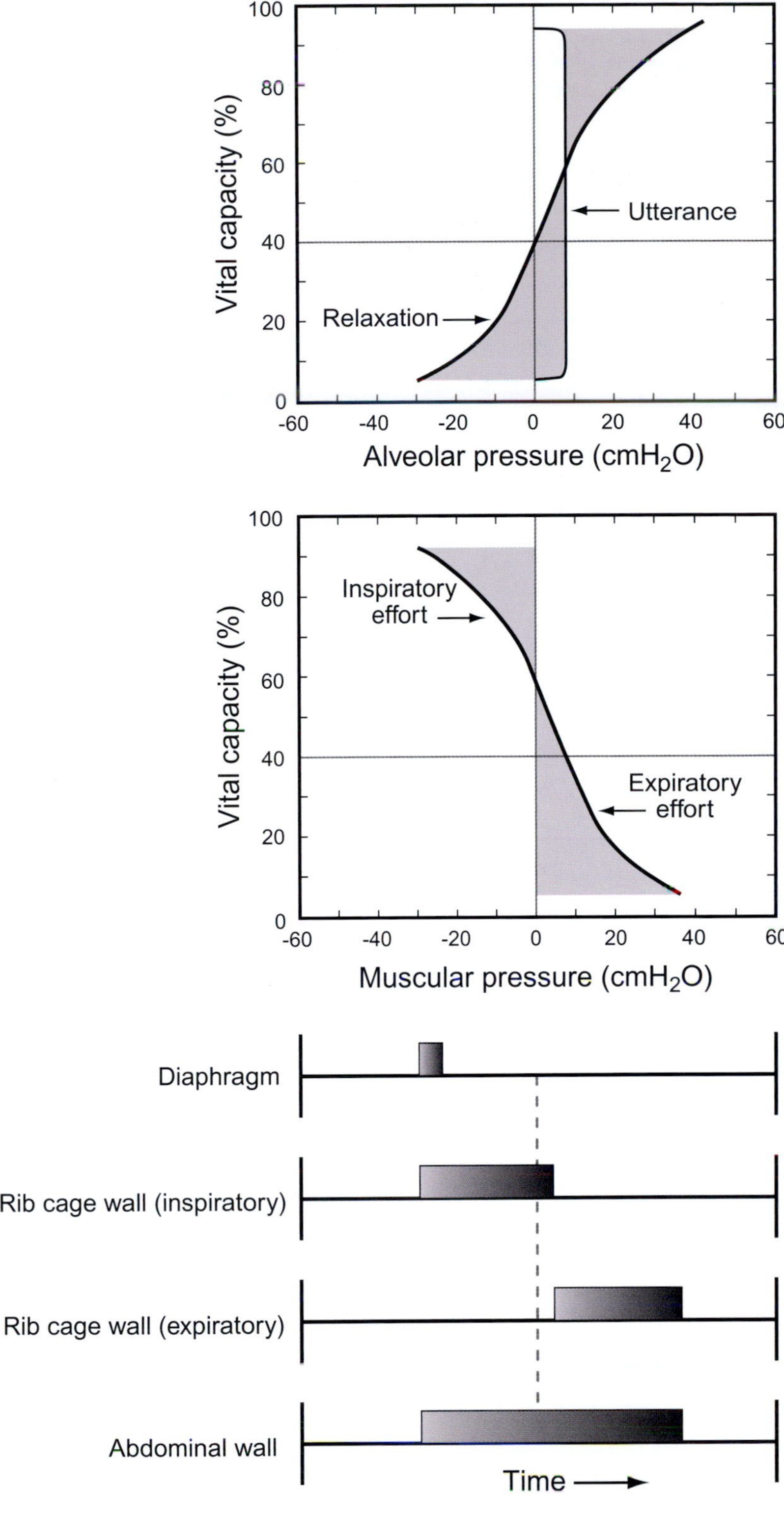

Figure 2–27. Relaxation pressure, targeted alveolar pressure, muscular pressure, and temporal activity of chest wall components for a sustained vowel produced in the upright body position. From *Evaluation and management of speech breathing disorders: Principles and methods* (p. 59), by T. Hixon and J. Hoit, 2005, Tucson, AZ: Redington Brown. Copyright 2005 by Thomas J. Hixon and Jeannette D. Hoit. Modified and reproduced with permission.

Complete Relaxation

Complete relaxation isn't as easy as it sounds. When you attempt to relax your breathing muscles for observations like those discussed in the text, nobody knows for sure how successful you are. Some people are able to quiet the electrical activity of their major breathing muscles. But, that isn't evidence of complete relaxation, because it's not feasible to monitor the electrical activity of all the muscles of breathing. Respiratory physiologists consider people to be "excellent relaxers" if they're able to produce repeatable relaxation pressures throughout the vital capacity without any feedback other than the usual sensations associated with the task. Such people are also thought to be excellent bets for "complete relaxation" because their data correspond well with those obtained during studies of drug-induced paralysis in humans. How would you like to be in one of those studies? Not we. We're content with not knowing if we can completely relax.

representing the resting level of the breathing apparatus. Recall that the resting level is the level at which the breathing apparatus is in a mechanically neutral position and alveolar pressure is the same as atmospheric pressure, or zero. Note that the relaxation pressure is positive at lung volumes larger than the resting level and negative at lung volumes smaller than the resting level. The targeted alveolar pressure is shown to be constant throughout the lung volume (this is analogous to the pressure tracing from Figure 2–26, oriented vertically instead of horizontally).

The middle panel of Figure 2–27 shows the muscular pressure required to achieve the targeted alveolar pressure. At large lung volumes (near the beginning of the utterance), a negative (inspiratory) muscular pressure is required to counteract the high positive (expiratory) relaxation pressure. In the mid-lung-volume range, a slight positive muscular pressure is required to achieve the targeted alveolar pressure. And, at small lung volumes (near the end of the utterance), increasingly greater positive muscular pressure is required. By studying the top two panels of Figure 2–27, it should be clear that it is possible to specify the required muscular pressure by knowing the targeted alveolar pressure and the relaxation pressure at the prevailing lung volume. In this example, the targeted alveolar pressure for an extended steady utterance of normal loudness is 8 cmH_2O. The targeted alveolar pressure is higher for louder utterances and lower for softer utterances. For higher targeted alveolar pressures (loud speech), less negative muscular pressures are required at large lung volumes and more positive muscular pressures are required at small lung volumes. In contrast, for lower targeted alveolar pressures (soft speech), more negative muscular pressures are required at large lung volumes and less positive muscular pressures are required at small lung volumes.

The bottom panel of Figure 2–27 illustrates the activities of the different components of the breathing apparatus in the generation of muscular pressure.[1]

[1]This panel is based on the work of Hixon et al. (1976) and was distilled by Hixon and Hoit (2005) into the simple graphic display shown. The actions of the rib cage wall, diaphragm, and abdominal wall portrayed in the panel are based on different strain-stress (volume-pressure) analyses, which enabled the determination of the individual muscular pressure contributions of different components of the chest wall. The data required for these analyses included rib cage wall volume, abdominal wall volume, and lung volume (estimated via respiratory magnetometers—devices described in this chapter), as well as pleural pressure, abdominal pressure, and transdiaphragmatic pressure (estimated from catheter-balloon devices swallowed into the esophagus and stomach and connected to pressure transducers). The data of Hixon et al. do not specify how individual muscles contribute to the muscular pressure generated by each chest wall part (except for the diaphragm,

The solid horizontal bars indicate when the different components of the chest wall are active. The darker the shading within the bars, the greater the magnitude of the muscular pressure being generated. Reading from left to right, the panel shows that the diaphragm (inspiratory), the inspiratory rib cage wall component, and the abdominal wall (expiratory) component are active at the beginning of the utterance. The diaphragm and the inspiratory rib cage wall component generate the negative pressure required to counteract the positive relaxation pressure in this large lung volume range. However, the diaphragm shuts off very quickly and the inspiratory rib cage wall component alone assumes the role of "braking" against the high expiratory relaxation pressure. At the instant the inspiratory rib cage wall component shuts off, the expiratory rib cage wall component becomes active and remains active until the end of the utterance. Note that the abdominal wall component is active throughout the utterance.

Thus, extended steady utterance is produced using a continuously changing combination of relaxation pressure and muscular pressure, and a continuously changing activation of different chest wall components. Relaxation pressure goes from substantially positive to substantially negative. Muscular pressure follows an opposite pattern, going from substantially negative to substantially positive. The inspiratory muscles of the rib cage wall do nearly all of the inspiratory work at large lung volumes and the expiratory muscles of the rib cage wall and abdominal wall muscles do all of the expiratory work. Interestingly, the abdominal wall muscles are active throughout the utterance, even at times when a net negative pressure is required.

Why do the inspiratory muscles of the rib cage wall do most of the inspiratory braking rather than the diaphragm? The answer to this question is a mechanical one and is illustrated in Figure 2–28. When the inspiratory muscles of the rib cage wall contract and the diaphragm is inactive, the rib cage wall expands and pleural and abdominal pressures decrease. The decrease in abdominal pressure causes the liquid-filled abdominal content to place a downward hydraulic pull on the undersurface of the diaphragm. This hydraulic pull creates a stable base against which the inspiratory muscles of the rib cage wall can contract, without the diaphragm having to contract to stay in position. In effect, the hydraulic pull of the abdominal content enables the inspiratory muscles of the rib cage wall to simultaneously elevate the rib cage wall and pull downward on the diaphragm. There is no need to activate two sets of muscles under this circumstance, because the inspiratory muscles of the rib cage wall can effectively perform the function of two chest wall components. As discussed below, this mechanism does not work in downright body positions.

Why do the muscles of the abdominal wall remain active throughout extended steady utterance, even when a net inspiratory muscular pressure is required (at large lung volumes)? The answer appears to be that activation of the abdominal wall enhances the precision and control of speech breathing. When the diaphragm is inactive (as it is throughout almost all of extended steady utterance production), any pressure change is manifested identically across both the rib cage wall and abdominal wall (the breathing apparatus becomes a single compartment functionally). Whether such pressure resolves into movement of the rib cage wall, abdominal wall, or both, depends on the relative impedance of the two structures. If one part has relatively high impedance (due to muscle activation) and the other has relatively low impedance (due to absence of muscle activation), then alveolar pressure change will initially result in movement of the low impedance part.

Hixon and Hoit (2005) have suggested a simple analogy that is useful in attempts to more fully understand the concepts just discussed. This analogy is portrayed in Figure 2–29 and discussed in the following quote from their work.

> The inefficiencies that would result from not using simultaneous activity in the two parts can be appreciated by performing some simple maneuvers on a long inflated balloon (representing the breathing apparatus) containing

where there is only a single muscle in the part). Such data as are available on how individual muscles function have come from the use of electromyography, a method that senses the electrical activity of muscles through the use of metal electrodes placed over them or inserted directly into them. Available data of this type are piecemeal, incomplete, and, in some cases, are known to be invalid (Hixon & Weismer, 1995).

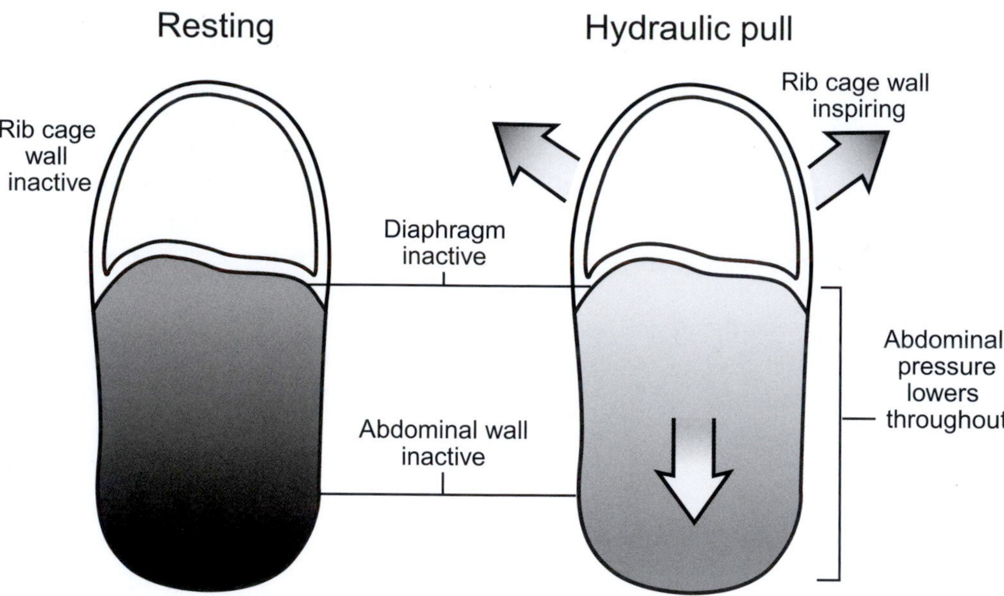

Figure 2–28. Mechanism of hydraulic pull of the abdominal content on the diaphragm.

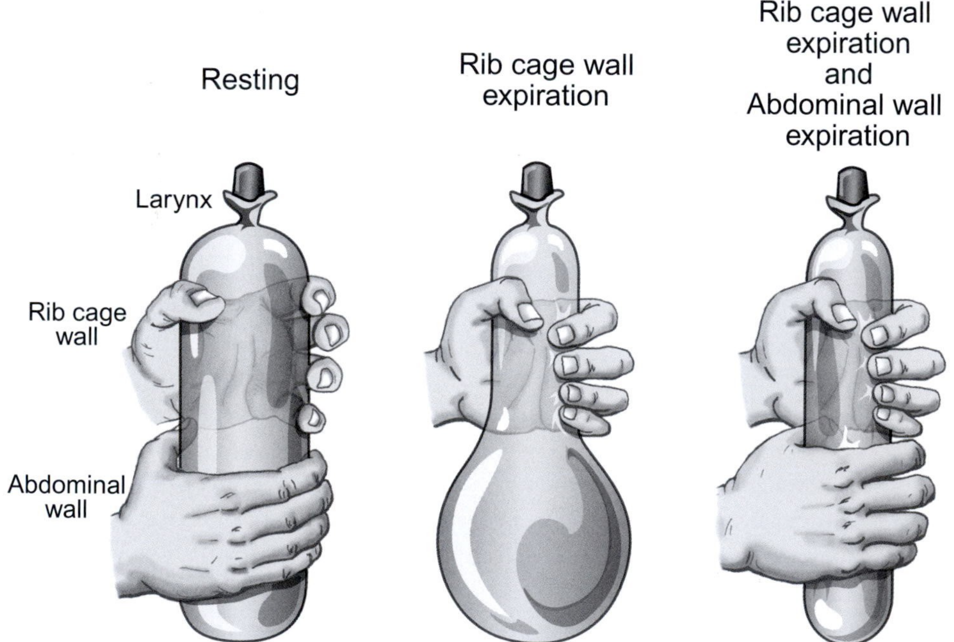

Figure 2–29. Balloon analogy of breathing apparatus control.

a squeaker in its neck (representing the larynx). If the half of the balloon nearest the squeaker (representing the rib cage wall) is squeezed (to simulate a decreasing rib cage wall volume achieved by a decreasing rib cage wall inspiratory effort), pressure inside the balloon (representing alveolar pressure) will increase and cause the other half of the balloon (representing the abdominal wall) to move outward. However, if both halves of the balloon are squeezed simultaneously (representing decreases in rib cage wall volume and abdom-

> inal wall volume), less extensive and slower movement is required of the half representing the rib cage wall to achieve an equivalent pressure adjustment. This also means that an unproductive outward (paradoxical) movement of the half of the balloon representing the abdominal wall is avoided. When both halves of the balloon are moved inward simultaneously, it is possible to have greater precision of control over the pressure inside the balloon (p. 63).

Breathing in Running Speech Activities

Running speech activities present different demands and require a different set of muscular strategies than extended steady utterances. Running speech activities include reading aloud, extemporaneous speaking, conversational speaking, and other activities that demand relatively continual utterance production. As with the discussion for extended steady utterances, running speech activities are considered here following the earlier conceptualizations and elaborations of Hixon (1973), Hixon and Hoit (2005), Hixon et al. (1976), and Weismer (1985).

Volume, pressure, and shape events associated with running speech activities are much more varied than those associated with extended steady utterances. This is because running speech is characterized by variations in phonetic content (sounds that differ in voicing and manner of production), prosody (utterances that differ in rate, intonation, loudness variation, and linguistic stress), and voice quality (utterances that differ in breathiness and timbre).

Volume events during running speech activities usually occur in the midrange of the vital capacity. As illustrated in Figure 2–30, conversational

What's Your Sign?

Speech is usually produced on expiration. But it's possible to produce it on inspiration. Try it. It's a bit awkward and difficult at first and your voice may sound higher in pitch and be more harsh than usual. But, you should be able to produce quite intelligible speech during inspiration, especially if you whisper. Once in a while, a person is encountered who uses inspiratory speech production. For example, we've seen people who produce voice more easily on inspiration than expiration following surgical reconstruction of a damaged larynx. Some people become so proficient at inspiratory speech production that you can be tricked into believing you're observing expiratory speech production (with a voice quality disorder). Never take a speaker's sign for granted.

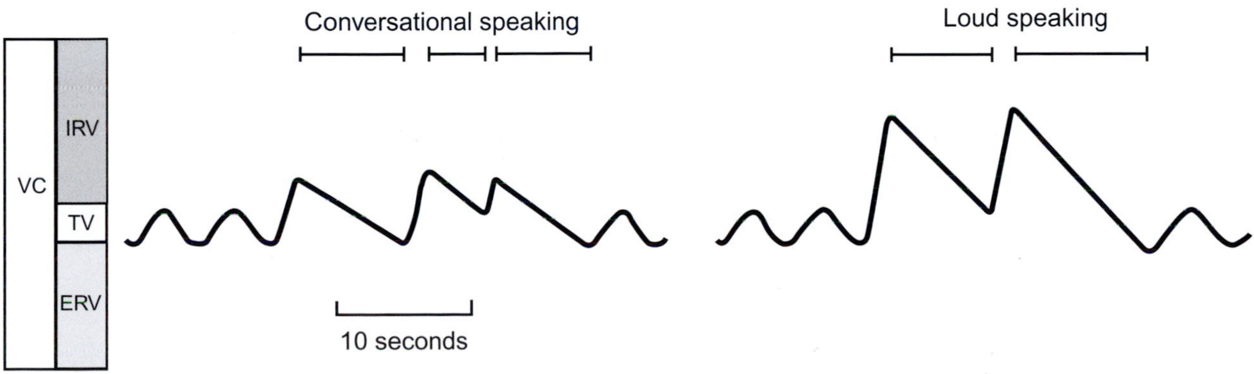

Figure 2–30. Volume events during running speech production.

speech production generally starts at twice resting tidal breathing depth (or less) and continues to near the resting level of the breathing apparatus, although at times it may encroach upon the expiratory reserve volume. There are mechanical advantages to speaking in this lung volume range. To begin, the breathing apparatus is not as stiff and the relaxation pressure is not as extreme as at very large and very small lung volumes. Furthermore, the relaxation pressure is positive for most running speech production (because relaxation pressure is positive at lung volumes larger than the resting level of the breathing apparatus) and this positive pressure is used to supplement the positive muscular pressure required. When speech production encroaches upon the expiratory reserve volume, muscular pressure must be exerted against a negative relaxation pressure.

Alveolar pressure is relatively steady during running speech production. Small variations in pressure are typically associated with linguistic stress, wherein stressed (relatively more prominent) syllables are generated by momentary pressure increases. Sometimes alveolar pressure declines slightly at the ends of breath groups, particularly at the ends of declarative sentences where loudness and pitch tend to decrease.

Rib cage wall and abdominal wall volumes generally decrease throughout the breath group in running speech activities. In most people, rib cage wall volume decreases at a much faster rate than abdominal wall volume. Recall that the rib cage wall covers a much larger surface of the lungs than does the abdominal wall (indirectly, through the diaphragm). Thus, the rib cage wall is well suited for effecting lung volume change for running speech activities.

Both relaxation pressure and muscular pressure contribute to the production of running speech breathing. Most of the time, the targeted alveolar pressure is higher (more positive) than the prevailing relaxation pressure. Therefore, positive muscular pressure must be added to the relaxation pressure throughout the breath group. To maintain the targeted alveolar pressure, the magnitude of the positive muscular pressure increases as the breath group proceeds because the relaxation pressure becomes increasingly less positive, and might even become negative if the breath group continues through lung volumes that are smaller than the resting level of the breathing apparatus. There is usually not a need to use inspiratory muscular pressure during running speech production, unless utterance is initiated at a larger-than-usual lung volume, and then inspiratory braking might be required briefly.

For running speech activities that are louder or softer than normal, targeted alveolar pressures are higher or lower, respectively, than those used to generate usual running speech. Thus, higher-than-normal muscular pressure is required for louder speech and lower-than-normal muscular pressure is required for softer speech at the prevailing lung volume. Nevertheless, as illustrated in Figure 2–30, it is important to note that louder speech is often initiated at larger lung volumes, where the prevailing relaxation pressure is greater.

The expiratory phase of most running speech is produced with expiratory rib cage wall and abdominal wall muscular pressures, the latter predominating. The inspiratory phase of the running speech breathing cycle is driven by the diaphragm. Interestingly, expiratory muscles of the rib cage wall and abdominal wall maintain a low level of activity during inspiration. This enables them to be in a state of readiness to begin driving expiration (speech production) as soon as inspiration has ended.

The abdominal wall plays an important role in running speech breathing. It generates most of the expiratory muscular pressure during speech production. It is also responsible for imposing the general background configuration assumed by the chest wall throughout the speech breathing cycle. As it turns out, there are important advantages to having the abdominal wall play such a prominent role in running speech breathing.

Figure 2–31 illustrates these advantages in the context of the shape of the chest wall for running speech activities. Inward displacement of the abdominal wall (by its own muscular action) has important consequences for the diaphragm and rib cage wall. As the abdominal wall moves inward, the diaphragm is pushed headward such that its radius of curvature increases and its principal muscle fibers elongate. This positions the diaphragm so that it can produce the quick and powerful inspirations that are critical for minimizing interruptions during running speech activities. Inward displacement of the abdominal wall also lifts the rib cage wall. This stretches the expiratory muscles of the rib cage wall,

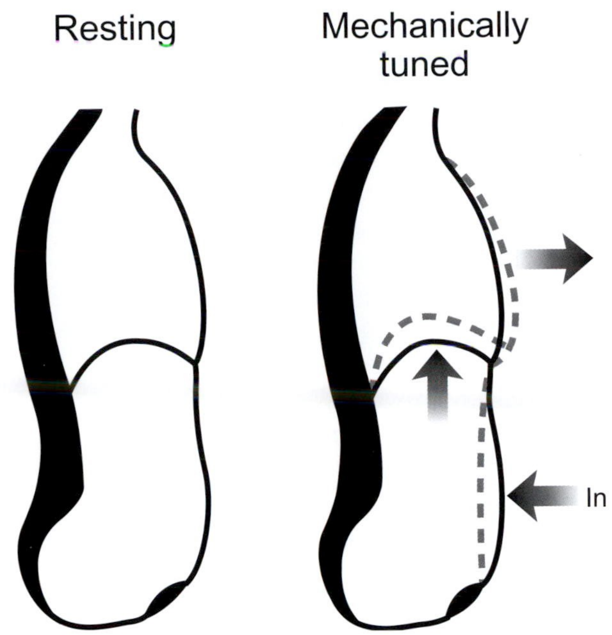

Figure 2–31. Shape of the chest wall for running speech activities.

thereby increasing their potential for generating the quick expiratory pulses needed to produce linguistic stress and loudness change. Also, with the abdominal wall held firmly inward, expiratory efforts by the rib cage wall can be fully resolved into pressure change. If the abdominal wall were not held firmly in place, expiratory efforts of the rib cage wall would be resolved into outward movement of the abdominal wall before a pressure change could be effected (recall the balloon analogy provided above). Thus, the activation of abdominal wall muscles and the resultant inward displacement serve to "mechanically tune" the breathing apparatus for inspiration and expiration during running speech breathing. When the abdominal wall muscles are impaired, speech breathing is predictably impaired (recall the Scenario at the start of the chapter and see the continuation of it at the end of the chapter).

Finally, a good deal of information about volume, pressure, and shape events for running speech activities is carried in the speech (acoustic) signal. Thus, it is possible for a listener to gather clues about running speech breathing by just listening to a person's speech. Breath group length provides clues about volume events. In general, the longer the breath group, the larger the volume excursion. Loudness provides clues about alveolar pressure, because the two are strongly positively correlated. Thus, as a general rule, the louder the speech produced, the higher the alveolar pressure. Finally, inspiratory duration and the rate of loudness change provide clues about the shape of the chest wall. When the chest wall is configured appropriately for speech production (larger-than-relaxed rib cage wall and smaller-than-relaxed abdominal wall), inspirations are short and loudness changes for linguistic stress are quick.

Adaptive Control of Speech Breathing

Although speech breathing is usually carried out in the ways described above, there are many other ways it can be performed. This means that speech breathing can be adapted when the circumstances call for change.

Adaptive control is not unique to speech breathing, but occurs in essentially all motor control systems. For example, if a violinist breaks a string during a performance, he may decide not to stop, but rather to continue playing by reprogramming his usual fingering (Wolff, 1979). In a skilled violinist, this reprogramming can be done instantly and without much effort. This is adaptation par excellence. The violinist adapts by allowing the "motor idea" to control the performance. The goal is the important thing, not the way it is attained.

Adaptive control is commonplace in speech breathing as well. For example, a speaker must adapt when body position changes, when ventilatory drive changes (as with exercise or a change in elevation), when a tight-fitting belt restricts chest wall movement, or when the air temperature is extremely hot or cold. There are many such examples of changing circumstances that occur in everyday life and that demand adaptive control of speech breathing. And experimental work has provided interesting documentation as to how speech breathing can be changed without compromising its output goals (Bouhuys, Proctor, & Mead, 1966; Hixon et al., 1973; Hixon & Weismer, 1995; Warren, Morr, Rochet, & Dalston, 1989).

For example, by increasing the effective relaxation pressure of the breathing apparatus (by using a device to lower the pressure at the airway opening),

What's Your Opinion?

It was a student party. People were in a good mood. A vacation was just around the corner. Most people were well into the food and libation. The band was loud to a fault. One couple slipped off into another room. Things happened. Different reports were given to the police. His version was that it involved sex by mutual consent. He said neither was under the influence. Her version was different. She said things started out innocently, but that he was drunk and forced her. She called it rape and reported it several days later. He claimed that she never cried out for help. Nobody who was in the adjacent room reported hearing anything. She claimed that he pinned her down and that his weight made it impossible for her to scream because she couldn't breathe. What's your forensic opinion? Could she have screamed or not?

it is possible to change the usual strategy for braking against high positive relaxation pressure at large lung volumes. Whereas a person usually brakes solely with the inspiratory muscles of the rib cage wall (when in an upright body position), the diaphragm will supplement the braking effort of the rib cage wall when relaxation pressure is made to be abnormally high.

As another example, although the usual background shape of the chest wall is relatively constant, it is possible to produce speech with a constantly changing chest wall shape. This can be demonstrated by moving the abdominal wall in and out repeatedly while sustaining a vowel and maintaining a constant alveolar pressure (voice loudness).

Another example is one that involves interaction with another part of the speech production apparatus, the velopharynx. When a velopharyngeal leak is created experimentally (by "talking through the nose"), a person will expire more air than usual while speaking. This adaptation serves to maintain adequate levels of oral pressure to achieve suitable consonant production.

A final example is one that happens in many everyday situations. A person in an upright body position usually performs running speech activities using a chest wall shape in which the rib cage wall is larger and the abdominal wall is smaller than their respective sizes during rest at the prevailing lung volume. However, when the arms are folded across the front of the rib cage wall, the same person will use a chest wall shape that involves a smaller-than-usual rib cage wall size and a larger-than-usual abdominal wall size. What happens is that the abdominal wall surrenders to the heavy mechanical load imposed by the folded arms.

Body Position and Speech Breathing

A change in body position may alter the mechanical behavior of the breathing apparatus, primarily because gravity has such a strong influence on this massive structure. Thus, with each new body position, a new mechanical solution may need to be found for speech breathing. Most of this section is devoted to discussion of the supine body position (as contrasted to the upright body position discussed above), but other body positions are considered as well. As with the sections on extended steady utterances and running speech activities, the discussion here is based on conceptualizations and elaborations of Hixon (1973), Hixon and Hoit (2005), and Hixon et al. (1976).

Figure 2–32 depicts the influence of gravity on different parts of the chest wall in the upright and supine body positions. In the upright body position, gravity acts in the expiratory direction on the rib cage wall, tending to reduce its size, whereas gravity acts in the inspiratory direction on the abdominal wall, tending to increase its size. When a shift is made to the supine body position, gravity acts in

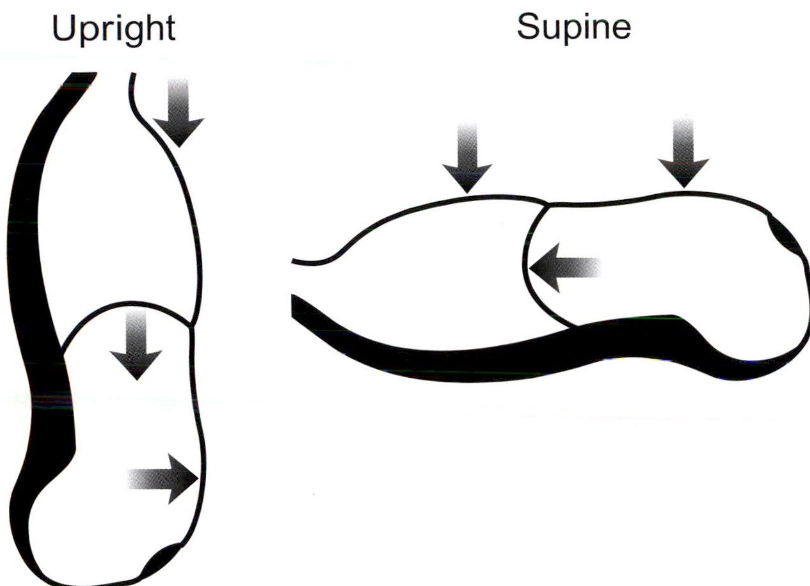

Figure 2–32. Gravitational effects on the breathing apparatus.

Flat Out

Two terms that get more than their fair share of misuse are "supine" and "prone." Supine means lying on your back (usually face up). The easy way to remember this is to consider the spelling of supine. Take out its second letter and you have "spine." On your spine is on your back. So-called couch potatoes spend a lot of time supine in front of their television sets. Prone, also called procumbent, means lying on your front (usually face down). Take its first three letters and you have the first three letters of the word "prostrate" (as in face down submission or adoration). Shooters often spend time lying prone (on their front) when practicing with a rifle on a firing range. The confusion encountered when using the terms supine and prone arises because both involve being flat out. The memory devices suggested here should make it easy to keep the two body positions straight (pun intended).

the expiratory direction on both the rib cage wall and abdominal wall. This causes the relaxation pressure to be greater at any given lung volume in the supine body position than in upright body position. The expiratory gravitational force exerted on the abdominal wall pushes the diaphragm headward, causing the resting level of the breathing apparatus to decrease to about 20 %VC from its upright value of about 40 %VC. These changes in the mechanical status of the breathing apparatus have an effect on speech breathing.

Extended Steady Utterances in the Supine Body Position

Figure 2–33 represents a sustained vowel of normal loudness produced throughout the vital capacity in the supine body position, and is analogous to

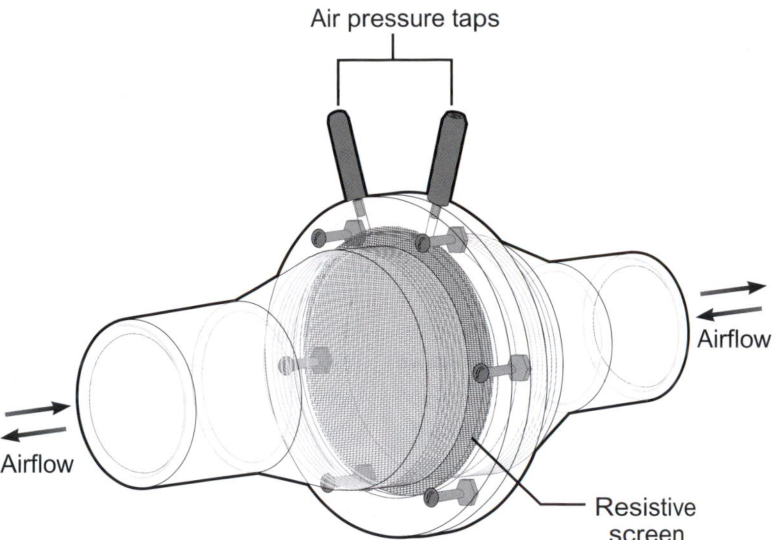

Figure 2–39. Pneumotachometer. From *Evaluation and management of speech breathing disorders: Principles and methods* (p. 162), by T. Hixon and J. Hoit, 2005, Tucson, AZ: Redington Brown. Copyright 2005 by Thomas J. Hixon and Jeannette D. Hoit. Modified and reproduced with permission.

Where's the Border?

Borders may or may not be important. Ride your Harley-Davidson motorcycle around the monument at the Four Corners junction from Arizona through New Mexico through Colorado to Utah (for the geographically challenged, this is a continuous left turn) without wearing a helmet and there will be times you're breaking the law and times you're not. You need to know each state's law and identify each border to know your status. But the border between the rib cage wall and the abdominal wall is another story. When the two structures move, it's hard to identify where their two edges meet. The respiratory magnetometers discussed in the text make it so that you don't have to fret such delineation. Magnetometers have the advantage that their coils can be placed at the center of the surfaces being monitored and far away from their edges. Where's the border? Who cares? It's not important to know when using respiratory magnetometers.

Figure 2–40 portrays respiratory magnetometers as they might be positioned to make volume measurements. Pairs (front and back mates) of electromagnetic coils are used to sense anteroposterior diameter changes of the rib cage wall and abdominal wall. The rib cage wall and abdominal wall each displace volume as they move and together they displace a volume equal to that displaced by the lungs. Thus, one need only sum the output signals from the two pairs of electromagnetic coils to obtain a measurement of lung volume change at the body surface. Respiratory magnetometers generate low

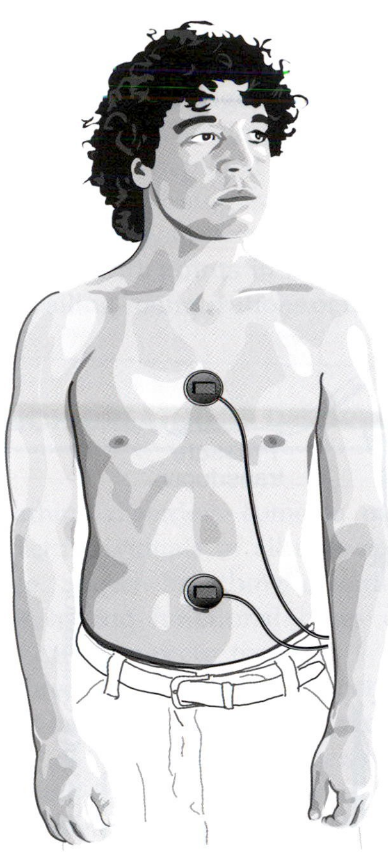

Figure 2–40. Respiratory magnetometers. From *Evaluation and management of speech breathing disorders: Principles and methods* (p. 167), by T. Hixon and J. Hoit, 2005, Tucson, AZ: Redington Brown. Copyright 2005 by Thomas J. Hixon and Jeannette D. Hoit. Modified and reproduced with permission.

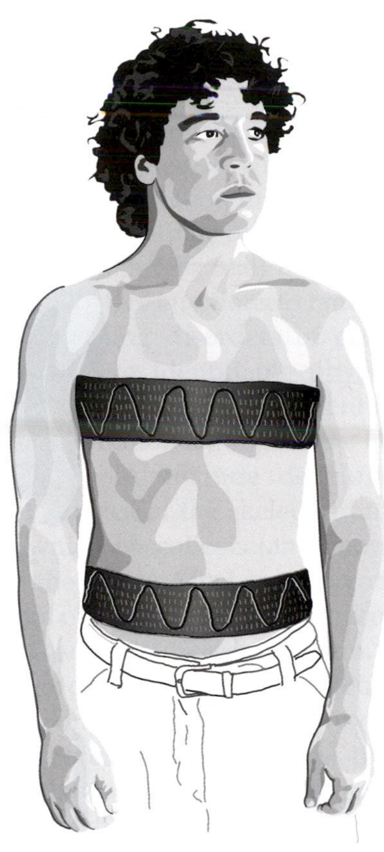

Figure 2–41. Respiratory inductance plethysmographs. From *Evaluation and management of speech breathing disorders: Principles and methods* (p. 168), by T. Hixon and J. Hoit, 2005, Tucson, AZ: Redington Brown. Copyright 2005 by Thomas J. Hixon and Jeannette D. Hoit. Modified and reproduced with permission.

power electromagnetic fields that are safe for clinical use. Nevertheless, it is prudent to avoid using respiratory magnetometers on pregnant females or on anyone with an implanted electronic pacemaker.

Figure 2–41 depicts respiratory inductance plethysmographs as they might be positioned to make volume measurements. Broad elastic bands with embedded electrical wires are used to sense average cross-sectional areas of the rib cage wall and abdominal wall. Again, as with respiratory magnetometers, the rib cage wall and abdominal wall each displace volume as they move and the summed displacement equals that of the lungs. In this case, one need only sum the output signals from the two elastic sensing bands (average cross-sectional areas) to arrive at a measurement of lung volume change at the body surface.

Pressure Measurement

The most important pressure for speech breathing is alveolar pressure. Alveolar pressure cannot be measured directly during speech production. The problem is that speech production is characterized by various obstructions and constrictions along the larynx and pharyngeal-oral apparatus that preclude access to the alveoli. Nevertheless, alveolar pressure can be estimated from oral pressure during the production of a particular type of speech sample.

As shown in the upper panel of Figure 2–42, a small polyethylene pressure sensing tube is placed at one corner of the mouth just behind the front teeth so that one of its ends is perpendicular to the flow of air out of the mouth. The other end of the tube production. *Journal of Speech and Hearing Research, 10*, 49–56.

Weismer, G. (1985). Speech breathing: Contemporary views and findings. In R. Daniloff (Ed.), *Speech science* (pp. 47–72). San Diego, CA: College-Hill Press.

Western, P., & Patrick, J. (1988). Effects of focusing attention on breathing with and without apparatus on the face. *Respiration Physiology, 72*, 123–130.

Whalen, D., & Kinsella-Shaw, J. (1997). Exploring the relationship of inspiration duration to utterance duration. *Phonetica, 54*, 138–152.

Wilder, C. (1983). Chest wall preparation for phonation in female speakers. In D. Bless & J. Abbs (Eds.), *Vocal fold physiology: Contemporary research and clinical issues* (pp. 109–123). San Diego, CA: College-Hill Press.

Winkworth, A., Davis, P., Adams, R., & Ellis, E. (1995). Breathing patterns during spontaneous speech. *Journal of Speech and Hearing Research, 38*, 124–144.

Winkworth, A., Davis, P., Ellis, E., & Adams, R. (1994). Variability and consistency in speech breathing during reading: Lung volumes, speech intensity, and linguistic factors. *Journal of Speech and Hearing Research, 37*, 535–556.

Wolff, P. (1979). Theoretical issues in the development of motor skills. *Symposium on developmental disabilities in the pre-school child*. Chicago: Johnson and Johnson Baby Products.

Wyke, B. (1974). Respiratory activity of intrinsic laryngeal muscles: An experimental study. In B. Wyke (Ed.), *Ventilatory and phonatory control systems* (pp. 408–429). New York: Oxford University Press.

3

Laryngeal Function and Speech Production

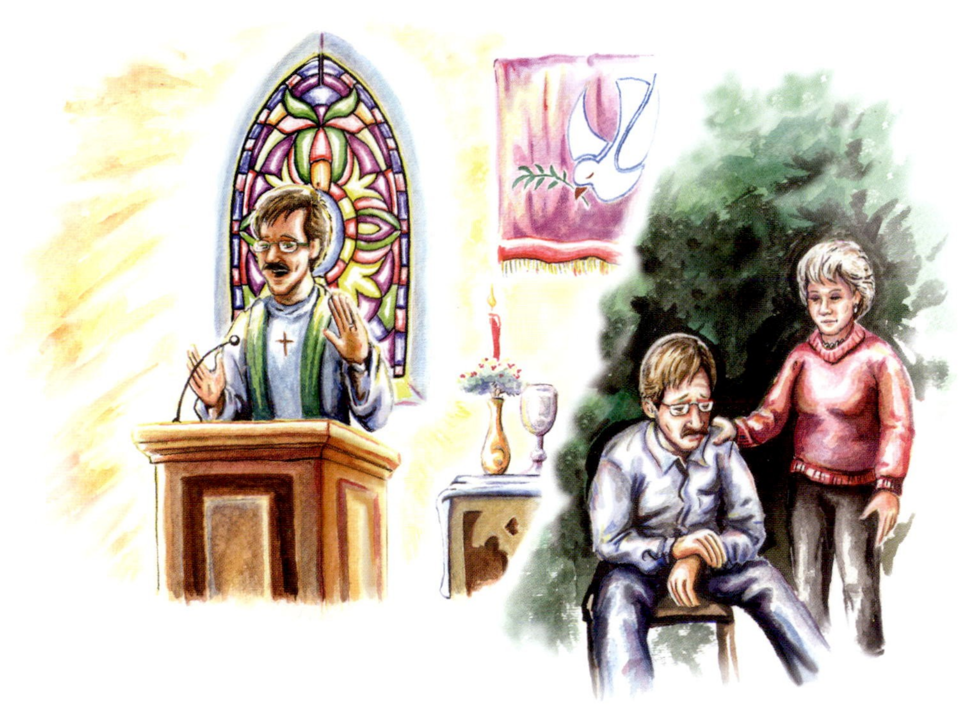

Scenario

His voice was his livelihood and in many ways his life. At age 42, he was at the top of his ecumenical game. As a member of the clergy, he was outstanding by any metric. The members of his large church were extremely fond of him and looked to him for guidance. He had a very successful weekly radio ministry that broadcasted his influence well beyond the walls of his church and the territory of his local congregation. His wife was a rock of his life. She cared for their family that included a girl 18 years old, and two boys, 16 and 15. She also was an accomplished musician and directed the church choir. The children were all interested in horses, 4-H, and music, although somewhat different from the music of their mother.

The daughter left in the fall to attend her first semester of college. She had chosen a small college with religious affiliation. The choice was at the urging of her parents. The mother was saddened by the daughter's departure, but things went on pretty much as usual. The daughter's first-semester grades were not impressive (poor would be more accurate), especially given her track record in high school. The sons had turned their interests to cars and motorcycles. The father had been hoping their interests would follow something in team sports, but this did not meet their fancy. Near the end of the year, the mother underwent surgery for breast cancer.

It was in the spring that the father first noticed a "catch" in his voice. During an episode of his radio ministry, he experienced some difficulty that went away after he cleared his throat several times and drank some water. He thought no more of it. Then, during a sermon at his church, he suddenly experienced a feeling of being momentarily frozen in his speech. It happened three times over the course of 30 minutes. He disguised this embarrassment from those in attendance. He mentioned it to his wife after the service. Neither knew what to make of it. Within the next week, the problem grew. He had difficulty speaking on the phone, at the church board meeting, and even to his wife and sons. He telephoned his physician, a member of the church, and told him about the problem. The physician offered that he might be under more stress than usual.

The problem continued to worsen and quickly so. Within 2 weeks of noticing the first "catch," he had developed a hoarse voice that had a strained-strangled quality to it and that seemed to interrupt his speech under its own free will. He had to ask the assistant pastor of the church to do his radio show for the week and despite his thinking that he would somehow be able to deliver his Sunday sermon, he finally realized that he could not do it. A substitute was quickly recruited.

The situation had become desperate and the physician from his church managed to get him in to see an ear, nose, and throat specialist (otorhinolaryngologist) on short notice. No diagnosis was made, but the specialist thought there might be some sort of neurological problem and referred the minister to a neurologist. It took longer to get this appointment, but it too was not fully enlightening. The neurologist found nothing suggestive of neural disease.

What could turn the life of a healthy 42-year-old man around in such a short time and be so utterly debilitating? This once articulate, fluent, verbally engaging individual had been rendered functionally speechless, unable to administer to his congregation, completely stymied as to the cause of his problem and his fate. It was a terrible turn of events that nobody seemed to understand.

INTRODUCTION

The larynx is an air valve located within the front of the neck. This valve is positioned vertically between the trachea (windpipe) and pharynx (throat) and can be adjusted to vary the amount of coupling between the two. The larynx serves a variety of functions, including speech (inclusive of voice) production.

This chapter begins with a discussion of the fundamentals of laryngeal structure and function. This is followed by consideration of laryngeal function for speech production, measurement of laryngeal function, laryngeal disorders that affect speech production, and clinical professionals who evaluate and manage such disorders. The chapter ends with a review and a closing scenario.

FUNDAMENTALS OF LARYNGEAL FUNCTION

This section covers topics fundamental to the understanding of laryngeal function. These include (a) anatomy of the laryngeal apparatus, (b) forces and movements associated with its actions, (c) adjustments resulting from its actions, (d) control variables involved in its behaviors, (e) neural substrates of laryngeal control, and (f) laryngeal functions.

Anatomy of the Laryngeal Apparatus

The skeleton of the larynx, its joints, and its internal topography are considered in this section. Muscular components are discussed below under the section on active forces.

Skeleton

Figure 3–1 depicts the skeletal framework of the laryngeal apparatus. This framework consists of bone, cartilage, ligament, and tendon. The flexibility of this superstructure changes with age, being soft and pliable in childhood and hard and more rigid in adulthood.

Thyroid Cartilage. The thyroid cartilage is the largest of the laryngeal cartilages and forms most of the front and sides of the laryngeal skeleton. This cartilage provides a shieldlike housing for the larynx and offers protection for many of its structures.

Figure 3–2 shows the thyroid cartilage. Two quadrilateral plates, called the thyroid laminae, are fused together at the front of the thyroid cartilage and diverge widely (more so in women than in men) toward the back. The configuration of the two thyroid laminae resembles the bow of a ship. The line of fusion between the two plates is called the angle of the thyroid. The upper part of the structure contains a prominent V-shaped depression that is termed the thyroid notch and can be palpated at the front of the neck. This notch is located just above the most forward projection of the cartilage, an outward jutting called the thyroid prominence or Adam's apple.

The back edges of the thyroid laminae extend upward into two long horns and downward into two short horns. The upper horns, called the superior cornua, are coupled to the hyoid bone (discussed below). The lower horns, termed the inferior cornua, have facets (areas where other structures join) on their lower inside surfaces. These facets provide for the formation of joints with the cricoid cartilage. The inferior cornua straddle the cricoid cartilage like a pair of legs.

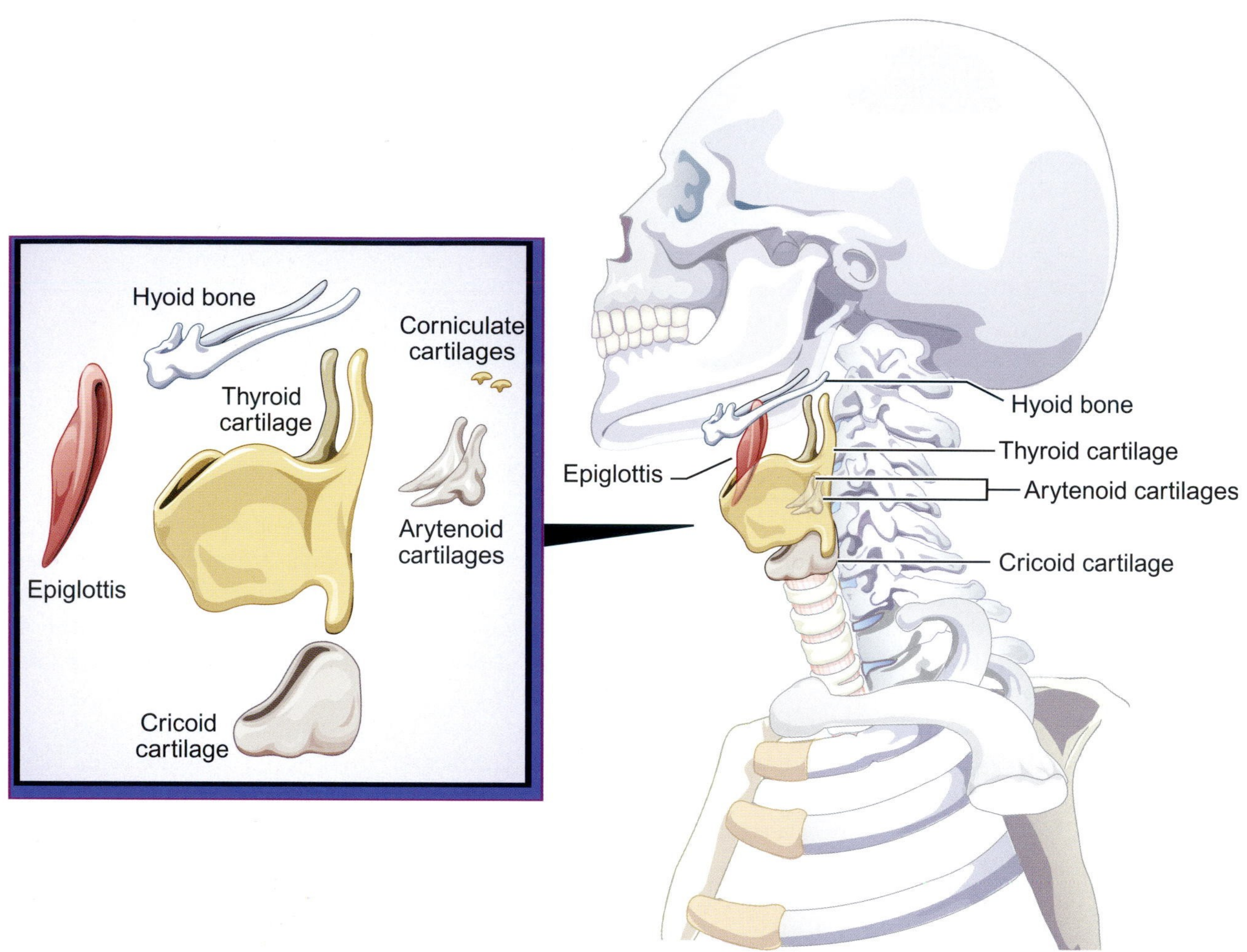

Figure 3–1. Skeletal framework of the laryngeal apparatus.

Sizing Things Up

There's a tendency when viewing anatomical drawings, photographs, and video images of structures of the larynx to overestimate the size of things. The trachea looks long and large in cross-section. The glottis seems to be a big hole. The vocal folds appear to be massive lips. The vocal ligaments look like pencils. And the vibratory movements of the vocal folds (when slowed down) give the impression of a flag blowing in a stiff wind. Some calibration may be helpful. Your trachea is about as long and big around as your middle finger. Your wide-open glottis is about the size of a dime. Your approximated vocal folds have a surface area about the size of your thumbnail (well trimmed). The vocal ligaments are about as thick as wooden matchsticks. And your vocal folds only move about the length of the cuticle on your thumbnail. If you're like us, you'll find all this to be surprisingly small. Yes?

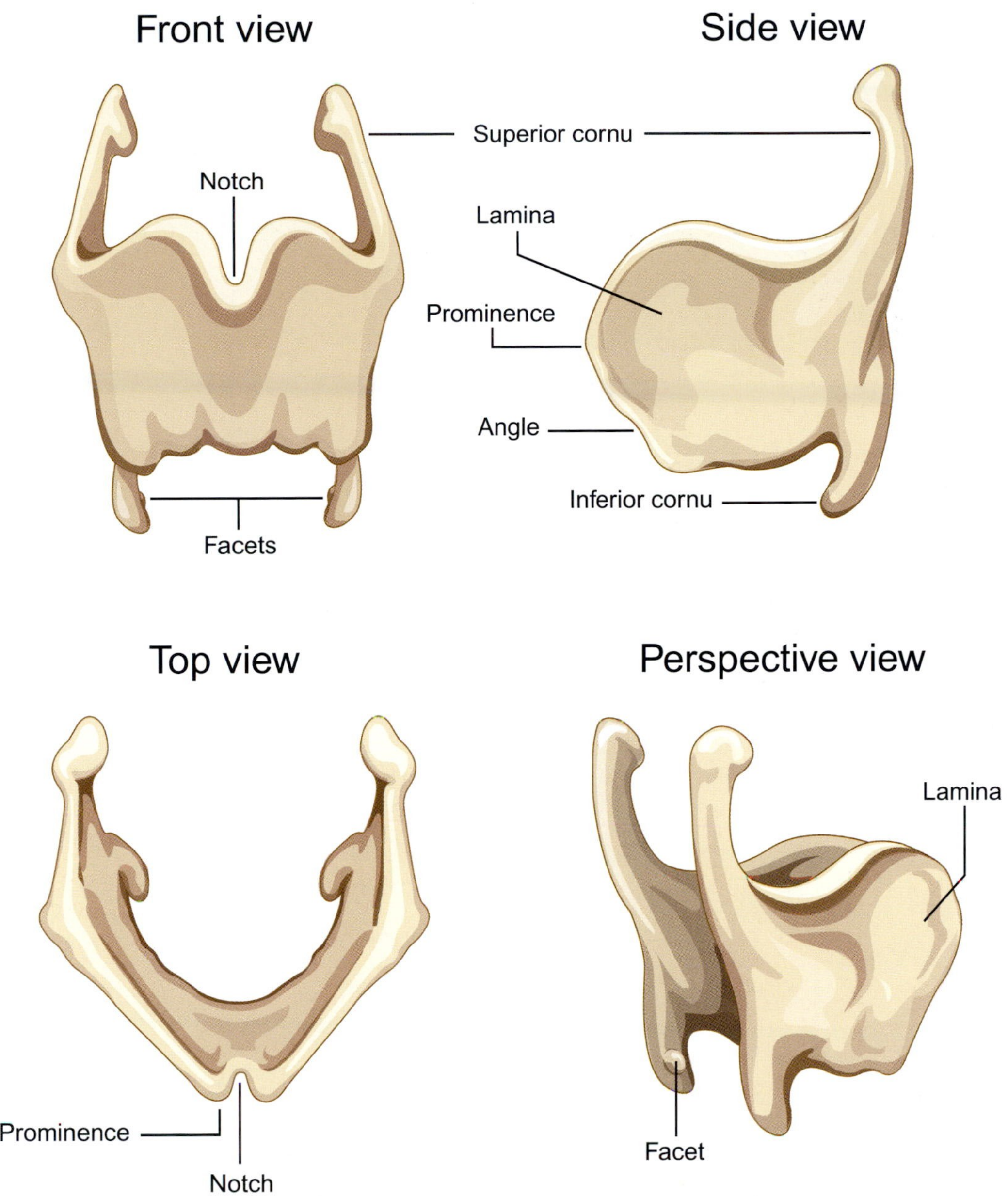

Figure 3–2. Thyroid cartilage.

Cricoid Cartilage. The cricoid cartilage forms the lower part of the laryngeal skeleton. It is a ring-shaped structure located above the trachea. As shown in Figure 3–3, the cricoid cartilage has a thick plate at the back, the posterior quadrate lamina, which resembles a signet on a finger ring. A semicircular structure, called the anterior arch, forms the front of the cricoid cartilage and is akin to a band on a finger ring.

Four facets are located on the cricoid cartilage. The lower two facets, one on each side at the same level, are positioned near the junction of the posterior quadrate lamina and anterior arch. Each of these facets articulates with a facet on one of the inferior cornua of the thyroid cartilage.

The upper two facets of the cricoid cartilage, one on each side at the same level, are located on the sloping rim of the posterior quadrate lamina. Each

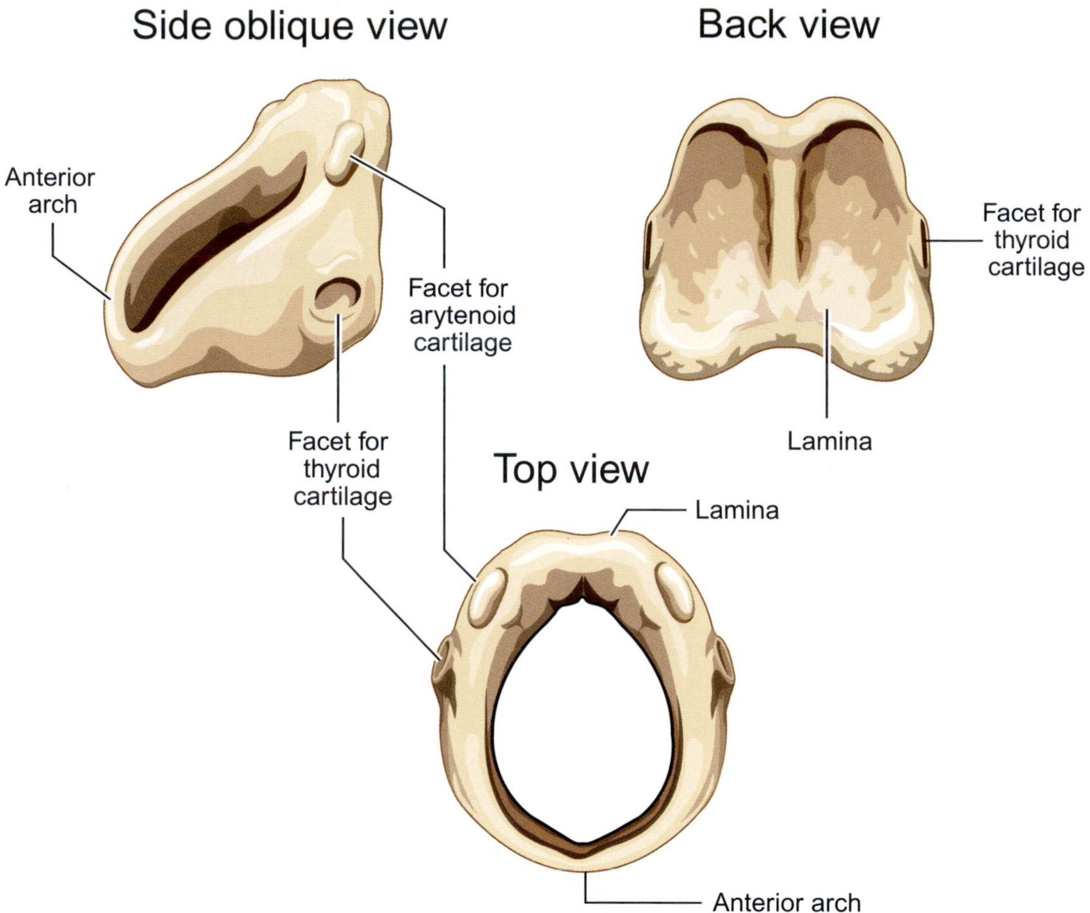

Figure 3–3. Cricoid cartilage.

of these facets articulates with a facet on the undersurface of one of the arytenoid cartilages.

Arytenoid Cartilages. There are two arytenoid cartilages. Each is located atop one side of the sloping rim of the posterior quadrate lamina of the cricoid cartilage. As shown in Figure 3–4, each arytenoid cartilage has a complex shape that includes an apex, base, and three sides. The apex of each cartilage is capped with another small cone-shaped cartilage called a corniculate cartilage that is often fused to the arytenoid cartilage. The base of each arytenoid cartilage has a flexible pointed projection that extends toward the front and is designated the vocal process. The base also includes a rounded stubby projection that extends toward the back and side and is referred to as the muscular process. The undersurface of each muscular process has a facet that articulates with one of the upper facets of the cricoid cartilage.

Epiglottis. Figure 3–5 depicts the epiglottis. The epiglottis is a single cartilage that is positioned behind the hyoid bone (discussed below) and root of the tongue. The upper part of the epiglottis, its body, is broad and resembles the distal end of a forward-curving shoehorn. The front and back surfaces of this part of the structure are referred to as its lingual (tongue) and laryngeal (larynx) surfaces, respectively. The lingual surface attaches to the hyoid bone. The lower part of the cartilage tapers downward into a stalk called the petiolus (little leg) and attaches to the inside of the thyroid cartilage just below the thyroid notch.

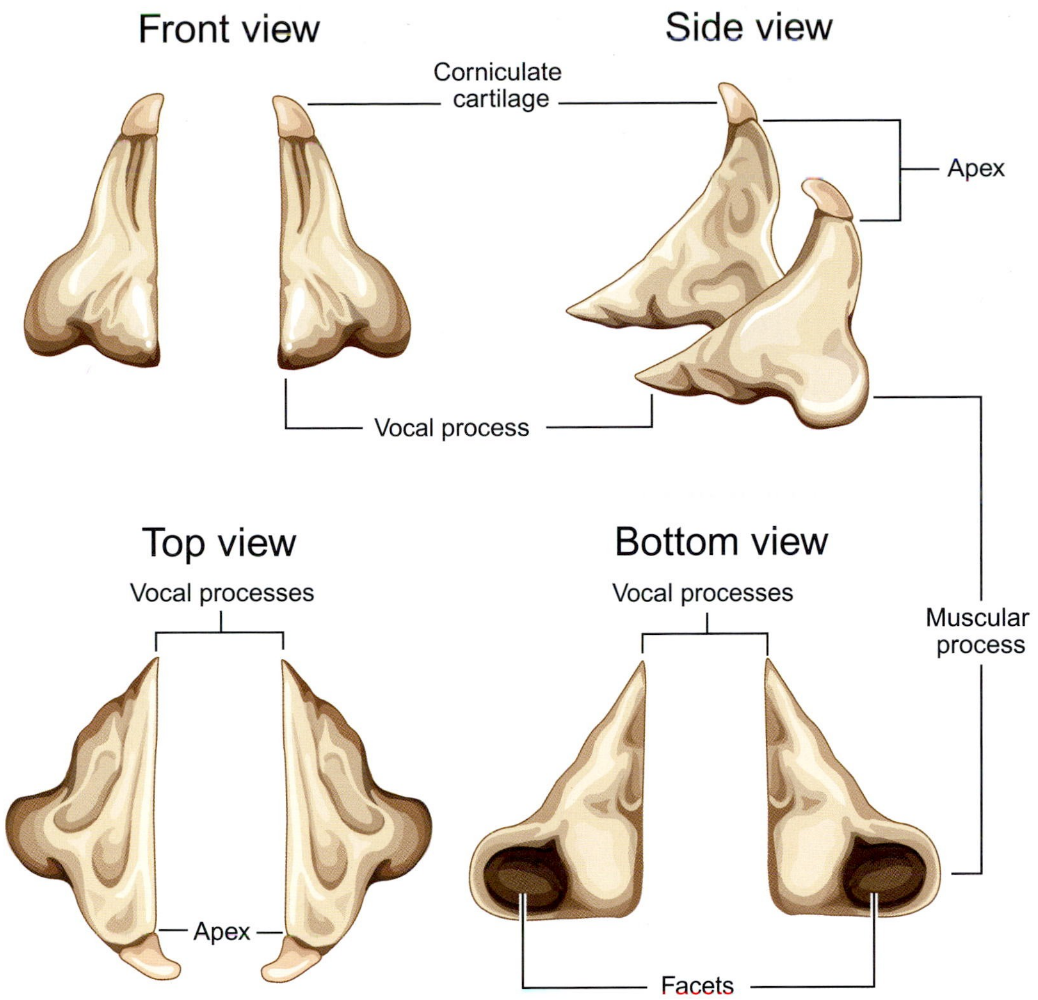

Figure 3–4. Arytenoid cartilages.

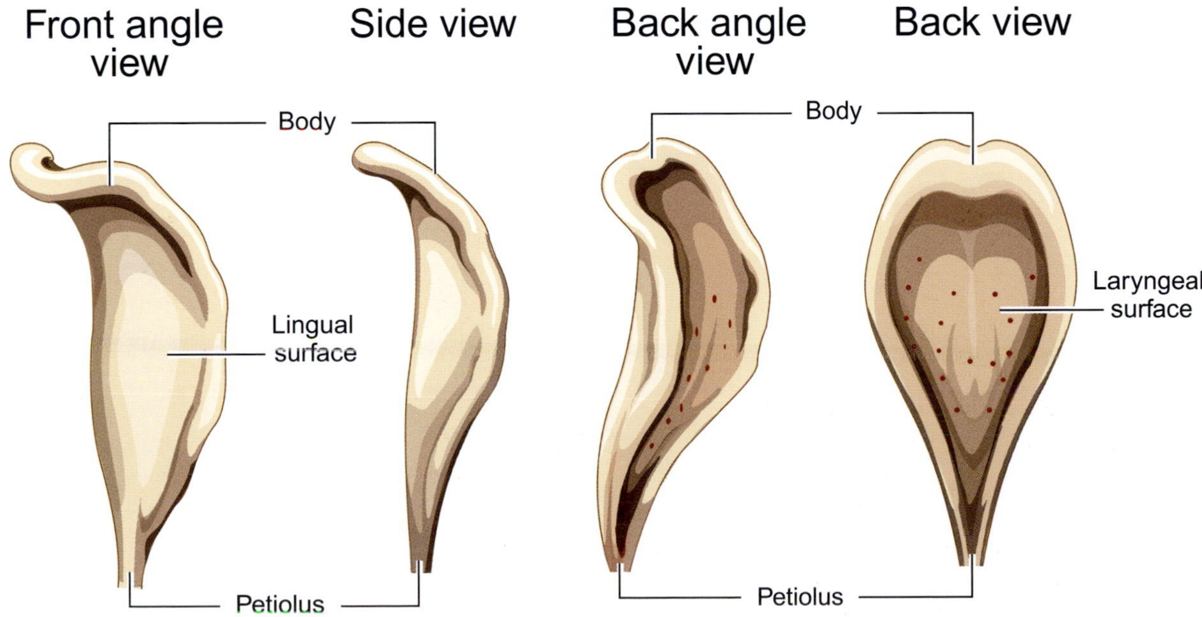

Figure 3–5. Epiglottis.

Hyoid Bone. Figure 3–6 depicts the hyoid bone (tongue bone). Technically, the hyoid bone is not a part of the larynx. Nevertheless, it serves as an integral component in many laryngeal functions. Thus, it is commonly afforded a prominent place in discussion of the laryngeal skeleton.

The hyoid bone is free-floating in the sense that it is not attached to any other bone. It is a U-shaped structure that is positioned horizontally within the neck, its open end facing toward the back. The hyoid bone consists of a body and two pairs of greater and lesser horns (cornua) that project upward. The greater cornua are located toward the back of the structure and join with the superior cornua of the thyroid cartilage. The lesser cornua extend from the body of the structure and may be capped by tiny cone-shaped cartilages. The hyoid bone is positioned at the top of the larynx and suspends it from above through various connections.

Laryngeal Joints

There are two pairs of joints in the larynx. One pair is between the cricoid and thyroid cartilages on each side. The other pair is between the cricoid and arytenoid cartilages on each side. Movements at these joints are conditioned by the nature of the facets on their articulating cartilages and the arrangement of surrounding ligaments.

Cricothyroid Joints. Figure 3–7 depicts the cricothyroid joints. These joints are positioned on the sides of the larynx and involve articulations between facets on the outer surfaces of the lower part of the cricoid cartilage and the inner surfaces of the inferior cornua of the thyroid cartilage. The cricothyroid joints are encapsulated by membranes that secrete synovial fluid. This fluid serves as a lubricant.

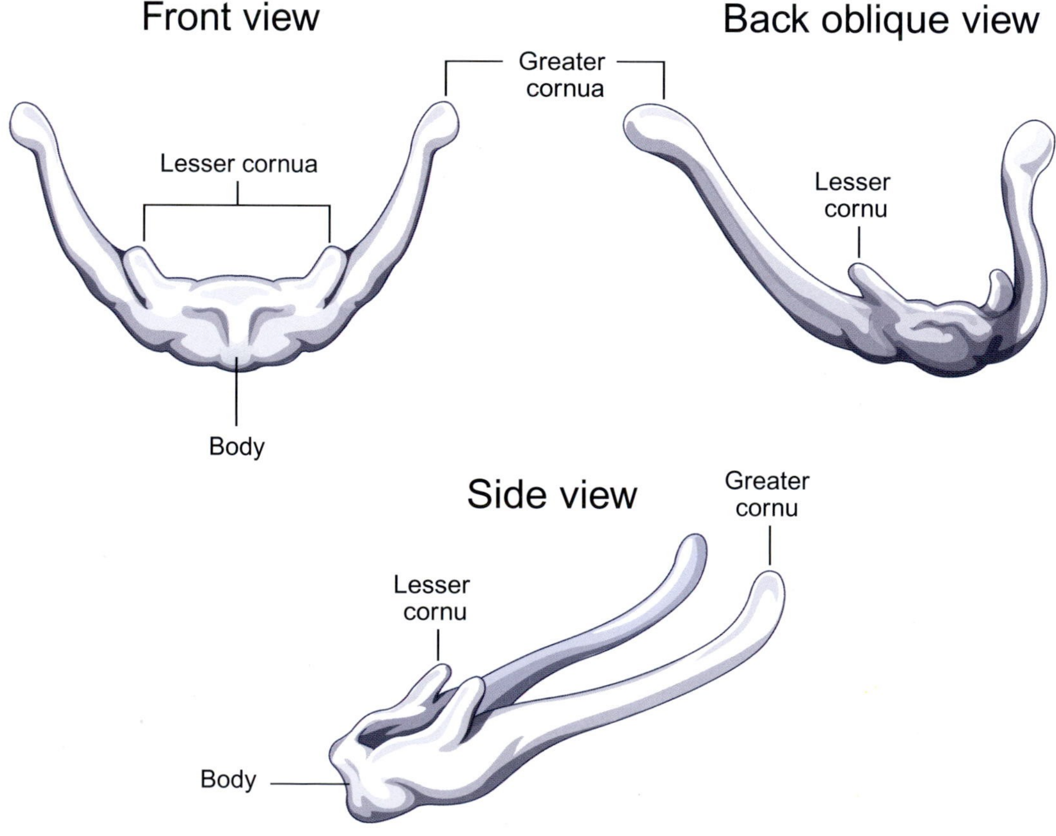

Figure 3–6. Hyoid bone.

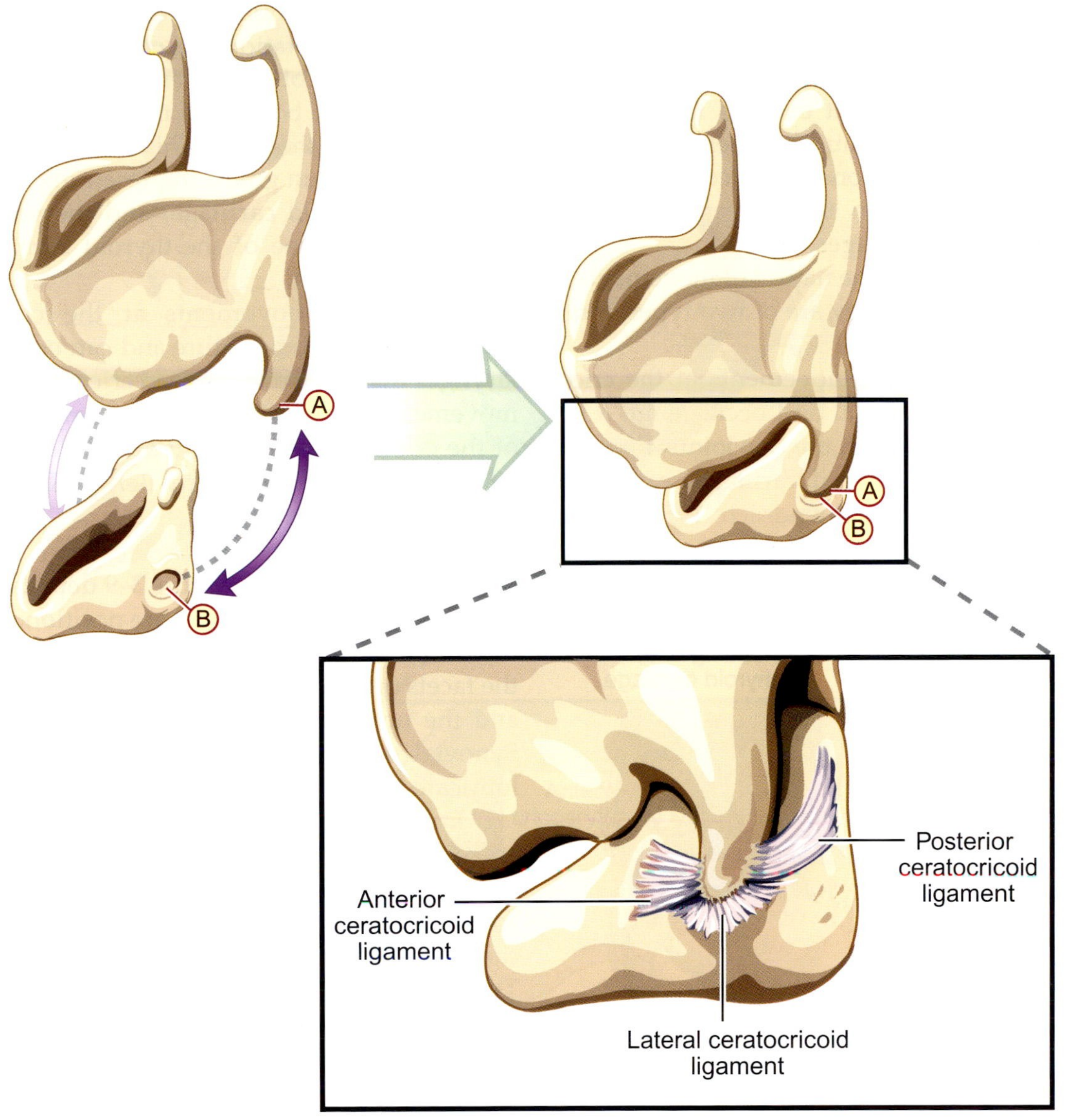

Figure 3–7. Cricothyroid joints.

Facets on the cricoid and thyroid cartilages vary from larynx to larynx and from side to side within the same larynx (Dickson & Maue-Dickson, 1982). Those on the cricoid cartilage generally face upward, toward the side, and backward. They are usually round or oval in shape and are concave. Facets on the thyroid cartilage typically face downward, toward the midline, and forward. They are usually round in shape and are convex. Occasionally a larynx will have cricothyroid joint facets that are rudimentary. Then the articulation between the cricoid and thyroid surfaces is formed by fibrous connective tissue (Zemlin, 1998).

Three ligaments extend between the side and back surfaces of the cricoid cartilage and the lower outside surfaces of the inferior cornu of the thyroid cartilage on each side. These three ligaments encircle most of the corresponding cricothyroid joint and are referred to as the anterior, lateral, and posterior ceratocricoid (cerato meaning horn) ligaments. The

Active Force. The active force of the laryngeal apparatus results from the contraction of muscles. Laryngeal muscles can be categorized as intrinsic, extrinsic, or supplementary. Muscles categorized as intrinsic have both ends attached within the larynx, whereas muscles categorized as extrinsic have one end attached within the larynx and one end attached outside the larynx. Muscles categorized as supplementary do not attach to the larynx directly but influence it by way of attachments to the neighboring hyoid bone.

The function described below for individual muscles assumes that the muscles of interest are engaged in shortening (concentric) contractions, unless otherwise specified as being engaged in lengthening (eccentric) contractions or fixed-length (isometric) contractions. The influence of individual muscle actions may also be conditioned by whether or not other muscles are active.

Intrinsic Laryngeal Muscles. Figure 3–15 depicts the intrinsic muscles of the larynx. These muscles

Two Worlds

Technical and colloquial definitions of terms can sometimes be quite different. Take, for example, the term "elastic." In a physical sense, something that's elastic returns to its original shape following deformation. Throw a golf club on the floor and it will deform and then return to its original shape. And you can predict what that shape will be. But consider the waistband of your underwear. Throw your underwear on the floor and its waistband will not assume a shape you can predict. That's because, in a physical sense, it's inelastic—it doesn't return to its original shape following deformation. So, although you might think of the waistband of your underwear as being elastic, a physicist would think just the opposite. Both of you are right in your colloquial and technical uses of the term "elastic," but you need to know which world you're talking in before you consider something to be "elastic" or not.

Motorboat

Probably as a child you played "motor boat" with friends by rapidly pounding your fists on their chests or backs while they sustained "ah." The variation in loudness that sounded to you like an idling motorboat was caused by rapid changes in alveolar pressure. Pound on someone's chest or back and with each blow their lungs compress a small amount and the air pressure inside them goes up momentarily. Pound at different rates and you change the perceived speed of your imaginary motor noise. The basis of all this fun is that the laryngeal apparatus and the voice are sensitive to adjustments in the breathing apparatus. You don't necessarily need to have a friend pounding on you to appreciate this sensitivity. Try to talk while driving a car down a cross-rutted dirt road or while sitting atop a trotting horse. The road and the horse will effectively do the pounding for you by bouncing your gut up and down and changing your alveolar pressure.

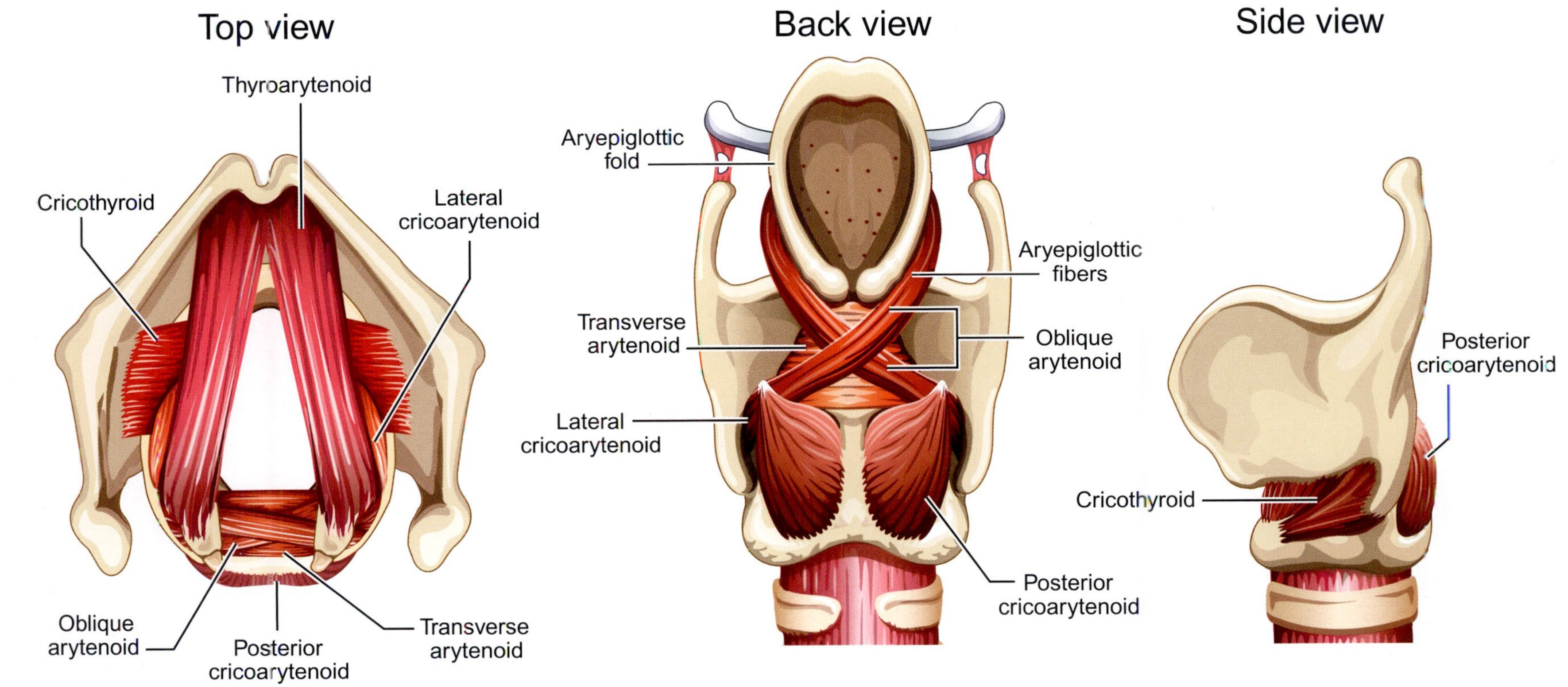

Figure 3–15. Intrinsic muscles of the larynx.

are responsible for changing the position and mechanical status of structures that form the walls of the laryngeal cavity. They are the ***thyroarytenoid***, ***posterior cricoarytenoid***, ***lateral cricoarytenoid***, ***arytenoid***, and ***cricothyroid*** muscles.

The ***thyroarytenoid*** muscle forms most of each vocal fold. This muscle extends between the inside surface of the thyroid cartilage (near the angle) and the arytenoid cartilage on the corresponding side. The front attachment of the muscle lies to the side of the front attachment of the corresponding vocal ligament. Fibers run generally parallel to the vocal ligament to insert on the front and outer sides of the arytenoid cartilage. Upper fibers run a straight course from front to back, whereas lower fibers twist in their course and swing off in an outward, backward, and upward direction (Broad, 1973; Zemlin, 1998). A small number of fibers toward the side of the muscle depart from the predominant front-to-back orientation of the others and course upward to the aryepiglottic fold, the side of the epiglottis, and into the region of the ventricular fold on the same side (Zemlin, 1998). The effects of contraction of different parts of the ***thyroarytenoid*** muscle are portrayed in Figure 3–16. Contraction of the longitudinal fibers of the ***thyroarytenoid*** muscle shortens it and reduces the distance between the thyroid and arytenoid cartilages. The reduction in distance between the two cartilages is typically effected as a forward pull on the arytenoid cartilage that rocks it toward the midline. Fixed-length (isometric) or lengthening (eccentric) contractions of the ***thyroarytenoid*** muscle (with other intrinsic muscles opposing) increase its internal tension (force per unit length). Contraction of vertical fibers of the ***thyroarytenoid*** muscle near the sidewall of the larynx may have an influence on the position and configuration of the corresponding ventricular fold (Reidenbach, 1998).

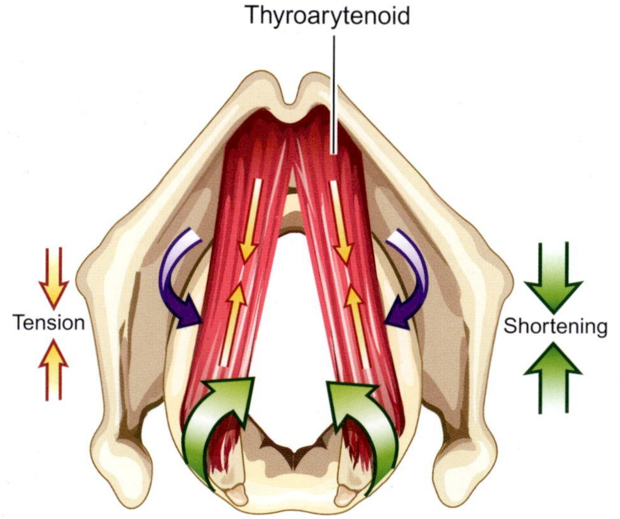

Figure 3–16. Effects of contractions of different parts of the ***thyroarytenoid*** muscles.

The ***thyroarytenoid*** muscle is sometimes described as having two distinct parts (Dickson & Maue-Dickson, 1982; van den Berg & Moll, 1955; Wustrow, 1953), called the ***external thyroarytenoid*** muscle (***thyromuscularis***) and the ***internal thyroarytenoid*** muscle (***thyrovocalis*** or ***vocalis***). As depicted schematically in Figure 3–17, the ***external thyroarytenoid*** muscle lies nearest the laryngeal wall and to the side of the ***internal thyroarytenoid*** muscle. The ***internal thyroarytenoid*** muscle flanks the vocal ligament. The ***internal thyroarytenoid*** muscle and the vocal ligament are sometimes referred to as the vocal cord, as distinguished from the vocal fold, although the terms vocal cord and vocal fold are also used interchangeably. The term vocal fold is more descriptive of the entire shelf-like structure and is preferred.

The notion of a two-part ***thyroarytenoid*** muscle, although embraced by many, is not accepted universally. Some argue that dissections have failed to reveal a separating fascial sheath within the ***thyroarytenoid*** muscle that would support the notion of two distinct anatomical parts (Mayet, 1955; Zemlin, 1998). Others argue that, with or without such a separating fascial sheath, the ***thyroarytenoid*** muscle is capable of differential actions in what is conceptualized to be its ***thyromuscularis*** and ***thyrovocalis*** subdivisions (Broad, 1973; Sonesson, 1960). These presumed differential actions (discussed below in another section) are believed by some to have salience in the control of voice production (Kahane, 2007; Orlikoff & Kahane, 1996; Titze, 1994).

Anatomical evidence is beginning to accumulate in support of differential actions of the two subdivisions of the ***thyroarytenoid*** muscle. For example, the ***thyrovocalis*** muscle appears to have distinct sub-compartments in which muscle fibers are differentially packed, suggesting that they function independently (Sanders, Rai, Han, & Biller, 1998).

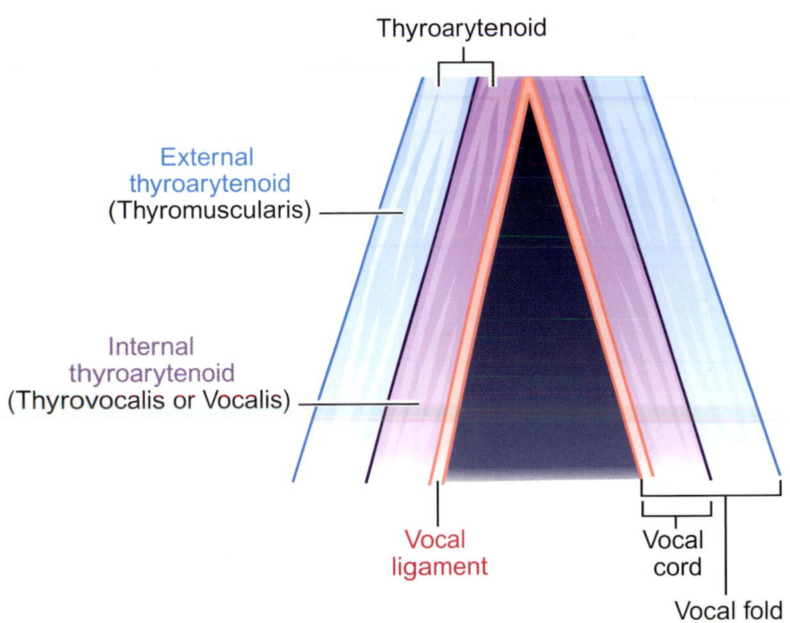

Figure 3–17. ***Thyromuscularis*** and ***thyrovocalis*** subdivisions of the ***thyroarytenoid*** muscles.

And, for another example, slow tonic muscle fibers have been found within the ***thyrovocalis*** muscle, but not within the ***thyromuscularis*** muscle (Han, Wang, Fischman, Biller, & Sanders, 1999). Contractions of these muscle fibers are prolonged, stable, precisely controlled, and fatigue resistant, all desirable characteristics for adjusting the background mechanical properties of the inner part of the vocal fold. Current evidence suggests that slow tonic muscle fibers are not present in other mammals (including primates) and, therefore, may be a unique human specialization (Han et al., 1999).

The ***posterior cricoarytenoid*** muscle is a fan-shaped muscle located on the back surface of the cricoid cartilage. The muscle originates on the cricoid lamina and courses upward and toward the side in a converging pattern to insert on the upper and back surfaces of the muscular process of the arytenoid cartilage. Contraction of the ***posterior cricoarytenoid*** muscle rocks the arytenoid cartilage away from the midline as illustrated in Figure 3–18. This rocking is effected mainly by fibers located laterally within the muscle and that insert on the upper surface of the muscular process. Forceful contraction of these fibers may also slide the arytenoid cartilage upward and backward along the sloping rim of the cricoid cartilage. Contraction of fibers from the medial part of the ***posterior cricoarytenoid*** muscle that inserts on the back surface of the muscular process stabilizes the arytenoid cartilage against other forces that are directed forward (Zemlin, Davis, & Gaza, 1984).

The ***lateral cricoarytenoid*** muscle is a small fan-shaped muscle that originates from the upper rim of the cricoid cartilage. Fibers of the muscle extend upward and backward to insert on the muscular process and front surface of the arytenoid cartilage. As depicted in Figure 3–19, contraction of the ***lateral cricoarytenoid*** muscle rocks the arytenoid cartilage toward the midline. Activation of the ***lateral cricoarytenoid*** muscle may also slide the arytenoid cartilage forward and toward the side along the downward sloping path of the long axis of the cricoid facet of the cricoarytenoid joint.

The ***arytenoid*** muscle (also called the ***interarytenoid***) extends from the back surface of one arytenoid cartilage to the back surface of the other arytenoid cartilage. The ***arytenoid*** muscle is a complex structure that is considered to have two distinct and separate subdivisions, one designated as the ***transverse arytenoid*** muscle and one designated as the ***oblique arytenoid*** muscle. The ***transverse arytenoid*** muscle arises from the back surface and side of one arytenoid cartilage and courses horizontally to insert on the back surface and side of the other

the level of the vocal folds, this region of the larynx is the foremost contributor to laryngeal airway resistance. The ventricular folds are a secondary contributor. Thus, by adjusting the cross-sectional area and/or length of the internal larynx in the region of the vocal folds and ventricular folds, the laryngeal airway resistance will likely change. Resistance increases with increasing constriction and length of constriction.

It is important to note that laryngeal airway resistance is airflow dependent. This is portrayed in Figure 3–31 and means that even at fixed cross-sectional areas and/or lengths of the laryngeal airway, the value of resistance is influenced by how fast air is moving (van den Berg, Zantema, & Doornenbal, 1957). Laryngeal airway resistance is not measurable, but is calculated from the quotient of translaryngeal air pressure (in cmH_2O) to translaryngeal airflow (the flow of air through the larynx, in LPS).

The range of potential airway resistance values is large and can go from a very low resistance (wide open airway) to infinity (airtight closure of the airway). It is common to conceptualize laryngeal airway resistance in terms of a value that represents the average opposition to airflow through the laryngeal valve. This average opposition is often taken to reflect the magnitude of coupling between the trachea and pharynx during the activity of interest (Smitheran & Hixon, 1981).

Glottal Size and Configuration

The size and configuration of the glottis can be adjusted in a variety of ways. Such adjustments are reflected in changes in physical dimensions such as length, diameter, area, and shape in the horizontal plane, although vertical aspects (depth and shape) are also important.

Figure 3–32 shows examples of contrasting glottal sizes and configurations. Panel A of the figure (repeated from Figure 3–27) illustrates a large glottis of maximum length, diameter, and area, that diverges toward the back. This glottis is attendant to full abduction of the vocal folds and a maximally opened airway. Panel B (repeated from Figure 3–13) illustrates a glottis of medium size that is of lesser diameter and area than for full abduction and is typical of a glottis associated with resting tidal breathing. Panel C illustrates a small glottis com-

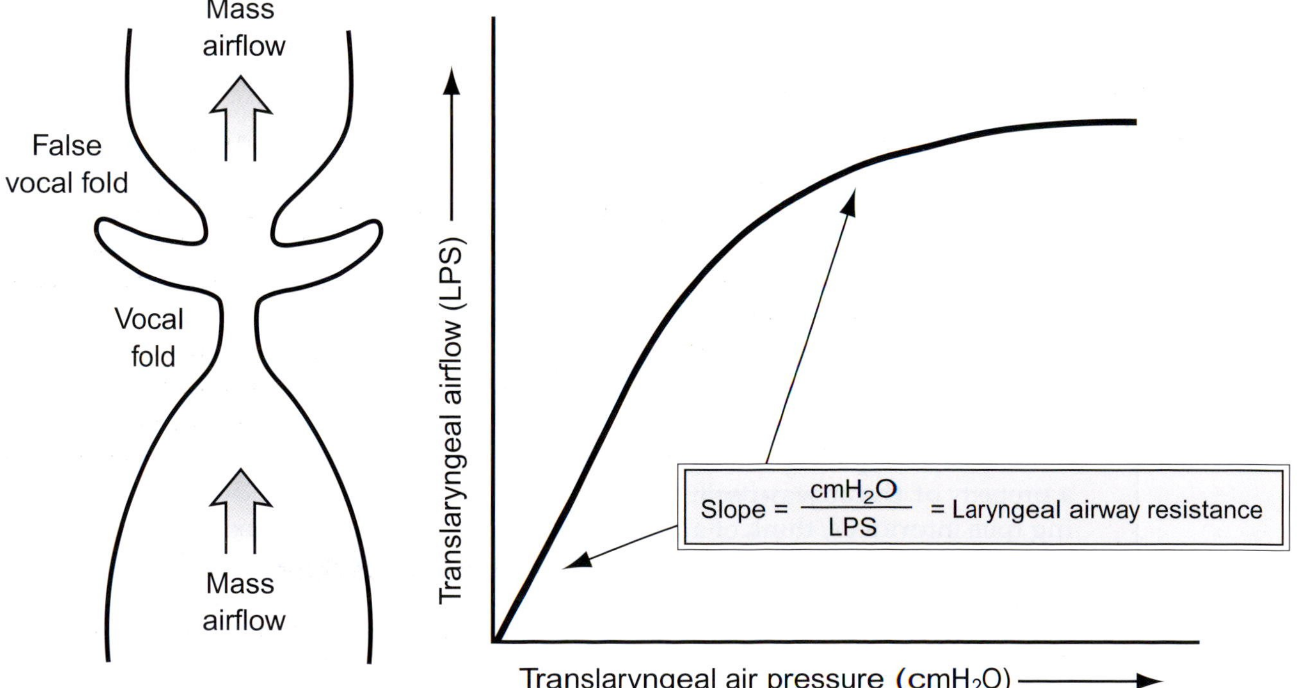

Figure 3–31. Laryngeal airway resistance adjustment.

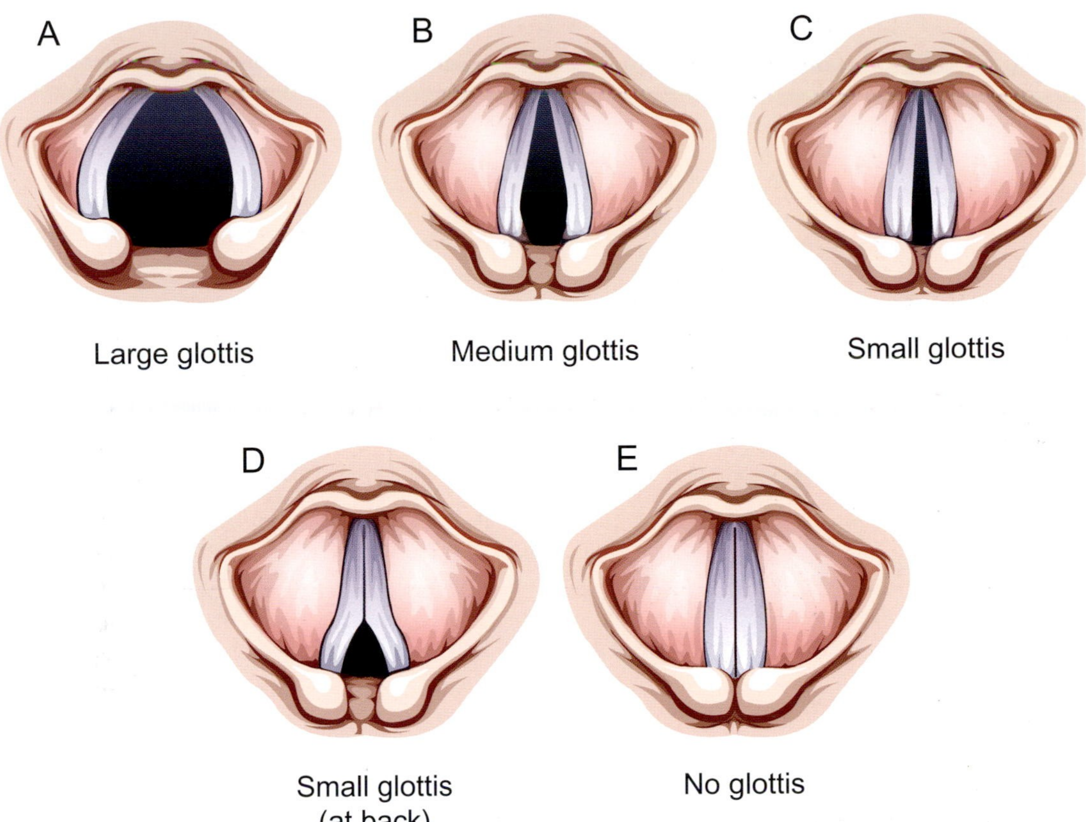

Figure 3–32. Contrasting glottal sizes and configurations.

pared to the diameters and areas of those portrayed in Panels A and B and shows a somewhat constricted airway. Panel D illustrates another small glottis, this one located at the back of the larynx. And Panel E (repeated from Figure 3–26) illustrates an airway that is closed airtight and has no glottis.

Abduction and adduction of the vocal folds are the main contributors to glottal size and configuration changes. When the glottis extends the entire length of the vocal folds, abduction and adduction influence glottal size mainly through side-to-side movements of the free margins of the vocal folds. During breathing, these free margins are widely separated, but typically go through an abduction-adduction cycling that corresponds to the cycling of inspiration-expiration. Maximum glottal size can be achieved during very deep inspiration following panting (Sekizawa, Sasaki, & Takishima, 1985).

Abduction of the vocal folds increases glottal size, whereas adduction of the vocal folds decreases it. Active and/or passive forces can cause abduction of the vocal folds. Active abduction of the vocal folds results mainly from contraction of the ***posterior cricoarytenoid*** muscles, with secondary abduction forces resulting from downward stretching of the conus elasticus. Active adduction is brought about by contraction of the ***lateral cricoarytenoid*** muscles and ***arytenoid*** muscles (***transverse*** and ***oblique*** subdivisions). When just the ***lateral cricoarytenoid*** muscles are activated, the arytenoid cartilages are made to toe inward and the front portions of the vocal folds are in apposition and full adduction, whereas the back portions remain somewhat separated, such that only a small-size opening exists (see Panel D in Figure 3–32).

Stiffness of the Vocal Folds

Figure 3–33 portrays factors that can adjust the stiffness of the vocal folds. Stiffness of the vocal folds is an indication of their rigidity or tautness. Stiffness is the reciprocal of compliance and in physical terms

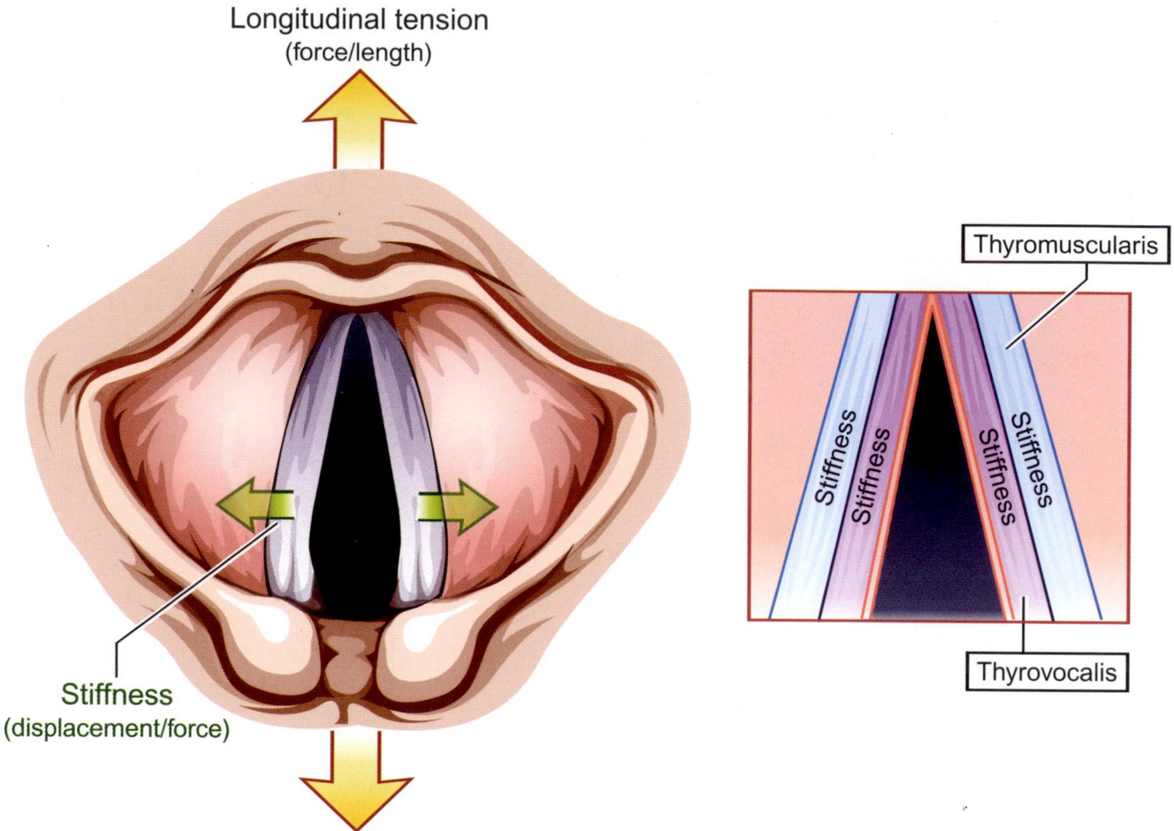

Figure 3–33. Vocal fold stiffness adjustment.

conveys an indication of how much the vocal folds move for a given force applied to them. The stiffness of the vocal folds may differ somewhat from one location to another within the vocal folds. For example, the folds may be stiffer nearer their points of attachment to the thyroid and arytenoid cartilages than at their midpoints.

The most important component of vocal fold stiffness is manifested perpendicular to the long axes of the vocal folds (Titze, 1994). Vocal fold stiffness can be changed by contractions of muscles external to the vocal folds that tend to stretch them and/or pull them more taut from end to end and by contractions of muscles internal to the vocal folds that modify their internal mechanical status.

Stretching of the vocal folds and/or pulling them more taut from end to end is accomplished by muscle actions that increase the distance between the two ends of the vocal folds (the inner surface of the thyroid cartilage and the tips of the vocal processes of the arytenoid cartilages) and/or increase the longitudinal tension (force per unit of length) operating along them lengthwise. These actions are similar to the stretching of a guitar string by the turning of its tuning peg to tighten and tense the string. The tensile strength of the vocal ligaments along the medial edges of the vocal folds is the limiting factor as to how much the vocal folds can be stretched and how much longitudinal tension can be applied.

Contraction of muscles within the vocal folds themselves can also change their stiffness. A more forceful contraction results in greater stiffness, whereas a less forceful contraction results in lesser stiffness. Contractions of muscle fibers that lie within the lateral portions of the vocal folds (the ***thyromuscularis*** muscles) mainly stiffen those parts of the vocal folds, and contractions of the muscle fibers that lie within the medial portions of the vocal folds (the ***thyrovocalis*** muscles) mainly affect those portions.

Effective Mass of the Vocal Folds

Mechanisms for changing the length of the vocal folds are discussed above. However, the length set by these mechanisms may or may not be the "effective" length employed for some activities. That is, the full mass of the vocal folds may not participate in certain activities and a lesser "effective" mass may participate. This is illustrated in Figure 3–34.

Full mass and effective mass are the same when the vocal folds are fully abducted, maximally elongated, and have unencumbered free margins along their lengths. Full mass and effective mass are different, however, when the full mass of the vocal folds is partitioned by action that encumbers the vocal folds at some intermediate point along their lengths. An example can be seen in the form of adductory adjustments of the vocal folds that are mediated through the cricoarytenoid joints, activated by the ***lateral cricoarytenoid*** muscles, and manifested as medial compression between the tips of the vocal processes of the arytenoid cartilages. When the vocal processes of the arytenoid cartilages are made to toe inward sufficiently (see section above on glottal size and configuration), the membranous portions of the vocal folds are approximated and their cartilaginous portions remain separated. Under this circumstance, the vocal folds are partitioned longitudinally into two masses having very different functional potentials. The membranous portion of the configuration blocks the flow of air through the larynx, whereas the cartilaginous portion allows the free passage of air.

Considering this example further, different levels of activation of the ***lateral cricoarytenoid*** muscles generate different magnitudes of medial compression. Once the tips of the vocal processes are approximated, increasingly forceful contractions of the ***lateral cricoarytenoid*** muscles can further reduce the effective mass of the membranous portions of the vocal folds by forcing the tips of the vocal processes to make additional more forceful and forward contact in association the downward and forward rocking of the vocal processes of the arytenoid cartilages.

Neural Substrates of Laryngeal Control

Laryngeal movement is controlled by the nervous system. The nature of such movement and the nature of its control are different for different activities. For example, control of the laryngeal apparatus is different for coughing, throat clearing, crying, singing,

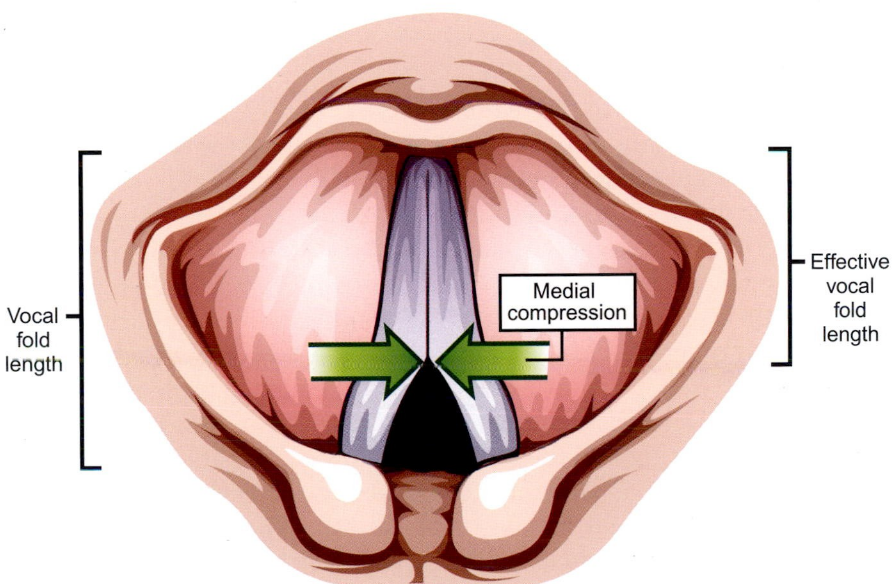

Figure 3–34. Effective vocal fold length adjustment.

speaking, and swallowing. These and other activities involve a range of laryngeal adjustments, some of which are reflexive and others of which are precisely monitored and voluntarily controlled. Speaking and swallowing are the two most important activities for the purposes of this book. Control for swallowing is discussed in Chapter 12.

All control commands to the laryngeal apparatus are sent through cranial nerves and cervical spinal nerves. Cranial nerves originate in the brainstem, whereas cervical spinal nerves originate within the uppermost segments of the spinal cord. These nerves course outward to provide motor innervation to the intrinsic, extrinsic, and supplementary muscles of the laryngeal apparatus. As shown in Table 3–1, motor innervation to the laryngeal apparatus is effected by five cranial nerves and three spinal nerves. Cranial nerve innervations include cranial nerves V (trigeminal), VII (facial), X (vagus), XI (accessory), and XII (hypoglossal), and spinal nerve innervations include cervical spinal segments C1, C2, and C3.

Innervation to the five intrinsic muscles of the larynx is through cranial nerves X and XI. Some consider cranial nerve X to be primary (Zemlin, 1998), whereas others consider the bulbar branch of cranial nerve XI to be primary (Dickson & Maue-Dickson, 1982; Orlikoff & Kahane, 1996). There is general agreement that two branches of cranial nerve X are critical to vocal fold function. The recurrent laryngeal branch (also called the inferior laryngeal branch) provides motor supply to four intrinsic muscles, the ***thyroarytenoid***, ***posterior cricoarytenoid***, ***lateral cricoarytenoid***, and ***arytenoid*** muscles. The remaining intrinsic muscle of the larynx, the ***cricothyroid*** muscle, receives its motor supply from the external branch of the superior laryngeal nerve. There is variation among larynges concerning the way specific nerves branch on their way to the larynx and how they interconnect with other nerves (Sanders, Wu, Mu, & Biller, 1993; Sanudo et al., 1999). For example, the recurrent laryngeal nerve has been shown to bifurcate or trifurcate before entering into the left or right sides of the larynx in more than one-third of larynges studied (Beneragama & Serpell, 2006).

Innervation of the three extrinsic muscles of the larynx is provided differentially via cranial nerves X, XI, and XII and cervical spinal nerves C1, C2, and C3. A mixture of cranial nerve and cervical spinal nerve supply is provided for the ***sternothyroid*** and ***thyrohyoid*** muscles, whereas the ***inferior constrictor*** muscle of the pharynx is supplied by cranial nerves X and XI.

The eight supplementary muscles of the laryngeal apparatus receive their motor innervation in various combinations through cranial nerves V, VII, and XII and cervical spinal nerves C1, C2, and C3. The ***sternohyoid***, ***omohyoid***, ***geniohyoid***, ***hyoglossus***, and ***genioglossus*** muscles are supplied by cranial nerve XII, with the ***sternohyoid*** and ***omohyoid*** muscles also receiving motor supply from C1, C2, C3. The remaining three supplementary muscles are

Table 3–1. Summary of the Cranial and Segmental Origins of the Motor Nerve Supply to the Muscles of the Laryngeal Apparatus. Cranial nerves include V (trigeminal), VII (facial), X (vagus), XI (accessory), and XII (hypoglossal). Spinal nerves include the first three cervical spinal nerves (C1, C2, C3). Muscles are categorized as intrinsic, extrinsic, or supplementary.

MUSCLE	INNERVATION
INTRINSIC	
Thyroarytenoid	X, XI
Posterior cricoarytenoid	X, XI
Lateral cricoarytenoid	X, XI
Arytenoid	X, XI
Cricothyroid	X, XI
EXTRINSIC	
Sternothyroid	XII, C1, C2, C3
Thyrohyoid	XII, C1, C2
Inferior constrictor	X, XI
SUPPLEMENTARY	
Sternohyoid	XII, C1, C2, C3
Omohyoid	XII, C1, C2, C3
Digastric	V, VII
Stylohyoid	VII
Mylohyoid	V
Geniohyoid	XII
Hyoglossus	XII
Genioglossus	XII

Note: All of the intrinsic muscles of the larynx are innervated by the recurrent laryngeal branch (also called the inferior laryngeal branch) of cranial nerve X, except for the cricothyroid muscle, which is innervated by the external branch of the superior laryngeal nerve.

innervated by cranial nerves V and/or VII. The ***digastric*** muscle receives motor innervation from both cranial nerves, its ***anterior*** belly from cranial nerve V and its ***posterior*** belly from cranial nerve VII (Dickson & Maue-Dickson, 1982). The other of the remaining supplementary muscles, the ***stylohyoid*** and ***mylohyoid*** muscles, receive motor innervation from cranial nerve VII and cranial nerve V, respectively.

Laryngeal adjustments are not executed without information about their consequences. This is especially true for activities in which rapid and precise movements are at a premium, such as those that are characteristic of vocal fold adjustments. Sensory information is critical to the control of such movements. This information comes from several sources, the relative importance of which depends on the activity being performed. These sources have in common some type of mechanoreceptor that converts a mechanical event into a neural signal that is then transmitted along a sensory nerve to the central nervous system.

Mechanoreceptors are distributed throughout the larynx in its muscles, joints, and mucosal coverings. Included among these are receptors that provide information about muscle lengths and their rates of change (Konig & von Leden, 1961b; Okamura & Katto, 1988; Sanders, Han, Wang, & Biller, 1998), joint movements (Jankovskaya, 1959; Kirchner & Wyke, 1965), and mucosal deformations (Kirchner & Suzuki, 1968; Konig & von Leden, 1961a; Sampson & Etyzaguirre, 1964). Such information is used to determine the mechanical status of the larynx and to elicit certain reflexive behaviors. There remains much to be known about the contribution of mechanoreceptors during laryngeal adjustments. Presumably they function as part of an integrated laryngeal feedback system (Orlikoff & Kahane, 1996). For laryngeal adjustments that target sound production, such a system would also have to take into account information provided by another type of mechanoreceptor, hair cells within the cochlea of the auditory system (via cranial nerve VIII).

Less than full agreement exists about which cranial and spinal nerves and branches convey sensory information from different structures of the larynx to the central nervous system (Dickson & Maue-Dickson, 1982). Most agree that the internal branch of the superior laryngeal nerve carries sensory information from the mucosa that covers the supraglottal region of the laryngeal cavity, including the base of the tongue, epiglottis, aryepiglottic folds, and backs of the arytenoid cartilages. This nerve is also believed to transmit information from mechanoreceptors in the muscles of the larynx that respond to stretch (Duffy, 2005). There is general agreement that the recurrent laryngeal nerve carries sensory information from the mucosa of the subglottal region of the laryngeal cavity and structures that are located below the vocal folds. Sensory information from the extrinsic and supplementary muscles travels via several different nerves. For example, the ***mylohyoid*** and ***stylohyoid*** muscles are served by sensory components of cranial nerves V and VII, respectively, whereas the ***digastric*** muscle is served by sensory components of both cranial nerves V and VII.

Laryngeal Functions

The larynx performs a variety of functions. Those considered here relate to (a) degree of coupling between the trachea and pharynx, (b) protection of the pulmonary airways, (c) containment of the pulmonary air supply, and (d) sound generation.

Degree of Coupling Between the Trachea and Pharynx

Actions of the larynx determine the degree of coupling between the trachea (windpipe) and pharynx (throat). For the most part, changing the positions of the vocal folds changes the connectivity between these two components of the airway. For example, the laryngeal airway is open during breathing to enable the movement of air to and from the lungs (ventilation). The degree of coupling for breathing events depends on the depth of breathing, rate of breathing, force of breathing, and phase of breathing (inspiratory or expiratory).

Coupling between the trachea and pharynx is also important in certain special acts of breathing (discussed in Chapter 2). For certain of these acts, the laryngeal airway is held open so that the full force of tracheal pressure and airflow can be delivered to downstream structures (such as the tongue and lips) or to devices placed in the oral cavity or at the airway opening (such as the mouthpieces of wind instruments).

Protection of the Pulmonary Airways

The pulmonary airways are a major part of the respiratory lifeline and the maintenance of their integrity is critical. The larynx is positioned at the juncture between the pulmonary airways and the so-called upper airway (pharyngeal cavity, oral cavity, nasal cavities). As such, the larynx is strategically located as a valve to protect the pulmonary airways from the intake of foreign matter.

The main food channel (from the mouth to the esophagus) and the main air channel (from the nose and mouth to the larynx) cross paths in the lower pharynx. Thus, the laryngeal airway must be closed during swallowing to prevent food or liquid from entering the trachea. This closure is accomplished by approximation of the vocal folds and ventricular folds and includes a period of apnea (breath holding) during swallowing (see Chapter 12 for details).

Containment of the Pulmonary Air Supply

Closure of the laryngeal valve is important to containment of the pulmonary air supply for activities that require the generation of high pressures at different locations within the torso (abdominal, pleural, alveolar, tracheal) and/or the fixation of structures of the torso (rib cage wall, diaphragm, abdominal wall). Closure of the laryngeal valve is critical to the initiation and/or maintenance of forceful acts such as coughing, vomiting, defecation, urination, parturition (child birth), and the lifting of heavy objects.

Sound Generation

Much of the interest in the present chapter is with sound generation. Sound generation at the level of the larynx can be of several types, three of which are most relevant to the concerns of this chapter. They are: (a) transient (popping) sound, in which the airstream is momentarily obstructed and then abruptly released; (b) turbulence (hissing) sound, in which air is forced through a narrowed airway; and (c) quasi-periodic (buzzing) sound, in which the vocal folds are forced into vibration and move rapidly to and fro to interrupt the airstream repeatedly. The last of these generates voice and is what gives the larynx its popular designation as the "voice box."

LARYNGEAL FUNCTION IN SPEECH PRODUCTION

Laryngeal function in speech production is complex and takes many forms. Three of these forms are (a) transient utterances, (b) extended sustained utter-

Get Thee Out

Reflexive coughing is our friend. It serves to clear the breathing airway via a powerful and violent explosion or series of such explosions. Your own experience with uncontrollable coughing is evidence of just how dedicated the pulmonary apparatus and laryngeal apparatus are to keeping things out of your lungs. Enormous air pressures and airflows are generated during reflexive coughing that cause violent movements of the vocal folds. Excessive reflexive coughing can be abusive to the larynx, lead to unpleasant symptoms, and result in voice disorders. Less violent coughing done voluntarily and repeatedly over long periods can have similar cumulative effects. Then there is the equally notorious family cousin, the bad habit of continual throat clearing. Less outgoing than its other two relatives (pun intended), frequent throat clearing can be grating on the vocal folds. Abuse not thy larynx.

ances, and (c) running speech activities. Understanding the principles that underlie these forms of laryngeal function enables extrapolation to other forms.

Transient Utterances

A transient (very brief duration) utterance can be produced at the level of the larynx in the form of a sudden explosive burst. This constitutes a glottal stop-plosive that is analogous to the downstream production of the voiceless stop-plosives consonants /p/, /t/, and /k/. As depicted in Figure 3–35, glottal stop-plosive production involves an initial blockage of the laryngeal airstream by full adduction of the vocal folds. Air pressure then builds up within the tracheal space. This is followed by an abrupt release of the vocal fold adductory force and a simultaneous abrupt release of the pent-up air (Rothenberg, 1968; Stevens, 2000).

The speed with which air flows through the rapidly opening laryngeal airway is very high and gives rise to the generation of a brief burst of noise that excites the pharyngeal-oral airway. The entire act is somewhat like that of a weak voiceless cough in which the sudden release of pent-up air results in an impulse-like popping sound at the glottis (Broad, 1973). The release phase bears analogy to the discharge of an electrical capacitor through a time-varying resistance (Fant, 1960). The noise excitation during the release causes the pharyngeal-oral airway to vibrate throughout its entire length and to produce a plosive utterance that is distinctly lower in "pitch" than the pitches associated with other stop-plosives generated downstream.

Sustained Utterances

Two types of sustained utterances are discussed in this section. One is turbulence noise production and the other is voice production. The first relies on the flow of air through a relatively stable or slowly changing constriction, whereas the second has to do with vibration of the vocal folds that is faster than the naked eye can follow.

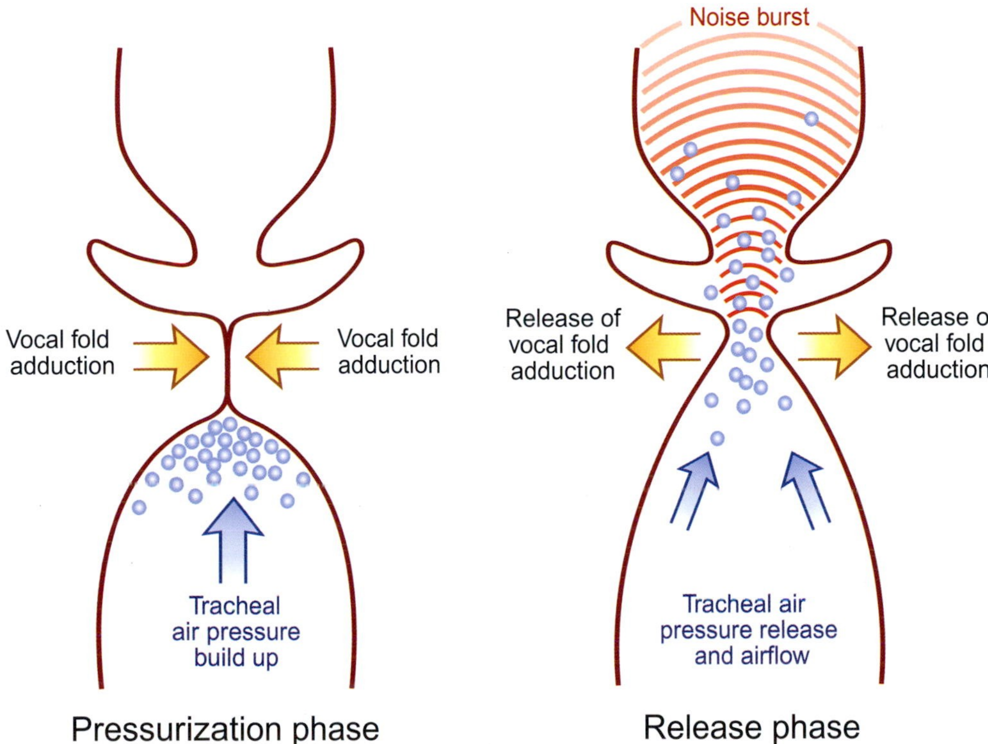

Figure 3–35. Glottal voiceless stop-plosive production.

Turbulence Noise Production

Air flowing from the breathing apparatus may encounter constrictions within the laryngeal airway. The most important of these usually occur at the level of the glottis, where inward movements of the vocal folds reduce the size and/or change the configuration of the airway.

Major constrictions cause air to flow turbulently. This means that air tumbles on itself, forming eddies (back flows), burbles (bubbles), and other irregularities. This agitation of air results in the generation of turbulence (friction) noise that contains a broad range of frequencies. The specific spectrum (frequency and sound pressure level content) of this noise depends on the nature of the interaction between the airstream and the constriction (Fant, 1960; Hixon, 1966; Minifie, 1973; Stevens, 2000).

Sustained noise is associated with sustained voiceless sound production in the larynx. One example is the production of the glottal fricative /h/, as illustrated in Figure 3–36. Glottal fricative production is achieved by positioning the vocal folds well inward to form a long slit-like constriction.

The act of whispering is another example of sustained noise production. Whispering can also be accomplished with a long slit-like constriction, but is often accompanied by other glottal configurations. One of the most frequent of these is a rearward-facing Y configuration. In this configuration, the membranous front parts of the vocal folds are firmly approximated (as in Figure 3–34), loosely approximated, or not approximated at all (Monoson & Zemlin, 1984; Rubin, Praneetvataku, Gherson, & Moyer, 2006; Solomon, McCall, Trosset, & Gray, 1989; Zemlin, 1998), and the cartilaginous rear parts of the vocal folds are relatively far apart. This configuration is achieved by contracting the ***lateral cricoarytenoid*** muscles so that the vocal processes of the arytenoid cartilages toe inward, while leaving the ***arytenoid*** muscles less active or inactive.

Quiet whispering and loud whispering (also called stage whispering) have been reported by some to be associated with different laryngeal adjustments (Monoson & Zemlin, 1984; Pressman & Keleman, 1955; Sawashima & Hirose, 1983). However, the most comprehensive study done of laryngeal configurations during whispering failed to find a consistent

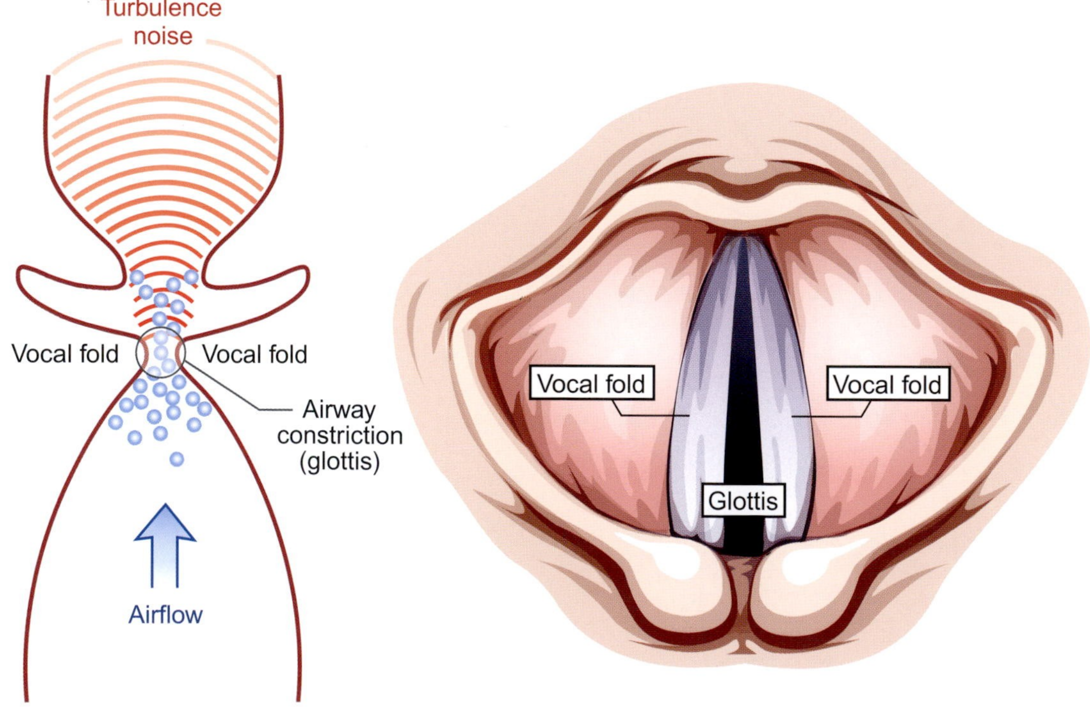

Figure 3–36. Glottal voiceless fricative production.

set of patterned adjustments for different types of whispering across speakers (Solomon et al., 1989). This suggests that the size of the glottis, rather than its specific configuration, may be the more important variable of the two (along with turbulent airflow) in the production of whispering of all types.

Under conditions of the sustained production of /h/ or whispering, the size and configuration of the glottis remain relatively fixed. Therefore, changes in the frequency content and sound pressure level of the noise are most influenced by the magnitude of the tracheal air pressure generated by the breathing apparatus and the resultant flow of air through the larynx (Hixon, Minifie, & Tait, 1967). When compared to usual voice production, quiet whispering has been shown to be produced using lower tracheal air pressure, higher translaryngeal airflow, and lower laryngeal airway resistance (Stathopoulos, Hoit, Hixon, Watson, & Solomon, 1991).

Voice Production

Voice results from vibration of the vocal folds. Such vibration modulates (chops up) the airstream into a series of air puffs. As depicted in Figure 3–37, the disturbances that constitute the voice source correspond to the series of abrupt closures of the laryngeal airway in association with the terminations of these air puffs. That is, the repeated, sudden decreases in airflow are what acoustically excite the upper airway (pharyngeal, oral, and nasal cavities) during voice production (Gauffin & Sundberg, 1989; Rothenberg, 1983). This section discusses the nature of vocal fold vibration during sustained voice production, how voice production is initiated, and various other aspects of voice, including fundamental frequency, sound pressure level, fundamental frequency-sound pressure level profiles, spectrum, and registers.

Vocal Fold Vibration. Once vibration is established in the vocal folds, it proceeds in a relatively steady quasi-periodic fashion. Each vibration consists of lateral and medial excursions of the vocal folds that rapidly and repeatedly valve the expiratory airstream. Movements of the vocal folds under this condition are passive and akin to the movements of the lips when air is blown between them. (Try it. Moisten your lips, pucker up slightly, gently blow air through them, and feel them vibrate.)

Each vibration of the vocal folds (or lips) is not caused by muscular contractions that pull them apart and force them back together again. Muscular forces are important, but only in the sense that they "set" the vocal folds (or lips) in position to be able to passively move to and fro when aeromechanical forces are applied to them. Thus, a key element of the laryngeal adjustment for sustained vocal fold vibration is to position and hold the vocal folds in the airway so that vibration can be established and maintained by air pressures and airflows acting on the vocal folds (van den Berg, 1958). The conditions

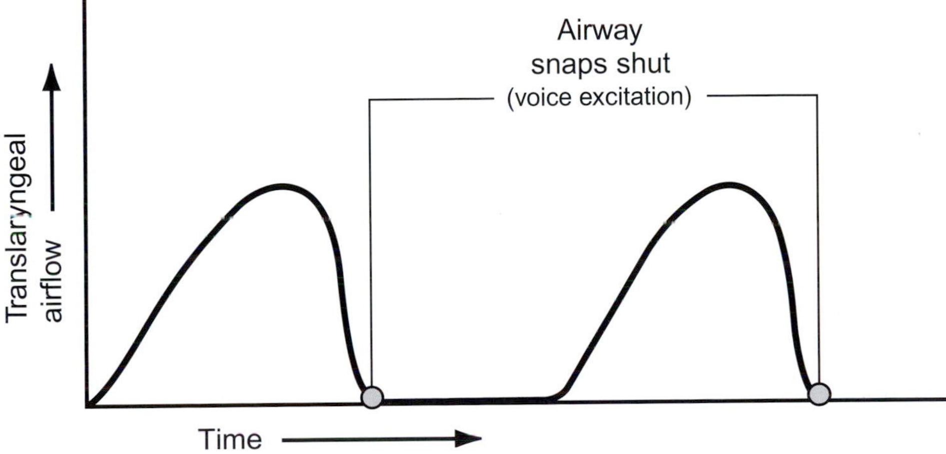

Figure 3–37. Voice source generation through abrupt closures of the laryngeal airway and sudden airflow declination.

To or Fro and To and Fro

Is this title a misprint? No. It's about oscillation and vibration. Many writers use the terms oscillation and vibration as if they were interchangeable. Some dictionaries do likewise. But, in the strictly correct use of the two terms, they are not synonymous. An oscillation is a movement in one direction (either to or fro), whereas a vibration is a double oscillation in two directions (to and fro). Consider the name of the oscilloscope, which is a device that can display signal change in one direction (or two, if you like). It's not called a vibroscope. And consider your summer electrical fan that turns side to side. Read the box it came in and you'll see that it's called a double-oscillation fan. It could just as well be called a single-vibration fan. So, the next time someone says they saw an oscillation of a vocal fold, ask which way it went, because an oscillation doesn't need to make a round trip like a vibration does.

Every Which Way

Despite current understanding of how the vocal folds vibrate to produce voice, it was only within the earlier part of the last century that scholars were unenlightened about many aspects of the process. Some scholars argued that voice resulted from up and down movements of the two vocal folds in opposite directions. Other scholars believed that vocal fold movements during voice production were strictly horizontal and akin to stiff shutters that slid together and apart repeatedly. These incorrect "guesses" about how the vocal folds functioned during voice production were dispelled by data obtained with high-speed motion picture filming of the larynx. This technology enabled the study of the rapid movements of the vocal folds in precise detail. Thus, what earlier in the last century seemed to be "every which way" of vocal fold movement during voice production, has settled down to the way things are as described in the adjacent text.

needed to sustain vocal fold vibration, once established, are a steady source of energy from the breathing apparatus and some form of nonlinear interaction with the structures being vibrated, namely, the vocal folds. As well, such vibration can be sustained only if the energy source exerts a force on the moving vocal folds that changes with the direction of the velocity of movement (Titze, 1994).

For most forms of voice production, the cover of each vocal fold moves somewhat like a horizontal ribbon that is loosely tethered at both ends (by the thyroid and arytenoid cartilages) and whose middle portion twists (flutters back and forth) as air is driven past it (Titze, 1994). Taking closure of the larynx (full approximation of the edges of the vocal folds) as a starting point, movement begins when the air pressure below the vocal folds (tracheal air pressure) rises and forces the bottom edges of the two folds apart.

As depicted in Figure 3–38, the vocal folds continue to separate as the tracheal pressure bubbles upward through the larynx. This pattern of lateral

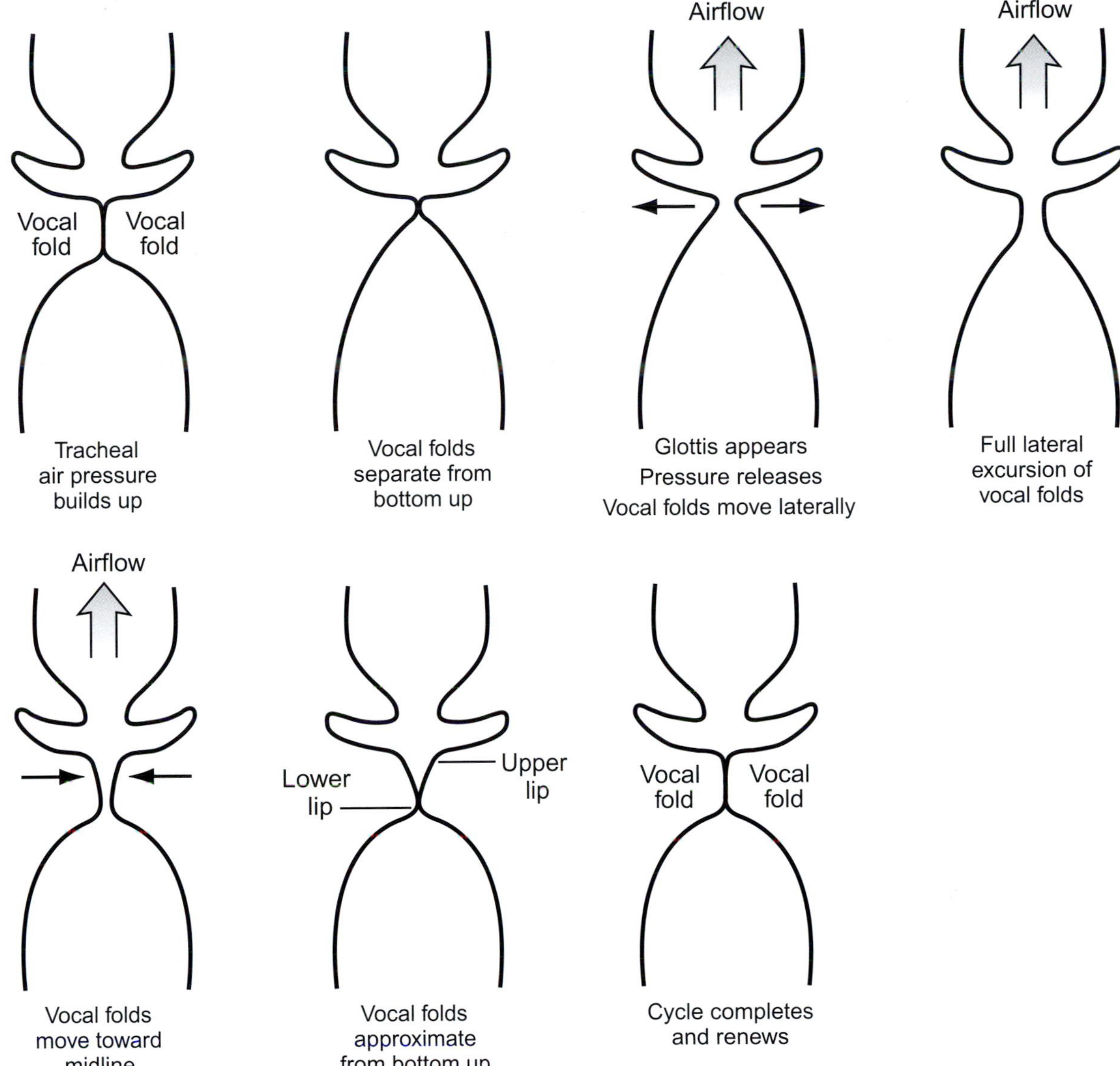

Figure 3–38. Vertical phase difference in side-to-side excursion of the vocal folds during voice production.

excursion of the vocal folds exhibits a so-called vertical phase difference in which lower points on the medial surfaces of the vocal folds are displaced earlier than points above them. A vertical phase difference is also manifested as the vocal folds move back together again. That is, lower points on the medial surfaces of the vocal folds move together before points on the upper surfaces move together (Hirano, Yoshida, & Tanaka, 1991; Schonharl, 1960; Timcke, von Leden, & Moore, 1958). These types of movements of the medial surfaces of the vocal folds occur because the covers of the vocal folds are relatively loosely coupled to their muscular bodies (Story & Titze, 1995). Such movements have been described as to and fro undulations of the surfaces of the vocal folds that are of a vertical-elliptical-horizontal nature (Baer, 1981) or as vertically propagating mucosal waves (like surface waves on water) that progress within the covers of the vocal folds and whose rippling effects can be seen on the top surfaces of the vocal folds (Berke & Gerratt, 1993; Hirano, Kakita, Kawasaki, Gould, & Lambiase, 1981).

Air pressure from below pushes the vocal folds laterally (apart). Elastic restoring forces in the vocal folds move them medially (back inward toward the midline). Air flowing through the larynx also plays an important role in lateral and medial excursions of the vocal folds when the folds are separated and a glottis exists. As the vocal folds move toward the sides, the vertical configuration of the glottis creates a converging airstream, whereas as they move toward the midline, the glottis creates a diverging airstream (Ishizaka & Matsudaira, 1972; McGowan, 1991; Titze, 1988c).

The average air pressure within the glottis is greater for a converging glottal configuration than for a diverging glottal configuration (Scherer & Titze, 1983). This asymmetry between converging and diverging configurations is key to making sustained vibration of the vocal folds possible. The fact that the outgoing and incoming paths of vocal fold movements are not mirror images is one of the important conditions that allows vocal fold vibration to be sustained (Titze, 1994). A great deal of research has been devoted to details of the aeromechanical coupling between the forces of breathing and the vocal folds during voice production and the mechanical coupling between different regions of the vocal folds (Orlikoff & Kahane, 1996). Consideration of these details is beyond the scope of this book and can be found in comprehensive and detailed form elsewhere (Titze, 2006a).

Initiation of Voice. A number of events precede the sustained quasiperiodic vibrations of the vocal folds that generate voice. These include adjustments of the larynx that preset the voice production apparatus and determine the form of vibration at voice onset.

Presetting adjustments of the larynx occur in advance of actual voice production (Faaborg-Andersen, 1957; Hirano, Kiyokawa, & Kurita, 1988) and are coordinated with adjustments of the breathing apparatus (Faaborg-Andersen, Yanagihara, & von Leden, 1967; Hixon, Watson, Harris, & Pearl, 1988). Presetting adjustments of the larynx may have influences on the laryngeal opposing pressure, laryngeal airway resistance, glottal size and/or configuration, vocal fold stiffness, and effective vocal fold mass. The adjustments chosen depend on the nature of the ensuing voice production. For example, different fundamental frequencies, sound pressure levels, and voice registers will condition the nature of the presetting adjustments. Laryngeal presetting is accomplished before any acoustic feedback having to do with the voice is available (Orlikoff & Kahane, 1996). This means that the larynx is mechanically "tuned" by the nervous system (as are other subsystems of the speech production apparatus) prior to the production of voice.

The intricate details of voice onset are manifested in the manner in which the larynx and breathing apparatus interact to generate the first few cycles of vocal fold vibration. This phase of vocal fold adjustment is often designated as the vocal attack phase (Daniloff, Schuckers, & Feth, 1980; Koike, 1967; Koike, Hirano, & von Leden, 1967; Moore, 1938). The most frequently used system for classifying vocal attack includes three different interplays between the laryngeal apparatus and the breathing apparatus. These are depicted in Figure 3–39 and include (a) simultaneous action of the laryngeal apparatus and breathing apparatus, (b) action of the laryngeal apparatus preceding action of the breathing apparatus, and (c) action of the breathing apparatus preceding action of the laryngeal apparatus.

Simultaneous vocal attack (sometimes labeled usual or normal) is characterized by the synchronous generation of expiratory airflow and the approximation of the vocal folds along their length. This form of vocal attack is characterized by a gradual increase in tracheal air pressure and voice onset that stabilizes relatively rapidly into the quasiperiodic pattern typical of sustained vocal fold vibration.

Vocal attack in which laryngeal action precedes that of the breathing apparatus is often designated as a hard vocal (or glottal) attack or so-called coup de glotte. Laryngeal opposing pressure is very high during hard glottal attack and "squeezes" the vocal folds firmly against one another prior to any significant rise in tracheal air pressure. Action of the breathing apparatus raises tracheal air pressure to a level that is sufficient to overcome the laryngeal opposing pressure. Vibration of the vocal folds begins abruptly and with greater amplitude initially than is characteristic of simultaneous vocal attack and its accompanying lower tracheal air pressure.

Vocal attack in which breathing action leads laryngeal action is designated as breathy (sometimes called aspirate or soft). In this form of vocal attack, expiratory airflow begins before the vocal folds are

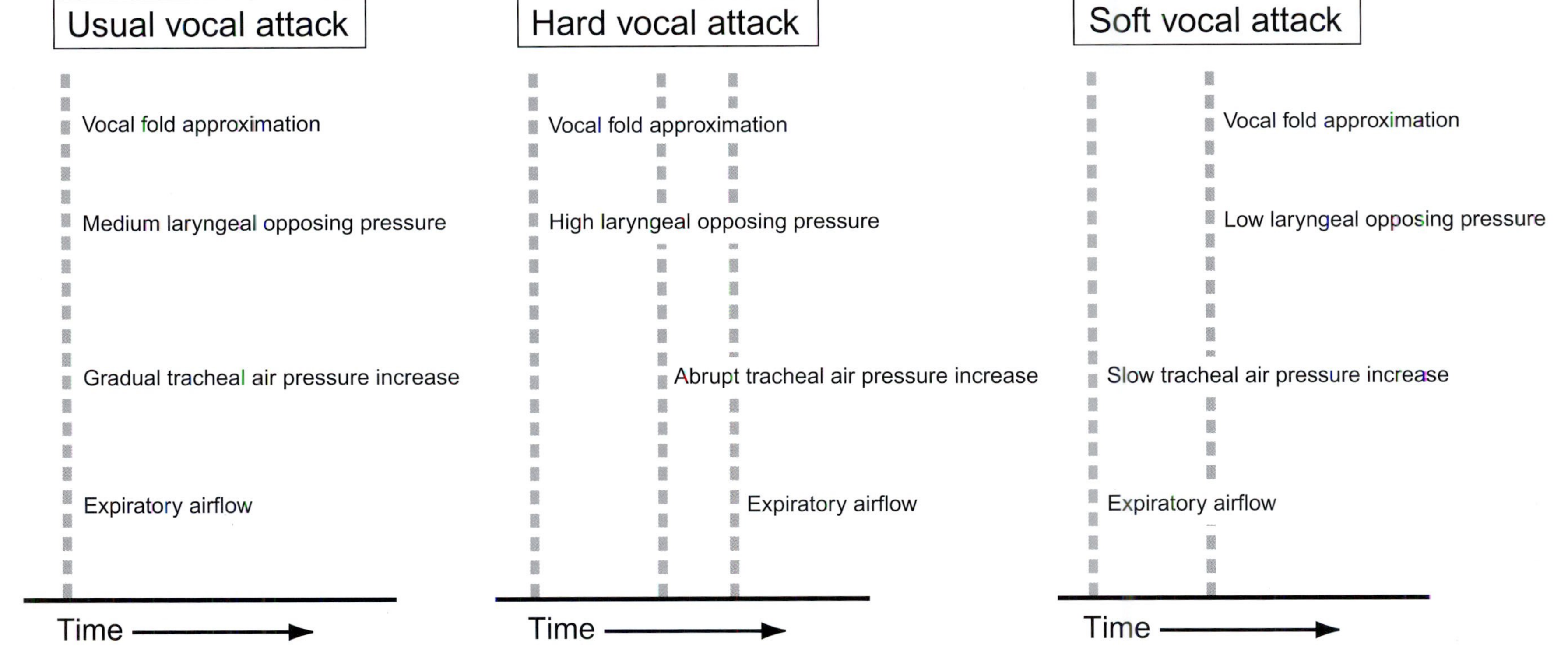

Figure 3–39. Three types of vocal attack.

moved to the midline. Movement of the vocal folds into the airstream may cause noise to be generated initially. As the vocal folds approach one another and constrict the airway, vibration begins. Fast flowing air lowers the air pressure between the vocal folds and pulls them toward the midline. This inward pulling force is opposed by elastic recoil of the vocal folds that tends to restore their set position. These two medial-lateral forces alternate such that momentum increases with each successive vibration. The vocal folds move closer and closer together with successive vibrations until they approximate and a regular and even cycle of movement is established. An analog to this form of vocal attack can be demonstrated with the lips and an airstream. (Try it. Moisten your lips. Take a deep breath and then expire briskly through your lips while slowly moving them together. They should vibrate with increasing amplitude until a continuous steady vibratory pattern is established.)

Vocal fold vibration will not begin without sufficient drive from the breathing apparatus. The preset laryngeal apparatus will simply sit in position until breathing force is adequate to set the vocal folds into vibration. The onset of vibration is conditioned largely by tracheal air pressure and translaryngeal airflow. The threshold where such air pressure and airflow come into play (and voicing begins) depends on the prevailing laryngeal opposing pressure. The threshold (minimum) tracheal air pressure needed to produce voice (sometimes called the phonation threshold pressure) typically ranges in the neighborhood of 2 to 3 cmH_2O. This air pressure is required to overcome the muscular opposing pressure, surface tension, and gravitational force operating to maintain closure of the laryngeal airway at the level of the glottis. There is a slight hysteresis (force direction difference) in the rise and fall of tracheal air pressure and the threshold pressure for voice production. This is shown in a clear effect for voice production to cease at a slightly lower tracheal air pressure than the air pressure it takes to just get it started (Hixon, Klatt, & Mead, 1970; Plant, Freed, & Plant, 2004).

Fundamental Frequency. The fundamental frequency of the voice (or of vocal fold movement) is related to the average rate of vocal fold vibration (cycles of movement). The fundamental frequency can be changed over a very wide range, typically about three octaves for a young adult (Fairbanks, 1960). Fundamental frequency is usually expressed on a continuum in units of cycles per second or Hertz. It is also sometimes expressed on a musical scale in semitones (Baken & Orlikoff, 2000).

The fundamental frequency of the human voice depends to a considerable extent on the sex of the individual and the size of the larynx. Men are more likely to exhibit lower average fundamental frequencies than women, and women are more likely

Rest in Peace

You may wonder why we don't use the term "subglottal pressure" in the text. The reason is that we believe the term has problems. Consider the following. The "sub" part of the term isn't specific to a location. Bronchial and alveolar pressures are also "sub" glottal. The "glottal" part of the term is also troublesome. Glottis means hole. There are times during voice production when the vocal folds are in apposition and the larynx is closed. How during those times can anything be "sub" glottal. You can't be below a hole when there isn't one. Respiratory physiologists use tracheal pressure to refer to the pressure of interest. Tracheal pressure designates the site of the pressure and is accurate regardless of whether the laryngeal airway is open or closed. Using the term tracheal pressure also removes ambiguity involved in the use of "sub" as a location. The term subglottal pressure should be buried. Rest in peace.

to exhibit lower average fundamental frequencies than children.

The strongest auditory-perceptual correlate of fundamental frequency is the pitch of the voice. Pitch is the subjective impression of the relative position of a sound along a musical scale. Sound pressure level and spectral content of the voice also influence the perception of pitch, but to far less important degrees than does the fundamental frequency. Thus, for the most part, a higher pitch is associated with a higher fundamental frequency and a lower pitch is associated with a lower fundamental frequency.

Control of the fundamental frequency is vested mainly in adjustments of the vocal folds and breathing apparatus. Adjustments of the vocal folds are of primary importance in changing fundamental frequency, whereas adjustments of the breathing apparatus have a supporting role.

Three laryngeal factors influence the rate of vocal fold vibration during sustained voice production. These include (a) the stiffness of the vocal folds, (b) their effective vibrating mass, and (c) the tautness of their covers as influenced by vertically applied force. These three factors may work singly or in different combinations to influence the fundamental frequency, and may do so differently in different portions of the fundamental frequency range.

The stiffness of the vocal folds is generally the most important of the three laryngeal factors that influence the rate of vocal fold vibration (Stevens, 2000). The general mechanism for controlling the stiffness of the vocal folds is discussed above and illustrated in Figure 3–33. Stiffness of the vocal folds can be adjusted through either or both external or internal forces applied to the vocal folds. With regard to the rate of vocal fold vibration during sustained voice production, a major factor in the adjustment of the stiffness of the vocal folds is the application of external force by the ***cricothyroid*** muscles, which, through their actions, tend to stretch the vocal folds and/or increase the force per unit of length (tension) along them. The effect of such actions can be to reduce the cross section and thickness of the vocal folds and to stiffen them such that they vibrate at a faster rate.

Internal force, applied by the vocal folds themselves, can also increase their stiffness during sustained voice production. This force is exerted by way of contraction of the ***thyroarytenoid*** muscles, which, through their actions, tend to make the vocal folds more rigid, especially in relation to forces applied at right angles to their long axes. As a consequence, the vocal folds vibrate at a faster rate.

During sustained voice production, the adjustment of stiffness of the vocal folds can vary depending on the fundamental frequency (low, intermediate, or high) and the extent to which different parts of the cross sections of the vocal folds move during vocal fold vibration (muscular bodies versus covers or both). For example, ***cricothyroid*** muscle activity may increase the fundamental frequency of the voice by applying an external stretching force to the vocal folds over a limited range of fundamental frequencies and then ***thyroarytenoid*** muscle activity may further adjust fundamental frequency by exerting an internal force on the vocal folds. The nature of this internal force depends on whether the ***thyromuscularis*** portion, ***thyrovocalis*** portion, or both portions of the ***thyroarytenoid*** muscle are activated. Once the upper limit of a particular external adjustment in stiffness is reached, the ***cricothyroid*** muscle increases its level of activity to set the next externally generated stiffness range and the ***thyroarytenoid*** muscle further adjusts internally to meet the stiffness demands of the fundamental frequency target. This alternation of activity is often referred to as a stair-step adjustment of stiffness, coming partly from outside the vocal folds and partly from within the vocal folds (Hollien, 1960b). This two-part adjustment is also referred to as loading the vocal folds (from without) through isotonic or isometric ***cricothyroid*** muscle activity and tuning of the vocal folds (from within) through isometric ***thyroarytenoid*** muscle activity (Arnold, 1961).

Thus, the combined activities of the ***cricothyroid*** and ***thyroarytenoid*** muscles are responsible for setting the prevailing stiffness of the vocal folds. This is true whether the fundamental frequency is changed in discrete steps up or down or continuously as when sliding up or down in fundamental frequency during a glissando. How the ***cricothyroid*** and ***thyroarytenoid*** muscles cooperate to achieve different fundamental frequencies differs in different parts of the overall fundamental frequency range (for example, the ***cricothyroid*** contribution predominates at high fundamental frequencies), but these two muscles are almost invariably cooperating players in adjusting the fundamental frequency of the voice (Shipp & McGlone, 1971; Titze, 1994).

The fundamental frequency of the voice can also be changed through changes in the effective vibrating mass of the vocal folds (Stevens, 2000). The general mechanism for controlling the effective vibrating mass of the vocal folds is discussed above and illustrated in Figure 3–34. This mechanism is achieved by adjusting the effective vibrating length of the vocal folds. During sustained voice production, the effective vibrating length of the vocal folds can be altered through actions of the ***lateral cricoarytenoid*** muscles that vary the medial compression of the vocal folds in the area of approximation of the tips of the vocal processes. This mechanism for effecting fundamental frequency change is usually considered to be a secondary or ancillary mechanism of control.

Studies of air-driven excised larynges, in which medial compression has been experimentally manipulated, have shown that increases in medial compression result in increases in fundamental frequency (van den Berg & Tan; 1959; van den Berg et al., 1960). The suspected mechanism is a decrease in the effective vibrating mass of the vocal folds by stopping their vibration in the region of the tips of the arytenoid processes (Honda, 1995). This mechanism has been likened to the pressing of a guitar string against a fret so that only the part of the string nearer the sounding box of the guitar is permitted to vibrate (Broad, 1973). The action of increasing medial compression may also serve to stiffen the vocal folds in the vicinity of the forceful adduction and further shorten the vocal folds as the tips of the vocal processes are rocked inward and forward. The collective effects of stopping the vibration of the back parts of the vocal folds and shortening and stiffening the remaining front parts (the membranous parts) results in a more rapid rate of vibration of the vocal folds.

Allowing only a fraction of the mass of the vocal folds to vibrate longitudinally during voice production may not be the only way in which segmental function of the vocal folds can influence the fundamental frequency of the voice or other features of voice. Although not well understood, it is believed that the ***thyroarytenoid*** muscles are able to differentially activate in ways that can influence the thickness, configuration, and regional stiffness of the vocal folds, and even establish conditions in which only the free margins of the vocal folds participate in the vibratory pattern (Hollien & Curtis, 1962). The ***thyrovocalis*** portion of the ***thyroarytenoid*** muscle may have an especially important role in adjusting the free margin of the vocal fold and could influence the effective mass of the vocal fold in the lateral-medial dimension (Story & Titze, 1995).

Still another mechanism that influences the fundamental frequency of the voice relates to the elevation of the larynx (sometimes referred to as its

The Cattle Are Lowing

An effective method for teaching certain principles of voice production involves the use of an excised cow larynx. The cow larynx is large compared to the human larynx and is different in some respects. The cow larynx does not have false vocal folds, nor is it richly endowed with mucous glands for lubricating the vocal folds. After all, cows don't produce voice for long periods like people do. A cow larynx can be made to vibrate by attaching the blower end of a vacuum cleaner to the tracheal end of the larynx and then manually adjusting such factors as medial compression and longitudinal tension of the vocal folds. Fundamental frequency, sound pressure level, and source spectrum changes are easily made. Placing an inverted container (the size of a coffee pot) above the larynx roughly simulates the resonance contribution of the missing upper airway. When all is done right, the experience is both instructive and "mooooving" to students.

vertical height). As high fundamental frequencies are generated, there is a tendency for the larynx to rise in the neck, especially near the upper extreme of the fundamental frequency range. This elevation is probably accomplished by activation of the ***thyrohyoid*** muscles (Faaborg-Andersen & Sonninen, 1960; Sonninen, 1968). Elevation of the larynx is believed to invoke a secondary mechanism for further increasing the stiffness of the vocal folds once major effort has been exerted to increase stiffness through activation of the ***thyroarytenoid*** and ***cricothyroid*** muscles. Elevation of the larynx results in a downward pull on the undersurface of the vocal folds mediated through the conus elasticus (interior elastic lining of the larynx in the subglottal region). This pull further stiffens the covers of the vocal folds (especially at the free margins of the vocal folds), by placing a vertical tug on them, and increases the rate at which the vocal folds vibrate (Ohala, 1972). This mechanism is usually the last biomechanical adjustment invoked to reach the highest fundamental frequencies possible. As with the case for changing the effective vibrating mass of the vocal folds, laryngeal elevation is considered a secondary or ancillary mechanism of fundamental frequency control.

Not all fundamental frequency control is vested in the larynx. The breathing apparatus also makes adjustments in association with changes in fundamental frequency. The most consistent of these adjustments is a tendency for tracheal air pressure to increase with increases in fundamental frequency (Shipp & McGlone, 1971). This is believed to relate to the need for a higher driving pressure in the face of both increasing laryngeal opposing pressure and laryngeal airway resistance (Kunze, 1962). This higher tracheal air pressure is needed to initiate voicing and maintain it under the conditions of increased stiffness of the vocal folds. In one sense, it is a cost placed on the breathing apparatus as a result of the laryngeal adjustment to achieve a higher fundamental frequency (Plant & Younger, 2000). The magnitude of this cost has been found to increase the most toward the upper end of the fundamental frequency range, suggesting that increments in the stiffness of the vocal folds may be especially large in that region (Kunze, 1962; Shipp & McGlone, 1971).

Adjustment of the breathing apparatus alone under conditions of a fixed laryngeal adjustment is not a very viable means of adjusting fundamental frequency of the voice (except in the loft voice register, discussed below). This is because increases in tracheal air pressure result in only small increases in fundamental frequency (Rubin, 1963; van den Berg, 1957). Typical magnitudes of change are only 2 to 4 Hz in fundamental frequency per cmH_2O of air pressure (Hixon et al., 1970). Thus, a change in fundamental frequency for a one octave change in an adult male (perhaps 120 Hz to 240 Hz) would require a 30 to 60 cmH_2O pressure change (an exorbitant cost) if effected solely through a breathing adjustment.

Mechanisms for lowering fundamental frequency, when decreases involve changes from frequencies that are above the usual fundamental frequency, are somewhat the inverse of those for raising fundamental frequency. That is, vocal fold stiffness and/or tracheal air pressure may be decreased. However, when fundamental frequency is lowered below its usual value, other mechanisms appear to come into play.

The first mechanism is to reduce vocal fold stiffness by contraction of the ***thyromuscularis*** (lateral) portions of the ***thyroarytenoid*** muscles. This contraction shortens the vocal folds and causes a slackening of the vocal ligaments and the ***thyrovocalis*** (medial) portions of the ***thyroarytenoid*** muscles (Zemlin, 1998). The second frequency-lowering mechanism entails a lowering of the larynx within the neck that further decreases the stiffness of the vocal folds by removing some of the usual traction placed on their undersurfaces. This is brought about through activation of the ***sternothyroid*** and ***sternohyoid*** muscles, which pull downward on the laryngeal housing (Atkinson, 1978; Honda, 1995; Ohala, 1972; Ohala & Hirose, 1970; Zemlin, 1998).

Sound Pressure Level. The sound pressure level of speech (the acoustic signal) is a measure of its physical magnitude (Baken & Orlikoff, 2000). This magnitude is related to the amplitude of the sound emanating from the upper airway and is generically referred to as the intensity of the signal (although technically sound pressure level and intensity are different quantities and the latter is more difficult to measure).

The sound pressure level (SPL) of speech is expressed on a continuum in ratio units of decibels (dB) and can be changed over a wide range, typically by about 40 dB for a young adult (Coleman, Mabis, & Hinson, 1977). Sound pressure level can be measured on different physical scales that are weighted to account for the relative prominence of different concentrations of energy.

The sound pressure level depends on the nature of the speech being produced and the location of the microphone relative to the lips. A vowel produced at a typical level and measured 30 cm from the lips (a standard distance) might be 65 dB, whereas a vowel produced at a shouting level might be in excess of 100 dB.

The strongest auditory-perceptual correlate of sound pressure level is loudness. Loudness is the subjective sensation of the relative magnitude of sound. This perception relies mainly on sound pressure level, but is influenced to lesser degrees by the fundamental frequency and spectral content of the sound produced. Generally, the higher the sound pressure level, the greater the magnitude of the perceived loudness.

Control of the sound pressure level of speech is vested in adjustments of the breathing apparatus, laryngeal apparatus, and pharyngeal-oral apparatus. These adjustments are usually executed simultaneously across these three subsystems, as depicted in Figure 3–40.

Breathing behavior influences sound pressure level of the voice through changes in tracheal air pressure, which correspond closely to changes in alveolar air pressure. That is, increases and decreases in tracheal air pressure cause increases and decreases in sound pressure level (Cavagna & Margaria, 1965; Hixon & Minifie, 1972; Isshiki, 1964; Ladefoged & McKinney, 1963; Titze, 1994; van den Berg, 1956). A doubling of tracheal air pressure for usual voice production might result in an increase in sound pressure level in the neighborhood of 8 to 12 dB (Broad, 1973; Daniloff et al., 1980; Stevens, 2000). The precise linkage between change in tracheal air pressure and change in sound pressure level depends on the prevailing sound pressure level of the voice. For example, the influence of a 1 cmH_2O

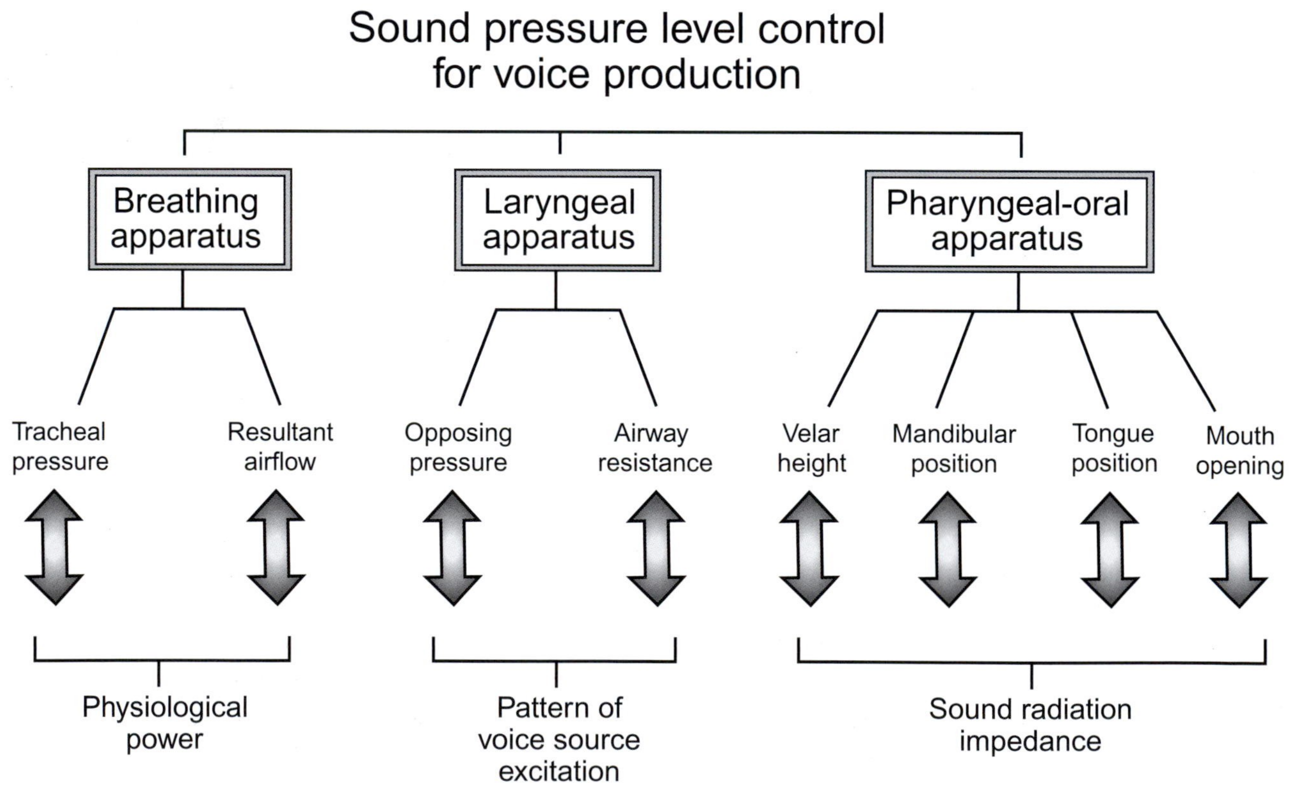

Figure 3–40. Breathing apparatus, laryngeal apparatus, and pharyngeal-oral apparatus control of sound pressure level.

change in tracheal air pressure during the production of a soft voice will result in as much as a 3 dB change in sound pressure level, whereas the same change in tracheal air pressure during the production of a loud voice will result in only a 0.5 dB change in sound pressure level (Hixon & Minifie, 1972).

Laryngeal opposition also plays a role in changing sound pressure level. Both laryngeal opposing pressure and laryngeal airway resistance increase with increases in the sound pressure level of the voice (Isshiki, 1964; Kunze, 1962). Increases in opposing pressure, effected by increasingly forceful contractions of the ***lateral cricoarytenoid*** and ***arytenoid*** muscles (***transverse*** and ***oblique*** subdivisions), are needed to contain the increased tracheal air pressure and prevent it from escaping uselessly (Daniloff et al., 1980). Increases in laryngeal airway resistance, also effected by contractions of the adductory muscles, relate to a reduction in average glottal size (Holmberg, Hillman, & Perkell, 1988).

The combined increase in tracheal pressure and heightened opposition provided by the larynx results in a change in the pattern of vocal fold vibration and excitation of the upper airway. For speech of higher sound pressure level, the vocal folds separate faster, return to the midline faster, and remain in approximation at the midline for a longer period during each cycle of vocal fold vibration (Minifie, 1973). The vocal folds also often separate to a greater extent during the generation of higher sound pressure levels (Kent, 1997).

Two underlying features of laryngeal behavior are critically important to how efficiently energy from the breathing apparatus is converted into acoustic energy (Titze, 1988b, 1994, 2006b). One of these is the abruptness with which the vocal folds return to the midline and airflow declines (referred to as the airflow declination rate or glottal area declination rate). The abruptness of this decline relates to the strength of the acoustic excitation of the upper airway (Dromey, Stathopoulos, & Sapienza, 1992; Holmberg et al., 1988; Titze, 2006b). The other important feature of laryngeal behavior is the average size of the glottis during the attempt to produce a higher sound pressure level. Exploration with computer modeling suggests that the optimal acoustic power is generated when the average glottal size is about midway between that for tight adduction of the vocal folds, as associated with a pressed voice, and that for loose adduction of the vocal folds, as associated with a breathy voice (Titze, 1994).

Although the breathing apparatus and laryngeal apparatus contribute most to sound pressure level changes, the pharyngeal-oral apparatus also influences sound pressure level of the voice. In general, it tends to blossom open more and more with successive increases in sound pressure level. This general opening up of the apparatus achieves an effect that is somewhat akin to that provided by

Listen My Children and You Shall Hear

Some people are loud and then some people are really loud. The conversion of aerodynamic power to acoustic power is better in some than in others and some of the best at it have been listed as celebrities in different folk sources. Different hollering, yelling, screaming, shouting, and loud voice champions have been crowned around the world. The *Guinness Book of Records* (Folkard, 2006) lists Jill Drake as the reigning screaming champion at 129 dB and Annalisa Wray as the reigning shouting champion at 121.7 dB. Alan Myatt, the town crier of Gloucester, England, once was touted in the *Guinness Book of Records* as having the world's loudest voice, an ear-piercing 112.8 dB. Had Paul Revere been so endowed as a town crier he wouldn't have had to knock on so many doors and he might have been able to awaken all of Lexington, Massachusetts on a single breath. Well, maybe not all, but at least much of the South Side.

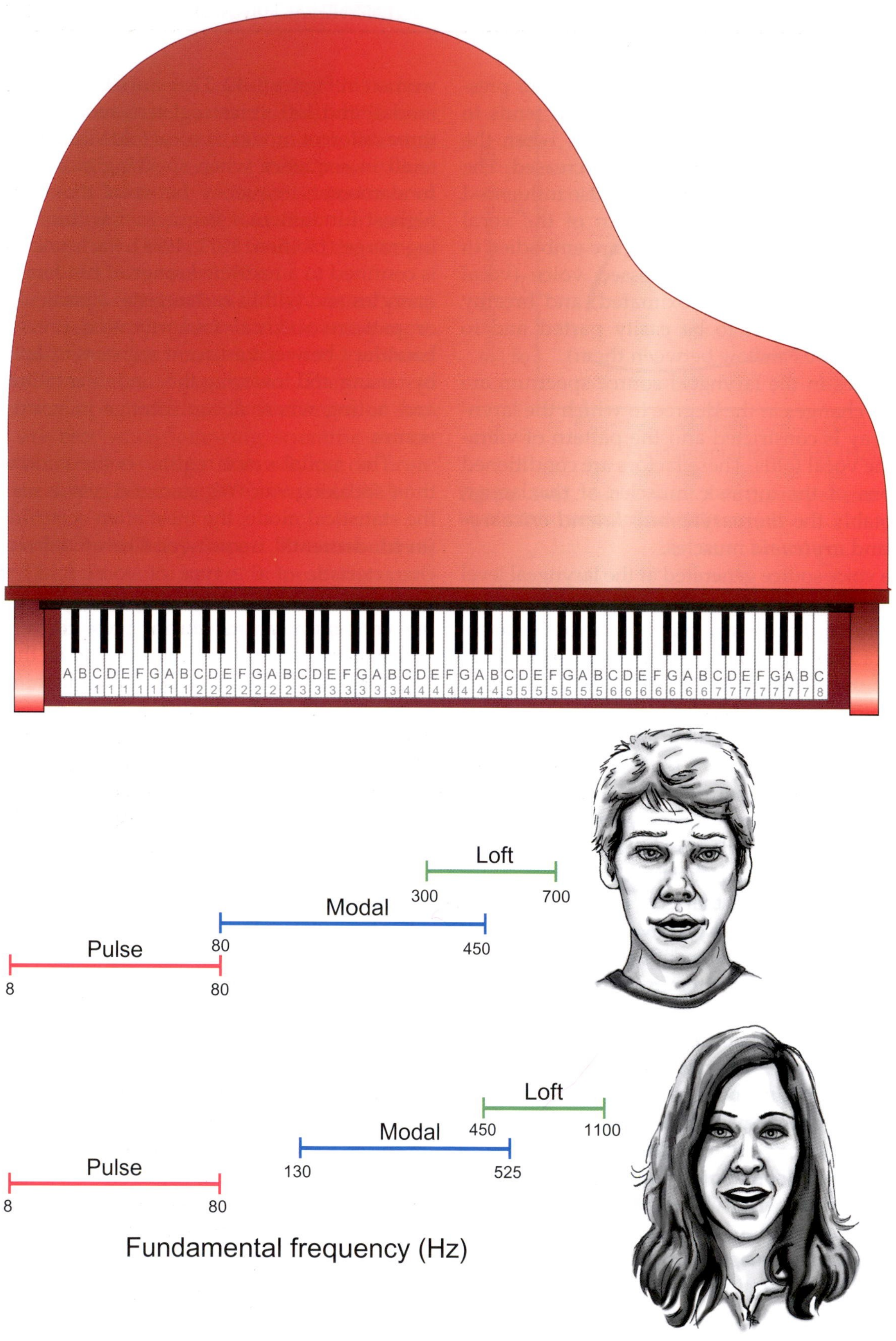

Figure 3–42. Voice registers along the fundamental frequency scale.

appearances of a small glottis. The pulse produced in association with this short-lived glottis is relatively rich in harmonic structure, but low in sound pressure level. Fundamental frequency and sound pressure level tend to change together in the pulse register and do not have the relative independence found in modal voice register (Murry & Brown, 1971a, 1971b).

Voice production in the pulse voice register is generated with moderate or low values of tracheal air pressure and translaryngeal airflow (Allen & Hollien, 1973; Holmberg, Hillman, & Perkell, 1989; McGlone, 1967; McGlone & Shipp, 1971; Murry, 1971; Murry & Brown, 1971b). The vocal folds are short, thick, slack, and compliant (Allen & Hollien, 1973; Hollien, Damste, & Murry, 1969) and medial compression is moderate (McGlone & Shipp, 1971). The tracheal air pressure bubbles up through the relatively lax vocal folds, creating a significant vertical phase difference. Lateral vocal fold movements are moderate and usually not along the entire length of the membranous portion of the vocal folds (Orlikoff & Kahane, 1996). The prolonged approximation phase of vocal fold vibration results in a near-total damping of upper airway excitation with each pulse of activity (Coleman, 1963; Titze, 1988a; Wendahl, Moore, & Hollien, 1963). The voice source, therefore, is a series of nearly discrete excitations to the upper airway that gives the listener the perception that the voice is a string of tiny pops (like those that can be made by applying repeated bursts of pressure behind the lips when they are thickly puckered and gently held together).

The loft voice register is the highest of the three speaking voice registers and gets it name from its high placement within the fundamental frequency range. This register is also called the falsetto voice register. The quality of the voice produced in this register is sometimes described as thin, flutelike, and breathy, with acoustic characteristics that resemble a pure tone.

The vibration of the vocal folds in the loft voice register is somewhat simpler than that for the modal and pulse voice registers. Excursions of the vocal folds are relatively small and the glottis is narrow. The vibratory pattern of the vocal folds entails little or no vertical phase difference. Rather, movements are mainly horizontal and confined to the vicinity of the free margins of the vocal folds. Such movements take on the appearance of vibrating strings alternately moving horizontally away from and toward one another. Approximation of the vocal folds is not obligatory for voice production in the loft register. When the vocal folds do approximate, the contact between them is usually light (involves low adductory forces). The voice source produced in conjunction with loft voice register contains less high harmonic energy than that for modal voice register

Not an Island Unto Itself

The behavior of the larynx is not independent of its surrounds. When transitioning back and forth across the boundary between the modal and loft voice registers, the boundary between the two registers will differ somewhat in fundamental frequency from one transition to another. This is because the larynx is coupled to the breathing apparatus and the breathing apparatus has resonance properties that interact with the mode of vibration of the vocal folds. These resonance properties change when there are different amounts of air in the lungs. Thus, transitioning back and forth across the boundary between the modal and loft voice registers occurs at different fundamental frequency breaking points when the lung volume is different. The lesson contained in this observation is that a neighbor can influence the behavior of the larynx. It is not an island unto itself.

(Colton, 1972) and the sound pressure level of the voice is lower in the loft register than in the modal register (Orlikoff & Kahane, 1996).

Voice production in the loft voice register is generated with moderately high tracheal air pressure and translaryngeal airflow (Large, Iwata, & von Leden, 1970; McGlone, 1970; Shipp & McGlone, 1971; Shipp, McGlone, & Morrisey, 1972), elongated and thin vocal folds that are under great longitudinal tension (Hollien & Moore, 1960), and very high stiffness of the mucosal covers of the vocal folds (Gay, Hirose, Strome, & Sawashima, 1972; Hirano, 1974; Hirano, Vennard, & Ohala, 1970). Changes in fundamental frequency and sound pressure level in the loft register are significantly influenced by changes in tracheal air pressure and airflow through the larynx (Colton, 1973; Isshiki, 1964, 1965; van den Berg et al., 1960; Yanagihara & Koike, 1967), with acoustic variables following directional changes in aeromechanical variables (Hollien, 1972). For example, increases in airflow through the larynx result in increases in both fundamental frequency and sound pressure level of the resulting laryngeal tone (van den Berg et al., 1960).

Running Speech Activities

The larynx is a critical participant in running speech activities. During inspiration, the vocal folds abduct and dilate the laryngeal airway to allow air to flow freely into the pulmonary apparatus. During expiration, the vocal folds sometimes abduct and dilate the airway to enable the full impact of expiratory air pressures and airflows to reach downstream structures for oral consonant articulations (Hixon & Abbs, 1980; Netsell, 1973). Also during expiration, the vocal folds act as an articulator by moving in and out of the airway to valve the flow of air during glottal stop-plosive and fricative consonant productions (Hirose, 1977; Lofqvist & Yoshioka, 1984; Orlikoff & Kahane, 1996; Sawashima, Abramson, Cooper, & Lisker, 1970).

The larynx is most widely thought of for its generation of the laryngeal tone during speech production. This tone is the carrier of speech and has an important influence on speech intelligibility. It also conveys information about the speaker's age, sex, physical stature, health status, emotional status, identity, and other factors.

Adjustments of the laryngeal tone are the main concern of this section. Consideration is given to the articulatory functions of the larynx in Chapter 5 where the articulatory functions of pharyngeal-oral structures are discussed. The focus here is on adjustments in fundamental frequency, sound pressure level, and spectrum of the laryngeal tone. These adjustments can be made individually or in different combinations and may occur within individual speech sounds or extend across two or more sounds. Such adjustments are used to convey different meanings with the voice, disambiguate certain aspects of the communication, emphasize certain parts of the flow of speech over others, provide information through different voice shadings and nuances, establish certain affects (impressions), and affirm roles in relationships.

Fundamental Frequency

Fundamental frequency change is prominent during running speech activities and can range as much as two octaves (Fairbanks, 1960). Fundamental frequency is often measured and displayed in a tracing called a fundamental frequency contour, which tracks change in fundamental frequency over time. Such a contour is shown in Figure 3–43 for a spoken sentence.

Listening to fundamental frequency change in the voice evokes a perception of time-varying pitch

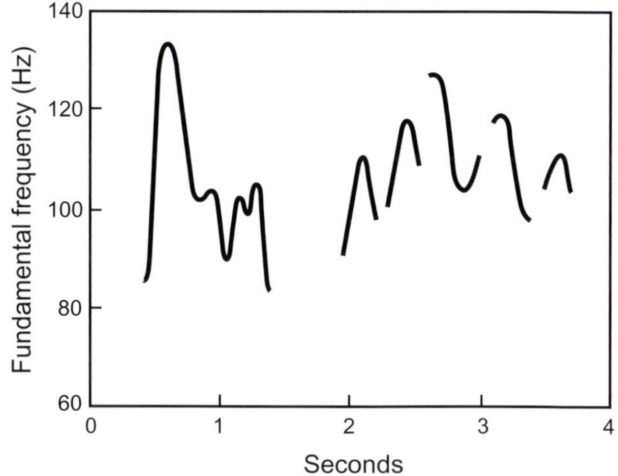

Figure 3–43. Fundamental frequency contour for a spoken sentence of an adult male.

change that is referred to as an intonation contour. Perceptions of intonation contours are influenced by sensitivity to pitch inflections and pitch shifts. Inflections are modulations in pitch during voiced segments, whereas shifts are changes in pitch from the end of one voiced segment to the beginning of the next (Fairbanks, 1960). The intonation contour underlies what the listener comes to consider as the melody or tunefulness of speech. This contour operates around a mode (the most often sensed pitch) that determines what the listener judges to be the characteristic pitch level of the voice.

The mechanism for changing fundamental frequency during running speech activities is different from that described above for changing fundamental frequency from one sustained utterance to another. Recall that for sustained voice production, increases and decreases in tracheal air pressure are accompanied by corresponding increases and decreases in fundamental frequency. In contrast, running speech activities usually involve a relatively steady tracheal air pressure, except for a decline toward the ends of breath groups involving declarative statements.

Adjustments in fundamental frequency during running speech activities are vested mainly in laryngeal actions. These laryngeal actions rely, in large part, on interplay between contractions of the ***cricothyroid*** and ***thyroarytenoid*** muscles, along with bracing actions of the ***posterior cricoarytenoid*** muscles, which adjust the stiffness of the vocal folds. (Atkinson, 1978; Gay et al., 1972; Hirano, Ohala, & Vennard, 1969; Netsell, 1969). Actions of the ***cricothyroid*** muscles are more strongly correlated with the fundamental frequency of the voice than are the actions of other intrinsic muscles of the larynx, as long as the ***cricothyroid*** muscles are not functioning near their maximum output (Atkinson, 1978; Titze, 1994). This means that changes in the longitudinal tension of the vocal folds are of prime importance to the control of the fundamental frequency of the voice during running speech events.

Sound Pressure Level

Like fundamental frequency, sound pressure level also changes significantly during running speech activities. This is true of the average sound pressure level associated with different speaking situations (soft, normal, or loud speech) and rapid variations from the average level (such as accompany varying levels of linguistic stress). A routine conversation might find the sound pressure level to swing as much as 25 to 30 dB. The magnitude of sound pressure level and its directional changes can be measured and displayed in a tracing referred to as a sound pressure level contour, one of which is shown for a sentence production in Figure 3–44.

Changes in sound pressure level over time, as illustrated in Figure 3–44, give rise to a subjective impression of a loudness contour that embodies percepts of an average loudness and variations about it. Vowels are the main contributors to loudness judgments in running speech activities. Adjustment in vowel and consonant sound pressure levels, while usually moving in the same direction, find vowel sound pressure level to change more than consonant sound pressure level (Hixon, 1966; Stevens, 2000). This is due to a tendency to open up the pharyngeal-oral apparatus more to accomplish vowel increases, and a tendency to constrict the apparatus more to accomplish consonant increases. These two competing tendencies result in a tradeoff in sound pressure level change, in which the vowel dominates because of its more prominent carrying power (Fairbanks & Miron, 1957).

Perceived loudness contours convey what is judged to be the forcefulness or effort used to generate the acoustic product. Such contours are strongly related to actual sound pressure level contours, but do not bear a one-to-one correspondence

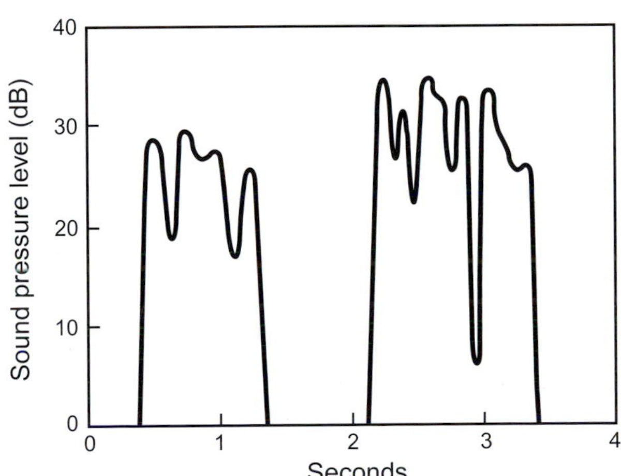

Figure 3–44. Sound pressure level contour for a spoken sentence of an adult male.

to them. For example, when counting from one to ten, the syllables tend to sound equally loud to the listener despite the differences in sound pressure levels across the different vowels in the series. Indeed, certain sounds have intrinsically higher or lower sound pressure levels than other sounds. This is a distinction that is not usually appreciated by the casual listener.

Control of sound pressure level for running speech activities is conditioned by adjustments of the breathing apparatus, laryngeal apparatus, and pharyngeal-oral apparatus. The most important breathing apparatus adjustment has to do with changing the magnitude of the average tracheal air pressure and with effecting small increases in that pressure to emphasize certain speech segments (Netsell, 1969). These background level and pulsatile tracheal air pressure events are the result of muscular pressure adjustments by the chest wall (Hixon, Mead, & Goldman, 1976).

Laryngeal participation in sound pressure level control for running speech activities usually involves heightened vocal fold adductory forces that manifest as increases in the laryngeal opposing pressure. These forces enable the buildup of tracheal air pressure and increase as speech becomes progressively louder or contrastive stress levels become greater from one syllable to another (Hirano et al., 1969; Netsell, 1969, 1973). The muscles implicated in heightening vocal fold adductory forces are primarily the ***lateral cricoarytenoid*** and ***arytenoid*** muscles, although muscles that stiffen the vocal folds (the ***thyroarytenoid*** and ***cricothyroid*** muscles) may also contribute.

Pharyngeal-oral adjustments are often associated with changes in the sound pressure level of running speech. These adjustments tend to be characterized by increased mouth opening, because increased mouth opening reduces the acoustic radiation impedance during running speech activities. Thus, the pharyngeal-oral apparatus tends to open more and more with successive increases in the sound pressure level to enhance transmission of acoustic energy generated at the glottis (Daniloff et al., 1980; Netsell, 1973).

Spectrum

The spectrum of the laryngeal source changes rapidly and often during running speech activities. Such changes are associated with changes in the fundamental frequency or sound pressure level of the voice and with other changes in the pattern of vocal fold vibration. Slower changes in the spectrum of the laryngeal tone may result from prolonged use of the vocal folds, transient abuse of the vocal folds, so-called laryngeal fatigue, or a reduction in hydration of the laryngeal apparatus.

Source spectrum changes may give rise to changes in voice quality, a perceptual attribute that

Tick Tock

Anyone who has played music to the beat of a metronome knows how maddening it can be. When just learning the music, it's a challenge to keep up. Then, once you have the music mastered, it seems like you have to slow down to be on pace. But something has to set the pace, like a conductor of an orchestra. The larynx usually does this during speech production. It's the metronome of the speech production apparatus. The movements of other speech production structures are constrained by what the larynx does. It does no good to get to a position before the larynx because then you'll just have to wait. And, if you arrive at a position later than the time specified by the larynx, you have big problems. It's not quite as simple as we've portrayed, but it's close enough to give you the idea. Maybe you've heard the nursery rhyme "Hickory, dickory, dock, the voice box is the clock." Well, maybe not, because it was just written.

pertains to the sound of the voice beyond its pitch and loudness characteristics (Behrman, 2007). Depending on the speaking situation, the spectrum can change in ways that cause the listener to perceive voice qualities that range from breathy to pressed or are labeled by a great variety of other descriptors (Minifie, 1973; Stevens, 2000). The diversity of descriptors applied to different voice qualities reflects both the personal preferences of individual listeners and the difficulties involved in getting groups of listeners to arrive at a consensus.

All of the intrinsic muscles of the larynx can influence the laryngeal source spectrum during running speech activities, because all of them have influences on the nature of vocal fold vibration. Those with the most significant influence, however, are thought to be the ***thyroarytenoid, lateral cricoarytenoid,*** and ***arytenoid*** muscles.

Development and Laryngeal Function in Speech Production

Between the birth cry and adulthood, about two decades pass. During this time, laryngeal structure and function undergo significant change, as does the voice they produce. This section considers salient developmental changes and some of their influences on voice production.

The structure of the larynx undergoes relocation and remodeling during the developmental period. This includes changes in its positioning within the neck, and in its size, configuration, and mechanical properties.

The newborn larynx rides high within the neck, such that the lower edge of the cricoid cartilage is positioned between the third and fourth cervical vertebrae. The larynx and velopharynx are close companions in this arrangement. The epiglottis contacts the velum and nasal breathing is obligatory early on. This mechanical arrangement facilitates the nursing needs of the infant while simultaneously ensuring an adequate airway for ventilation (Laitman & Crelin, 1976; Sasaki, Levin, Laitman, & Crelin, 1977). By 4 to 6 months of age, this arrangement begins to change and is present mainly only during swallowing. This is part of a transitional period in which the infant switches from nasal to oral breathing (Kent & Vorperian, 1995).

As the infant grows, the larynx descends from its initial high position (Wind, 1970). By the end of the first year of life, the lower edge of the cricoid cartilage has descended to the middle of the fourth cervical vertebra. By age 3 years, the descent has reached to the middle of the fifth cervical vertebra, and by age 5 years it has reached the middle of the sixth cervical vertebra. Downward migration continues to the region of the seventh cervical vertebra between 10 and 20 years of age.

The framework of the larynx also undergoes significant developmental change. The thyroid cartilage, for example, is contiguous with the hyoid bone at birth and then separates from it vertically. The laminae of the thyroid cartilage form a somewhat semicircular structure in the infant larynx and proceed to a more angular form in the larynx of the older child (Kahane, 1975). The angle formed by the thyroid laminae narrows to a more prominent configuration, especially in older male children (Kahane, 1978; Malinowski, 1967).

The framework of the infant larynx is destined to triple in size during the developmental period (Bosma, 1985). Growth of the laryngeal cartilages is generally more linear in the female than the male, with the most rapid changes in the size of the male laryngeal framework occurring during the pubertal growth spurt (Dickson & Maue-Dickson, 1982; Kahane, 1978). With the exception of the front of the male thyroid cartilage, the growth of the laryngeal cartilages has been characterized as involving an increase in size and weight while configuration is generally maintained (Kahane, 1978, 1982). Structural differences in the framework of male and female larynges have been reported to exist as early as 3 years of age (Crelin, 1973). However, predominant thought has it that the most significant framework differences between male and female larynges are demonstrated somewhat later in development, with the greatest contrasts in sexual dimorphism occurring around puberty (Kahane, 1982).

The structures of the laryngeal framework are soft and pliable at the beginning of life and proceed to become firm and less flexible with age (Tucker & Tucker, 1979). Ossification (turning to bone) of the hyoid begins at about 2 years of age. Cartilages of the larynx begin to show signs of ossification much later in life, usually during the first couple of decades of adulthood (Aronson, 1990).

Age and Laryngeal Function in Speech Production

Once the structure and function of the larynx are fully matured, they are subject to additional modifications throughout adulthood. Some of these changes lead to changes in the voice.

The lower edge of the cricoid cartilage has descended to the upper edge of the seventh cervical vertebra by young adulthood. Thereafter, it continues to descend to reach the middle and then the bottom of the seventh cervical vertebra as aging continues into senescence. The larynx, in fact, continues to lower slightly even throughout senescence (Wind, 1970).

The framework of the larynx also undergoes modification during the adult years. Some of the cartilages of the larynx gradually ossify (turn to bone), whereas others gradually calcify (turn to salt). These modifications make the framework of the aging adult larynx increasingly stiff and brittle as time goes on (Zemlin, 1998).

Ossification is confined to components of the framework that are constituted of a hyaline matrix and manifests sequentially in the thyroid, cricoid, and arytenoid cartilages of the larynx. Ossification begins in these three cartilages during the early decades of adulthood (a little earlier in men than in women) and is relatively complete by the time senescence begins (Hately, Evison, & Samuel, 1965; Zemlin, 1998). Calcification is confined to components of the framework that are formed by an elastic matrix. Such calcification occurs later in senescence (more pronounced in men than in women) and is exhibited in the epiglottis, corniculate cartilages, cuneiform cartilages, and parts of the arytenoid cartilages (Kent & Verporian, 1995; Malinowski, 1967). The arytenoid cartilages are unique as components of the laryngeal scaffolding because they are made of a hyaline matrix in some parts and an elastic matrix in other parts (Kahane, 1980, 1983; Sato, Kurita, Hirano, & Kiyokawa, 1990). Thus, the arytenoid cartilages are subjected to hardening twice during the aging process, early in adulthood by ossification and late in adulthood by calcification.

The joints of the larynx also change with advancing age in adulthood. The cricoarytenoid joints, for example, undergo changes in both their joint capsules and articular surfaces (Kahane & Hammons, 1987; Kahn & Kahane, 1986; Segre, 1971). Changes at the articular surfaces include abrasion, ossification, erosion, and deformation, all of which influence movements at the joints. Most important is that the movement of the arytenoid cartilages around the cricoarytenoid joints can be reduced in older individuals, which, in turn, can limit the degree to which the vocal folds can be approximated (Kahane, 1988).

The vocal folds and structures that control them also undergo change during aging in adulthood. This includes nerve fiber loss and muscle atrophy that lead to losses in mass and muscle strength (Aronson, 1990; Cooper, 1990; Ferreri, 1959). Other changes with aging include a loss of tissue elasticity in the vocal folds, dehydration of the laryngeal mucosa, edema, and alteration in the density of different fibers constituting the structural matrices of the vocal folds (Aronson, 1990; Benjamin, 1988; Kahane & Beckford, 1991; Keleman & Pressman, 1955; Kent & Vorperian, 1995; Linville, 1995; Mueller, Sweeney, & Baribeau, 1985).

Histological age-related changes in the vocal folds may have important functional consequences for voice production. With advanced age, not only is muscle tissue lost within the body of the vocal fold, connective tissue is gained (Kahane, 1983). Simultaneously, the cover of the vocal fold undergoes modification, with different layers of the lamina propria changing in different ways with advancing age (Hirano et al., 1983; Kahane, 1983; Kahane, Stadlin, & Bell, 1979). The superficial layer thickens, becomes swollen with fluid, and declines in fiber density. The intermediate layer thins out as elastic fibers wane in size and number. And the deep layer thickens (especially in males over 50 years of age) as collagenous fibers increase in size and density. These age-related changes in the lamina propria may cause the vocal folds to take on a bowed configuration (Honjo & Isshiki, 1980; Mueller et al., 1985), develop surface irregularities along their free margins (Kahane, 1983), and stiffen (Kent, 1997).

The variety of changes attendant to the aging of the framework, muscle, and fiber matrices of the larynx have implications for its function. These changes and their consequences may be somewhat different for men and women, as discussed in the section below on sex and laryngeal function in speech production.

Finally, it should be noted that nearly everything known about the influence of aging on laryngeal structure and function is based on the use of chronological age (easy to quantify) as the primary temporal marker (Shipp & Hollien, 1969). However, it may be that physiological age (more difficult to measure) is, in fact, a more relevant temporal marker. Beyond this distinction, it is also believed that health status has important implications and must be taken into account when attempting to understand voice changes across adulthood (Ramig & Ringel, 1983)

Sex and Laryngeal Function in Speech Production

The structure and function of the larynx are different in some ways between the sexes. Certain dissimilarities have an influence on voice production.

During infancy and early childhood, the structure and function of the larynx are relatively similar in males and females. Later in childhood, differences between the sexes start to emerge, especially during puberty. This period of major laryngeal mutation for males causes abrupt changes in voice that manifest as secondary sex characteristics. The most prominent of these is a lowering of the fundamental frequency of the male voice by about an octave. The sexual dimorphism in the structure and function of the larynx seen in early adolescence are maintained across the adult life span.

Ossification and calcification of the larynx occur earlier chronologically in males than in females. Ossification in males begins in the third decade of life, whereas in females it starts in the fourth decade. The female larynx may, in some cases, never completely ossify (Claassen & Kirsch, 1994).

The vocal folds also show differences in structure between the sexes across adulthood. Male vocal folds lengthen, whereas female vocal folds maintain a relatively constant length into senescence (Kazarian et al., 1978).

Men usually demonstrate full approximation of the vocal folds during voice production, whereas women usually do not. This difference is portrayed in Figure 3–46. Young women often show an opening between the vocal folds during voice production, especially in the cartilaginous segment (Behrman, 2007; Biever & Bless, 1989; Sodersten & Lindestad, 1990). Elderly women, in contrast, often show an opening during voice production in the membranous segment of the vocal folds or show a spindle-shaped opening that runs the entire length of the vocal folds (Linville, 1992). Reasons for male-female differences in vocal fold approximation are speculative. Factors that have been suggested include differences in the arrangement of the cricoarytenoid

They Didn't Quite Get It

She had a beautiful coloratura soprano voice and after years of formal training was just about to begin an operatic career. It ended abruptly on a ski slope when a careless youngster crashed into her and slammed her headfirst into a tree. She suffered facial lacerations, blunt trauma to the larynx, and temporomandibular joint damage. She never again had full singing ability. Jaw movement was especially a problem and very painful. She could no longer meet the demands of operatic roles. Forensic testimony concluded that she was 100% impaired because she could not perform a full operatic role. The career for which she had prepared was lost. The jury decided otherwise and awarded her little more than her medical expenses. The twisted logic was revealed in an interview with the foreman of the jury following the trial. "We didn't see why she couldn't just sing country songs instead. They're short and not as demanding." They didn't quite get it.

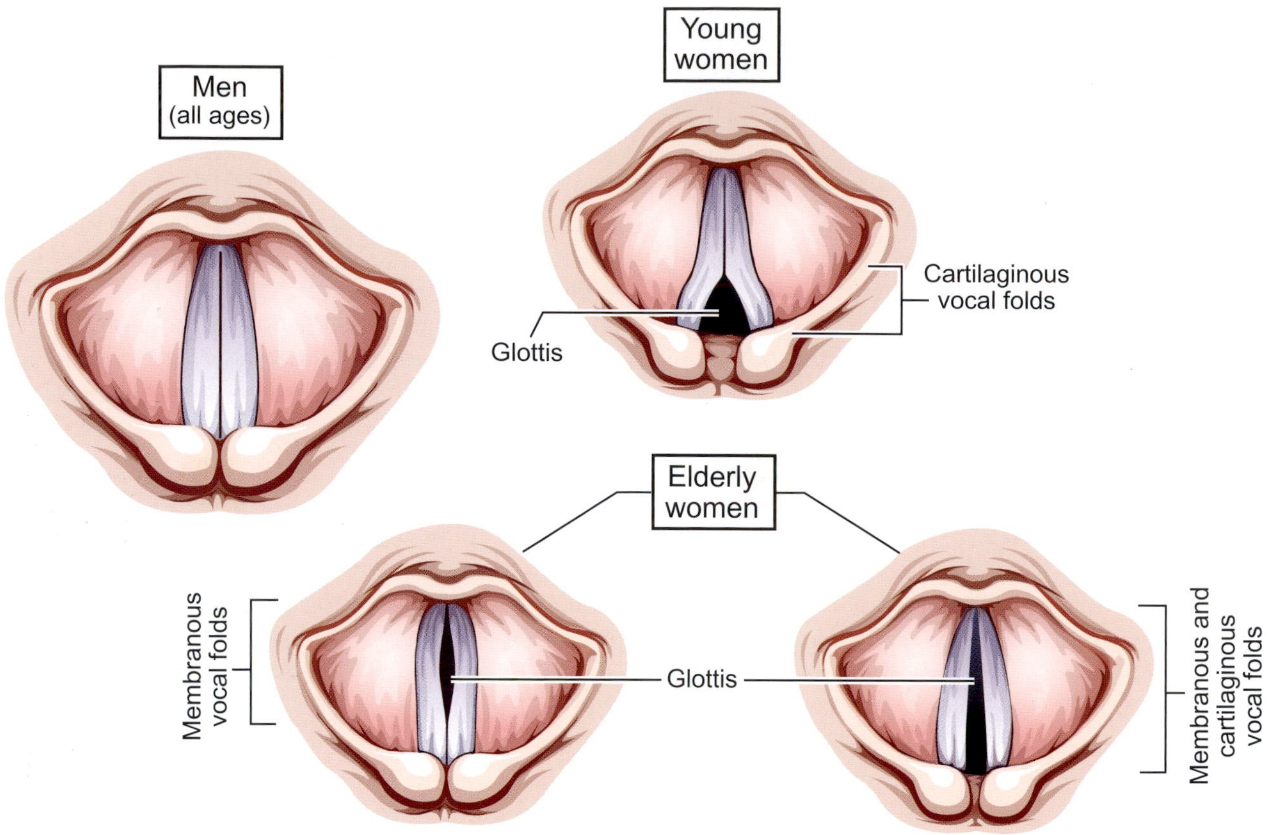

Figure 3–46. Male and female vocal fold approximations during voice production.

joints, differences in the muscle mass of the body of the vocal folds, and differences in the covers of the vocal folds (Hirano et al., 1988; Hirano, Kiyokawa, Kurita, & Sato, 1986). Cultural factors may also be at play, with a breathy voice quality being a more desirable characteristic of a female voice than a male voice (Linville, 1992).

Continuing from the adolescent period, differences in the fundamental frequencies of males and females persist throughout adulthood. However, as shown in Figure 3–47, males and females appear to evidence different patterns of age-related change across adulthood. The patterns shown from a collection of cross-sectional studies suggest that older men have a higher fundamental frequency than younger men (Hollien & Shipp, 1972; Honjo & Isshiki, 1980; Mueller et al., 1985), whereas older women have a lower fundamental frequency than younger women (Awan & Mueller, 1992; Benjamin, 1981; Honjo & Isshiki, 1980; Linville, 1987; Linville & Fisher, 1985; Mueller et al., 1985; Russell, Penny, & Pemberton, 1995; Stoicheff, 1981).

Menopause is one factor in the lowering of fundamental frequency in women prior to senescence. This is suggested by the fact that significantly lower fundamental frequencies have been found in women who have completed menopause than in women of the same age who have not completed menopause (Stoicheff, 1981). Data of this nature have prompted some to suggest that a male-female coalescence model of aging voice production may have currency (Hollien et al., 1994). In such a model, the hormone-related factors that cause differences to occur between males and females in adolescence are counteracted to some degree by hormone-related factors associated with menopause in women. The directional shift in fundamental frequency with menopause is consistent with this model.

The narrowing of fundamental frequency differences with advancing age has different mechani-

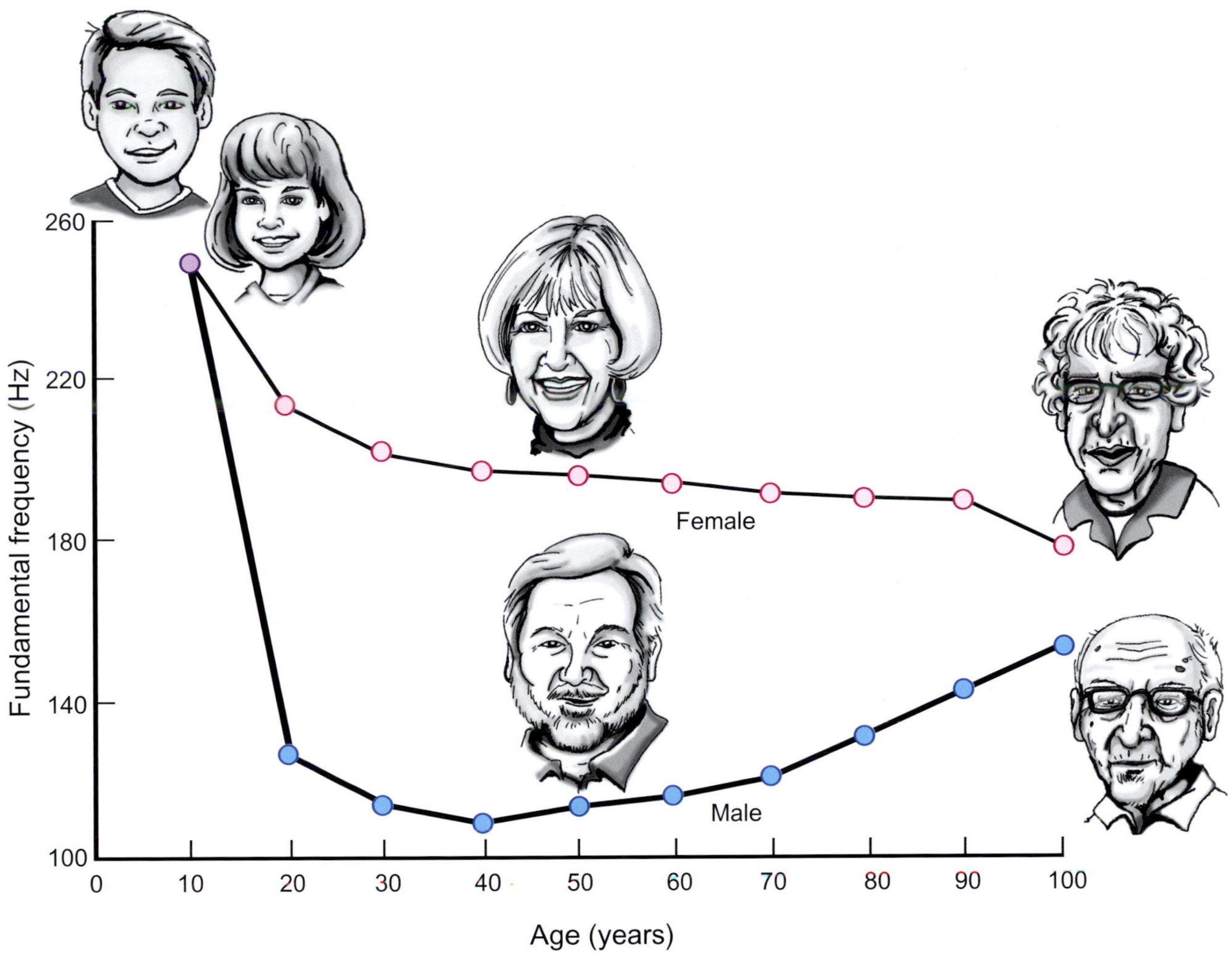

Figure 3–47. Fundamental frequency changes from ages 10 to 100 years in males and females. Data obtained from many published sources and rounded to the nearest decade for each sex.

cal roots for the two sexes. Age effects on the larynx tend to be more significant in men than in women and to have a greater influence on function (Linville, 1995). In men, the increase in fundamental frequency may have roots in muscle atrophy, thinning of the lamina propria, and general loss of mass (Hirano, Kurita, & Sakaguchi, 1989; Kahane, 1987; Segre, 1971), factors that would tend to move the fundamental frequency upward. In women, the decrease in fundamental frequency (very late in life) may have roots in an age-related increase in edema (Ferreri, 1959; Honjo & Isshiki, 1980), a factor that would tend to move the fundamental frequency downward. Fundamental frequency changes with advanced age may help to explain why it is sometimes difficult to tell whether the voice on a telephone is that of a relatively high-pitched elderly man or a relatively low-pitched elderly woman. Life, as conveyed in the voice, would appear to have come full circle to anyone who has struggled to discern whether it is 6-year-old boy or a 6-year-old girl who just picked up the telephone and said "Hello."

Men and women demonstrate different average values in laryngeal airway resistance during voice production. This is due mainly to differences in the size of their laryngeal airways. A reasonable rule of thumb is that adult men and women who have not reached senescence will demonstrate laryngeal airway resistance values during vowel production of about 35 cmH_2O/LPS and 50 cmH_2O/LPS, respectively (Hoit & Hixon, 1992; Smitheran & Hixon, 1981).

Laryngeal airway resistance remains relatively similar across adulthood for men and for women (Hoit & Hixon, 1992; Holmes, Leeper, & Nicholson, 1994; Melcon, Hoit, & Hixon, 1989) until the eighth decade of life when men begin to show a lowering of resistance compared to men of younger ages. This lowering of resistance is accompanied by a significant increase in airflow through the larynx (Melcon et al., 1989). In contrast, women in their ninth decade of life do not show a decrease in resistance compared to younger women (Hoit & Hixon, 1992). It would appear that any lessening of laryngeal valving economy, if it occurs, is significantly delayed in women compared to men.

MEASUREMENT OF LARYNGEAL FUNCTION

Laryngeal function can be measured using different types and levels of observation. This section considers four measurement approaches that are often used in clinical environments. They are endoscopy, electroglottography, aeromechanical observations, and acoustical observations.

Endoscopy

Visualization of the larynx is one of the most important tools available for determining its status and quantifying its actions. Such visualization usually entails examination of the larynx from above and may be accomplished by the insertion of a viewing device through either the oral or nasal cavities (Dailey, Spanou, & Zeitels, 2007; Sataloff et al., 1988). This method, called endoscopy, includes some form of illumination of the larynx and some form of optical device that gathers the laryngeal image (Baken & Orlikoff, 2000).

As illustrated in the upper panel of Figure 3–48, visualization via the oral route is most often done with a device called a rigid endoscope that is positioned along the upper surface of the tongue (with the tongue tip pulled forward and out of the way) and into the oropharynx. The image can be viewed through an eyepiece or recorded by one of several different optical recording systems. The rigid endoscope provides an excellent image of the larynx, but has some limitations. One limitation is that the client might find the positioning of the device to be awkward and uncomfortable. Another limitation of the rigid endoscope is that it interferes with movements of pharyngeal-oral structures so that only

Being One with Your Larynx

Many aspects of laryngeal measurement show an uncanny "oneness" with the metric system. Titze (1994) suggests that this realization is helpful in making calculations off the top of your head when you don't have references at hand. A partial listing of items that he recommends be committed to memory for self-reference includes (a) the mass of a vocal fold is about 1 g, (b) the length of a vibrating vocal fold is about 1 cm, (c) the excursion of a vibrating vocal fold is about 1 mm, (d) the shortest period of vocal fold vibration is about 1 ms, (e) the surface wave velocity on a vibrating vocal fold is about 1 m/s, (f) the maximum peak-to-peak airflow through a vibrating larynx is about 1 L/s, (g) the maximum acceleration of airflow through a vibrating larynx is about 1 m^3/s, and (h) the maximum aerodynamic power generated by a vibrating larynx is about 1 J/s. We suggest you make it a goal to memorize these before you go to sleep tonight.

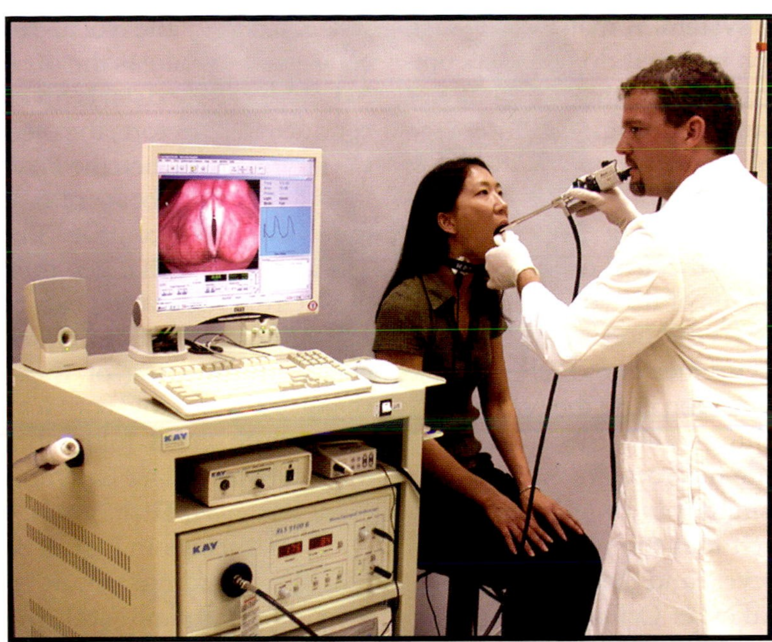

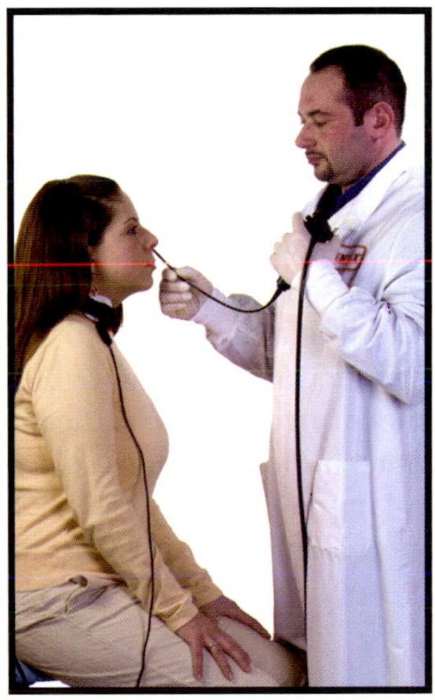

Figure 3–48. Visualization of the larynx via endoscopy. Upper panel illustrates oral approach with a rigid endoscope. Lower panel illustrates nasal approach with a flexible endoscope. Images provided courtesy of KayPENTAX, Lincoln Park, NJ. Reproduced with permission.

sustained utterances can be examined (Lofqvist & Oshima, 1993).

As illustrated in the lower panel of Figure 3–48, visualization via the nasal route is accomplished by inserting a device called a flexible endoscope through one side of the nose (usually the more open side) over the upper surface of the velum and into the pharynx. The flexible endoscope has positional controls so that its distal tip can be oriented to obtain an unobstructed view of the vocal folds (Hirano & Bless, 1993; Karnell, 1994). The image can be viewed through an eyepiece or recorded

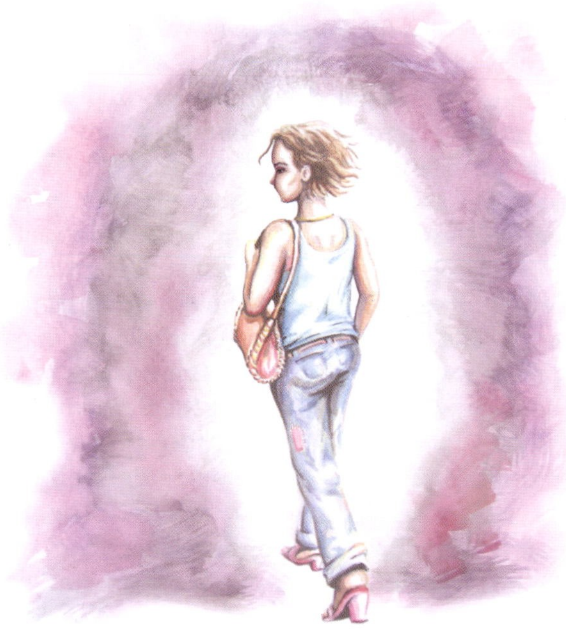

REFERENCES

Allen, E., & Hollien, H. (1973). Vocal fold thickness in pulse (vocal fry) register. *Folia Phoniatrica, 25*, 241–250.

Ardran, G., & Kemp, F. (1966). The mechanism of the larynx, I: The movements of the arytenoid and cricoid cartilages. *British Journal of Radiology, 39*, 641–654.

Arnold, G. (1961). Physiology and pathology of the cricothyroid muscle. *Laryngoscope, 71*, 687–753.

Aronson, A. (1990). *Clinical voice disorders: An interdisciplinary approach* (3rd ed.). New York: Thieme.

Atkinson, J. (1978). Correlation analysis of the physiological factors controlling fundamental voice frequency. *Journal of the Acoustical Society of America, 63*, 211–222.

Awan, S., & Mueller, P. (1992). Speaking fundamental frequency characteristics of centenarian females. *Clinical Linguistics & Phonetics, 6*, 249–254.

Baer, T. (1981). Observation of vocal fold vibration: Measurement of excised larynges. In K. Stevens & M. Hirano (Eds.), *Vocal fold physiology* (pp. 199–133). Tokyo, Japan: University of Tokyo Press.

Baken, R., & Orlikoff, R. (2000). *Clinical measurement of speech and voice* (2nd ed.). San Diego, CA: Singular.

Behrman, A. (2007). *Speech and voice science*. San Diego, CA: Plural.

Beneragama, T., & Serpell, J. (2006). Extralaryngeal bifurcation of the recurrent laryngeal nerve: A common variation. *ANZ Journal of Surgery, 76*, 928–931.

Benjamin, B. (1981). Frequency variability in the aged voice. *Journal of Gerontology, 36*, 722–736.

Benjamin, B. (1988). Changes in speech production and linguistic behaviors with aging. In B. Shadden (Ed.), *Communication behavior and aging: A sourcebook for clinicians* (pp. 162–181). Baltimore: Williams & Wilkins.

Berke, G., & Gerratt, B. (1993). Laryngeal biomechanics: An overview of mucosal wave mechanics. *Journal of Voice, 7*, 123–128.

Biever, D., & Bless, D. (1989). Vibratory characteristics of the vocal folds in young adult and geriatric women. *Journal of Voice, 3*, 120–131.

Boone, D., & McFarland, S. (1994). *The voice and voice therapy* (5th ed.). Englewood-Cliffs, NJ: Prentice-Hall.

Bosma, J. (1985). Postnatal ontogeny of performance of the pharynx, larynx, and mouth. *American Review of Respiratory Disease, 131*, 10–15.

Broad, D. (1973). Phonation. In F. Minifie, T. Hixon, & F. Williams (Eds.), *Normal aspects of speech, hearing, and language* (pp. 127–167). Englewood-Cliffs, NJ: Prentice-Hall.

Bruel & Kjaer, Inc. (2007). *Sound level meters and PC software for sound level meters*. Naerum, Denmark.

Casiano, R., Zaveri, V., & Lundy, D. (1992). Efficacy of videostroboscopy in the diagnosis of voice disorders. *Otolaryngology-Head and Neck Surgery, 107*, 95–100.

Catten, M., Gray, S., Hammond, T., Zhou, R., & Hammond, E. (1998). Analysis of cellular location and concentration in vocal fold lamina propria. *Otolaryngology-Head and Neck Surgery, 118*, 663–667.

Cavagna, G., & Margaria, R. (1965). An analysis of the mechanics of phonation. *Journal of Applied Physiology, 20*, 301–307.

Charpied, G., & Shapshay, S. (2004). *Anatomy and histology of the pars media of the cricothyroid muscle: A comparative study*. Paper presented at the International Conference on Voice Physiology and Biomechanics, Marseille, France.

Childers, D., Hicks, D., Moore, G., Eshenazi, L., & Lalwani, A. (1990). Electroglottography and vocal fold physiology. *Journal of Speech and Hearing Research, 33*, 245–254.

Childers, D., & Krishnamurthy, A. (1985). A critical review of electroglottography. *Critical Review of Biomedical Engineering, 12*, 131–161.

Childers, D., Smith, A., & Moore, G. (1984). Relationships between electroglottography, speech, and vocal cord contact. *Folia Phoniatrica, 36*, 105–118.

Classen, H., & Kirsch, T. (1994). Temporal and spatial localization of type I and II collagens in human thyroid cartilage. *Anatomy and Embryology, 189*, 237–242.

Coleman, R. (1963). Decay characteristics of vocal fry. *Folia Phoniatrica, 15*, 256–263.

Coleman, R., Mabis, J., & Hinson, J. (1977). Fundamental frequency—sound pressure level profiles of adult male and female voices. *Journal of Speech and Hearing Research, 20*, 197–204.

Colton, R. (1972). Spectral characteristics of the modal and falsetto registers. *Folia Phoniatrica, 24*, 337–344.

Colton, R. (1973). Vocal intensity in the modal and falsetto registers. *Folia Phoniatrica, 25*, 62–70.

Colton, R., & Casper, J. (1996). *Understanding voice problems: A physiological perspective for diagnosis and treatment* (2nd ed.). Baltimore: Williams & Wilkins.

Colton, R., & Conture, E. (1990). Problems and pitfalls of electroglottography. *Journal of Voice, 4*, 10–24.

Cooper, D. (1990). *Maturation, characteristics, and aging of laryngeal muscles*. Paper presented at the Pacific Voice Conference, San Francisco, CA.

Crelin, E. (1973). *Functional anatomy of the newborn*. New Haven, CT: Yale University Press.

Curry, E. (1946). Voice changes in male adolescents. *Laryngoscope, 56*, 795–805.

Dailey, S., Spanou, K., & Zeitels, S. (2007). The evaluation of benign glottic lesions: Rigid telescopic stroboscopy versus suspension microlaryngoscopy. *Journal of Voice, 21*, 112–118.

Damste, H. (1970). The phonetogram. *Practica Oto-Rhino-Laryngologica, 32*, 185–187.

Daniloff, R., Shuckers, G., & Feth, L. (1980). *The physiology of speech and hearing*. Englewood-Cliffs, NJ: Prentice-Hall.

D'Antonio, L., Netsell, R., & Lotz, W. (1988). Clinical aerodynamics for the evaluation and management of voice disorders. *Ear, Nose, and Throat Journal, 67*, 394–399.

de Melo, E., Lemas, M., Filho, J., Sennes, L., Saldiva, P., Tsuji, D. (2003). Distribution of collagen in the lamina propria of the human vocal fold. *Laryngoscope, 113*, 2187–2191.

Dickson, D., & Maue-Dickson, W. (1982). *Anatomical and physiological bases of speech*. Boston: Little, Brown and Company.

Dromey, C., Stathopoulos, E., & Sapienza, C. (1992). Glottal airflow and electroglottographic measures of vocal function at multiple intensities. *Journal of Voice, 6*, 44–54.

Duffy, J. (2005). *Motor speech disorders: Substrates, differential diagnosis, and management* (2nd ed.). New York: Mosby.

Faaborg-Andersen, K. (1957). Electromyographic investigation of intrinsic laryngeal muscles in humans. *Acta Physiologica Scandinavica, 41*(Suppl. 140), 1–150.

Faaborg-Andersen, K., & Sonninen, A. (1960). The function of the extrinsic laryngeal muscles at different pitch: An electromyographic and roentgenologic investigation. *Acta Otolaryngologica, 51*, 89–93.

Faaborg-Andersen, K., Yanagihara, N., & von Leden, H. (1967). Vocal pitch and intensity regulation: A comparative study of electrical activity in the cricothyroid muscle and the airflow rate. *Archives of Otolaryngology, 85*, 448–454.

Fairbanks, G. (1960). *Voice and articulation drillbook*. New York: Harper & Row.

Fairbanks, G., Herbert, E., & Hammond, J. (1949). An acoustical study of vocal pitch in seven- and eight-year-old girls. *Child Development, 20*, 71–78.

Fairbanks, G., & Miron, M. (1957). Effect of vocal effort upon the consonant-vowel ratio within the syllable. *Journal of the Acoustical Society of America, 29*, 621–626.

Fairbanks, G., Wiley, J., & Lassman, F. (1949). An acoustical study of vocal pitch in seven- and eight-year-old boys. *Child Development, 20*, 63–69.

Fant, G. (1960). *Acoustic theory of speech production*. Hague, Netherlands: Mouton.

Ferreri, G. (1959). Senescence of the larynx. *Italian General Review of Otorhinolaryngology, 1*, 640–709.

Fink, B. (1975). *The human larynx: A functional study*. New York: Raven Press.

Fink, B., Basek, M., & Epanchin, V. (1956). The mechanism of opening of the human larynx. *Laryngoscope, 66*, 410–425.

Flanagan, J. (1972). *Speech analysis, synthesis, and perception*. New York: Springer-Verlag.

Folkard, C. (2006). *Guinness book of records*. New York: Bantam Books.

Fourcin, A. (1974). Laryngographic examination of vocal fold vibration. In B. Wyke (Ed.), *Ventilatory and phonatory control systems* (pp. 315–326). London, UK: Oxford University Press.

Frable, M. (1961). Computation of motion at the cricoarytenoid joint. *Archives of Otolaryngology, 73*, 551–556.

Gauffin, J., & Sundberg, J. (1989). Spectral correlates of glottal voice source waveform characteristics. *Journal of Speech and Hearing Research, 32*, 556–565.

Gay, T., Hirose, H., Strome, M., & Sawashima, M. (1972). Electromyography of the intrinsic laryngeal muscles during phonation. *Annals of Otology, Rhinology, and Laryngology, 81*, 401–409.

Glaze, L., Bless, D., Milenkovic, P., & Susser, R. (1988). Acoustic characteristics of children's voice. *Journal of Voice, 2*, 312–319.

Glottal Enterprises, Inc. (2007). *Two-channel electroglottograph and microphone preamplifier, Model EG2–PC*. Syracuse, NY.

Gramming, P. (1991). Vocal loudness and frequency capabilities of the voice. *Journal of Voice, 5*, 144–157.

Gramming, P., & Sundberg, J. (1988). Spectrum factors relevant to phonetogram measurement. *Journal of the Acoustical Society of America, 83*, 2352–2360.

Han, Y., Wang, J., Fischman, D., Biller, H., & Sanders, I. (1999). Slow tonic muscle fibers in the thyroarytenoid muscles of human vocal folds: A possible specialization for speech. *Anatomical Record, 256*, 146–157.

Hasek, C., Singh, S., & Murry, T. (1980). Acoustic attributes of children's voices. *Journal of the Acoustical Society of America, 68*, 1252–1265.

Hately, B., Evison, G., & Samuel, E. (1965). The pattern of ossification in the laryngeal cartilages: A radiological study. *British Journal of Radiology, 38*, 585–591.

Hirano, M. (1974). Morphological structures of the vocal cord as a vibrator and its variations. *Folia Phoniatrica, 26*, 89–94.

Hirano, M. (1981). *Clinical examination of voice*. New York: Springer-Verlag Wien.

Hirano, M., & Bless, D. (1993). *Videostroboscopic examination of the larynx*. San Diego, CA: Singular.

Hirano, M., Kakita, Y., Kawasaki, H., Gould, W., & Lambiase, A. (1981). Data from high-speed motion picture studies. In K. Stevens & M. Hirano (Eds.), *Vocal fold physiology* (pp. 85–93). Tokyo, Japan: University of Tokyo Press.

Hirano, M., Kiyokawa, K., & Kurita, S. (1988). Laryngeal muscles and glottal shaping. In O. Fujimura (Ed.), *Vocal physiology: Voice production, mechanisms, and functions* (pp. 49–65) New York: Raven Press.

Hirano, M., Kiyokawa, K., Kurita, S., & Sato, K. (1986). Posterior glottis: Morphological study in excised larynges. *Annals of Otology, Rhinology, and Laryngology, 95*, 576–581.

Hirano, M., Kurita, S., & Nakashima, T. (1983). Growth, development and aging of human vocal folds. In D. Bless & J. Abbs (Eds.), *Vocal fold physiology: Contemporary research and clinical issues* (pp. 22–43). San Diego, CA: College-Hill Press.

Hirano, M., Kurita, S., & Sagaguchi, S. (1989). Aging of the vibratory tissue of the human vocal folds. *Acta Otolaryngologica, 107*, 428–433.

Hirano, M., Ohala, J., & Vennard, W. (1969). The function of the laryngeal muscles in regulating fundamental frequency and intensity of phonation. *Journal of Speech and Hearing Research, 12*, 616–628.

Hirano, M., & Sato, K. (1993). *Histological color atlas of the human larynx*. San Diego, CA: Singular.

Hirano, M., Vennard, W., & Ohala, J. (1970). Regulation of register, pitch and intensity of voice. *Folia Phoniatrica, 22*, 1–20.

Hirano, M., Yoshida, T., & Tanaka, S. (1991). Vibratory behavior of human vocal folds viewed from below. In J. Gauffin & B. Hammarberg (Eds.), *Vocal fold physiology: Acoustic, perceptual, and physiological aspects of voice mechanisms* (pp. 1–6). San Diego, CA: Singular.

Hirose, H. (1977). Laryngeal adjustments in consonant production. *Phonetica, 34*, 289–294.

Hixon, T. (1966). Turbulent noise sources for speech. *Folia Phoniatrica, 18*, 168–182.

Hixon, T. (2006). *Respiratory function in singing: A primer for singers and singing teachers.* Tucson, AZ: Redington Brown.

Hixon, T., & Abbs, J. (1980). Normal speech production. In T. Hixon, L. Shriberg, & J. Saxman (Eds.), *Introduction to communication disorders* (pp. 42–87). Englewood-Cliffs, NJ: Prentice-Hall.

Hixon, T., Klatt, D., & Mead, J. (1970). *Influence of forced transglottal pressure change on vocal fundamental frequency.* Paper presented at the Fall Meeting of the Acoustical Society of America, Houston, TX.

Hixon, T., Mead, J., & Goldman, M. (1976). Dynamics of the chest wall during speech production: Function of the thorax, rib cage, diaphragm, and abdomen. *Journal of Speech and Hearing Research, 19*, 297–356.

Hixon, T., & Minifie, F. (1972). *Influence of forced transglottal pressure change on vocal sound pressure level.* Paper presented at the Convention of the American Speech and Hearing Association, San Francisco, CA.

Hixon, T., Minifie, F., & Tait, C. (1967). Correlates of turbulent noise production for speech. *Journal of Speech and Hearing Research, 10*, 133–140.

Hixon, T., Watson, P., Harris, F., & Pearl, N. (1988). Relative volume changes of the rib cage and abdomen during prephonatory chest wall posturing. *Journal of Voice, 2*, 13–19.

Hoit, J., & Hixon, T. (1992). Age and laryngeal airway resistance during vowel production in women. *Journal of Speech and Hearing Research, 35*, 309–313.

Hollien, H. (1960a). Some laryngeal correlates of vocal pitch. *Journal of Speech and Hearing Research, 3*, 52–58.

Hollien, H. (1960b). Vocal pitch variations related to changes in vocal fold length. *Journal of Speech and Hearing Research, 3*, 150–156.

Hollien, H. (1962). Vocal fold thickness and fundamental frequency of phonation. *Journal of Speech and Hearing Research, 5*, 237–243.

Hollien, H. (1972). Three major vocal registers: A proposal. In A. Rigault & R. Charbonneau (Eds.), *Proceedings of the Seventh International Congress of Phonetic Sciences* (pp. 320–331). Hague, Netherlands: Mouton.

Hollien, H. (1974). On vocal registers. *Journal of Phonetics, 2*, 125–143.

Hollien, H., Brown, W., & Hollien, K. (1971). Vocal fold length associated with modal, falsetto and varying vocal intensity phonations. *Folia Phoniatrica, 23*, 66–78.

Hollien, H., & Colton, R. (1969). Four laminagraphic studies of vocal fold thickness. *Folia Phoniatrica, 21*, 179–198.

Hollien, H., & Curtis, J. (1960). A laminagraphic study of vocal pitch. *Journal of Speech and Hearing Research, 3*, 362–371.

Hollien, H., & Curtis, J. (1962). Elevation and tilting of vocal folds as a function of vocal pitch. *Folia Phoniatrica, 14*, 23–36.

Hollien, H., Damste, H., & Murry, T. (1969). Vocal fold length during vocal fry phonation. *Folia Phoniatrica, 21*, 257–265.

Hollien, H., Green, R., & Massey, K. (1994). Longitudinal research on adolescent voice change in males. *Journal of the Acoustical Society of America, 34*, 80–84.

Hollien, H., & Moore, P. (1960). Measurements of the vocal folds during changes in pitch. *Journal of Speech and Hearing Research, 3*, 157–163.

Hollien, H., & Shipp, T. (1972). Speaking fundamental frequency and chronological age in males. *Journal of Speech and Hearing Research, 15*, 155–159.

Holmberg, E., Hillman, R., & Perkell, J. (1988). Glottal airflow and transglottal air pressure measurements for male and female speakers in soft, normal, and loud voice. *Journal of the Acoustical Society of America, 84*, 511–529.

Holmberg, E., Hillman, R., & Perkell, J. (1989). Glottal airflow and transglottal air pressure measurements for male and female speakers in low, normal, and high pitch. *Journal of Voice, 3*, 294–305.

Holmes, L., Leeper, H., & Nicholson, I. (1994). Laryngeal airway resistance of older men and women as a function of vocal sound pressure level. *Journal of Speech and Hearing Research, 37*, 789–799.

Honda, K. (1995). Laryngeal and extra-laryngeal mechanisms of Fo control. In F. Bell-Berti & L. Raphael (Eds.), *Producing speech: Contemporary issues—For Katherine Safford Harris* (pp. 215–245). New York: American Institute of Physics.

Honjo, I., & Isshiki, N. (1980). Laryngoscopic and voice characteristics of aged persons. *Archives of Otolaryngology, 106*, 149–150.

Howard, D., Brereton, J., Welch, G., Himonides, E., DeCosta, M., Williams, J., & Howard, A. (2007). Are real-time displays of benefit in the singing studio? An exploratory study. *Journal of Voice, 21*, 20–34.

Ishii, K., Zhai, W., Akita, M., & Hirose, H. (1996). Ultrastructure of the lamina propria of the human vocal fold. *Acta Otolaryngologica, 116*, 778–782.

Ishizaka, K., & Matsudaira, M. (1972). Fluid mechanical considerations of vocal cord vibration. *Speech Communications Research Laboratory (Santa Barbara, CA), Monograph Number 8*, 1–72.

Isshiki, N. (1964). Regulatory mechanism of voice intensity variation. *Journal of Speech and Hearing Research, 7*, 17–29.

Isshiki, N. (1965). Vocal intensity and air flow rate. *Folia Phoniatrica, 17*, 92–104.

Isshiki, N. (1985). Clinical significance of a vocal efficiency index. In I. Titze & R. Scherer (Eds.), *Vocal fold physiology: Biomechanics, acoustics, and phonatory control* (pp. 230–238). Denver, CO: The Denver Center for the Performing Arts.

Isshiki, N., & von Leden, H. (1964). Hoarseness: Aerodynamic studies. *Archives of Otolaryngology, 80*, 206–213.

Jankovskaya, N. (1959). The receptor innervation of the perichondrium of the laryngeal cartilages. *Arkhiv Anatomii, Gistologii l'Enbriologii, 37*, 70–75.

Kahane, J. (1975). *The developmental anatomy of the human prepubertal and pubertal larynx.* Doctoral Dissertation, University of Pittsburgh, Pittsburgh, PA.

Kahane, J. (1978). A morphological study of the human prepubertal and pubertal larynx. *American Journal of Anatomy, 151*, 11–20.

Kahane, J. (1980). Age related histological changes in the human male and female laryngeal cartilages: Biological and functional implications. In V. Lawrence (Ed.), *Transcripts of the Ninth Symposium: Care of the Professional Voice*, Part I (pp. 11–20). New York: The Voice Foundation.

Kahane, J. (1982). Growth of the human prepubertal and pubertal larynx. *Journal of Speech and Hearing Research, 25*, 446–455.

Kahane, J. (1983). A survey of age-related changes in the connective tissue of the human adult larynx. In D. Bless & J. Abbs (Eds.), *Vocal fold physiology: Contemporary research and clinical issues* (pp. 44–49). San Diego, CA: College-Hill Press.

Kahane, J. (1987). Connective tissue changes in the larynx and their effects on voice. *Journal of Voice, 1*, 27–30.

Kahane, J. (1988). Age-related changes in the human cricoarytenoid joint. In O. Fujimura (Ed.), *Vocal physiology:*

van den Berg, J., & Tan, T. (1959). Results of experiments with human larynxes. *Practica Oto-Rhino-Laryngologica, 21*, 425–450.

van den Berg, J., Vennard, W., Berger, D., & Shervanian, C. (1960). *Voice production* (Black and white 16 mm sound motion picture film). Utrecht, Netherlands: SFW-UNFI.

van den Berg, J., Zantema, J., & Doornenbal, P. (1957). On the air resistance and the Bernoulli effect of the human larynx. *Journal of the Acoustical Society of America, 29*, 626–631.

Vennard, W. (1967). *Singing: The mechanism and the technic.* New York: Carl Fischer.

von Leden, H., & Moore, P. (1961). The mechanics of the cricoarytenoid joint. *Archives of Otolaryngology, 73*, 541–550.

Walker, W. (1977, May). Demonstrating resonance by shattering glass with sound. *Physics Teacher*, pp. 294–296.

Wang, R. (1998). Three-dimensional analysis of cricoarytenoid joint motion. *Laryngoscope, 108*, 1–17.

Wendahl, R., Moore, P., & Hollien, H. (1963). Comments on vocal fry. *Folia Phoniatrica, 15*, 251–255.

Wilson, K. (1979). *Voice disorders in children.* Baltimore: Williams & Wilkins.

Wind, J. (1970). *On the phylogeny and the ontogeny of the human larynx.* Groningen, Netherlands: Wolters-Noordhoff.

Wustrow, F. (1953). Bau und funktion des menshlichne musculus vocalis. *Zeitschrift fur Anatomie und Entwicklungsgeschichte, 116*, 506–522.

Yanagihara, N., & Koike, Y. (1967). The regulation of sustained phonation. *Folia Phoniatrica, 19*, 1–18.

Zemlin, W. (1998). *Speech and hearing science: Anatomy and physiology.* Boston: Allyn & Bacon.

Zemlin, W., Davis, P., & Gaza, C. (1984). Fine morphology of the posterior cricoarytenoid muscle. *Folia Phoniatrica, 36*, 233–240.

Zenker, W. (1964). Questions regarding the function of external laryngeal muscles. In D. Brewer (Ed.), *Research potentials in voice physiology* (pp. 20–40). New York: State University of New York.

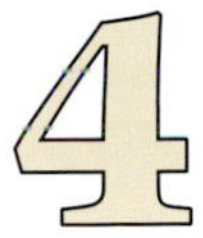

4

Velopharyngeal-Nasal Function and Speech Production

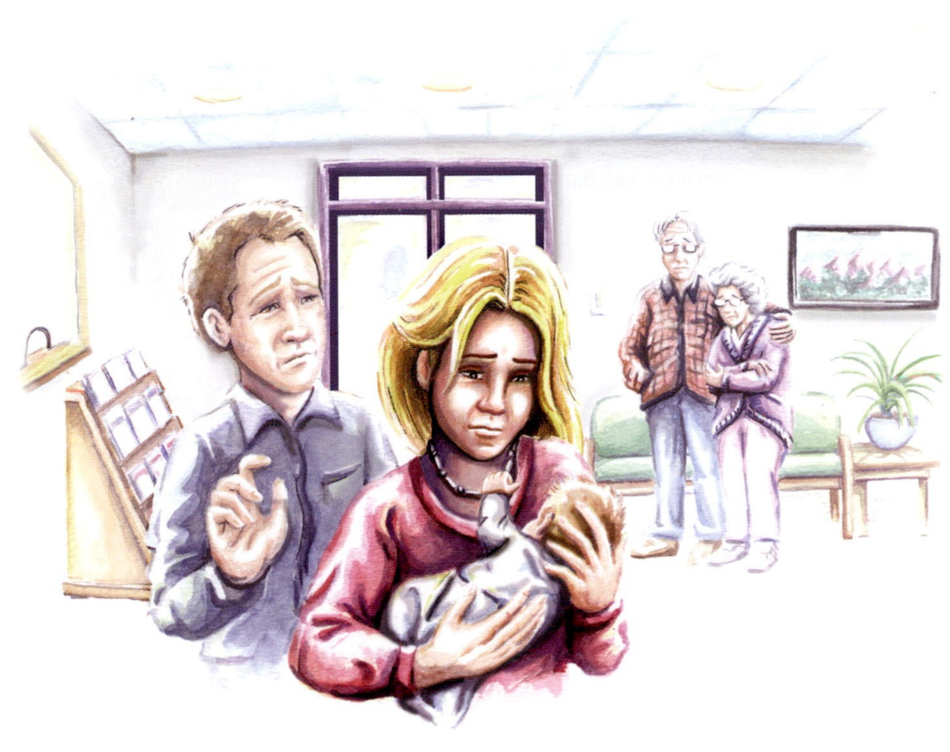

Scenario

It was to be their first baby and anticipation was running high. They were somewhat older parents who had chosen to focus initially on careers rather than on starting a family during the first decade of their marriage. The prospective grandparents (retired Ohio-Florida snowbirds) on the mother's side of the family had come south 3 weeks earlier than usual with the expectation of being helpful. A nursery was readied, routines were sketched out for a planned first month of parenthood, and the hopeful grandfather had managed to get his hands on two boxes of Cuban cigars for his son-in-law to distribute once the official celebration was begun. All was going well.

The pregnancy was full term and the delivery started out uneventfully, although labor turned out to be somewhat difficult. Finally the moment arrived and it was a boy. There was no need to elicit a cry. The new member of the family announced himself voluntarily and with intensity. However, his announcement had a bit of a strange quality to the ear of the obstetrician and other medical staff. The mother was understandably dazed and not fully cognizant, but she managed a smile at the obstetrician's declaration that it was a boy. Then she slumped into relief and exhaustion.

The obstetrician was the first to see the problem. The umbilical cord was cut and the newborn was handed to the delivery nurse. Nothing needed to be said to her. The father was comforting the mother as the obstetrician examined the baby more closely. The baby appeared to be physically normal, with one major exception. There was a cleft of both the lip and palate. The obstetrician took the father aside and explained the circumstances. A few minutes later, when the mother awoke, the same message was delivered.

The parents, especially the mother, seemed to collapse psychologically under the weight of the words. There was stunned silence and anguish. Then questions came in a flood, along with a flood of emotions. How could this be? Why did it happen? Had they done anything to cause this? Why had prenatal examinations not detected the problem? What did this mean for the baby? Was he mentally retarded? Could he go home? Would he be able to breast-feed? What should they do? Did he have to have surgery? When would it be done? Would he ever look normal? During these moments their dreams seemed shattered. It was overwhelming. Each tried to support the other, while trying to cope with feelings for each other and the baby. It was not the day they had envisioned in their rehearsals. The father talked with his wife's parents and then telephoned his own parents in Seattle.

A team of specialists in cleft palate and craniofacial disorders was called in to develop a management program. The management was expected to be lengthy. When the baby was 3 months of age, surgery was done to close the cleft of the lip. Then, when he was 12 months of age, another surgery was performed to close the cleft of the palate.

Middle ear infections proved to be a problem and were treated with antibiotics and the insertion of tubes to drain the middle-ear cavities. Speech development was monitored periodically and on the child's second birthday was found to have progressed to syllable and word utterances. Nasal emission of air could be heard during voiceless consonants and moderate hypernasality was perceived during vowels. Visualization of the velopharynx through nasoendoscopy revealed that the velopharynx was not closed for oralized speech production. This was confirmed via measures of nasal airflow. The management team recommended secondary surgery as the course to be taken. Two options were being considered, further surgery on the palate itself or the surgical construction of a pharyngeal flap. However, as it turned out, the management team did not have an opportunity to exercise either option.

Marital problems of the parents had led to divorce with the mother being awarded custody of the child. She and the child moved to another part of the country and severed ties with the child's father and the management team. She was depressed and after the move she distanced herself from her parents and friends. The mother and child lived a life of relative seclusion, his contact with other children being infrequent. Except for occasional visits to a pediatrician for earaches, his other health care needs were on hold.

INTRODUCTION

The velopharyngeal-nasal apparatus is located within the head and neck and comprises a system of valves and air passages. This system interconnects the throat and the atmosphere through the nose. Although most chapters concerned with velopharyngeal-nasal function and speech production focus on the velopharyngeal part of this system, the present chapter discusses the entire velopharyngeal-nasal apparatus as a single functional entity. This leads to a more comprehensive understanding of normal and abnormal function and a fuller appreciation for the principles involved in making evaluation and management decisions.

The chapter begins by discussing the fundamentals of velopharyngeal-nasal function, and then turns to consideration of velopharyngeal-nasal function and speech production. Subsequent sections cover measurement of velopharyngeal-nasal function, velopharyngeal-nasal disorders in speech production, and clinical professionals who work with velopharyngeal-nasal disorders in speech production. The chapter concludes with a review and the completion of its opening scenario.

FUNDAMENTALS OF VELOPHARYNGEAL-NASAL FUNCTION

This section considers the fundamentals of velopharyngeal-nasal function and lays the groundwork for subsequent consideration of velopharyngeal-nasal function in speech production. Topics include the anatomy of the velopharyngeal-nasal apparatus, forces and movements of the velopharyngeal-nasal apparatus, adjustments of the velopharyngeal-nasal apparatus, control variables of velopharyngeal-nasal function, neural substrates of velopharyngeal-nasal control, and ventilation and velopharyngeal-nasal function.

Anatomy of the Velopharyngeal-Nasal Apparatus

The valves and air passages of the velopharyngeal-nasal apparatus are linked together such that some of the components are arranged in mechanical series (one after another) and some are arranged in mechanical parallel (side by side). This section

Duane C. Spriestersbach

Spriestersbach had a distinguished career as a clinical investigator of the communication problems of children with cleft palate and craniofacial disorders. "Sprie," as he is affectionately called, served for many years as the program director of a large federally funded research grant on cleft palate at the University of Iowa. His leadership fostered much of the research done over 2 decades on normal velopharyngeal function for speech production and on the mechanisms involved in control of the velopharyngeal apparatus in individuals with velopharyngeal incompetence. Many of the names in the reference list to this chapter cut their research teeth under his guidance. Spriestersbach is an exceptional thinker. He has had an enormous impact on translating the products of research into practical clinical applications for those with speech disorders caused by cleft palate. He is now retired and lives in Iowa City, Iowa, where he continues to play a legendary mean hand of poker.

begins by discussing the skeletal superstructure that supports the velopharyngeal-nasal apparatus. From there, the section proceeds to separate discussions of the anatomy of the pharynx, velum, nasal cavities, and outer nose.

Skeletal Superstructure

Figure 4–1 depicts the skeletal superstructure of the velopharyngeal-nasal apparatus. This superstructure consists of the first six cervical vertebrae and various bones of the skull. The latter includes bones of the cranium (braincase) and facial complex (forehead, eyes, nose, mouth, and upper throat). These bones are individually complex structures that are rigidly joined together into a unified framework. This framework contributes to the walls, floor, and roof of the velopharyngeal-nasal apparatus through a system of structural processes, plates, and projections, and provides for the attachment of muscles of the velopharyngeal-nasal apparatus. Some of the most important bony structures of the apparatus (and selected of their contributions) include the temporal bones (sides of the lower braincase), frontal bone (front of the upper braincase), palatine bones (back of the floor of the nasal cavities), maxillary bones (front of the floor of the nasal cavities), sphenoid bone (back wall of the nasal cavities), ethmoid bone (upper side walls of the nasal cavities and upper part of their medial wall), vomer bone (lower part of the medial wall of the nasal cavities), inferior conchae (lower side walls of the nasal cavities), and nasal bones (bridge of the outer nose). The bony structures mentioned can be seen in various perspectives in Figure 4–1, in other figures in this chapter, and in depictions of the bony skeleton of the oral apparatus in Chapter 5.

Pharynx

Figure 4–2 depicts some of the salient structural features of the pharynx (throat). The pharynx is a tube of tendon and muscle that extends from the base of the skull to the cricoid cartilage in the front and to the sixth cervical vertebra in the back. The mix of tendon and muscle varies along the length of the pharynx. At the upper end of the structure, the makeup is solely connective tissue, called the pharyngeal aponeurosis, which effectively suspends the pharyngeal tube from above (the way the rim of a basketball goal suspends the net). Muscular tissue increases in proportion down the length of the pharynx, until it predominates. At the lower end, the pharynx is solely muscular and is continuous with the esophagus (gullet), where its front and back walls are in contact. This contact is broken during activities such as swallowing and regurgitation.

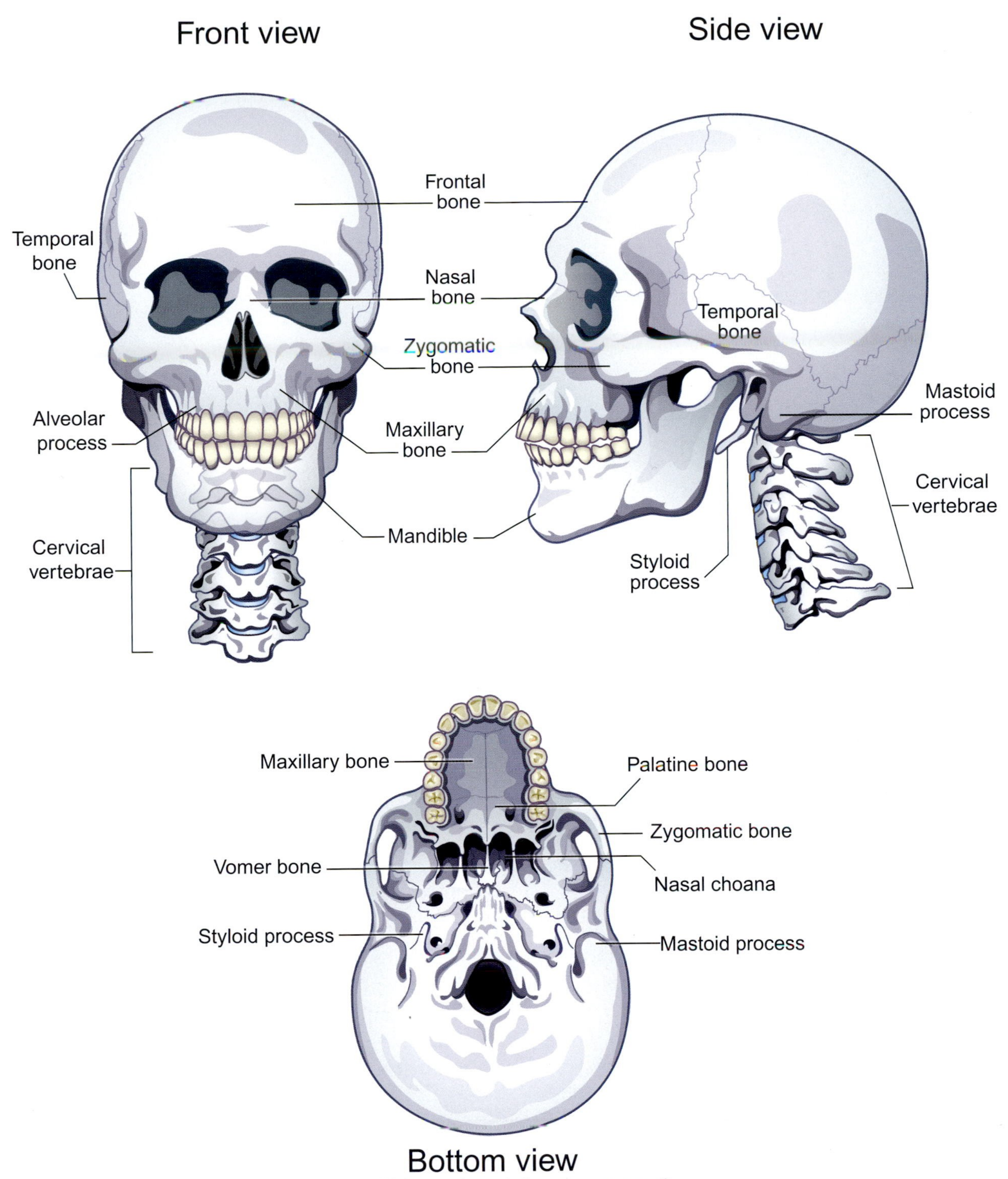

Figure 4–1. Skeletal superstructure of the velopharyngeal-nasal apparatus. The mandible (*lower jaw*) is shown for reference in front and side views. The bottom view has the mandible and vertebrae removed.

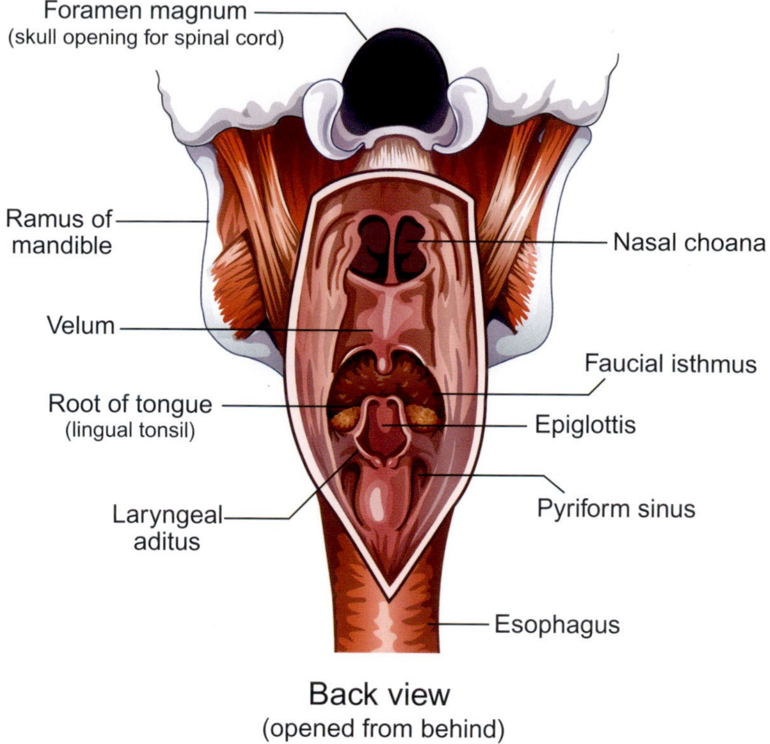

Figure 4–2. Salient features of the pharynx as revealed from a back view in which the posterior pharyngeal wall is opened from behind. The skull, mandible, and selected muscles are shown for reference.

The pharyngeal tube is widest at the top and narrows down its length. It is oval in cross section, being larger side to side than front to back. The front wall of the pharynx is partially formed by the back surfaces of the velum (defined below), tongue, and epiglottis. Otherwise, the structure is open at the front and connects, from top to bottom, with the nasal cavities, oral cavity, and laryngeal aditus (upper entrance to the larynx).

The pharynx comprises three cavities that are designated, from top to bottom, as the nasopharynx, oropharynx, and laryngopharynx. The boundaries of these cavities are shown in Figure 4–3. The nasopharynx lies behind the nose and above the velum. Because of the mobility of the velum, the lower boundary of the nasopharynx is somewhat arbitrary. A common convention is to specify this boundary operationally. For example, in midsagittal x-ray studies of the velopharyngeal-nasal apparatus, the boundary is often specified by a reference line extending between the upper surface of the hard palate and the most forward point on the uppermost vertebra.

The nasopharynx always remains patent, a feature that distinguishes it from the other subdivisions of the pharynx. The pharyngeal orifices of the eustachian (auditory) tubes are located on the lateral walls of the nasopharynx. These tubes enable pressure equilibration between the middle ears and atmosphere. Across the back surface of the nasopharynx, between the pharyngeal orifices of the eustachian tubes, lies a large mass of lymphoid tissue called the pharyngeal tonsil. This tissue is also referred to as the nasopharyngeal tonsil and, when abnormally enlarged, is designated as adenoid tissue (or just the adenoids). At the front, the nasopharynx connects to the nasal cavities through the nasal choanae (funnel-like openings). These are two oval-shaped apertures that are about twice as long (top to bottom) as they are wide (side to side) and are oriented in the verti-

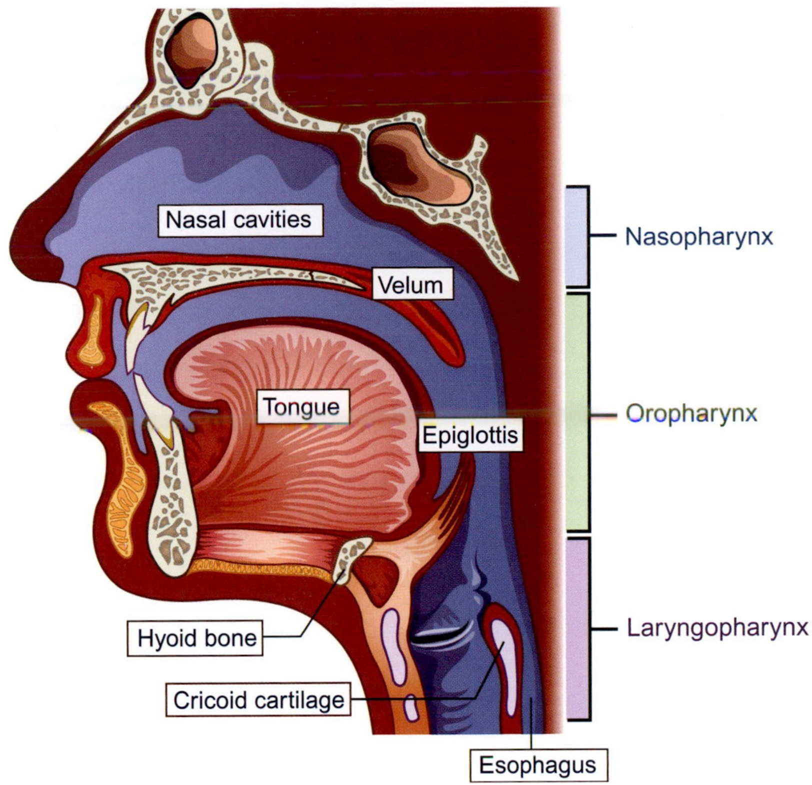

Figure 4–3. Boundaries of the nasopharynx, oropharynx, and laryngopharynx.

cal plane. The nasal choanae are also referred to as the posterior nares (nostrils) or internal nares and are somewhat like the breech ends of the barrels of a side-by-side double-barreled shotgun.

The oropharynx forms the middle part of the pharyngeal tube. The upper boundary of the oropharynx is coextensive with the lower boundary of the nasopharynx. The lower boundary of the oropharynx is the hyoid (tongue) bone. As shown in Figure 4–4, the front of the oropharynx opens into the oral cavity through the faucial isthmus (the narrow passage situated between the velum and the base of the tongue). This isthmus is bounded on the left and right sides by the anterior and posterior faucial pillars, pairs of muscular bands that resemble pairs of legs. The palatine tonsils are located between the anterior and posterior faucial pillars on each side of the isthmus. They are also often called the faucial tonsils and are "the" tonsils most often referred to colloquially. The back surface of the tongue is the site of still another tonsil, the so-called lingual tonsil. This tonsil is a broad aggregate of lymph glands distributed across much of the root of the tongue.

The oropharynx is the only subdivision of the pharynx that can be visualized without special equipment. The back wall of the oropharynx can be seen when looking at the pharynx through the faucial isthmus. Even more of the back wall can be observed when the velum is elevated, as in "open your mouth wide and say 'ah.'"

The laryngopharynx constitutes the lowermost part of the pharynx. The upper boundary of the laryngopharynx is the hyoid bone and the lower boundary is the base of the cricoid cartilage, where the pharynx is continuous with the esophagus. At the front, the laryngopharynx is bounded by the back surface of the tongue (and the lingual tonsil), the laryngeal aditus (formed by the epiglottis and aryepiglottic folds), and the pyriform sinuses (pear-shaped cavities located lateral to the aryepiglottic folds).

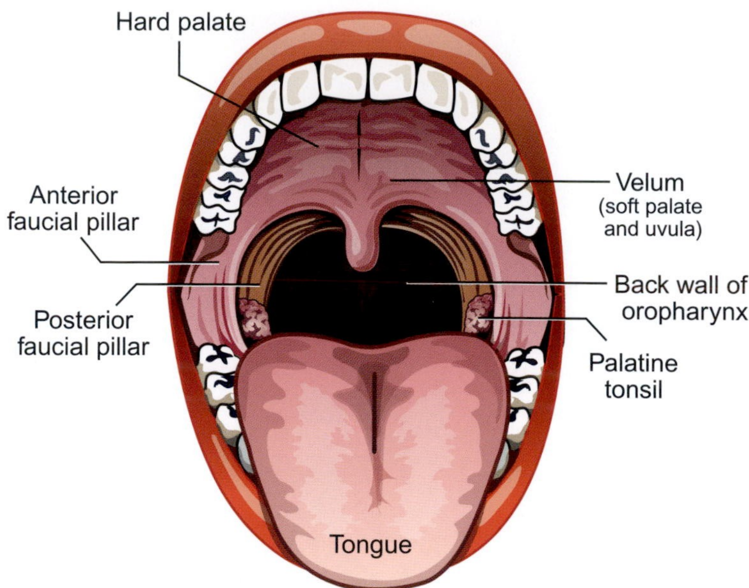

Figure 4–4. View of the oropharynx through the faucial isthmus.

Muscle tissue is an important part of the pharynx and encircles it, much like bands of cord encircle the casing (tread and sidewalls) of a radial automobile tire. In effect, the pharynx is an elongated structure that has the architecture of a sphincter. Its overall arrangement is similar to that of the gut. This should come as no surprise, because one of the duties of the pharynx involves its actions as a component of the digestive system.

Velum

The velum is a pendulous flap consisting of the soft palate and uvula. The word velum means "curtain." In this case, it is the curtain that hangs down from the back of the roof of the mouth, as illustrated in Figure 4–3 and Figure 4–4. A broad sheet of connective tissue, the palatal aponeurosis, forms a fibrous skeleton for the velum.

Despite a similar surface appearance throughout, the velum is not structurally homogeneous, but differs in composition from one region to another. These regional differences are manifested in layers of different types of tissues within the velum and differences in the distribution of muscle fibers within the structure.

Four tissue layers have been identified in the velum (Kuehn & Kahane, 1990). These include (a) a layer toward the under surface (oral surface) that is glandular (secreting) tissue with adipose (fat) tissue at the sides, (b) a middle layer of muscle tissue in which fibers run side to side in the central portion of the structure and front to back in its more superficial portion toward the upper surface (nasal surface), (c) an upper front layer consisting of connective tissue (tendon), and (d) a lower back layer consisting largely of glandular tissue.

Patterns of muscle fiber distribution differ along the length of the velum (Kuehn & Moon, 2005). These include (a) a front portion that is void of muscle fibers, (b) a middle one-third that is rich with muscle fibers that course in various directions (including across the midline) and include insertions into the lateral margins of the structure, (c) a proportioning of muscle fibers that tapers off toward the front and back of the structure, and (d) a uvular portion that is sparsely interspersed with muscle fibers.

In one sense, the uvula (meaning "little grape") is a pendulous structure suspended from another pendulous structure, the soft palate. One of several distinctions between the two is the nature of their blood supplies. The uvula has a richer vascular system than does the soft palate, a fact that has prompted the suggestion that this difference might serve to prevent excessive cooling of the smaller of the two structures (Moon & Kuehn, 2004).

Show Me Your Hand

They were twin girls. Each had speech that was a dead ringer for the other and was characterized by multiple misarticulations and hypernasality. What was the cause? Had they developed some sort of twin speech? Did one have a problem and the other was imitating it? Oral examinations revealed identical structural anomalies. Each girl had a short velum. Nasoendoscopic examinations further revealed that, for each girl, the velum elevated only occasionally during speech production, but never came close to the posterior pharyngeal wall. The girls' parents were with them and being interviewed by a student clinician and her supervisor. The moment the mother spoke there were suspicions. She had a severe speech disorder characterized by multiple misarticulations and hypernasality, and exhibited pronounced nasal grimacing when speaking. She allowed an oral examination. She had a short velum. It was three of a kind.

Nasal Cavities

The nasal cavities, also termed the nasal fossae (pronounced like posse), lie behind the outer nose. They constitute the inner nose and are two large chambers that run side by side (recall the double-barreled shotgun analogy suggested above). The two nasal cavities are separated from each other by the nasal septum, a partition in the midsagittal plane (although not often perfectly vertical). As shown in Figure 4–5, this partition has (a) a front part composed of cartilage, (b) an upper back part that is the perpendicular plate of the ethmoid (sieve-like) bone, and (c) a lower back part that is the vomer (ploughshare-like) bone. The floor of the nasal cavities is broad and slightly concave and formed by the hard palate. This floor consists of two sets of bones. The palatine processes of the maxillary bones (left and right upper jaws) form the front three-fourths of the hard palate, whereas the horizontal processes of the palatine bones form the back one-fourth of the structure (see Figure 4–1). The roof of the nasal cavities, in contrast to the floor, is quite narrow and formed by the cribriform plate of the ethmoid bone. The configuration of the two cavities is similar to the roofline of an A-frame house.

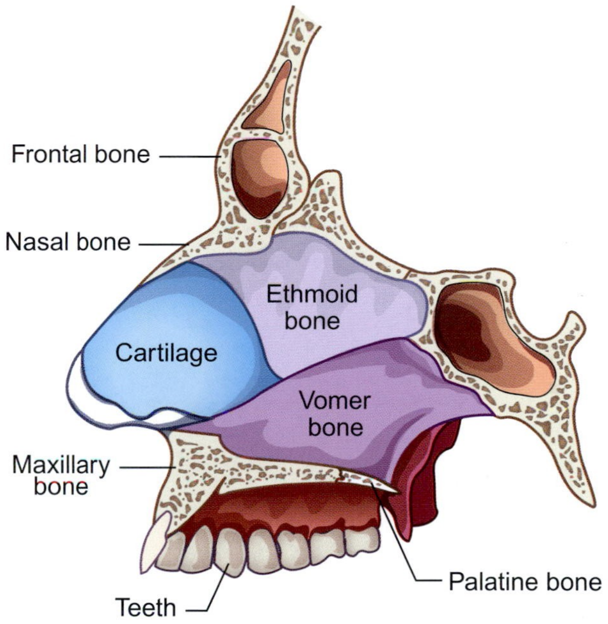

Figure 4–5. Components of the nasal septum. Selected other bones and teeth are shown for reference.

By far the most complex formations within the nasal cavities are located on its lateral walls. These formations are convoluted and labyrinthine and contain many nooks and crannies. Three shell-like structures give rise to this complexity. These structures are portrayed in Figure 4–6 and include the superior, middle, and inferior nasal conchae, formations that extend along the length of the nasal cavities. The nasal conchae, also called the nasal turbinates,

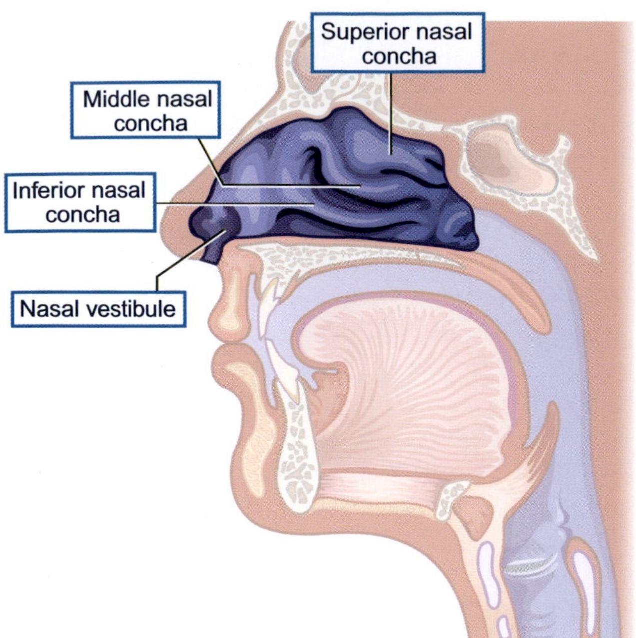

Figure 4–6. Superior, middle, and inferior nasal conchae.

have corresponding meatuses (passages) named for the conchae with which they are associated. The enfolding structure of the nasal cavities provides a large surface area to the inner nose and has a rich blood supply. A final structure of interest in each nasal cavity is the nasal vestibule, a modest dilation just inside the aperture of the anterior naris.

Outer Nose

Unlike the other components of the velopharyngeal-nasal apparatus, the parts of the outer nose are familiar to everyone, especially the surface features of the structure. The outer nose is, in fact, hard to ignore because it is in the center of the face and projects outward and downward conspicuously. The more prominent surface features of the outer nose include the root, bridge, dorsum, apex, alae, base, septum, and anterior nares, as shown in Figure 4–7.

The root (point of attachment) of the outer nose is to the bottom of the forehead. Following downward along the centerline are the bridge (upper bony part), dorsum (prominent upper surface), and apex (tip). The alae (wings) form much of the sides of the nose and contribute significantly to its general shape. The base of the nose constitutes the bottom of the structure, partitioned down the middle (more or less) by the lowermost part of the nasal septum, and including the anterior nares (nostrils). The anterior nares are also referred to as the external nares and are somewhat pear-shaped apertures that are typically about twice as long (front-to-back) as they are wide (side-to-side). The orientation of the plane of the apertures of the anterior nares varies among individuals, but most often ranges from horizontal to upwardly oblique toward the side. The two anterior nares are somewhat akin to the muzzle ends of the barrels of a side-by-side double-barreled

Disposing of Things

Mucus (a slimy substance) is formed in the nose to the tune of about half a pint a day (more when you have a cold). Particles filtered by the nose are collected in a blanket of mucus and moved through the nose by the action of cilia (tiny hair cells that collectively form a fringe). Things that get trapped are moved along toward the back of the throat and then swallowed into the stomach. Some material dries before reaching the back of the throat and fractionates into pieces containing filtered particles. This happens at different spots within the nose and in residues of various consistencies. Prim and proper folks refer to these residues as nasal exudates or pieces of dried nasal mucus. Most of us refer to them as "boogers." They are best gently blown into a tissue to rid them from the nose, but we all know other manual methods that are commonly practiced.

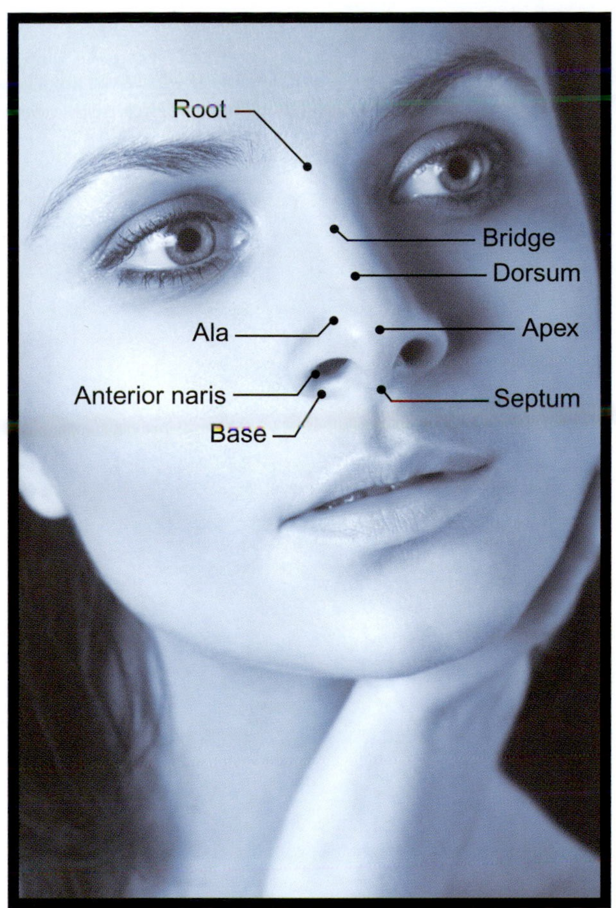

Figure 4–7. Surface features of the outer nose.

shotgun. Margins of the anterior nares include stiff hairs, called vibrissae. These hairs arrest the passage of particles riding on air currents.

Forces and Movements of the Velopharyngeal-Nasal Apparatus

Much of the functional potential of the velopharyngeal-nasal apparatus lies in its capacity for movement. This movement is caused by forces applied to and by different components of the apparatus.

Forces of the Velopharyngeal-Nasal Apparatus

The forces operating on the velopharyngeal-nasal apparatus are of two types—passive and active. Passive force is inherent and always present (although subject to change), whereas active force is applied depending on the will and ability of the individual. The passive and active forces operating on the velopharyngeal-nasal apparatus make up the total force functioning at different locations.

Passive Force. The passive force of velopharyngeal-nasal function arises from several sources. These include the natural recoil of muscles, cartilages, and connective tissues, the surface tension between structures in apposition, the pull of gravity, and aeromechanical forces within the upper airway (throat, mouth, and nose).

The distribution, sign, and magnitude of passive force depend on the prevailing mechanical conditions, including the positions, deformations, and levels of activity of different components of the velopharyngeal-nasal apparatus. For example, the pull of gravity differentially influences velopharyngeal-nasal function when body position is changed. Such influences are considered in detail below in another section.

Active Force. The active force of velopharyngeal-nasal function arises from muscles distributed within different components of the velopharyngeal-nasal apparatus. This active force results from the contraction of muscle fibers. The contribution of specific muscles to such force generation is not completely understood. Nevertheless, based on individual muscle architecture, consequences of muscle activation, and observations of the electrical activity of muscles during various activities, the probable roles of specific muscles can be specified with reasonable certainty.

The function described here for individual muscles assumes that the muscle under consideration is activated and involved in a shortening (concentric) contraction. Actually, the influence of individual muscle actions depends on whether or not related muscles are active, the mechanical status of different components of the velopharyngeal-nasal apparatus, and the nature of the activity being performed. The muscles of the pharynx, velum, and outer nose are considered below.

Muscles of the Pharynx. Figure 4–8 portrays the muscles of the pharynx. Six muscles within and

Back view

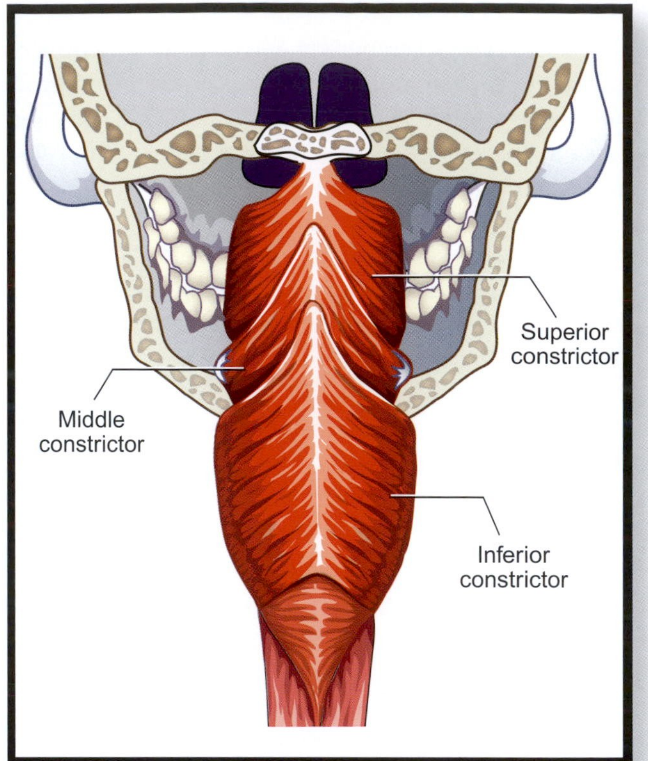

Side view

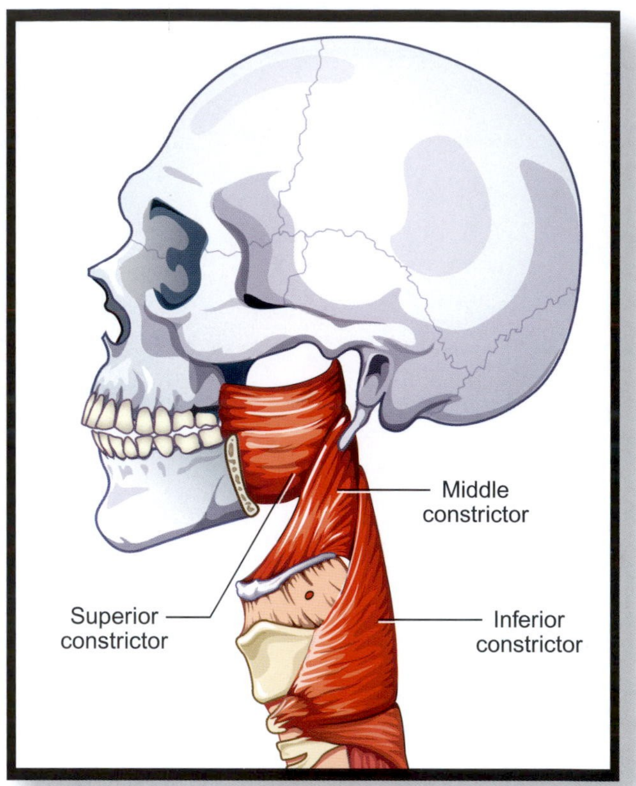

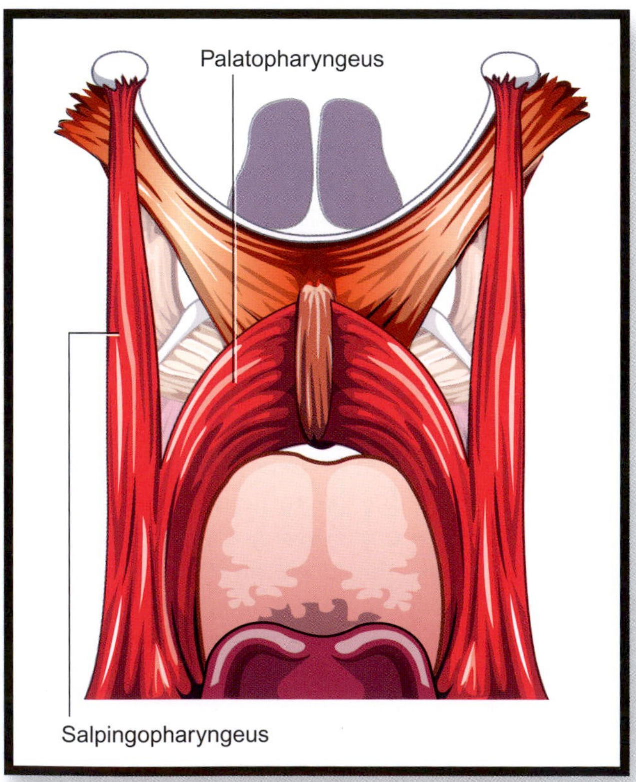

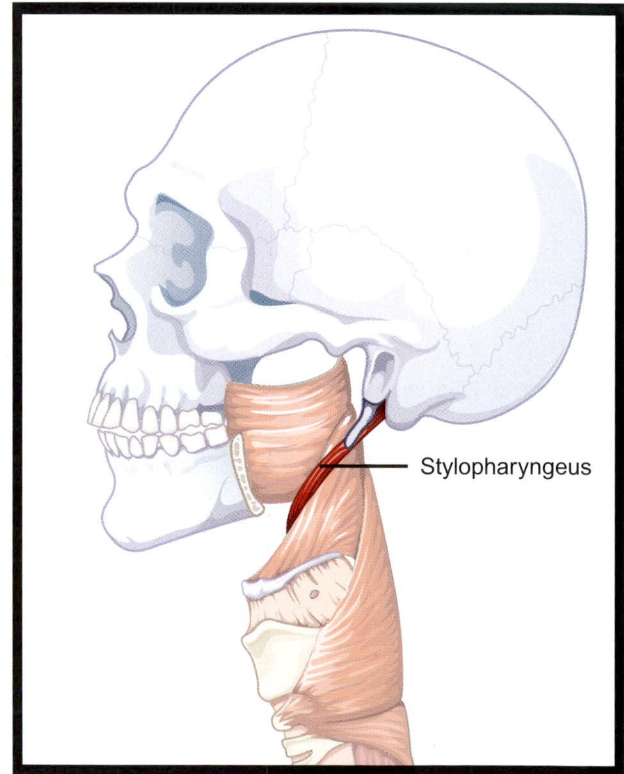

Figure 4–8. Muscles of the pharynx.

attached to the walls of the pharynx can influence the lumen of the pharyngeal tube (the cross section along its length). Of course, other structures along the front side of the pharynx can also influence the lumen of the pharynx through their adjustments (velum, tongue, and epiglottis).

The ***superior constrictor*** muscle is located in the upper part of the pharynx. It is a complex muscle with multiple origins that arise from the front of the pharyngeal tube. Front points of attachment include the medial pterygoid plate (of the sphenoid bone), the pterygomandibular ligament (a tendinous inscription between the ***superior constrictor*** muscle and the ***buccinator*** muscle, described in Chapter 5), the mylohyoid line (site of attachment of the ***mylohyoid*** muscle, described in Chapter 5, on the inner surface of the body of the mandible), and the side of the back part of the tongue. These multiple points of origin are sometimes used as a basis for conceptualizing the ***superior constrictor*** muscle as a cluster of four individual muscles. From top to bottom, these four are designated as the ***pterygopharyngeus***, ***buccopharyngeus***, ***mylopharyngeus***, and ***glossopharyngeus***. Fibers from the multiple origins of the ***superior constrictor*** muscle course backward, toward the midline, and upward to insert into the fibrous median raphe (seam) of the posterior pharyngeal wall. There, they join with fibers of the paired muscle from the opposite side. The uppermost fibers of the ***superior constrictor*** muscle are horizontal and located at the level of the velum. When the ***superior constrictor*** muscle contracts, it reduces the regional cross section of the pharyngeal lumen by forward movement of the posterior pharyngeal wall and forward and inward movement of the lateral pharyngeal wall. The paired ***superior constrictor*** muscles encircle the posterior and lateral walls of the upper pharynx (recall the radial tire analogy from above), so that their simultaneous contraction constricts the lumen of that part of the pharyngeal tube in the manner of a sphincter.

The ***middle constrictor*** muscle is a fan-shaped structure located midway along the length of the pharyngeal tube. Fibers of the muscle arise from the greater and lesser horns of the hyoid bone and the stylohyoid ligament (which runs between the downward and forward projecting styloid process of the temporal bone and the lesser horn of the hyoid bone) and radiate backward and toward the midline where they insert into the median raphe of the pharynx. The ***middle constrictor*** muscle is also sometimes conceptualized as comprising two muscles designated as the ***chondropharyngeus*** and ***ceratopharyngeus*** muscles. The uppermost fibers of the ***middle constrictor*** muscle course obliquely upward and overlap the lower fibers of the ***superior constrictor*** muscle, whereas the lowermost fibers of the muscle run obliquely downward beneath the fibers of the ***inferior constrictor*** muscle (discussed below). The middle fibers of the ***middle constrictor*** muscle run horizontally. The overlapping arrangement of the muscle fibers between the ***middle constrictor*** and ***superior constrictor*** muscles and between the ***inferior constrictor*** and ***middle constrictor*** muscles is akin to the way in which roof shingles partially overlap. When the ***middle constrictor*** muscle contracts, it decreases the cross section of the pharynx regionally, by virtue of forward movement of the posterior pharyngeal wall and forward and inward movement of the lateral pharyngeal wall. When the ***middle constrictor*** muscle acts in conjunction with its paired mate on the opposite side, the pharyngeal lumen is regionally constricted in the manner of a sphincter.

The ***inferior constrictor*** muscle is the most powerful of the three constrictor muscles of the pharynx. The fibers of this muscle arise from the sides of the thyroid and cricoid cartilages. The ***inferior constrictor*** muscle is sometimes thought of as consisting of two muscles. These are referred to as the ***thyropharyngeus*** and ***cricopharyngeus*** muscles. From the origins noted, fibers of the ***inferior constrictor*** muscle diverge in a fan-like configuration and course backward and toward the midline. There, they interdigitate with fibers from the ***inferior constrictor*** muscle of the opposite side at the median raphe of the pharyngeal tube. The middle and upper fibers of the ***inferior constrictor*** muscle ascend obliquely, whereas the lowermost fibers run horizontally and downward and are continuous with those of the esophagus. When the ***inferior constrictor*** muscle contracts, it draws the lower part of the posterior wall of the pharynx forward and pulls the lateral walls of the lower pharynx forward and inward. This action, in conjunction with that of the ***inferior constrictor*** muscle on the opposite side, constricts the lumen of the lower pharynx.

The ***salpingopharyngeus*** muscle is a narrow muscle that arises from near the lower border of the pharyngeal orifice of the eustachian tube. The fibers of the muscle course downward vertically and insert into the lateral wall of the lower pharynx where they blend with fibers of the ***palatopharyngeus*** muscle (discussed below). When the ***salpingopharyngeus*** muscle contracts, it pulls the lateral wall of the pharynx upward and inward. Acting simultaneously with its paired muscle from the opposite side, the effect achieved is one of decreasing the width of the pharynx.

The ***stylopharyngeus*** muscle is a slender muscle that runs a relatively long course. It originates from the styloid process of the temporal bone and runs downward, forward, and toward the midline. Most fibers of the muscle insert into the lateral wall of the pharynx at and near the juncture of the ***superior constrictor*** and ***middle constrictor*** muscles. Some fibers extend lower in the pharyngeal wall and insert into the thyroid cartilage. When the ***stylopharyngeus*** muscle contracts, it pulls upward on the pharyngeal tube and draws the lateral wall of the pharynx toward the side. Together with similar action of its paired mate from the opposite side, there results a widening of the lumen of the pharynx in the region where the muscle fibers insert into the lateral walls of the pharyngeal tube. There is also an upward pull placed on the larynx when the ***stylopharyngeus*** muscles contract.

The ***palatopharyngeus*** muscle runs the length of the pharynx and is a pharyngeal muscle. At the same time, it is also a muscle of the soft palate and in that context is called the ***pharyngopalatine*** muscle. The muscle is considered here from the pharyngeal perspective. The ***palatopharyngeus*** muscle arises mainly from the soft palate. The uppermost fibers are directed horizontally and intermingle with fibers of the ***superior constrictor*** muscle. A major fiber course is downward and toward the side through the posterior faucial pillar. Below the pillar, the fibers continue into the lower half of the pharynx and spread to the lateral wall of the structure and the thyroid cartilage. Some have suggested that the portion of the muscle that attaches to the thyroid cartilage be given recognition of its own as the ***palatothyroideus*** muscle (Cassell & Elkadi, 1995), whereas others disagree (Moon & Kuehn, 2004). When the velum is relatively stable, contraction of the ***palatopharyngeus*** muscle results in two movements. The uppermost fibers of the muscle draw the lateral pharyngeal wall inward to complement the action of the ***superior constrictor*** muscle of the pharynx, whereas the lowermost fibers of the muscle pull upward on the lateral pharyngeal wall and elevate the pharynx (attachments to the thyroid cartilage also effect an upward and forward pull on the larynx).

Figure 4–9 graphically illustrates the general force vectors for the six muscles of the pharynx discussed in this section. This illustration summarizes the potential active forces operating on the pharynx and shows the combinations of forces that could be in play at any moment to decrease or increase the lumen of the pharynx and/or change its positioning.

Having it Both Ways

A muscle is usually thought of as having an origin and an insertion. The origin is its anchored end and the insertion is its movable end. This is all well and good in textbooks, but in real life things are a bit more complicated. What may be the anchored end of a muscle for one activity may be the movable end of that muscle for another activity. A lot of it has to do with what neighboring muscles are doing. Thus, a muscle's function may change from time to time because various forces cause the mobility of its two ends to change in relation to one another. The convention adopted in the main text is to reflect such change by alternately labeling a muscle in accordance with its perceived primary function in a given context. Some purists may not embrace this convention, but it carries instructive power and simply points out that in the busy world of the muscle, turnabout is fair play.

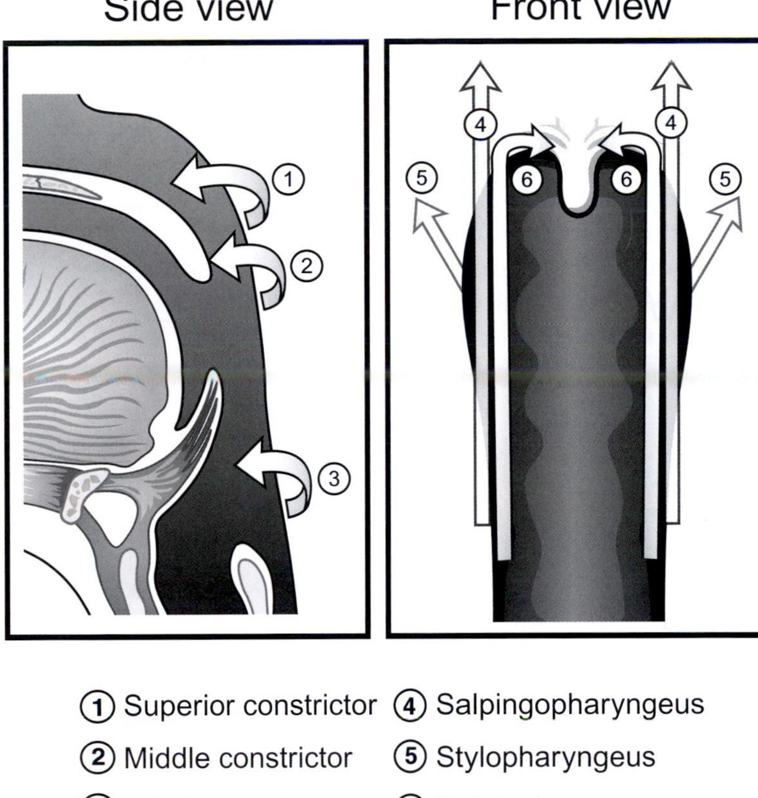

Figure 4–9. Summary of force vectors of the muscles of the pharynx.

Muscles of the Velum. Figure 4–10 illustrates the muscles of the velum. The five muscles shown can influence the positioning, configuration, and mechanical status of the structure.

The ***palatal levator*** muscle (also called the ***levator veli palatini*** muscle) forms much of the bulk of the velum. The ***palatal levator*** muscle is a cylindrical structure that arises from the petrous (hard) portion of the temporal bone and from the cartilaginous portion of the eustachian tube. From there, it courses downward, forward, and toward the midline, passing on the outside of the posterior naris. Fibers of the ***palatal levator*** muscle insert into the side of the velum and spread out where they join those of the ***palatal levator*** muscle from the opposite side. The spread of muscle fibers in each of the ***palatal levator*** muscles is to the midline and beyond to the other side of the velum (Kuehn & Moon, 2005). Fibers extend from behind the hard palate to the front of the uvula, encompassing approximately the middle 40% of the velum (Boorman & Sommerlad, 1985) or more (Kuehn & Kahane, 1990). The paired ***palatal levator*** muscles form a muscular sling from their cranial attachments through the velum. Each ***palatal levator*** muscle inserts into the velum at an angle of about 45°. When the ***palatal levator*** muscle contracts, it draws the velum upward and backward. Simultaneous contraction of the paired ***palatal levator*** muscles lifts the velum toward the posterior pharyngeal wall along an angular trajectory. Kuehn and Kahane (1990) have concluded that the force resulting from contraction of the ***palatal levator*** muscles is spread over a considerable distance within the soft palate. The significance of this observation is that it favors a potentially broad velum-to-pharynx contact area. Apposition between the velum and the posterior pharyngeal wall happens frequently and may involve significant contact forces. The upper surface of the velum consists of stratified squamous epithelium and is favorably composed to withstand such contact forces. Apposition between the velum and the posterior pharyngeal wall may also involve frictional forces associated with the velum sliding up and down the posterior

toward the middle of the velum. The hooked appearance of the velum results in identifiable landmarks during movement. The top of the hook (on the upper surface of the velum) is referred to as the velar eminence and the undersurface of the hook (on the lower surface of the velum) is designated as the dimple of the velum.

Movements of the Outer Nose. Movements of the outer nose result mainly from outward or inward movements of the nasal alae and may change the cross sections of the apertures of the anterior nares (nostrils). Under most circumstances, these movements are small. Exceptions occur during certain breathing events (see below), when signaling emotions (disdain, contempt, and anger), and when using the nares to slow the flow of air from the outer nose by increasing resistance at its exit ports.

Adjustments of the Velopharyngeal-Nasal Apparatus

The velopharyngeal-nasal apparatus is capable of many adjustments. The present discussion is limited to those adjustments that influence the degree of coupling between the oral and nasal cavities (through the velopharyngeal port) and between the nasal cavities and atmosphere (through the apertures of the anterior nares). Adjustments of lower parts of the pharynx are considered in Chapter 5 and Chapter 12.

Coupling Between the Oral and Nasal Cavities

The degree of coupling between the oral and nasal cavities can be adjusted. Such adjustment has a bearing on the size of the velopharyngeal port (the usual opening between the oral and nasal cavities). The range of possibilities extends from a fully open port to a fully closed port.

The velopharyngeal port is open most of the time to accommodate nasal breathing. Closure of the port can be brought about through action of the velum and/or pharynx. Combined action of the two structures is often described as a flap-sphincter action, the flap being movement of the velum and the sphincter being movement of the pharynx.

There is no universal pattern for achieving velopharyngeal closure. On the contrary, several movement strategies for achieving closure of the velopharyngeal port have been identified that involve different actions or combinations of actions of the velum, lateral pharyngeal walls, and posterior pharyngeal wall (Croft, Shprintzen, & Rakoff, 1981; Finkelstein et al., 1995; Poppelreuter, Engelke, & Bruns, 2000; Shprintzen, 1992; Skolnik, McCall, & Barnes, 1973). These movement strategies are illustrated in Figure 4–15 and include (a) elevation of the velum alone, (b) inward movement of the lateral pharyngeal walls alone, (c) elevation of the velum combined with inward movement of the lateral pharyngeal walls, and (d) elevation of the velum com-

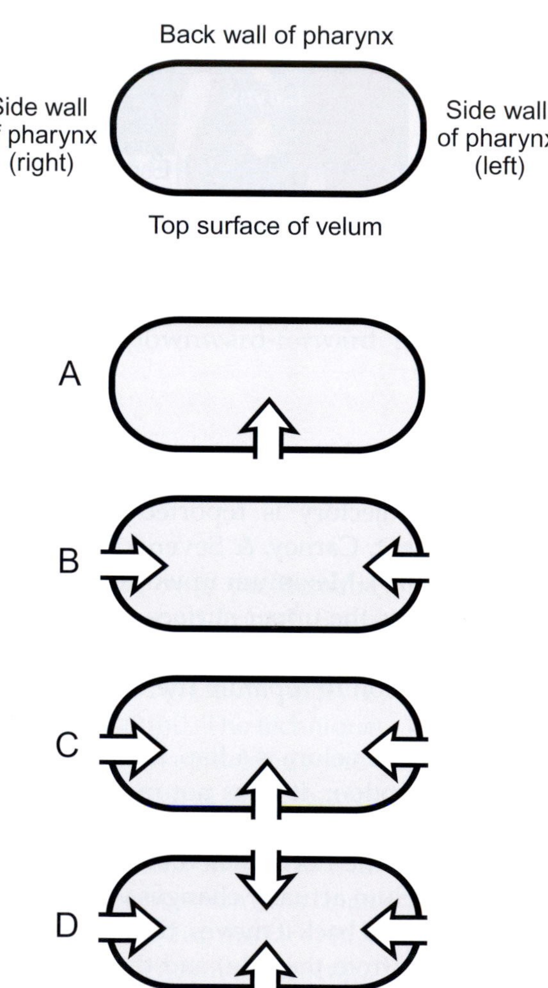

Figure 4–15. Patterns of velopharyngeal closure as seen from above.

bined with inward movement of the lateral pharyngeal walls and forward movement of the posterior pharyngeal wall.

The prevailing wisdom is that these different movement strategies for achieving closure are rooted in differences in anatomy of the velopharyngeal region (Finkelstein et al., 1995). For example, individuals with smaller front-to-back than side-to-side dimensions to the resting velopharyngeal port are more likely to use elevation of the velum alone as the strategy for achieving closure of the port than are individuals with other port configurations. Also, individuals with more nearly equal front-to-back and side-to-side dimensions to the velopharyngeal port are more likely to use inward movement of the lateral walls of the pharynx alone or simultaneous elevation of the velum and inward movement of the lateral walls of the pharynx as the strategy for achieving closure.

It should also be noted that different movement strategies for achieving closure of the velopharyngeal port are not fixed within individuals, but can change over time as velopharyngeal anatomy changes. For example, the nasopharyngeal tonsil (called the adenoids when abnormally enlarged) is often large in young children and enables closure to be achieved solely by elevation of the velum against its mass. This mass atrophies with age, however, and elevation of the velum without other adjustments of the pharynx may no longer be sufficient to achieve closure of the velopharyngeal port (Finkelstein, Berger, Nachmani, & Ophir, 1996; Siegel-Sadewitz, & Shprintzen, 1986). More is said about this under the section on the development of velopharyngeal-nasal function in speech production. For now, the important thing to know is that strategies for achieving velopharyngeal closure are subject to modification with changes in velopharyngeal anatomy.

The positioning of the velum in the adjustment of oral-nasal coupling is most often attributed to action of the ***palatal levator*** muscles (Dickson, 1972). Thought has typically been that lifting of the structure follows from the contractile force provided by these muscles and accounts for the midportion of the velum usually attaining the highest elevation during closure of the velopharyngeal port (Bell-Berti, 1976; Fritzell, 1963; Lubker, 1968; Seaver & Kuehn, 1980). Although action of the ***palatal levator*** muscles seems to be clearly associated with the flap component of the flap-sphincter closure adjustment, correlations between ***palatal levator*** activity and the elevation of the velum are weaker (albeit positive) than would be expected were the ***palatal levator*** muscles alone responsible for positioning the velum (Fritzell, 1979; Lubker, 1968). This suggests that other muscles must also be active in positioning the velum. Research, in fact, supports this inference.

Kuehn, Folkins, and Cutting (1982) made observations of the electrical activity of muscles of the velopharyngeal-nasal apparatus and related these observations to lateral x-ray images of the position of the velum. Muscles capable of exerting upward and downward force on the velum were among those studied. Kuehn et al. found that the different combinations of activity among the ***palatal levator***, ***glossopalatine***, and ***pharyngopalatine*** muscles were associated with the same positioning of the velum, suggesting a trading relationship among them.

The same three muscles have also been considered as a coordinative system in which function-based interaction rules prevail. Moon, Smith, Folkins, Lemke, and Gartlan (1994b), for example, studied the relative contributions of the ***palatal levator***, ***glossopalatine***, and ***pharyngopalatine*** muscles to a range of voluntary adjustments of the velopharynx performed as subjects visually monitored (via a phototransduction system) the relative opening of the velopharyngeal port. Based on multivariate statistical modeling, these authors concluded that these three velar muscles form a coordinative system in which voluntary adjustments of the velopharyngeal port are flexible and allow for different combinations of muscle activation. Clearly, classical notions of the velum being controlled by the ***palatal levator*** muscles alone are inadequate.

Finally, it is important to note that closing and opening adjustments of the velopharyngeal port are controlled by different factors. Closing adjustments are predominated by muscular forces that must overcome the passive forces of the velopharyngeal-nasal apparatus. Opening adjustments, in contrast, also involve muscular forces, but are usually aided by passive forces, such as the natural recoil of muscle and connective tissue and the pull of gravity (in upright body positions).

Coupling Between the Nasal Cavities and Atmosphere

The degree of coupling between the nasal cavities and atmosphere can be adjusted by changing the size of the anterior nares. The range of possibilities extends from fully open nares to fully closed nares. It is also possible to have different degrees of coupling for the two nares (one being open more than the other).

The anterior nares, like the velopharynx, are relatively open most of the time to accommodate nasal breathing. Dilation or constriction of the nares can be brought about through the actions of muscles of the outer nose. Such actions can be either opposed or supplemented by aeromechanical forces associated with breathing. For example, muscles that dilate the anterior nares may activate to resist the tendency of the nares to collapse in response to low pressures in their lumina. The need for such activation can be appreciated by sniffing briskly while watching the outer nose in a mirror. Both the nares and alae of the outer nose tend to be sucked inward by the lowering of nasal pressures. More forceful inspirations require increasingly forceful contractions of nasal dilators to maintain patent nares (Bridger, 1970).

Although dilation of the nares is more commonly associated with normal function than is constriction, there are times during expiration when the braking of airflow through the nose may be effected by constriction of the anterior nares. Such constriction is like putting "chokes" on the muzzle ends of the barrels in the double-barreled shotgun analogy mentioned above. An exaggerated version of such constriction is often observed in individuals with velopharyngeal incompetence. Referred to clinically as "nares constriction," this is often taken as a cardinal sign of velopharyngeal dysfunction and is thought to represent an attempt to valve the airstream to compensate for an inability to valve it at the velopharynx (Warren, Hairfield, & Hinton, 1985).

Control Variables of Velopharyngeal-Nasal Function

Several control variables are important in velopharyngeal-nasal function. Their relative significance depends on the particular activity being performed, whether it is breathing, speech production, singing, blowing, sucking, swallowing, gagging, whistling, wind instrument playing, or glass blowing, among others. For example, speech production involves control variables based on acoustical goals, whereas tidal breathing does not. And, for another example, the force with which the velopharynx is closed may be an important variable for an activity that calls for very high oral air pressure (glass blowing), but be a less important variable for an activity with low oral air pressure demands (whispering). For persons with a normally functioning velopharyngeal-nasal apparatus, the most significant features of control pertain to the velopharyngeal portion of the apparatus. There are times, however, when control of the outer nose can become important.

For purposes of this chapter, attention is devoted to three control variables that influence aeromechanical and acoustical aspects of velopharyngeal-nasal function. These include (a) the magnitude of the airway resistance offered by the velopharyngeal-nasal apparatus, (b) the magnitude of the muscular pressure exerted by the velopharyngeal sphincter to accomplish and maintain velopharyngeal closure, and (c) the magnitude of the acoustical impedance offered by the velopharyngeal-nasal apparatus.

Velopharyngeal-Nasal Airway Resistance

Resistance is defined, in a mechanical sense, as opposition to movement and results in a loss of energy through friction (similar to that of direct current in an electrical circuit). As portrayed in Figure 4–16, velopharyngeal-nasal airway resistance has to do with opposition to the mass flow of air (the breath) across the velopharyngeal port, nasal cavities, and outer nose.

Conceptualizing these three structures as resistors, adjustment of any of them can effect a change in airway resistance between the oral cavity and atmosphere through the nasal route. Thus, adjusting the cross section and/or length of the velopharyngeal port, changing the engorgement of the nasal cavities, or adjusting the cross section of the anterior nares, can all have consequences for the airway resistance across the velopharyngeal-nasal apparatus. Resistance is also airflow dependent. This means that it increases and decreases with increases and decreases in the rate at which air moves, even with-

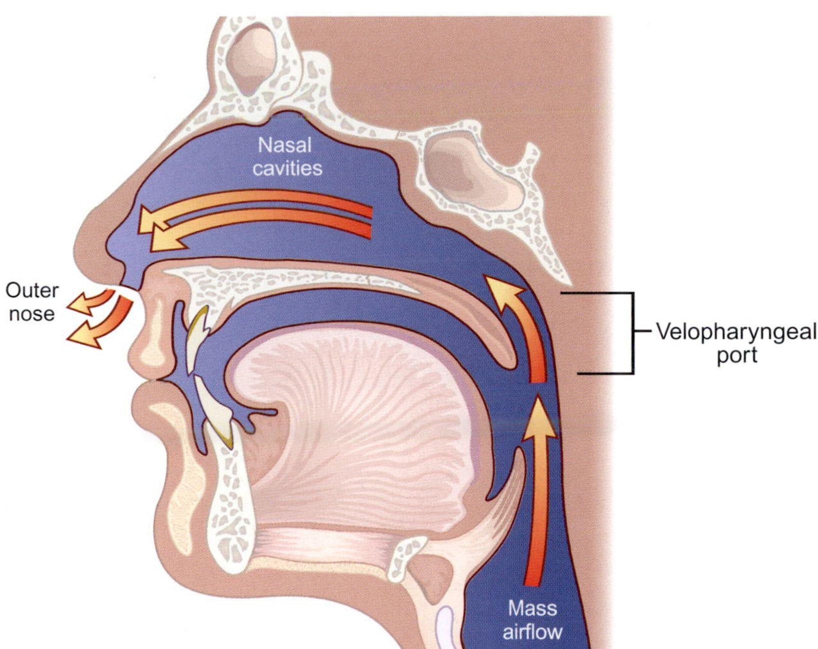

Figure 4–16. Components of velopharyngeal-nasal airway resistance.

out changes in the physical dimensions of the velopharyngeal-nasal airway.

The range of potential airway resistance values is large and can go from less than 1.0 cmH_2O/LPS (following the administration of a decongestant) to infinity (completely obstructed). Infinite airway resistance is usually effected through airtight closure of the velopharyngeal port. Obviously, once airtight closure is attained through airtight velopharyngeal closure, adjustments of the nasal cavities and outer nose have no further effect on the value of the resistance. Infinite velopharyngeal-nasal airway resistance can also be achieved in the case of an open velopharynx under circumstances where there is complete nasal blockage.

As should be clear from this discussion, the status of all parts of the velopharyngeal-nasal apparatus needs to be known to fully understand their influences on the movement of aeromechanical energy back and forth between the oral cavity and atmosphere via the nasal route. Historically, focus has been on the status of the velopharyngeal port alone, with little or no consideration given to the nasal cavities and outer nose in normal speakers. This limited focus is now known to have confounded certain interpretations of mechanism of velopharyngeal function and dysfunction.

Velopharyngeal Sphincter Compression

Once airtight velopharyngeal closure is attained, the force of that closure can be adjusted to meet the needs of the situation. This force, depicted in Figure 4–17, is represented by the compressive muscular pressure exerted to maintain the velopharyngeal sphincter in a closed configuration. The muscular pressure exerted at any moment must exceed the magnitude of the air pressure difference across the velopharyngeal sphincter (whether it be positive or negative) to prevent the velopharynx from being forced (blown or sucked) open. Thus, although the force required to effect airtight velopharyngeal closure for a minimally effortful activity may be low, that for an activity involving high positive oral air pressure must be high.

Certain individuals who routinely employ high oral air pressures are prone to develop stress-induced velopharyngeal incompetence. Woodwind and brass instrument players, who fall into this category, have a surprisingly high prevalence of velopharyngeal incompetence (Schwab & Schulze-Florey, 2004). Most frequently affected are those who play the oboe and clarinet (instruments with high oral air pressure and high oral airflow demands, respectively). Unfortunately, velopharyngeal incompetence in performing

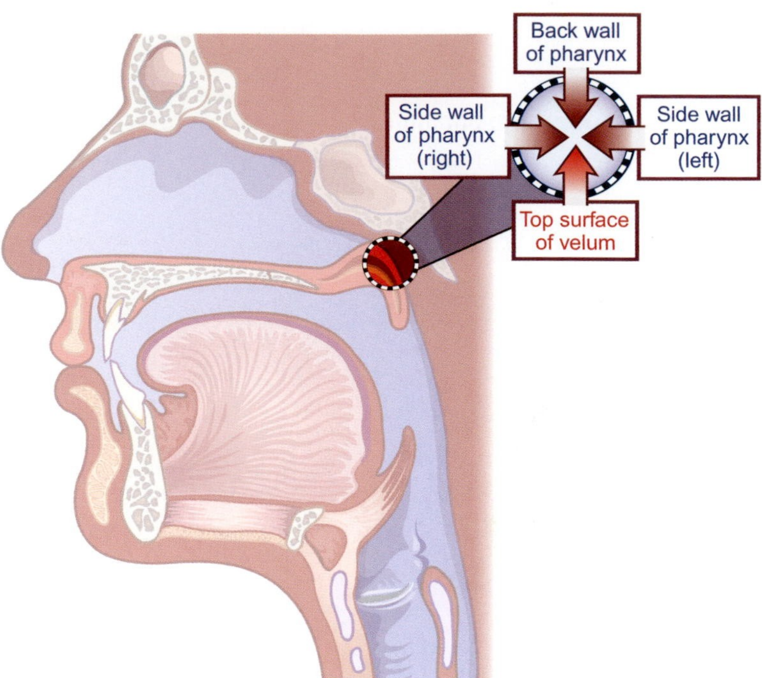

Figure 4–17. Compressive muscular pressure during velopharyngeal closure.

musicians often goes undiagnosed and is mistakenly rationalized as declining performance ability rather than a curable performance problem (Klotz, Howard, Hengerer, & Slupchynskj, 2001).

Velopharyngeal-Nasal Acoustic Impedance

Certain aspects of acoustic (sound) control are made possible through actions of the velopharyngeal-nasal apparatus. These actions influence acoustic impedance, which, like airway resistance, involves opposition to flow. In the case of acoustic impedance, however, the flow is of a different type and the opposition is frequency dependent (similar to that of an alternating current in an electrical circuit). The acoustic impedance offered by the velopharyngeal-nasal apparatus does not pertain to the mass flow of air but to the rapid to-and-fro bumping of air molecules in which each stays in a very restricted region and passes energy on to its neighbors. As portrayed in Figure 4–18, acoustic impedance influences flow propagation in waves (sounds, not breath). The acoustic impedance of concern here is that distributed across the velopharyngeal port, nasal cavities, and outer nose.

As discussed above, the velopharyngeal port can be adjusted to influence the degree of coupling between the oral and nasal cavities. When the port is closed, the pharyngeal-oral airway and nasal airway are separated. Thus, nearly all of the sound energy passes through the pharyngeal-oral airway and the acoustic impedance looking into the nasal cavities from their velopharyngeal end is nearly infinite. (A small amount of sound energy may be transmitted through the closed velopharynx via sympathetic vibration, such as when the velum acts like a drumhead.)

When the velopharyngeal port is open, the oral and nasal cavities are free to exchange sound energy and interact with one another acoustically, and sound energy may pass between the outer nose and atmosphere. Changes in the size of the velopharyngeal port are important to determining how sound energy is divided between the oral and nasal cavities. Also important are configurations of the oral and nasal cavities themselves and the extent to which each impedes the flow of sound energy. In the case of the nasal part of the system, degree of engorgement of the nasal cavities and status of the anterior nares are relevant factors.

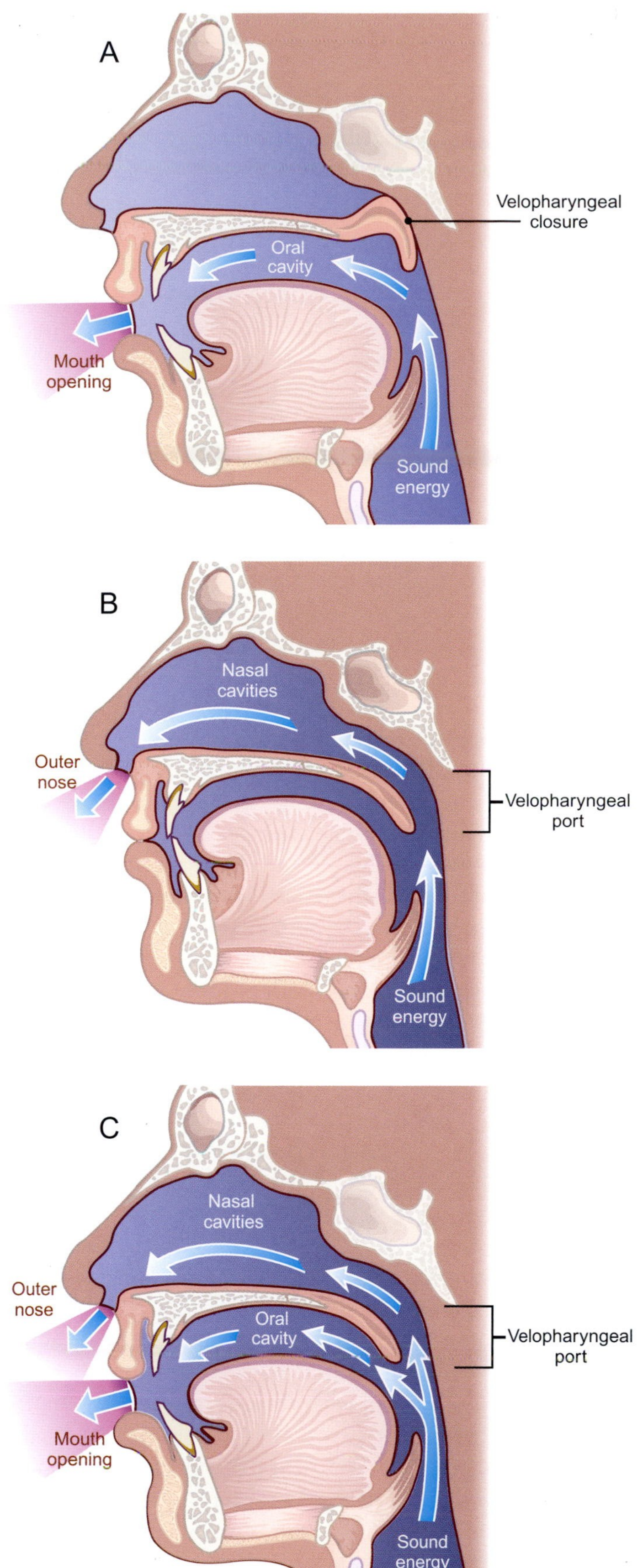

Figure 4–18. Oral-nasal sound wave propagation in relation to acoustic impedance.

Which Hunt

It is often stated that velopharyngeal incompetence or insufficiency allows air to pass into the nasal cavities causing hypernasality. This is a misconception. Significant quantities of air can pass into the nasal cavities through the velopharynx during utterance without there being a perception of hypernasality. As well, hypernasality may occur during utterance when no air is passing into the nasal cavities, such as when the covering tissue of a submucous cleft palate vibrates and excites the nasal cavities into sympathetic vibration. Flow of air into the nose does not cause hypernasality. In fact, hypernasality may be present when inspiratory speech is produced and airflow is passing through the nasal cavities in the opposite direction from usual. It's instructive to go through written discussions about velopharyngeal dysfunction and see which authors get it right and which authors get it wrong. Think of it as sort of a "which" hunt.

The greater proportion of sound energy will be directed through the airway (oral or nasal) having the lower acoustic impedance. Thus, the distribution of sound energy between the two airways will be inversely proportional to the ratio between their respective acoustic impedances (Curtis, 1968; Fant, 1960). This ratio will, of course, differ in accordance with the prevailing configurations of the two pathways and in relation to the spectral content of the sounds passing through. Chapter 8 provides a much more detailed discussion of the effects of oral-nasal coupling on speech.

Neural Substrates of Velopharyngeal-Nasal Control

Velopharyngeal-nasal movement is controlled by the nervous system, but the nature of that movement and the nature of its control differ with the activity being performed. That is, different parts of the nervous system take charge of different components of the velopharyngeal-nasal apparatus for different types of velopharyngeal-nasal activities. For example, neural control of the apparatus is different for sneezing, blowing, swallowing, and speaking. Control of velopharyngeal-nasal function in swallowing is covered in Chapter 12 and control of velopharyngeal-nasal function in speech production is discussed here.

Although different parts of the central nervous system are responsible for the control of the velopharyngeal-nasal activities, control commands are, nonetheless, sent through the same set of cranial nerves to muscles. These nerves originate in the brainstem and course outward to provide motor innervation to the pharynx, velum, and outer nose. As shown in Table 4–1, motor innervation of the pharynx and velum is effected through the pharyngeal plexus, a network that includes fibers from cranial nerves IX (glossopharyngeal), X (vagus), and possibly XI (accessory). An exception is found in the case of the ***palatal tensor*** muscle within the velum, whose motor innervation is provided by cranial nerve V (trigeminal). There may also be additional motor innervation to the pharynx and velum through cranial nerve VII (facial), especially related to the ***palatal levator*** and ***uvulus*** muscles. Motor innervation to the outer nose is effected by cranial nerve VII.

One might think that information about the motor nerve supply to different parts of the velopharyngeal-nasal apparatus would be straightforward and agreed upon. This is, indeed, the case for motor innervation to the outer nose, but not for motor innervation to the pharynx and velum. This

Table 4–1. Summary of the Motor and Sensory Nerve Supply to the Pharynx, Velum, and Outer Nose Components of the Velopharyngeal-Nasal Apparatus. The pharyngeal plexus is a network that includes cranial nerves IX (glossopharyngeal), X (vagus), and possibly XI (accessory). Other cranial nerves indicated in the table are V (trigeminal) and VII (facial).

	INNERVATION	
COMPONENT	MOTOR	SENSORY
Pharynx	Pharyngeal Plexus	V, VII, IX, X
Velum	Pharyngeal Plexus (except ***palatal tensor*** muscle, which is innervated by V)	V, VII, IX, X
Outer Nose	VII	V

Note: There may be additional motor innervation from cranial nerve VII to certain muscles of the pharynx and velum, especially the ***palatal levator*** muscle and ***uvulus*** muscle (Shimokawa, Yi, & Tanaka, 2005).

is because the linkage between specific cranial nerves and the motor supply to specific muscles is equivocal in some cases (Cassell & Elkadi, 1995; Dickson, 1972; Moon & Kuehn, 2004) and because conducting research on motor nerve function in the velopharyngeal-nasal region of human beings is extremely difficult (Kuehn & Perry, 2008).

Sensory innervation to the pharynx and velum is effected through cranial nerves V, VII, IX, and X. Sensory innervation to the outer nose is effected through cranial nerve V. Neural information traveling along the sensory nerve supply from the pharynx, velum, and outer nose comes from receptors that respond to various types of stimuli, including mechanical stimuli. For example, receptors located in the mucosa of the velum and pharynx respond to light touch and receptors located in and near the velopharyngeal-nasal muscles relay information about muscle length and tension.

Much of incoming information from the velopharyngeal-nasal apparatus is not sensed or perceived. This seems to be especially true for the velopharyngeal portion of the apparatus. For example, the potential for sensing the position of the velum in space (proprioception) and its movement (kinesthesia) is believed to be rudimentary or nonexistent. Empirical evidence for this can be found in studies in which normal speakers have been shown to have difficulty controlling velopharyngeal movements voluntarily (Ruscello, 1982; Shelton, Beaumont, Trier, & Furr, 1978). Thus, it seems likely that control of the velopharyngeal apparatus relies more heavily on other types of information, such as that associated with the sensing of air pressure and airflow (Liss, Kuehn, & Hinkle, 1994; Warren, Dalston, & Dalston, 1990) and that associated with the sensing of the acoustic signal (Netsell, 1990) via cranial nerve VIII (auditory).

Motor and sensory inputs are undoubtedly important for programming and controlling the velopharyngeal-nasal apparatus (Lubker, 1975). General models of motor skill acquisition and maintenance, in fact, rely heavily on motor and sensory substrates for control of the speech production apparatus (Kent, 1981; Schmitt, 1982). However, it is widely recognized that there is a need for additional information regarding the neural substrates of velopharyngeal-nasal control before there is a complete understanding of the motor and sensory capabilities of the normal apparatus (Kuehn & Perry, 2008; Liss, 1990).

Ventilation and Velopharyngeal-Nasal Function

Recall from Chapter 2 that ventilation is the movement of air in and out of the pulmonary apparatus for the purpose of gas exchange. This movement of air can be routed through the nose, the mouth, or both.

Resting tidal breathing usually occurs through the nose alone (unless there is obstruction in the velopharyngeal-nasal apparatus) in a rhythmical to-and-fro fashion. During inspiration, the nasal cavities function to warm, moisten, and filter air on its way from the atmosphere to the pulmonary apparatus. During expiration, the nasal cavities retain the warmth and moisture in air on its way from the pulmonary apparatus to the atmosphere. Three important aspects of velopharyngeal-nasal function for ventilation are nasal valve modulation, nasal cycling (side-to-side), and nasal-oral switching, and are discussed below.

Nasal Valve Modulation

The nose is a major source of resistance to the flow of air during breathing. This resistance is governed mainly by nasal patency and may be altered by many factors, including infection, trauma, emotion, air temperature, and eating hot food, among others (Bridger, 1970). Figure 4–19 suggests a novel solution for coping with one of the factors sometimes brought on when eating hot food, a runny nose.

In the normal upper airway, the greatest resistance to airflow occurs toward the front ends of the nasal passages in what are called the nasal valves. As portrayed in Figure 4–20, each nasal valve (left and right) comprises two components, an external valve and an internal valve.

The external nasal valve is contained in the vestibule of the nose and constitutes a vault formed by the nasal floor, nasal rim, and nasal septum. The nasal muscles can adjust the external valve in ways

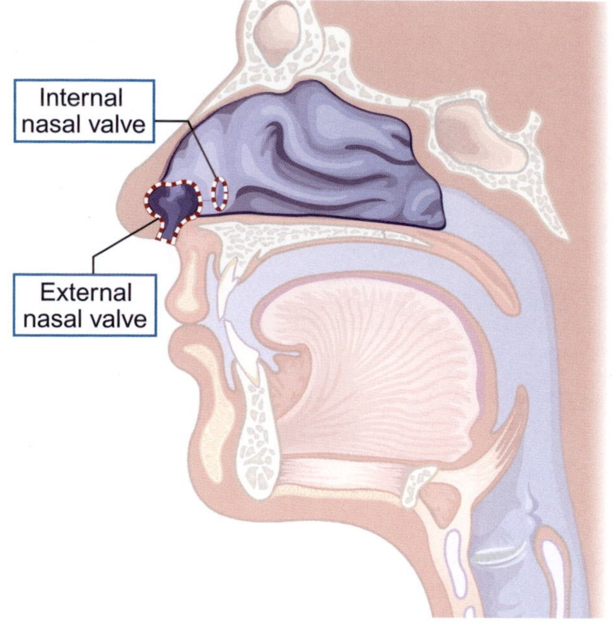

Figure 4–20. External and internal nasal valves.

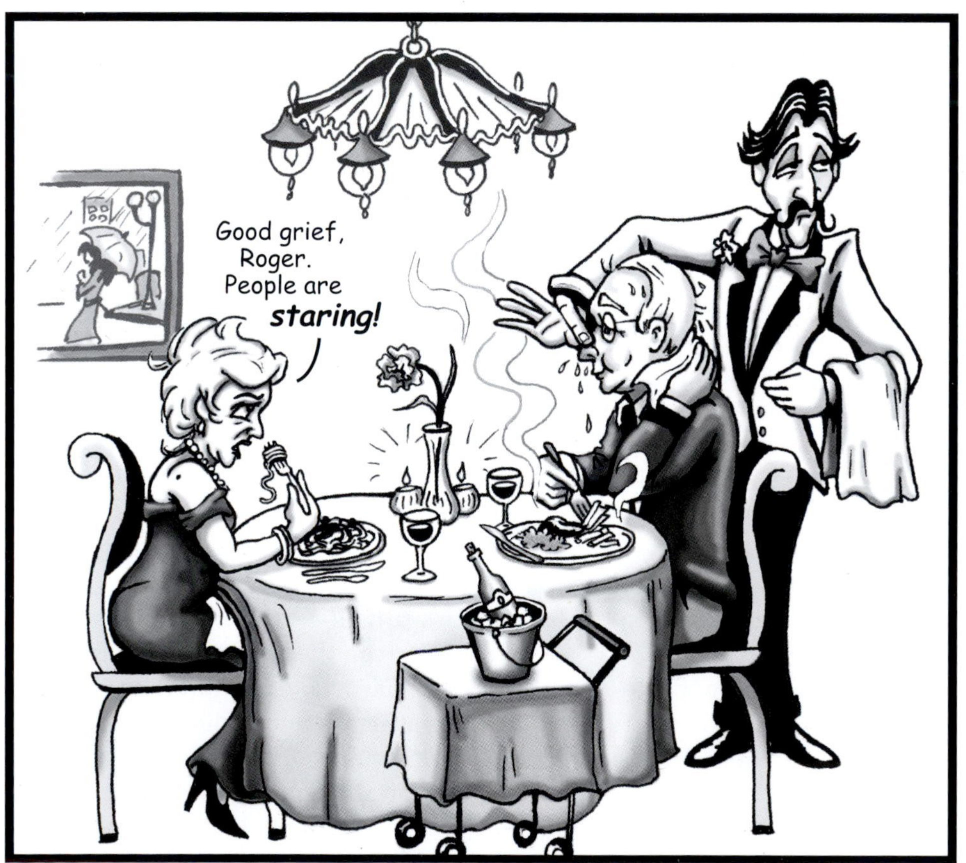

Figure 4–19. Cartoon showing a chic way to cope with a runny nose when eating hot food.

that dilate, constrict, and/or change its configuration. Either side of the outer nose is subject to collapse when the pressure difference across its ala is sufficiently negative. Nasal muscles that dilate an anterior naris increase the rigidity of the external valve and change the pressure that would close it to a more negative value, whereas nasal muscles that constrict an anterior naris make the critical pressure less negative (Bridger, 1970). Active dilation of the external valve occurs with inspiration and parallels active dilation in other parts of the breathing airway, such as the pharynx and larynx (Cole, 1976; Drettner, 1979).

The internal nasal valve is an orifice that forms the transition between the vestibule and the osseous nasal cavity (fossa) on each side just in front of the inferior nasal turbinate (Stoksted, 1953). The cross-sectional area of the internal nasal valve is the smallest found in the nasal airway and accounts for up to two-thirds of the resistance to airflow through the velopharyngeal-nasal apparatus during inspiration (Foster, 1962). Based on its anatomic (Proctor, 1982) and airflow-resistive (Hairfield, Warren, Hinton, & Seaton, 1987) characteristics, this valve is considered to be the main regulator of the nasal airway. The internal nasal valve is an active participant in tidal breathing. Specifically, it becomes larger during inspiration and smaller during expiration (Hairfield et al., 1987). This pattern is maintained when the external nasal valve is fixed in size by the insertion of relatively rigid tubing through the anterior nares into the nasal vestibules, indicating that adjustments of the anterior nares and alae are not responsible for the effect. The precise mechanism of regulation of the internal nasal valve is unknown.

Although the effort it takes to breathe is about three times greater through the nose than through the mouth, the nasal route typically prevails. This may be because nasal breathing is important to ensuring adequate alveolar gas exchange (Hairfield et al., 1987). It has been suggested that the larynx acts as an expiratory brake during tidal breathing to lengthen expiration and, thereby, enhance alveolar gas exchange (Gautier, Remmers, & Bartlett, 1973), and that an adequate brake also requires in-series braking by the nasal airway (Jackson, 1976). This may help to explain the paradoxical preference people have for breathing through their nose.

Nasal Cycling (Side-to-Side)

The rhythmic exchange of resting tidal breathing usually goes unnoticed. Also usually unnoticed, and even unknown, is the fact that the two sides of the nose behave differently during breathing. The fact of the matter is, everybody has two noses (somewhat like the two barrels of a side-by-side double-barreled shotgun).

For most people (estimates range up to 80%), these two noses (one on the left side and one on the right side) go through cycles of turbinate engorgement and deflation (Principato & Ozenberger, 1970; Stoksted, 1953). As portrayed in Figure 4–21, these cycles are typically 180° out of phase between the left and right sides and have identical periods. That is, as the left side is congesting (swelling), the right side is decongesting (shrinking), and vice versa. The reciprocal alternation between the left and right sides is characterized by similar changes in nasal cavity resistance, average airflow, and volume change. Cycling time varies from person to person and can range from as short as 30 minutes to as long as 5 hours or more. These alternating blockages and returns to patency go on throughout the day and night, without awareness on the part of the person breathing, despite the fact that the effective nasal airflow is at times almost entirely a function of the patent side (Principato & Ozenberger, 1970). The explanation for this lack of awareness on the part of the breather is that the total resistance to airflow remains relatively constant (Huang et al., 2003). Thus, despite large changes in the resistance to airflow from side to side, the total nasal resistance changes little because it reflects the resistance of the more patent nasal cavity. In fact, the total nasal resistance cannot vary any more than the difference between the minimal resistances of the individual sides of the nose (Principato & Ozenberger, 1970).

The purpose of nasal cycling appears to be to permit one side of the nose to go through a period of rest from the task of conditioning inspired air. Such turn taking allows for downtime wherein "house-cleaning" goes on. It has also been suggested that periodic congestion and decongestion of the nasal cavities provides a pumping mechanism for the generation of plasma exudate that serves as a vital line of defense against infection (Eccles, 1996).

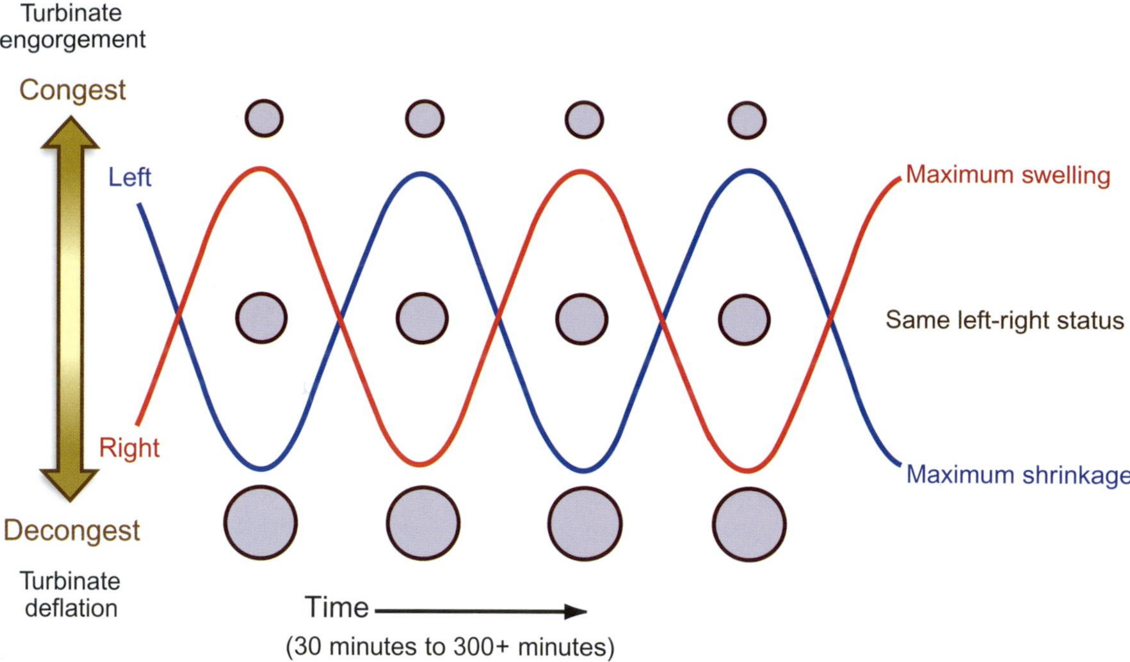

Figure 4–21. Left-right cycling of nasal airway resistance.

The pacemaker for the nasal cycle is thought to be the suprachiasmatic nucleus of the hypothalamus. This nucleus is considered to regulate autonomic tone of the left and right nasal vasculatures (Eccles & Eccles, 1981). Apparently, alternating actions by the sympathetic and parasympathetic portions of the autonomic nervous system result in vasoconstriction and decongestion, respectively. The pacemaker for the nasal cycle produces an ultradian (more frequent than once a day) rhythm that includes asymmetries in left-right cerebral electroencephalographic (EEG) activity (Werntz, Bickford, Bloom, & Shannahoff-Khalsa, 1983). This activity is such that greater EEG amplitudes are associated with decreased resistance to airflow in the nasal cavity of the opposite side.

It is interesting to note that the alternating rhythm associated with the nasal cycle is influenced by body position (Cole & Haight, 1986) and decreases with age (Mirza, Kroger, & Doty, 1997). The nasal cycle appears to be ablated in persons with high spinal cord lesions during the first year after injury. This is believed to be due to damage to the cervical sympathetic nerves supplying the nasal mucosa (Saroha, Bottrill, Saif, & Gardner, 2003). Surprisingly, individuals between 1 and 4 years out from such injuries demonstrate an irregular nasal cycle, whereas those more than 4 years out show a return to a normal alternating nasal cycle (Saroha et al., 2003). The mechanism of recovery is unknown.

Nasal-Oral Switching

Most breathing is done through the nose. Nasal breathing is desirable because it (a) converts the temperature of incoming air to that of the body, (b) adjusts the relative humidity of incoming air to an advantageous 80%, and (c) extracts dust, bacteria and other contaminants from incoming air. The last of these involves taking what is trapped and propelling it toward the pharynx through wavelike ciliary action in a mucous blanket. Eventually the debris collected is swallowed and passed on to the stomach for disposal. Less systematic "blowing of the nose" is also a method of disposal.

Breathing through the mouth is not uncommon (Niinimaa, Cole, & Mintz, 1981; Saibene, Mognoni, & LaFortuna, 1978; Vig & Zajac, 1993; Warren, Drake, & Davis, 1992). However, constant mouth breathing can be problematic because it does not accomplish the warming, moistening, and filtering functions of the nose. Only a small fraction of the population breathes through the mouth routinely (Niiminaa et al., 1981; Sabiene et al., 1978), and this is usually the result of nasal obstruction. It has been estimated that about 10% of all mouth breathing is habitual rather than obligatory (Warren, Hairfield, Seaton, & Hinton, 1988).

If the tidal breathing demand exceeds that associated with rest, it may become necessary to switch to mouth breathing or mouth breathing in combination with nose breathing. The key factor in such switching appears to be the prevailing nasal resistance. Nasal resistance values for healthy adults and children range from 1.0 to 3.5 cmH_2O/LPS for resting tidal breathing (Warren, Duany, & Fischer, 1969; Warren, Mayo, Zajac, & Rochet, 1996). Resistance values in excess 4.5 cmH_2O/LPS during tidal breathing are thought to constitute impairment (McCaffrey & Kern, 1979).

Who Nose?

As discussed in the text, we all have two noses that cycle side to side. We've emphasized that this involves a change in nasal resistance, but there's more to this story. Did you know that you alternate the sides you sleep on at night to alternate noses and breathe comfortably? Or did you know that nasal cycling is a marker for age-related nervous system changes? And did you know that your two noses can each sense different smells at the same time? Bet you didn't know that your spatial skills are better when you breathe through your left nostril and your verbal skills are better when you breathe through your right nostril? (Would you believe this book was written during right nostril breathing just to make it clearer? No. We didn't think you would.) Why there's even a reflex that can be elicited from your armpit (the crutch reflex) that makes your nose on the same side get congested. Isn't this amazing? Who nose what else could be going on?

The Masked Man's Nose

Nose masks are often used in research and clinical endeavors. Such masks must be sealed airtight against the face so that air doesn't leak around their edges. But therein lies a potential problem. How the face gets compressed beneath the edges of a mask can influence how air moves through the outer nose. Try the following. Breathe in and out through your nose to experience your usual nasal resistance to airflow. Next, touch your face below both your eyes and slowly slide that facial tissue toward the middle of your face—but don't touch your outer nose. Notice how it gets harder to breathe when you do this. How your facial tissue gets "scrunched" greatly influences your nasal resistance, even though you may not actually touch your outer nose. The same is true for how you position a mask on someone else. Be careful. Don't scrunch the facial tissue around the outer nose. Otherwise, you may raise nasal resistance to airflow.

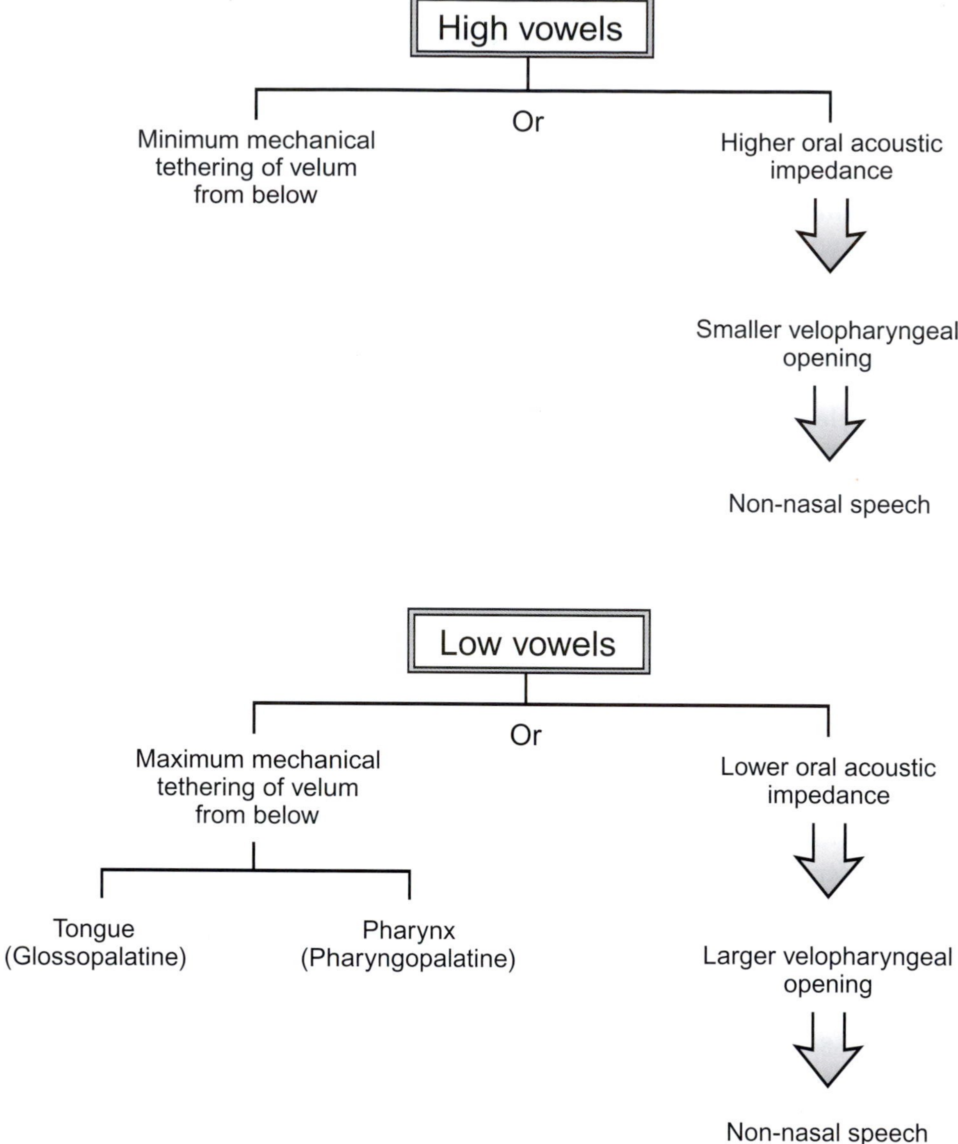

Figure 4–22. Possible velar height control mechanisms.

and nasals /m/ and /n/. In their aeromechanical studies of nasal airflow during speech production, Thompson and Hixon (1979) and Hoit et al. (1994) found airtight velopharyngeal closure on all sustained /s/ productions and essentially all sustained /z/ productions of 192 children and adults (ages 3 to 97 years). Airtight closure of the velopharyngeal port is clearly a priority on speech sounds that rely on the management of the oral airstream for their production. Support for this is also found in the x-ray study of Iglesias et al. (1980), wherein sustained production of /z/ had a higher velar elevation and more forward displacement of the posterior pharyngeal wall than did any of four sustained vowels that were studied.

Sustained nasal consonants are produced with large openings of the velopharyngeal port, as shown in Figure 4–23. Specifically, the position of the velum is the same (or slightly higher) for /m/ productions (Lubker, 1968) and /n/ productions (Iglesias et al., 1980) compared to that observed for resting tidal breathing through the nose. Furthermore, ***palatal***

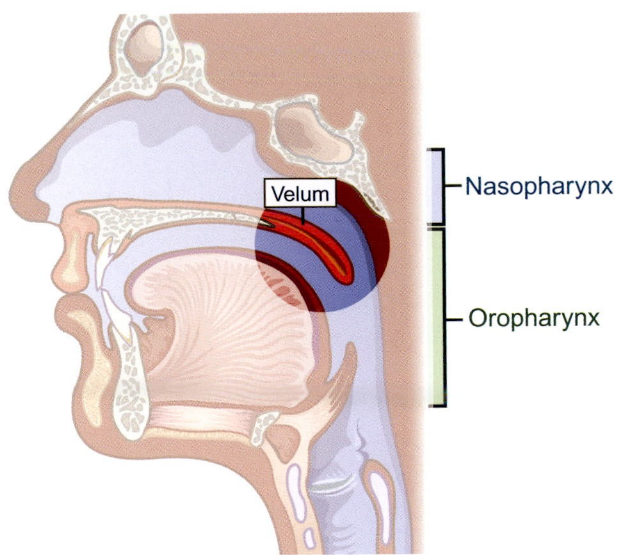

Figure 4–23. Velar position for nasal consonant production.

levator muscle activity during the production of sustained nasal consonants is not discernible (Lubker, 1968). Predictably, nasal airflow is substantial during nasal consonant productions (Hoit et al., 1994; Thompson & Hixon, 1979).

Function of the outer nose has also been documented during sustained utterances. Lansing, Solomon, Kossev, and Andersen (1991) recorded single motor unit discharges from nasal muscles of five adults during a variety of speaking and breathing activities. They found that certain nasal motor units discharged only during speech production and not during resting tidal breathing or voluntary inspirations. Some motor units were active only during the production of sustained vowels, some during sustained nasal consonants, but none during sustained voiced fricatives. Merely thinking about the production of a speech sound did not activate these units, nor did any of them activate during solitary nonspeech movements of the breathing apparatus, larynx, tongue, or velopharynx.

Lansing et al. (1991) suggested that such nasal muscle activity is evidence that the nasal muscles assist in valving the velopharyngeal-nasal airway during speech production and that the outer nose should be considered an articulator and as part of a coordinative structure along with other components of the speech production apparatus. Two aspects of this inclusion are important. One is that the outer nose could act, along with other components of the velopharynx and the breathing apparatus, larynx, mandible (lower jaw), tongue, and lips, to control air pressures and airflows for speech production. The other is that the outer nose could act to change the size, shape, and stiffness of the nasal resonating cavity and its walls, thus affecting the acoustic output. The research of Lansing et al. provides convincing evidence that the outer nose is a functional component of the velopharyngeal-nasal apparatus for speech production purposes.

Velopharyngeal-Nasal Function and Running Speech Activities

Running speech activities require rapid adjustments of the velopharyngeal-nasal apparatus. A few minutes spent watching x-ray images of running speech activities reveals that velopharyngeal articulation is every bit as fast and intricate as are movements of the mandible, tongue, and lips. During running speech production, the velopharyngeal port closes to various degrees for oral speech sounds and opens to various degrees for nasal speech sounds. The precise pattern of opening and closing and the degree to which the velopharyngeal port is opened or closed are matters having to do with the speech sounds in an utterance sequence and the rate at which that sequence is produced (Kent et al., 1974).

When consonants and vowels are combined as they are in running speech activities, primacy of control of the velopharyngeal-nasal apparatus is vested in consonant productions. The reason for this is that the production of many consonant elements relies heavily on appropriate management of the airstream. Sacrificing the aeromechanical requirements of these consonants may result in sacrificing the intelligibility of speech, whereas sacrificing closure for vowel productions may increase nasalization but has only a minimal affect on speech intelligibility. Those consonant elements that rely most on aeromechanical management of the airstream are often referred to as "the pressure consonants" because they are characteristically produced with high oral air pressure and little or no velopharyngeal opening. Stop-plosive, fricative, and affricate speech sounds (see Chapter 5) are categorized as pressure consonants. In contrast, nasal consonants

Playing by Her Own Rule

She was a young woman with a profound bilateral hearing loss. She'd received intensive behavioral therapy for imprecise articulation, but essentially no progress was being made. A puzzled speech-language pathologist made the referral. What was preventing improvement in speech? The answer was found in a recording of nasal airflow. A large burst of airflow was found to accompany each segment of speech that included a voiceless consonant. The young woman had apparently developed a production rule that said, "Only close your velopharynx for speech when your voice is on." It turned out to be a rule that could be changed by displaying nasal airflow for her to monitor on a storage oscilloscope so that she could see her rule in action and adopt a more appropriate one with some guidance. Her velopharynx cooperated and her articulation improved.

are produced with a low oral air pressure and a relatively wide-open velopharyngeal port.

The control of the velopharyngeal-nasal apparatus during running speech production is not simply a sequencing of separate and independent position and movement patterns for different speech sounds. To use an analogy, velopharyngeal adjustments for sequences of speech sounds are not like sequences of typewriter characters that are produced when each is called on to make an appearance (Hixon & Abbs, 1980). Rather, the position and movement patterns for two or more speech sounds may occur simultaneously, such that their productions actually overlap and intermingle. Part of this has to do with how the brain prepares in advance for velopharyngeal-nasal adjustments and part has to do with how the mechanical-inertial properties of the velopharyngeal-nasal apparatus influence its behavior. More is said about these principles in Chapter 5.

Underlying the assembling of velopharyngeal-nasal positions and movements is the principle that consonants influence the velopharyngeal-nasal adjustments of all speech sounds (consonants and vowels) within their interval of preparation. The precise influence depends on both the type of consonant and type of vowel. For example, the preparation period for oral consonants results in smaller velopharyngeal port openings for vowels that precede them, whereas the preparation period for nasal consonants results in larger velopharyngeal port openings for vowels that precede them (Warren & DuBois, 1964). Furthermore, when a nasal consonant is preceded by two consecutive vowels, the opening of the velopharyngeal port for the nasal consonant is initiated during the production of the first vowel in the sequence (Moll & Daniloff, 1971). Even the presence of a word boundary within a sequence does not affect this observation. The interactions between different speech sound adjustments of the velopharyngeal-nasal apparatus condition the position and movement patterns observed, such that, at any instant, the configuration of the apparatus may contain evidence of things that are coming and things that have already taken place.

Some models of velopharyngeal function have tried to account for variations in velar movement during speech production through a binary (on-off) scheme of velar function (Moll & Daniloff, 1971; Moll & Shriner, 1967). Although these models account for some of the phenomena observed in running speech activities, they do not adequately predict temporal relationships observed at the velopharyngeal-nasal periphery (Kent et al., 1974), nor do they conform to the observation that the electrical activity of muscles of the velum varies in a relatively continuous manner during speech production that correlates positively with velopharyngeal positioning (Lubker, 1968).

Adjustments of the outer nose have also been documented during running speech activities (Lansing et al., 1991) and demonstrate the importance of nasal structures in the function of the velopharyngeal-nasal apparatus. Specifically, Lansing et al. observed single motor unit discharges from nasal muscles during speech utterances. These motor units did not respond to large rapid, passive stretch of the skin around the mouth, cheeks, or eyes, thereby making it unlikely that the discharges during speech production were reflex responses produced by the contraction of facial muscles. The authors concluded that the single motor unit activity of nasal muscles was evidence that the nasal muscles may not only assist in actively valving the nasal airway for nasalized speech sounds, but may also act in concert with actions of other facial muscles during speech production.

Some have questioned the role of the velopharyngeal apparatus as an "articulatory" structure, contending that it simply remains "on" during running speech production unless a nasal consonant or a pause occurs (Moll & Shriner, 1967). Others have contested this view and argued that the velopharynx is very much an articulator that receives its commands at the same time as do other articulatory structures (mandible, tongue, and lips), even though such commands might not always be identified as being associated with individual speech sounds (Kent et al., 1974). Now it is known that not only is the velopharynx an articulator, but so is the outer nose (Lansing et al., 1991). What remains to be known are all of the synergies between the velopharyngeal and nasal parts of the velopharyngeal-nasal apparatus.

Gravity and Velopharyngeal-Nasal Function in Speech Production

Velopharyngeal-nasal function changes with changes in the spatial orientation of the velopharyngeal-nasal apparatus, primarily because of the influence of gravity. Each time the apparatus is reoriented within a gravity field, alternate mechanical solutions are required to meet the goals for adjusting the velopharyngeal port.

Reorientation in this context can result from a change in body position. For example, the usual upright (standing or seated) body position can be changed to semirecumbent, supine, prone, side-lying (left and right lateral), and head down, among others. Correspondingly, the orientation of the velopharyngeal-nasal apparatus will follow these changes.

On purely mechanical grounds, certain predictions can be made about the influence of body position on velopharyngeal-nasal function. These predictions are illustrated in Figure 4–24. When the apparatus is in an upright position, the pull of gravity is in a direction that tends to lower the velum. Muscle force associated with the elevation of the velum must overcome this pull. And any muscle force associated with the lowering of the velum augments this pull. Departure from an upright orientation results in gravity pulling on the structures of the velopharyngeal-nasal apparatus in different ways.

When in the supine body position, gravity acts to pull the velum toward the posterior pharyngeal wall. Thus, gravity functions in a direction that tends to move the velum toward the nasopharynx, contrary to what it does in the upright body position. Muscle force associated with movement of the velum toward the posterior pharyngeal wall augments the pull of gravity, and muscle force associated with moving the velum away from the posterior pharyngeal wall must overcome the pull of gravity. Reorientation of the velopharyngeal-nasal apparatus by changing body position from upright to supine may also result in new resting positions for structures of the apparatus and a different resting configuration to the velopharyngeal port (which is open in both circumstances).

Moon and Canady (1995) conducted a study of the effects of body position (and, therefore, gravity) on velopharyngeal muscle activity during speech production. They studied the activation levels (using electromyography) of the ***palatal levator*** and ***pharyngopalatine*** muscles in upright and supine body positions and hypothesized that activation would be modulated by gravitational effects. Lower peak activation levels were observed in the supine body position for the ***palatal levator*** muscle, suggesting that less activation was required when the pull of gravity was in the same direction (toward the posterior pharyngeal wall). Also, for most subjects, the activation level of the ***pharyngopalatine*** muscle was greater in the supine body position where the pull of gravity was counter to movement of the velum away from the posterior pharyngeal

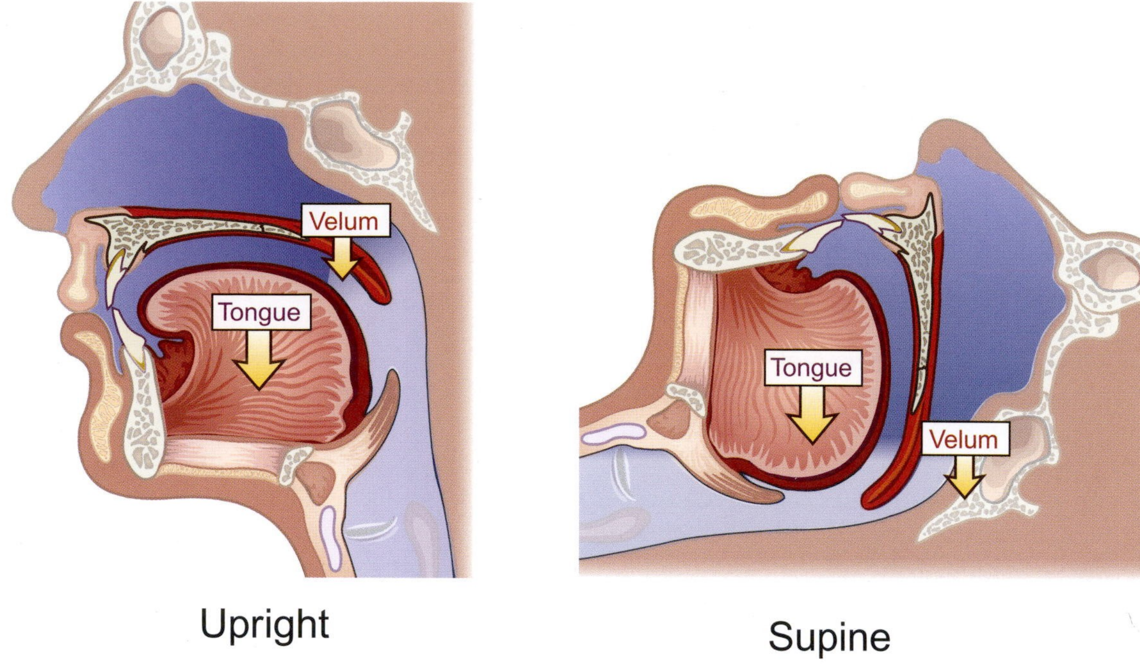

Figure 4–24. Predicted influences of body position on velopharyngeal-nasal function.

wall. Overall, the observations of Moon and Canady generally support the notion that levels of muscle activity in the velum are modulated in relation to the direction of the pull of gravity, with the effect being robust in the ***palatal levator*** muscle.

Reorientation of the velopharyngeal-nasal apparatus in space is not restricted to changes in body position. Reorientation can also mean that the body is maintained in a fixed position and the head is moved about different axes and, thus, the spatial orientation of the velopharyngeal-nasal apparatus follows. For example, the head can be pitched about a lateral axis, rolled about a longitudinal axis, and yawed about a vertical axis. As well, simultaneous adjustments can be made through more than one axis (pitching the head upward and yawing it to the right at the same time).

Rotation of the head about a lateral axis is an especially common activity that influences the spatial orientation of the velopharyngeal-nasal apparatus (nod your head yes to this statement). Full flexion and full extension of the neck (head rotated forward and backward, respectively) delimit the range of possible orientations associated with head rotation. Rotation through this range places maximally contrasting gravitational forces on the velopharyngeal-nasal apparatus, especially the velum. When the head is rotated downward from its usual position (toward a position where the mandible would rest on the rib cage wall), the pull of gravity on the velum is in a direction that tends to pull the structure away from the posterior pharyngeal wall. In contrast, when the head is rotated upward from its usual position (toward a position where the tip of the nose is maximally elevated), the pull of gravity on the velum is in a direction that tends to pull the velum toward the posterior pharyngeal wall.

Tilting the position of the body and rotating the head can have functionally similar outcomes in the context of a gravity field when the two actions reorient the velopharyngeal-nasal apparatus spatially in the same manner. Although changes in body position from upright to supine are pronounced, rotations of the head tend to be more subtle to the observer, even though they may involve significant reorientation of the velopharyngeal-nasal apparatus. Persons with structural-based or neuromotor-based borderline velopharyngeal competence present special cases that bear watching. In such persons, rotation of the head upward may enhance movement of the velum toward the posterior pharyngeal wall and, thereby, improve speech. In contrast, rotation of the head downward may do just the opposite.

Finally, gravitational influences are not limited to the velopharyngeal portion of the velopharyngeal-nasal apparatus. Reorientation of the velopharyngeal-nasal apparatus also affects the function of the nasal cavities. For example, it has been shown that nasal patency decreases and nasal airway resistance increases in downright as compared to upright body positions (Rudcrantz, 1969). This change in patency appears to relate to vascular changes associated with the assumption of downright body positions, including stroke volume, cardiac minute volume, and blood pressure increases. This is followed by a baroreceptor-mediated reflex that evokes a depression in blood pressure via a decrease in heart rate and the dilation of the peripheral blood vessels (Detweiler, 1973). Such dilation in the nasal region leads to engorgement (swelling) of the nasal mucosa, decrease in nasal patency, and an increase in nasal airway resistance. Also, because the nasal region is positioned above the heart in upright body positions and at the same level or below the heart in downright body positions, regional blood pressure changes. A higher blood pressure in downright body positions causes the blood vessels in the nasal mucosa to dilate and nasal congestion to increase (Hiyama, Ono, Ishiwata, & Kuroda, 2002).

Development of Velopharyngeal-Nasal Function for Speech Production

The birth cry is the first utterance for most human newborns. X-ray images of this first utterance have shown that it is made with an open velopharynx (Bosma, Truby, & Lind, 1965). Apparently, the "newborn instruction manual" has no entry about crying without hypernasality. So, what is the developmental schedule in getting from the birth cry (open velopharynx) to adult-like use of the velopharynx for speech purposes (mostly closed)?

In the first few months of life, the velum is in close proximity to the epiglottis, causing the infant to be an obligate nasal breather (Sasaki, Levine, Laitman, & Crelin, 1977). This configuration of upper airway structures has been identified as the reason that infant vocalization sounds nasalized (Kent, 1981). Acoustical and perceptual studies of infant vocalization have suggested that the velopharynx is open during cry (Wasz-Hockert, Lind, Vuorenkoski, Partanen, & Valanne, 1964) and noncry (Hsu, Fogel, & Cooper, 2000; Kent & Murray; 1982; Oller, 1986) vocalization up to about 4 months of age, and that the velopharynx probably closes for oral sound production sometime between 4 and 6 months of age. However, physiological data provided by Thom, Hoit, Hixon, and Smith (2006) have been interpreted to show that this is not the case.

Thom et al. (2006) studied six infants longitudinally from 2 to 6 months of age using a double-barreled nasal cannula to sense ram air pressure at the anterior nares. This device made it possible to determine the binary (open or closed) status of the velopharyngeal port during vocalization. The results showed that the velopharynx was open for precry windups, whimpers, and laughs, and closed for cries, screams, and raspberries at all ages studied. For syllable utterances, velopharyngeal closure increased with age, but was not complete and still undergoing development at 6 months of age (the highest age studied).

Thom et al. (2006) had hypothesized that the velopharynx would be consistently closed for oral sound production by 6 months of age, but this prediction was not supported. This leaves one in suspense, knowing only that consistent velopharyngeal closure for syllable utterances begins sometime after 6 months of age and before 3 years of age when airtight velopharyngeal closure during oral speech sound production has been documented in children (Thompson & Hixon, 1979). Although closure for syllable utterances was still not consistent at 6 months of age, it was also true that all infants were able to close the velopharynx for syllable productions as early as 2 months of age. Why, then, did infants not consistently close the velopharynx for oral utterances from that time on? It is probably because velopharyngeal closure is not necessarily required for vowel production, and vowels are by far the most prevalent speech-related utterances generated by infants. Sometime between 6 months and 3 years of age, and presumably closer to the former, children consistently use airtight velopharyngeal closure for oral speech sound production. Perhaps the purposive use of words on a regular basis is the critical point of consistent use of airtight velopharyngeal closure.

as prostheses and are custom fabricated to meet the needs of each individual. The prosthodontist is concerned with restoring impaired function, appearance, comfort, and health to individuals who need prosthetic devices to substitute for structures that have been affected by congenital anomalies, disease, trauma, or surgery. Individuals who require the services of a prosthodontist include those born with palatal clefts that are exceptionally wide and are managed through the fitting of a palatal obturator, a device that is fixed to the maxillary teeth and occludes the gap between the palatal shelves. Such a palatal obturator and combination denture is shown in Figure 4–31. Similarly, individuals who have large parts of the palate resected because of cancer may be fitted with an obturator as a replacement for the excised structure. A prosthodontist may fabricate customized velar-lift prostheses for persons who have paresis or paralysis of the velum. A velar-lift prosthesis consists of a plate that extends backward along the roof of the mouth to lift the velum to a horizontal plane and support its weight against the force of gravity. Persons with flaccid paresis or paralysis of the velum are often managed with this type of prosthetic device. The speech-language pathologist usually works with the prosthodontist to help evaluate the success of different prostheses on velopharyngeal-nasal function in relation to breathing, speaking, and swallowing.

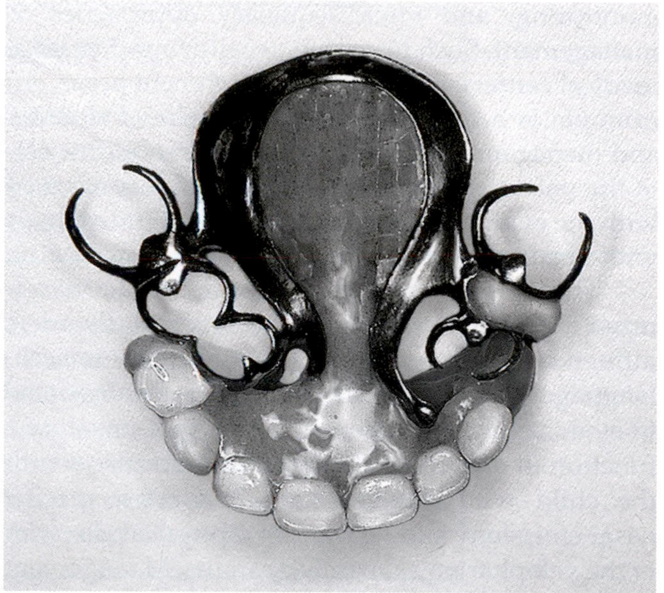

Figure 4–31. Photograph of a palatal obturator and combination denture as viewed from below. From *Cleft palate speech* (3rd ed., p. 324), by S. Peterson-Falzone, M. Hardin-Jones, and M. Karnell, 2001, St. Louis, MO: Elsevier Mosby. Copyright 2001 by Elsevier Mosby. Reproduced with permission.

A psychologist is an individual who has special expertise in helping individuals cope with significant problems of everyday living. The psychologist can play an important role for many individuals with

Wait Lifting

Occasionally a person fitted with a velar-lift prosthesis will wear it for several weeks or months and find that when it is removed the velum is able to move. Further evaluation will usually confirm that the velum is working better than it did before the prosthesis was fitted or even that it is working normally. How can this be? How can a paretic or paralyzed velum come back to life and start working again? Most likely the velum was nearly able to do its job to begin with, but its owner may have surrendered to gravity and not used whatever minimal strength was available. This, in turn, may have allowed the velum to become even weaker through disuse. Then, once in place, the prosthesis did part of the lifting work for the velum (probably the toughest part) and the velum was able to accomplish the rest on its own. Think of this as a sort of wait lifting (pun intended), if you will.

velopharyngeal-nasal disorders that affect speech production. For example, those who have undergone surgical ablation of different parts of the head and neck or who have neural disease that has resulted in their being unable to move normally for speech production purposes, are often in need of counseling to help them deal with the psychological processes attendant to their loss of function. Psychological depression, grief, and embarrassment are several factors often encountered in persons with acquired velopharyngeal-nasal disorders that manifest in speech production problems. In other cases, the psychologist plays an important role in helping families and loved ones cope with perceived losses or conditions surrounding velopharyngeal-nasal disorders. For example, the parents of a child born with a cleft of the palate may be overwhelmed with emotion (see the scenario at the beginning of this chapter) and need counseling and psychological support to help them deal with their situation and future.

REVIEW

The velopharyngeal-nasal apparatus is located within the head and neck and comprises a system of valves and air passages that interconnects the throat and atmosphere through the nose.

The velopharyngeal-nasal apparatus includes the pharynx, velum, nasal cavities, and outer nose.

Forces of the velopharyngeal-nasal apparatus are of two types—passive and active, the former arising from several sources and the latter arising from muscles distributed within different parts of the velopharyngeal-nasal apparatus.

Muscles of the pharynx include the ***superior constrictor***, ***middle constrictor***, ***inferior constrictor***, ***salpingopharyngeus***, ***stylopharyngeus***, and ***palatopharyngeus***.

Muscles of the velum include the ***palatal levator***, ***palatal tensor***, ***uvulus***, ***glossopalatine***, and ***pharyngopalatine***.

Muscles of the outer nose include the ***levator labii superioris alaeque nasi***, ***anterior nasal dilator***, ***posterior nasal dilator***, ***nasalis***, and ***depressor alae nasi***.

Movements of the pharynx enable its lumen to be changed along its length, either by constriction or dilation at different sites.

Movements of the velum involve shape changes of the structure and are mainly along an upward-backward or downward-forward path.

Movements of the outer nose influence the cross sections of the anterior nares and are involved in breathing events and the signaling of emotions.

Adjustments of the velopharyngeal-nasal apparatus can influence the degree of coupling between the oral and nasal cavities and between the nasal cavities and atmosphere.

Closure of the velopharyngeal port can be achieved through a variety of movement strategies that involve different actions or combinations of actions of the velum, lateral pharyngeal walls, and posterior pharyngeal wall, strategies that are conditioned by velopharyngeal anatomy.

Closing and opening adjustments of the velopharyngeal port are controlled by different factors, with closing being controlled by muscular forces and opening being controlled by passive forces and muscular forces.

Adjustments of the anterior nares are involved in different activities and play a prominent role in breathing to resist the tendency of the outer nose to collapse in response to low pressures in its lumina.

The control variables of velopharyngeal-nasal function include airway resistance offered by the velopharyngeal-nasal apparatus, muscular pressure exerted by the velopharyngeal sphincter to maintain closure, and acoustical impedance in opposition to the flow of sound energy.

Different parts of the nervous system are responsible for the control of different components of the velopharyngeal-nasal apparatus and different activities, with motor and sensory innervation being effected mainly through cranial nerves.

Nasal airflow is modulated by the nasal valve, which consists of external and internal parts, the latter of which is primarily responsible for the governing of nasal patency.

The two sides of the nose go through changes in which their respective nasal turbinates alternately engorge and constrict in a rhythmical cycle that varies from person to person and has implications for the conditioning of inspired air and protection against infection.

The warming, moistening, and filtering aspects of nasal function are important to health, and nasal breathing prevails until airway resistance becomes excessive, whereupon a switch is made to oral-nasal breathing.

The role of velopharyngeal-nasal function in speech production is to control the degree of coupling between the oral and nasal cavities and between the nasal cavities and atmosphere.

Both the velopharynx and outer nose are active during sustained utterances, the patterning depending on the speech sound being produced, and with high vowels showing greater velar height, greater velar contact with the posterior pharyngeal wall, and greater velopharyngeal sphincter compression than low vowels.

Running speech activities involve the combining of consonants and vowels with primacy of control being vested in consonant productions, especially those associated with high oral air pressure and little or no opening of the velopharyngeal port.

Position and movement patterns of the velopharyngeal-nasal apparatus may reflect the occurrence of two or more speech sounds simultaneously, such that their productions overlap and intermingle and show evidence of how the brain prepares in advance for velopharyngeal-nasal adjustments and how the mechanical properties of the velopharyngeal-nasal apparatus influence its behavior.

Gravity has effects on velopharyngeal-nasal function that are manifested through reorientation of the position of the body or rotation of the head about different axes, and are attributed to mechanical and cardiovascular factors.

Velopharyngeal-nasal function for speech production develops gradually, and sometime between 6 months and 3 years of age (presumably closer to the former) airtight velopharyngeal closure for oral speech sound production can be expected to occur.

There is no credible evidence that velopharyngeal-nasal function for speech production changes with age in the mature velopharyngeal-nasal apparatus.

The sex of the speaker appears to have an influence on certain details of velopharyngeal-nasal function during speech production, but it is not clear that these differences are functionally important or that they are relevant to clinical concerns.

The instrumental measurement of velopharyngeal-nasal function can be accomplished with several methods, including direct visualization, x-ray imaging, aeromechanical observations, and acoustical observations.

Velopharyngeal-nasal disorders can influence speech production to different degrees and may result from congenital, developmental, or acquired problems of the velopharyngeal-nasal apparatus that have functional or organic bases.

Different clinical professionals have roles in the evaluation and management of velopharyngeal-nasal disorders that affect speech production, including speech-language pathologists, plastic surgeons, otorhinolaryngologists, neurologists, prosthodontists, and psychologists.

Scenario

Six years had passed since that eventful morning in Florida. Time and distance had muted the mother's memories, but the realities were with her daily in the form of her son. He was about to begin an educational journey in which his mother would play a lesser role than she had to this point in his life. Others would now have things to say about the boy's welfare. The mother's inertia on health care needs for the child was about to be overturned by social forces.

It began with a first-grade teacher in conversation with the school's nurse and later in consultation with the school's psychologist. All had concerns for the child's social development and his problems with speech. He stood out among his classmates because of his shyness and reticence. The speech-language pathologist who serviced the school was asked to evaluate the boy. Her report indicated that he had speech sound misarticulations, a moderately hypernasal voice, and nares constriction on pressure consonants. She concluded that he showed signs consistent with a significant velopharyngeal leak during speech production and recommended that he be referred to the regional cleft palate and craniofacial disorders clinic for instrumental evaluation. The mother provided medical records from the previous management team at the time of clinical intake.

Evaluation showed velopharyngeal incompetence and a small anterior oronasal fistula that was difficult to discern visually because of its configuration. Measurements of the cross-sectional area of the velopharyngeal port, with and without occlusion of the fistula, indicated that the fistula contributed to the overall problem and needed to be closed along with secondary surgical management of the velopharynx. The size of the velopharyngeal port was calculated for stop-plosive sound production with the fistula occluded using aeromechanical techniques and found to be 15 mm^2. The surgical method of choice was a pharyngeal flap. Lateral pharyngeal wall movement was observed via ultrasound and found to be minimal during oral consonant productions. A relatively high-placed, broad, superiorly based pharyngeal flap was constructed. Closure of the anterior fistula and construction of the pharyngeal flap were done in one hospitalization.

Six-month follow-up evaluation of the child indicated that the closure of the anterior fistula was successful and the pharyngeal flap was functioning well. Velopharyngeal port size for stop-plosive production had reduced to 2.5 mm^2. Nasal breathing was not obstructed and the mother reported no snoring problems or sleep apnea in the child. Misarticulations persisted, hypernasality was reduced, and nares constriction was less obvious and inconsistent. The child was placed on a behavior modification program with the speech-language pathologist to deal with his remaining speech and speech production signs. He responded well and within a short period of time began to make consistent improvement.

The mother came to understand that her sheltering of the child had been detrimental, despite her protective intentions. She went through a period of self-healing that paralleled the progress made by her son. She contacted her parents and arranged a weeklong visit over the 4th of July. It was her first return to Ohio in several years and her son's first time ever to see his grandparents' horse farm. All that week he saddled up on Buster, a brown and white pony that seemed to have been waiting for him and carried a white cowboy hat on the horn of his saddle. Life was good that week in "The Buckeye State," especially in the vicinity of Canfield. There would be other fun-filled weeks in that area for years to come, including a time to show Buster at the Canfield Fair.

Netsell, R. (1990). Commentary. *Cleft Palate Journal, 27,* 58–60.

Niinimaa, V., Cole, P., & Mintz, S. (1981). Oronasal distribution of respiratory airflow. *Respiratory Physiology, 43,* 69–75.

Nusbaum, E., Foly, L., & Wells, C. (1935). Experimental studies of the firmness of the velar-pharyngeal occlusion during the production of the English vowels. *Speech Monographs, 2,* 71–80.

Oller, K. (1986). Metaphonology and infant vocalizations. In B. Lindblom & R. Zetterstrom (Eds.), *Precursors of early speech* (pp. 21–36). New York: Stockton Press.

Poppelreuter, S., Engelke, W., & Bruns, T. (2000). Quantitative analysis of the velopharyngeal sphincter function during speech. *Cleft Palate-Craniofacial Journal, 37,* 157–165.

Principato, J., & Ozenberger, J. (1970). Cyclical changes in nasal resistance. *Archives of Otolaryngology, 91,* 71–77.

Proctor, D. (1982). The upper airway. In D. Proctor & I. Andersen (Eds.), *The nose—upper airway physiology and the atmospheric environment* (pp. 23–44). Amsterdam, Netherlands: Elsevier Biomedical Press.

Quigley, L., Shiere, F., Webster, R., & Cobb, C. (1964). Measuring palatopharyngeal competence with the nasal anemometer. *Cleft Palate Journal, 1,* 304–313.

Rood, S., & Doyle, W. (1978). Morphology of tensor veli palatini, tensor tympani, and dilator tubae muscles. *Annals of Otology, Rhinology, and Laryngology, 87,* 202–210.

Rudcrantz, H. (1969). Postural variations of nasal patency. *Acta Otolaryngologica, 68,* 435–443.

Ruscello, D. (1982). A selected review of palatal training procedures. *Cleft Palate Journal, 19,* 181–193.

Saibene, F., Mognoni, P., & LaFortuna, C. (1978). Oronasal breathing during exercise. *Pleugers Archives, 378,* 65–69.

Saroha, D., Bottrill, I., Saif, M., & Gardner, B. (2003). Is the nasal cycle ablated in patients with high spinal cord trauma? *Clinical Otolaryngology and Allied Sciences, 28,* 142–145.

Sasaki, C., Levine, P., Laitman, J., & Crelin, E. (1977). Postnatal descent of the epiglottis in man. *Archives of Otolaryngology, 103,* 169–171.

Schmidt, R. (1982). The schema concept. In J. Kelso (Ed.), *Human motor behavior: An introduction* (pp. 219–235). Hillsdale, NJ: Lawrence Erlbaum.

Schwab, B., & Schulze-Florey, A. (2004). Velopharyngeal insufficiency in woodwind and brass players. *Medical Problems of Performing Artists, 19,* 21–25.

Seaver, E., Dalston, R., Leeper, H., & Adams, L. (1991). A study of nasometric values for normal nasal resonance. *Journal of Speech and Hearing Research, 34,* 715–721.

Seaver, E., & Kuehn, D. (1980). A cineradiographic and electromyographic investigation of velar positioning in non-nasal speech. *Cleft Palate Journal, 17,* 216–226.

Shelton, R., Beaumont, K., Trier, W., & Furr, M. (1978). Videopanendoscopic feedback in training velopharyngeal closure. *Cleft Palate Journal, 15,* 6–12.

Shimokawa, T., Yi, S., & Tanaka, S. (2005). Nerve supply to the soft palate muscles with special reference to the distribution of the lesser palatine nerves. *Cleft Palate-Craniofacial Journal, 42,* 495–500.

Shprintzen, R. (1992). Assessment of velopharyngeal function: Nasopharyngoscopy and multiview videofluoroscopy. In L. Brodsky, L. Holt, & D. Ritter-Schmidt (Eds.), *Craniofacial anomalies: An interdisciplinary approach* (pp. 196–207). St. Louis, MO: Mosby.

Shprintzen, R., McCall, G., Skolnick, L., & Lenicone, R. (1975). Selective movement of the lateral aspects of the pharyngeal walls during velopharyngeal closure for speech, blowing, and whistling in normals. *Cleft Palate Journal, 12,* 51–58.

Siegel-Sadewitz, V., & Shprintzen, R. (1986). Changes in velopharyngeal valving with age. *International Journal of Pediatric Otorhinolaryngology, 11,* 171–182.

Skolnick, M. (1970). Videofluoroscopic examination of the velopharyngeal portal during phonation in lateral and base projections—A new technique for studying the mechanics of closure. *Cleft Palate Journal, 7,* 803–816.

Skolnick, M., McCall, G., & Barnes, M. (1973). The sphincteric mechanism of velopharyngeal closure. *Cleft Palate Journal, 10,* 286–305.

Stoksted, P. (1953). Rhinometric measurements for determination of the nasal cycle. *Acta Otolaryngologica, Supplement 109,* 1–159.

Subtelny, J., & Koepp-Baker, H. (1956). The significance of adenoid tissue in velopharyngeal function. *Plastic and Reconstructive Surgery, 12,* 235–250.

Thom, S., Hoit, J., Hixon, T., & Smith, A. (2006). Velopharyngeal function during vocalization in infants. *Cleft Palate-Craniofacial Journal, 43,* 539–546.

Thompson, A., & Hixon, T. (1979). Nasal air flow during normal speech production. *Cleft Palate Journal, 16,* 412–420.

Tomoda, T., Morii, S., Yamashita, T., & Kumazawa, T. (1984). Histology of human eustachian tube muscles: Effect of aging. *Annals of Otology, Rhinology, and Laryngology, 93,* 17–24.

Tucker, L. (1963). *Articulatory variations in normal speakers with changes in vocal pitch and effort.* Master's Thesis, University of Iowa, Iowa City.

Vig, P., & Zajac, D. (1993). Age and gender effects on nasal respiratory function in normal subjects. *Cleft Palate-Craniofacial Journal, 30,* 279–284.

Warren, D. (1964). Velopharyngeal orifice size and upper pharyngeal pressure-flow patterns in normal speech. *Plastic and Reconstructive Surgery, 33,* 148–162.

Warren, D. (1967). Nasal emission of air and velopharyngeal function. *Cleft Palate Journal, 4,* 148–156.

Warren, D., Dalston, R., & Dalston, E. (1990). Maintaining speech pressures in the presence of velopharyngeal impairment. *Cleft Palate Journal, 27*, 53–58.

Warren, D., Dalston, R., Trier, W., & Holder, M. (1985). A pressure-flow technique for quantifying temporal patterns of palatopharyngeal closure. *Cleft Palate Journal, 22*, 11–19.

Warren, D., Drake, A., & Davis, J. (1992). Nasal airway in breathing and speech. *Cleft Palate-Craniofacial Journal, 29*, 511–519.

Warren, D., Duany, L., & Fischer, N. (1969). Nasal pathway resistance in normal and cleft lip and palate subjects. *Cleft Palate Journal, 6*, 134–140.

Warren, D., & DuBois, A. (1964). A pressure-flow technique for measuring velopharyngeal orifice area during continuous speech. *Cleft Palate Journal, 1*, 52–71.

Warren, D., Hairfield, W., & Hinton, V. (1985). The respiratory significance of the nasal grimace. *ASHA, 27*, 82.

Warren, D., Hairfield, W., Seaton, D., & Hinton, V. (1987). The relationship between nasal airway cross-sectional area and nasal resistance. *American Journal of Orthodontics and Dentofacial Orothopedics, 92*, 390–395.

Warren, D., Hairfield, W., Seaton, D., & Hinton, V. (1988). Relationship between the size of the nasal airway and nasal-oral breathing. *American Journal of Orthodontics and Dentofacial Orthopedics, 93*, 289–293.

Warren, D., Hairfield, W., Seaton, D., Morr, K., & Smith, L. (1988). The relationship between nasal airway size and nasal-oral breathing. *American Journal of Orthodontics and Dentofacial Orthopedics, 93*, 289–293.

Warren, D., Mayo, R., Zajac, D., & Rochet, A. (1996). Dyspnea following experimentally induced increased nasal airway resistance. *Cleft Palate-Craniofacial Journal, 33*, 231–235.

Wasz-Hockert, O., Lind, J., Vuorenkoski, V., Partanen, T., & Valanne, E. (1964). The infant cry: A spectrographic and auditory analysis. *Clinics in Developmental Medicine, Supplement 29*. London, UK: Heinemann.

Werntz, D., Bickford, R., Bloom, F., & Shannahoff-Khalsa, D. (1983). Alternating cerebral hemispheric activity and the lateralization of autonomic nervous function. *Human Neurobiology, 2*, 39–43.

Wilson, F., Kudryk, W., & Sych, J. (1986). The development of flexible fiberoptic video nasendoscopy (FFVN) clinical-teaching-research applications. *ASHA, 28*, 25–30.

Zajac, D. (1997). Velopharyngeal function in young and older adult speakers: Evidence from aerodynamic studies. *Journal of the Acoustical Society of America, 102*, 1846–1852.

Zajac, D. (2000). Pressure-flow characteristics of /m/ and /p/ production in speakers without cleft palate: Developmental findings. *Cleft Palate-Craniofacial Journal, 37*, 468–477.

Zajac, D., & Hackett, A. (2002). Temporal characteristics of aerodynamic segments in the speech of children and adults. *Cleft Palate-Craniofacial Journal, 39*, 432–438.

Zajac, D., & Mayo, R. (1996). Aerodynamic and temporal aspects of velopharyngeal function in normal speakers. *Journal of Speech and Hearing Research, 39*, 1199–1207.

5

Pharyngeal-Oral Function and Speech Production

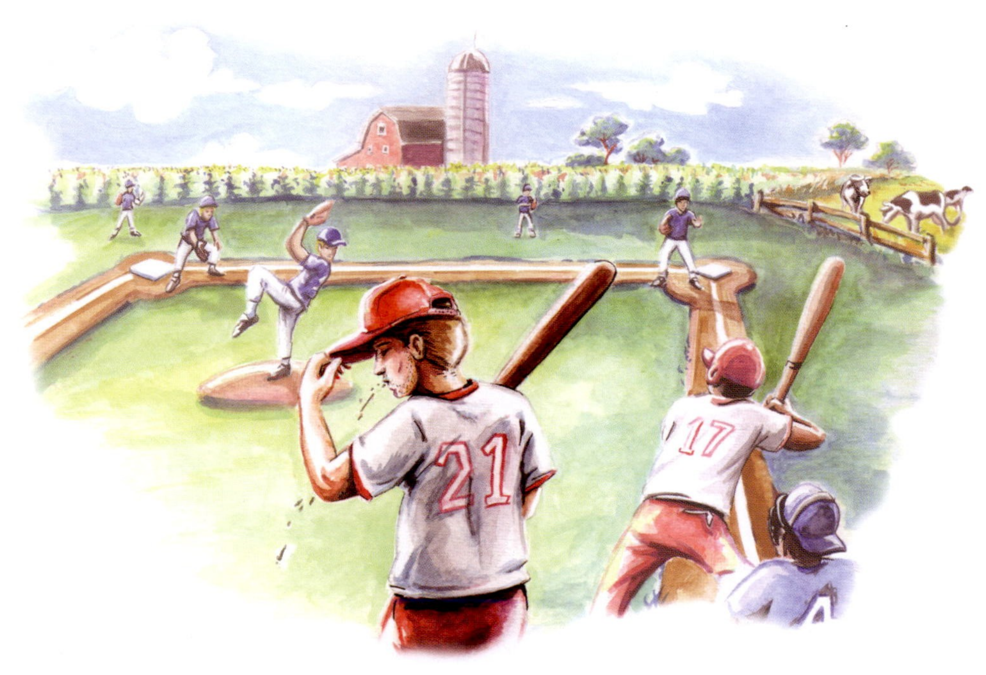

Scenario

His early life was good. He graduated from high school and was the first in his family to attend college. He made it through his sophomore year in agriculture and then his funds were drawn down. His parents were not people of means and could not help him. He took a job in a feed store to try to make enough money to continue his education. His intentions were good, but he never again saw the inside of a college classroom. It was partly because of the need to work and partly because a young woman captured his heart. After that, it was two children. He rose to become the manager at work.

One of his passions was baseball and he was very good at it. So good, in fact, that he once was given a tryout for a major-league farm team. He didn't make the team, but he was good enough to play during summers in a first-rate amateur baseball league in a nearby city. He could chew tobacco and spit with the best of them and the fans called him the vacuum cleaner because he would suck up any ball hit in the vicinity of third base. Little did he know, at the time, that his baseball habits would turn on him.

It was about a decade after his wedding that his life's burden fell on him. There was a feeling of fullness along the left side of his tongue. When he touched that side it felt different from the right side. He thought it might be the beginnings of a canker sore. He tried to look in his mouth with a mirror but he couldn't see anything special. It just felt different. He gargled with salt water, but his symptoms persisted. He thought they might eventually go away and so he procrastinated. It did him no good. The fullness remained.

He mentioned the problem to his wife and she insisted that he see a physician. The physician was suspicious. They discussed his history with chewing tobacco and she referred him to an otolaryngologist who performed a biopsy and did other tests that revealed cancer in his tongue. The problem was thought to be widespread and would require surgery to excise the cancerous tissue. The procedure would be extensive and had uncertainties that could only be resolved during the surgery itself. The waiting carried its own pain, took away sleep, and instilled increasing fear.

As he succumbed to anesthesia, his thoughts were pessimistic. When he awoke, it was worse than he had imagined. Spread of the cancer was such that his surgeon had to perform a total glossectomy (complete tongue removal) and also remove parts of his cheek and mandible on the left side. His oral cavity was empty down to the muscles that ran along the bottom of his mandible. His larynx was in clear view when he opened his mouth. The left side of his face was markedly disfigured. When he tried to speak to his wife, both were in disbelief. His voice sounded hollow and bizarre and his speech was unintelligible. He couldn't eat by mouth.

He came to feel desperate and sometimes cried when alone. He fell into psychological depression and lost a significant amount of weight. His spirit was broken. Physical recovery was painful and he felt embarrassment in front of his family and friends because of the way he looked and sounded. He came to believe that he would never again be able to speak in a social situation or be able to return to work. Life was grim for him and he felt isolated. He considered suicide on several occasions. His wife was also under stress. Fortunately, what seemed to be a certain dark future, turned out to have some bright spots.

Gone But Not Forgotten

Arm and leg amputations occurred in large numbers during the Civil War. Amputees from this era reported that pain or other sensations continued to arise from where their missing limbs had been. Some described them as sensory ghosts and many doctors of the time thought that those who reported them had mental problems. Not so. Phantom limb pain or other sensations are now recognized to be common following amputation of any body part and scientists have embraced a number of theories about their origins. Those who have had their tongues amputated (usually surgically and because of cancer) also report tongue pain or other sensations that are analogous to those associated with their better known phantom-limb counterpart. Ghost tongues are most prominent right after surgery and tend to fade away with time, although they are known to abruptly reappear on occasion. All of this is really quite haunting when you think about it.

INTRODUCTION

The pharyngeal-oral apparatus, together with the velopharyngeal-nasal apparatus (discussed in Chapter 4), forms the upper airway. The pharyngeal-oral part of this airway is critical to various activities. Especially important in the present context are its functions during speaking and swallowing.

This chapter considers the fundamentals of pharyngeal-oral function, followed by a discussion of speech production. Also discussed are methods for measuring pharyngeal-oral function. This is followed by consideration of the nature of pharyngeal-oral disorders and the clinical professionals who are concerned with such disorders. The chapter then proceeds to a review of its contents and the presentation of a closing scenario. The function of the pharyngeal-oral apparatus during swallowing is discussed in Chapter 12.

FUNDAMENTALS OF PHARYNGEAL-ORAL FUNCTION

This section is concerned with the principles underlying pharyngeal-oral function. It includes a discussion of the anatomy of the pharyngeal-oral apparatus, the forces and movements of the apparatus, and the potential adjustments of the apparatus. Next, the control variables of pharyngeal-oral function and the neural substrates of pharyngeal-oral control are addressed. Finally, attention is directed toward the range of functions that are performed by the pharyngeal-oral apparatus.

Anatomy of the Pharyngeal-Oral Apparatus

The pharyngeal-oral apparatus is a flexible tube that extends from the larynx to the lips. The fabric of this tube is formed mainly of bone and muscle. The apparatus undergoes an approximate 90-degree bend (like a plumber's elbow joint) at the level of the oropharynx. There, the shorter and vertical pharyngeal portion communicates through the oropharyngeal (faucial) isthmus with the longer and horizontal oral portion. Skeletal structure supports the pharyngeal-oral apparatus and provides the framework around which its internal topography is organized. Both this skeletal structure and its associated internal topography are considered below.

Skeleton

Figure 5–1 shows the skeletal superstructure of the pharyngeal-oral apparatus. This framework comprises the upper portion of the vertebral column and various bones of the skull.

Cervical Vertebrae. The upper portion of the vertebral column supports the skull and provides a scaffold for the neck. The cervical (neck) segments of the vertebral column lie behind the three subdivisions of the pharynx—laryngopharynx, oropharynx, and nasopharynx—and form part of the substance of their back walls (see Chapter 4).

Skull. The skull forms the framework of the head and comprises a large number of irregularly shaped bones. These are distributed in two major subdivisions. One is the cranium (braincase), which houses

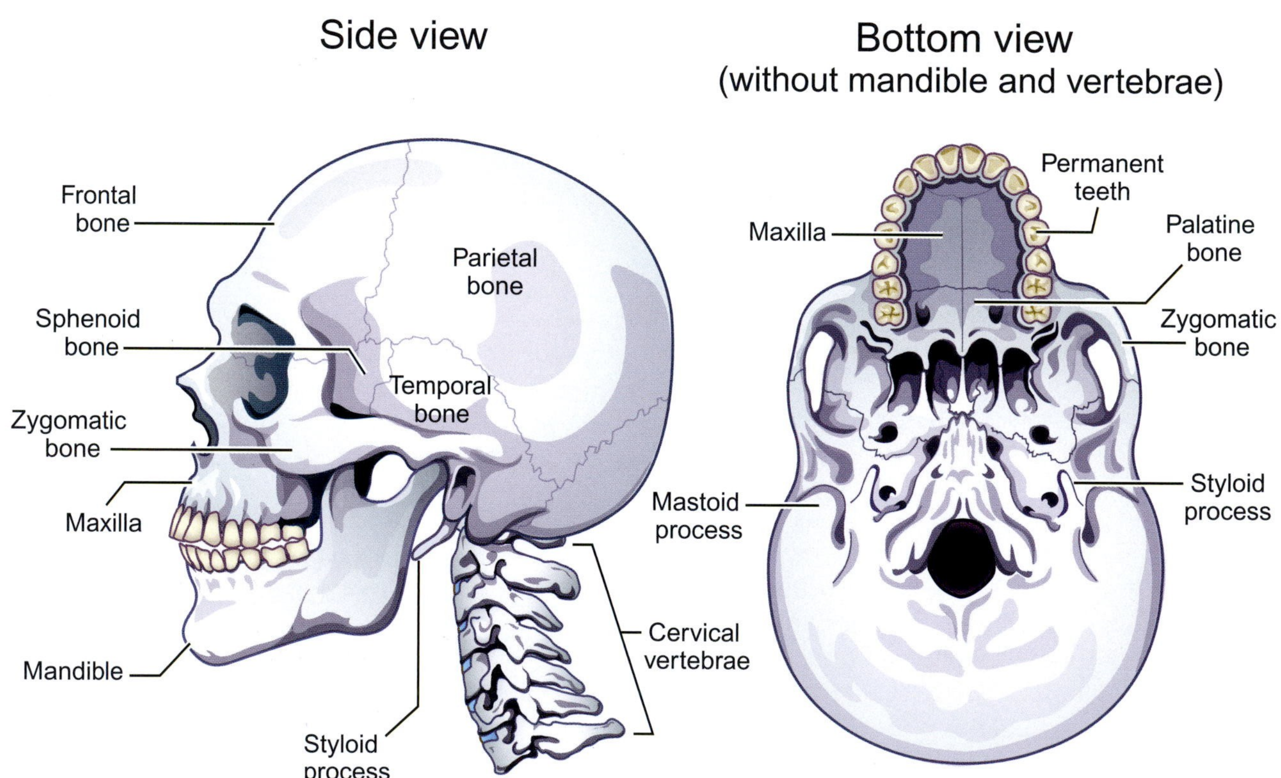

Figure 5–1. Skeletal superstructure of the pharyngeal-oral apparatus.

and protects the brain, and the other is the facial skeleton, which provides an underlying superstructure for much of the pharyngeal-oral apparatus. Certain parts of the facial skeleton are discussed in Chapter 4, in the context of the velopharyngeal-nasal apparatus, and are given further consideration here, along with other parts introduced below. The bones of the facial skeleton are especially important to the pharyngeal-oral apparatus in that they contribute to the formation of the roof, floor, and sides of the oral cavity.

Maxilla. Figure 5–2 depicts the maxilla. The maxilla forms the upper jaw and most of the hard palate. It consists of two complex bones (one on the left and one on the right) that combine at the midline. The maxilla lends strength to the roof of the oral cavity (as well as to the floor of the nasal cavities) and provides a buttress for the facial skeleton. Each bone of the maxilla has a palatine process that extends horizontally to the midline and joins with the palatine process from the opposite side to form the front three-fourths of the hard palate. The back one-fourth of the hard palate is formed by the much smaller palatine bones, which are closely associated with the palatine processes of the maxilla, and have horizontal processes that extend to the midline from each side to complete that part of the hard palate.

Other processes project from the maxilla. One of the most important of these is the alveolar process (sometimes called the alveolar arch). The alveolar process of the maxilla is a thick spongy projection that extends downward and houses the upper teeth. This process accommodates 16 permanent teeth (8 on each side)—6 molars, 4 premolars, 2 canines, and 4 incisors. Ten deciduous teeth (baby teeth or milk teeth) are typically found in infants and young children and are later replaced by the permanent teeth.

Mandible. Figure 5–3 shows the salient features of the mandible. The mandible (lower jaw) is a large horseshoe-shaped structure when viewed from above or below. Its open end faces toward the back. The front and sides of the mandible together form what is termed the body of the structure. The left and right halves of the mandible join at the front through a fibrous symphysis (line of union) that ossifies (turns to bone) during the first year of life. The tooth-bearing upper surface of the body of the mandible is termed its alveolar process (a counterpart to the lower surface of the maxilla). In the adult, the alveolar process of the mandible, like the alveolar process of the maxilla, accommodates 16 permanent teeth—6 molars, 4 premolars, 2 canines, and 4 incisors. Also, like the alveolar process of the maxilla, the alveolar process of the mandible usually holds 10 deciduous teeth (baby teeth or milk teeth) in infants and young children that are later replaced by permanent teeth.

On each side of the mandible toward the back, there is an upward projection. This part of the mandible is referred to as the ramus (meaning a branch from the body). The location along the bottom of the mandible where each ramus diverges upward

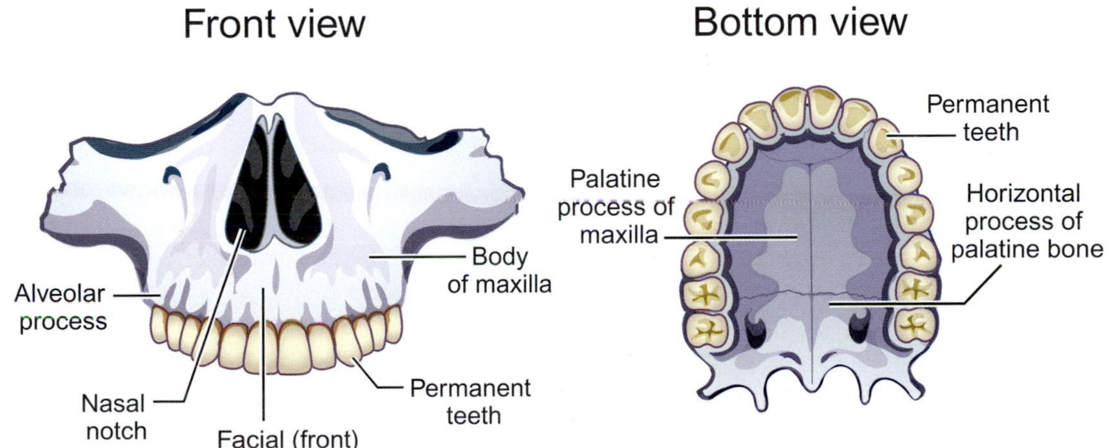

Figure 5–2. Maxilla.

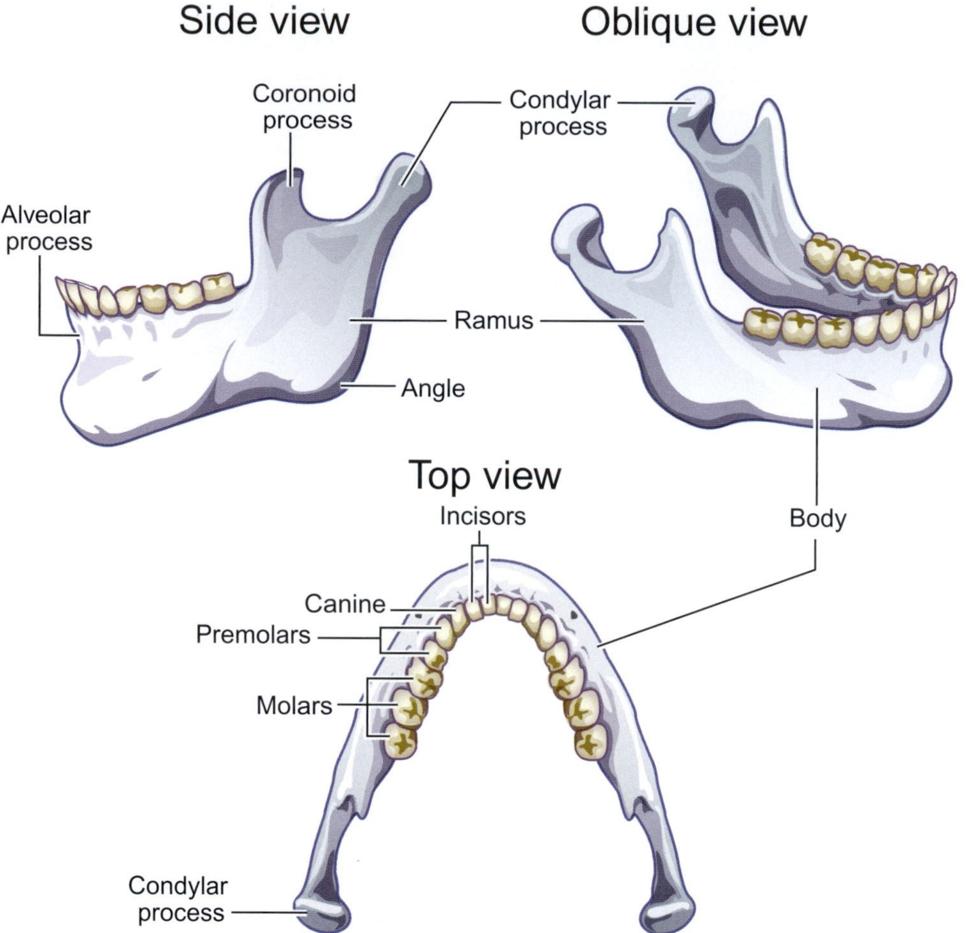

Figure 5–3. Mandible.

is designated as the angle. The upper part of each ramus has two projections, one at the front called the coronoid process and one at the back called the condylar process (also called the condyle). The coronoid process is somewhat rounded, whereas the condylar process has a neck and a prominent head.

Other Bones of the Skull. Other bones of the skull form important components of the pharyngeal-oral apparatus. These bones are some 20 in number and are individually complex structures joined together by immovable fibrous joints (sutures). These bones present a wide array of processes, plates, projections, and air chambers that provide for the purchase of muscles and for the formation of sinuses within the head. The sinuses are hollows within the skull that have connections to the nasal cavities, the most important of which are the so-called paranasal sinuses (frontal, maxillary, ethmoid, and sphenoid).

In addition to the maxilla and mandible, some of the most important bony structures of the skull include the frontal bone (front of the upper braincase), parietal bones (sides of the upper braincase), temporal bones (sides of the lower braincase), sphenoid bone (base of the front of the cranium), palatine bones (back of the roof of the mouth), and zygomatic bones (part of the bony cheeks). Bony structures associated with the velopharyngeal-nasal apparatus are discussed in Chapter 4. Consideration of all of the structural details of the bones of the cranium and facial skeleton is beyond the scope of this chapter. For the reader interested in more detail than that provided here, the illustrations and descriptions of the bones of the skull provided by Zemlin (1998) are recommended. The cartoon in Figure 5–4 offers the reader some inspiration in this regard and illustrates in its legend that anatomy and physiology are tightly linked.

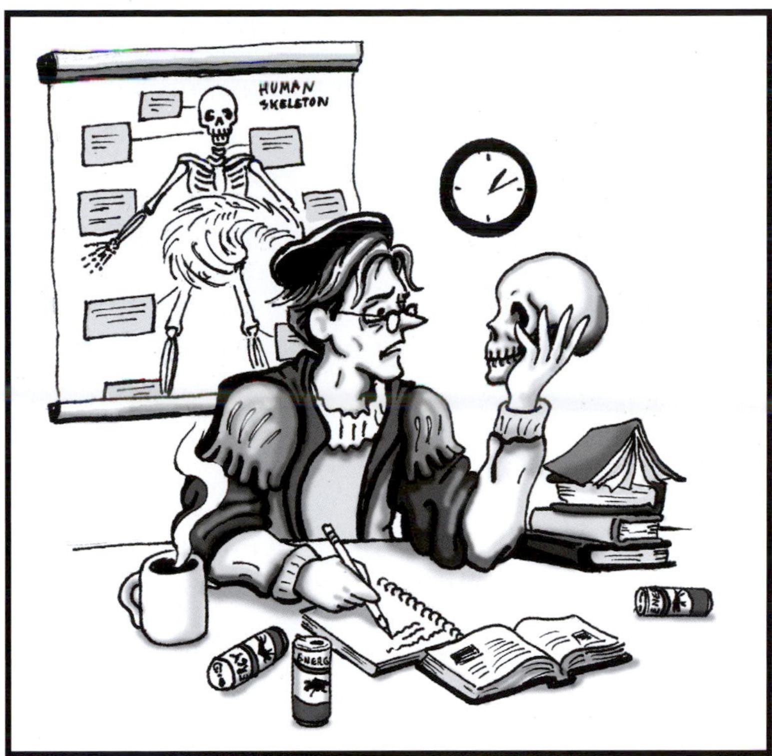

Figure 5–4. "That skull had a tongue in it, and could sing once." (Hamlet in *Hamlet*, Act 5, Scene 1, William Shakespeare).

Grant Fairbanks (1910–1964)

Fairbanks was a giant in speech science. He also trained others who became distinguished scientists. Fairbanks was a key figure in the development of speech science as a discipline and had a major influence in bringing it to the fore as an integrated science. One of his best-known works was the development of the notion that speech production was controlled in the manner of a servomechanism that relied on sensory feedback. His book titled *Voice and Articulation Drillbook* (Fairbanks, 1960) is a classic and contains the famous *Rainbow Passage* that has been used in more speech research studies than any other reading. Fairbanks died while on a flight between Chicago and San Francisco. The flight was diverted to Denver where the coroner ruled that he had choked to death while eating. Fairbanks was greatly admired as a scientist. The three of us are honored to be able to directly trace our professional lineages to him.

Temporomandibular Joints

The mandible (lower jaw) articulates with the left and right temporal bones along the sides of the skull to form the temporomandibular joints. As illustrated in Figure 5–5, these joints are located just in front of and below the ear canals. They can be palpated when the mandible is alternately raised and lowered. The temporomandibular joints are enclosed by

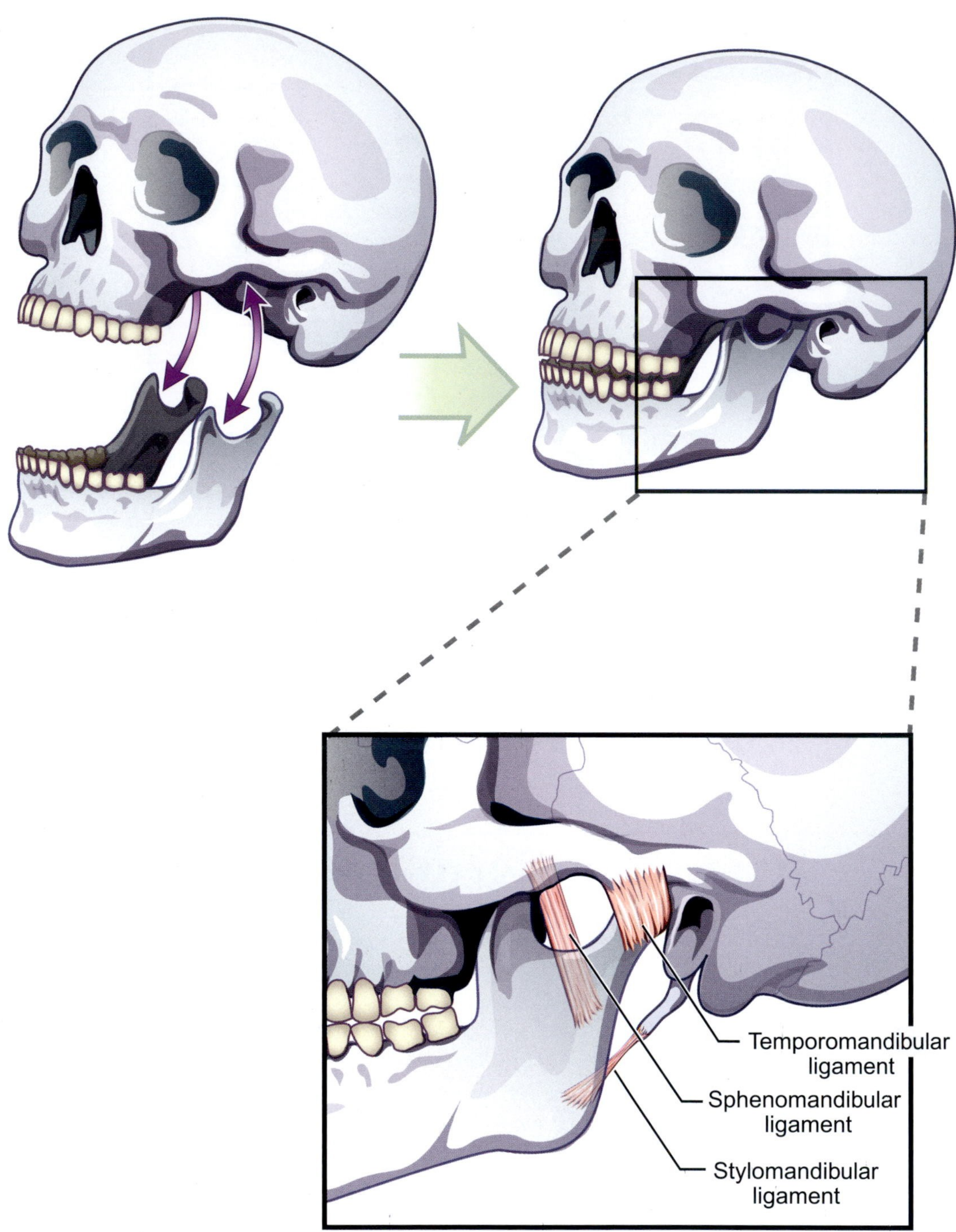

Figure 5–5. Temporomandibular joints and ligaments.

a fibrous capsule and lubricated by synovial fluid. Each joint is of the condyloid variety in that it consists of an ovoid (egg-shaped) process (the head of the condyle) that fits into an elliptical-shaped cavity within the temporal bone on the corresponding side (Dickson & Maue-Dickson, 1982).

The anatomical arrangement of each temporomandibular joint is such that the condyle of the mandible (the more rearward of its two processes) is separated from its receiving cavity by a cartilaginous meniscus (crescent) called the articular disk. The surfaces of the condyle and the temporal bone are themselves covered with fibrocartilage that is devoid of vascular tissue (Sicher & DuBrul, 1975).

Three ligaments influence the function of each temporomandibular joint (see Figure 5–5). These are the temporomandibular ligament, the sphenomandibular ligament, and the stylomandibular ligament. The temporomandibular ligament extends between the outer surface of the zygomatic arch and the outer and back surfaces of the neck of the condyle. This ligament limits the degree to which the condyle can be displaced downward and backward. The sphenomandibular ligament extends between the angular spine of the sphenoid bone and the inner surface of the ramus below the condyle. It limits downward and backward displacement of the mandible. The stylomandibular ligament extends between the styloid process of the temporal bone to near the angle of the mandible. This ligament limits downward and forward displacement of the mandible.

Temporomandibular Joint Movements

Movements at the temporomandibular joints are conditioned by the physical arrangements of the joints and their binding ligaments (both discussed above). The skull and mandible represent the articulating structures of the joint and the relative movement of these two dictates the nature of the action possible. For most activities, the skull is considered to be the more rigidly fixed member of the pair. Under some circumstances, however, the opposite is true. An example is when the chin is rested on the top of a table and the jaws are separated, such that the skull rotates upward and backward. Excluding such circumstances, movements at the temporomandibular joints are routinely conceptualized as movements of the mandible relative to a stabilized skull. This convention is followed here.

Movements of the mandible are mediated through its condylar processes and are determined by how these processes are oriented within the elliptical-shaped receiving cavities of the temporal bones. The mandible can be moved in several ways relative to the skull. As shown in Figure 5–6, it can be displaced upward and downward, forward and backward, and side to side. These three displacement possibilities are made possible by a hinge-like action, a forward and backward gliding action, and a side-to-side gliding action, respectively. The displacement possibilities depicted in Figure 5–6 are portrayed individually. This portrayal belies the fact that the movements at the temporomandibular joints are often multidimensional and very complex. This complexity is discussed below in other sections.

Internal Topography

The internal topography of the pharyngeal-oral apparatus is fashioned around a hollow tube that bends at a right angle at the junction between the pharyngeal and oral portions of the structure. The pharyngeal, oral, and buccal cavities and their mucous lining deserve individual consideration.

Pharyngeal Cavity. Recall from Chapter 4 that the pharynx (throat) is a tube of tendon and muscle that extends from the base of the skull to the larynx. This tube is widest at the top and narrows down its length and is larger side to side than front to back. The lower and middle parts of the pharyngeal tube are designated as the laryngopharynx and oropharynx, respectively, and are the parts of greatest interest in this chapter. Pharyngeal muscles ring the back and sides of the laryngopharynx and oropharynx. The lower part of the oropharynx is bounded by the tongue and epiglottis, whereas the upper part of the structure opens into the mouth at the front through the anterior faucial pillars (palatoglossal arch). The back wall of the upper part of the oropharynx can be seen when looking back through the faucial isthmus (see Figure 4–4).

Oral Cavity. Figure 5–7 depicts the oral cavity (mouth cavity). The oral cavity is bounded at the front and sides by the lips, teeth, and alveolar processes of the maxilla and mandible, above by the hard palate and velum, below by the floor of the mouth (mainly the tongue), and at the back by the anterior faucial pillars (palatoglossal arch). The front entryway to the oral cavity is designated as the oral vestibule and is defined to include the lips, cheeks, front teeth, and forward-most segments of the alveolar processes of the maxilla and mandible. The lips and/or front teeth form the front orifice of the oral cavity (oral airway opening). The palatoglossal arch forms an orifice at the back of the cavity.

The tongue is, of course, a prominent feature of the oral cavity. Although unitary in nature, it is sometimes subdivided into different regions. The subdivisions chosen may have either anatomical

Side view

Occlusion

Side view

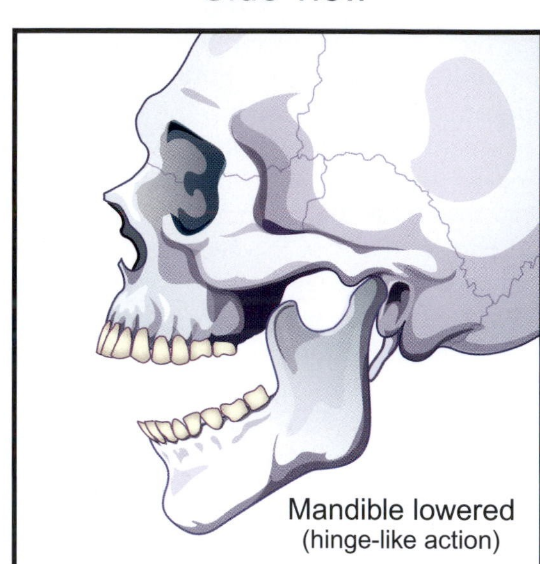

Side view

Mandible moved forward (gliding action)

Front view

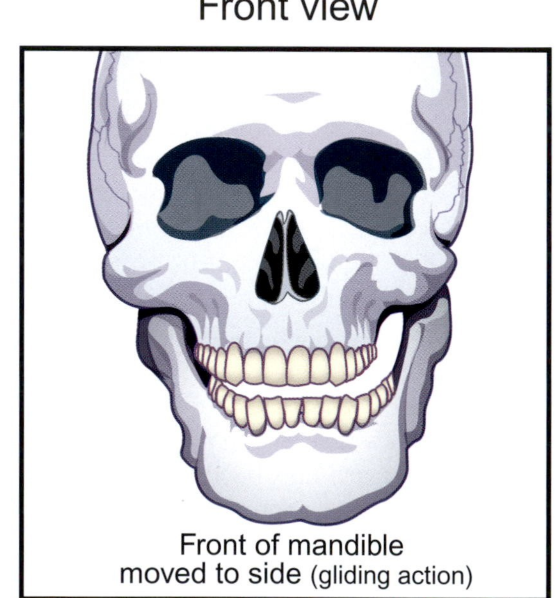

Figure 5–6. Temporomandibular joint movements.

or functional bases, depending on their purpose. Anatomical schemes usually recognize a root and a blade to the tongue, the former pertaining to the vertically oriented back wall of the structure (front wall of the laryngopharynx and oropharynx) and the latter pertaining to the horizontally oriented upper surface of the structure (floor of the oral cavity) (Zemlin, 1998). In contrast, functional schemes usually recognize regions of the tongue that are considered important for one or another functional behaviors of the structure (Kent, 1997). Figure 5–8 adopts a scheme that has relevance to the purposes of this chapter and those of Chapter 12 (Swallowing).

In Figure 5–8, the tongue is shown as consisting of five different components, termed the tip, blade, dorsum, root, and body. The tip of the tongue is the

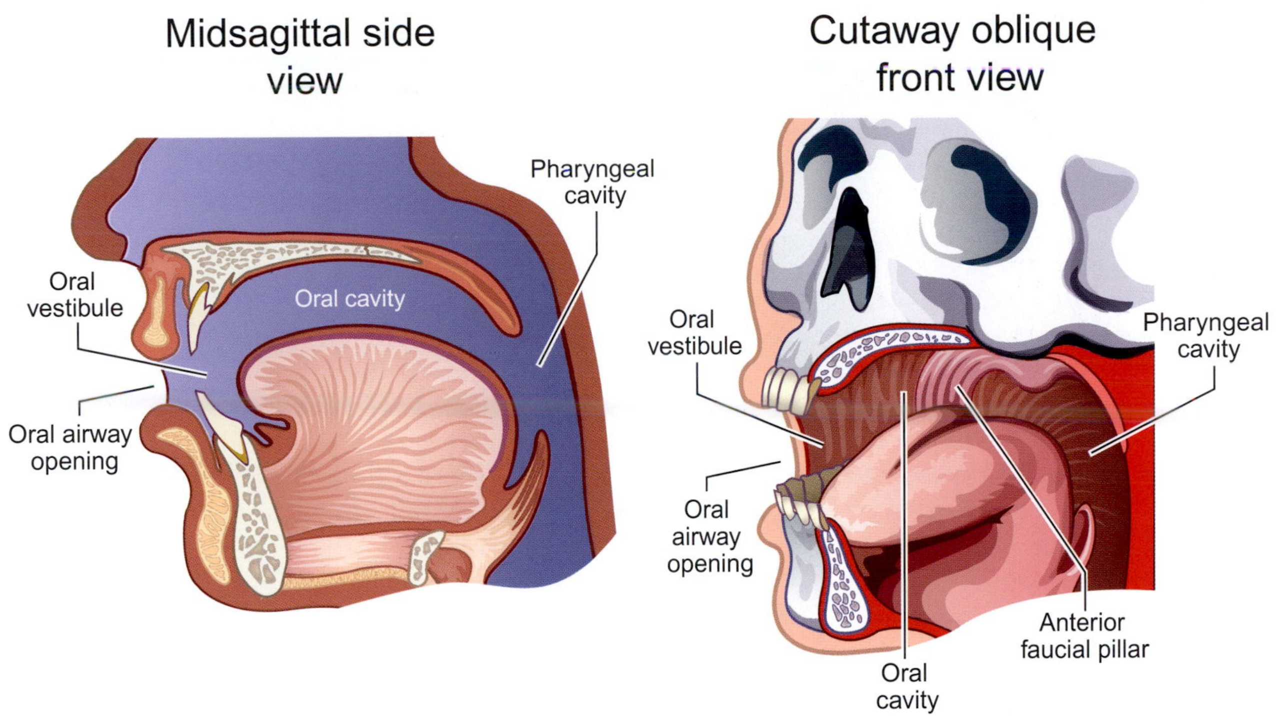

Figure 5–7. Oral cavity and oral vestibule.

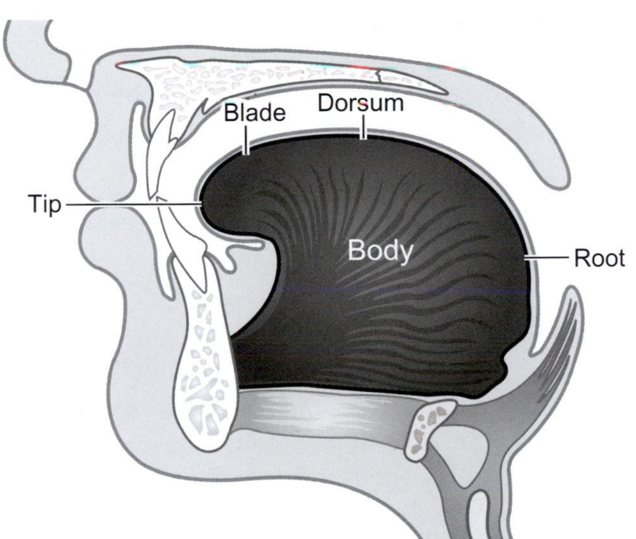

Figure 5–8. Functional scheme showing five components of the tongue.

part of its surface nearest the front teeth at rest. The blade is the part of its surface that lies behind the tip and below the alveolar ridge of the maxilla and the front part of the hard palate. The dorsum of the tongue constitutes the surface that lies behind the blade and below the back part of the hard palate and the velum. The root of the tongue designates the part of the surface of the structure that faces the back of the pharynx and the front of the epiglottis. And, the body of the tongue represents its central mass, which underlies the other four surface features discussed.

Buccal Cavity. The buccal cavity lies to the sides of the oral cavity. This cavity constitutes the small space between the gums (gingivae) and teeth internally and the lips and cheeks (buccae) externally. The buccal cavity connects to the oral cavity through spaces between the teeth and behind the last molars. The status of the lips and cheeks are major determinants of the size of the buccal cavity.

Mucous Lining. The pharyngeal-oral apparatus contains a mucous lining on its internal surfaces. This lining consists of an outer layer of epithelium and an inner layer of connective tissue (lamina propria). The details of this layering differ at different locations within the pharyngeal-oral apparatus, especially the outer layer of epithelium (Dickson & Maue-Dickson, 1982). The most prominent mucosa

Dancing in the Moonlight

He was a pleasant young man who was honorably discharged after serving in the military. He had made his way to a large Veterans Administration Medical Center. His only complaint was hearing loss, but the audiologist thought his speech was inconsistent with his hearing test results. The moment he said his name to the speech-language pathologist, there was suspicion that he had impairment of one or both cranial nerves serving the tongue. When asked to open his mouth, the beam of a flashlight revealed a shrunken and wrinkled tongue that seemed to dance around under the surface like a bagful of jumping beans. The signs were classic of lower motor neuron disease and a neurologist reported presumptive bilateral congenital agenesis (failure to develop) of the hypoglossal nerves (motor nerves to the tongue). How had this escaped detection during his physical examination for the military? Perhaps he was only asked to say "ah."

general lining has a shiny appearance and covers all of the soft tissues of the apparatus except the gums, hard palate, and tongue. A so-called masticatory mucosa covers the gums and the hard palate and has a collagen subflooring that causes its epithelium to hold firmly against adjacent bone. The upper surface of the tongue is covered with what is termed a specialized mucosa. This mucosa contains an array of small pockets and crypts that house taste buds.

Forces and Movements of the Pharyngeal-Oral Apparatus

Forces are responsible for movements of the pharyngeal-oral apparatus. Such forces and movements constitute the mechanical level of function of the apparatus.

Forces of the Pharyngeal-Oral Apparatus

Two types of forces are applied to the pharyngeal-oral apparatus, passive and active. Passive force is inherent and always present, but subject to change. Active force is applied in accordance with the will and ability of the individual.

Passive Force. The passive force of the pharyngeal-oral apparatus arises from several sources. These include the natural recoil of structures that line its walls, the surface tension between structures in apposition (lips, tongue, gums, hard palate, velum), the pull of gravity, and aeromechanical forces within the pharyngeal and oral portions of the apparatus (throat, mouth, oral vestibule). The distribution, sign, and magnitude of passive force depend on mechanical circumstances, including the positions, deformations, and levels of activity (if pertinent) of different components of the pharyngeal-oral apparatus.

Active Force. The active force of pharyngeal-oral function comes from the contraction of muscles. Some muscles are intrinsic, meaning that they have both ends attached within a component, and some are extrinsic, meaning that they have one end attached within a component and one end attached outside the component. Muscle actions within the pharyngeal-oral apparatus are not fully understood, but are known with reasonable certainty based on their architectures, the consequences of muscle activations, and observations of electrical activities.

The function portrayed here for individual muscles assumes that the muscle of interest is engaged in a shortening (concentric) contraction, unless otherwise specified as being involved in a lengthening (eccentric) contraction or a fixed-length (isometric) contraction. The tongue presents a somewhat more complex situation because of its special status as a muscular hydrostat (see below). The influence of individual muscle actions is also dependent on whether other muscles are active simultaneously, the mechanical status of different components of the apparatus, and the nature of the activity being performed.

Muscles of the Pharynx. The muscles of the pharynx are discussed in detail and portrayed in Chapter 4. These are located within the laryngopharynx, oropharynx, and nasopharynx. For the purposes of this chapter, those within the laryngopharynx and oropharynx are of primary interest and are reviewed here briefly.

Muscles of the laryngopharynx and oropharynx can influence the lumen of the pharynx (the cross section along its length) in the region that lies behind the tongue, epiglottis, and oral cavity (the back wall of which is easily visualized through the faucial isthmus). The lumen of the pharynx in this region can also be influenced by adjustments of the tongue and epiglottis. Muscles that attach to the laryngopharynx and oropharynx fabric proper (within the posterior and lateral pharyngeal walls) are revisited here. These include the ***inferior constrictor*** muscle, ***middle constrictor*** muscle, and ***stylopharyngeus*** muscle.

The ***inferior constrictor*** muscle of the pharynx is located toward the bottom of the structure. Fibers of the muscle arise from the sides of the thyroid and cricoid cartilages and diverge in a fan-like configuration as they course backward and toward the midline. There they interdigitate with fibers of the paired mate from the opposite side. The middle and upper fibers of the muscle ascend obliquely, whereas the lowermost fibers run horizontally and downward and are continuous with those of the esophagus. When the ***inferior constrictor*** muscle contracts, it pulls the lower part of the back wall of the pharynx forward and draws the sidewalls of the lower pharynx forward and inward. These actions cause the lumen of the lower pharynx to reduce in cross section.

The ***middle constrictor*** muscle of the pharynx is located midway along the length of the pharyngeal tube. Fibers of the muscle arise from the greater and lesser horns of the hyoid bone and the stylohyoid ligament and course backward and toward the midline where they insert into the median raphe of the pharynx. The uppermost fibers of the ***middle constrictor*** muscle course obliquely upward and overlap the lower fibers of the ***superior constrictor*** muscle, whereas the lowermost fibers of the muscle run obliquely downward beneath the fibers of the ***inferior constrictor*** muscle. Recall that this fiber arrangement is akin to the way in which roof shingles partially overlap. When the ***middle constrictor*** muscle contracts, it decreases the cross-sectional area of the oropharynx by pulling forward on the posterior pharyngeal wall and forward and inward on the lateral pharyngeal wall. Simultaneous contraction of the left and right ***middle constrictor*** muscles causes the pharyngeal lumen to constrict regionally in the manner of a sphincter.

The ***stylopharyngeus*** muscle extends between the styloid process of the temporal bone and the lateral wall of the pharynx near the juncture of the ***superior constrictor*** and ***middle constrictor*** muscles of the pharynx. Its fibers run downward, forward, and toward the midline. When the ***stylopharyngeus*** muscle contracts, it pulls the pharyngeal tube upward and draws the lateral wall of the pharynx toward the side. Together with similar action of its paired mate from the opposite side, there results a widening or dilation of the lumen of the pharynx, especially in the region of the oropharynx, but also elsewhere along the length of the pharyngeal tube.

Muscles of the Mandible. Seven muscles provide active forces that operate on the mandible. These muscles are depicted in Figure 5–9 and are responsible for positioning the mandible in accordance with the movements allowed by the temporomandibular joints. Included among these muscles are the ***masseter, temporalis, internal pterygoid, external pterygoid, digastric, mylohyoid,*** and ***geniohyoid***.

The ***masseter*** muscle is a flat, quadrilateral structure that covers much of the outer surface of the ramus of the mandible. Fibers of the muscle are in two layers. An outer layer forms the bulk of the muscle and courses from an aponeurosis along the front two-thirds of the zygomatic arch downward and backward to insert on the angle and nearby outer surface of the ramus of the mandible. An inner layer of fibers courses from the entire length of the zygomatic arch downward and forward to insert into the outer surface of the upper half of the ramus and its coronoid process. Contraction of the outer layer of the ***masseter*** muscle results in elevation of the

the form of a dense felt-like network of fibrous elastic tissue that lies below the epidermis and constitutes an encapsulating structural bag around the tongue (Zemlin, 1998). It is through this special soft skeleton of the tongue that various muscles are able to bring about the wide variety of tongue movements that are possible (see discussion below).

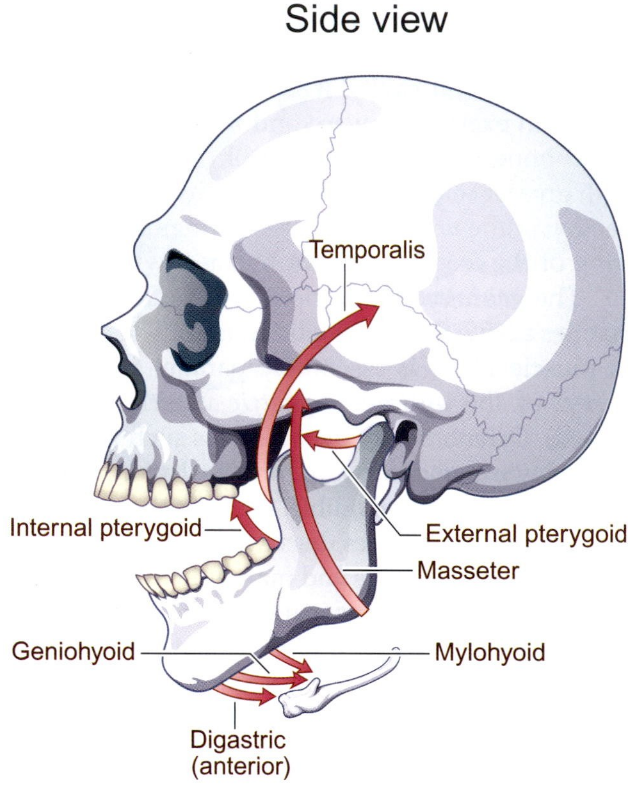

Figure 5–10. Actions of muscles of the mandible.

Eight muscles are responsible for movements of the tongue. These include four intrinsic muscles (having both their origins and insertions within the tongue) and four extrinsic muscles (having their origins in adjacent structures and their insertions in the tongue).

The intrinsic muscles of the tongue include the ***superior longitudinal, inferior longitudinal, vertical,*** and ***transverse*** muscles. These muscles are depicted in Figure 5–11.

The ***superior longitudinal*** muscle is a broad, flat muscle that lies just beneath the expansive upper surface (dorsum) of the tongue. Fibers originate within the root of the tongue from the hyoid bone and course forward in an imbricated pattern (like overlapping fish scales) along the long axis of the tongue. Forward attachments of the muscle are in the region of the front edges of the tongue and the upper surface of the tongue tip. Fibers near the midline course downward to their attachments, whereas fibers toward the side course obliquely toward the lateral boundary of the tongue. Contraction of the entire ***superior longitudinal*** muscle can shorten the tongue and increase its convexity from front to back. Because the muscle is composed of a series of short imbricated fibers, it can also activate

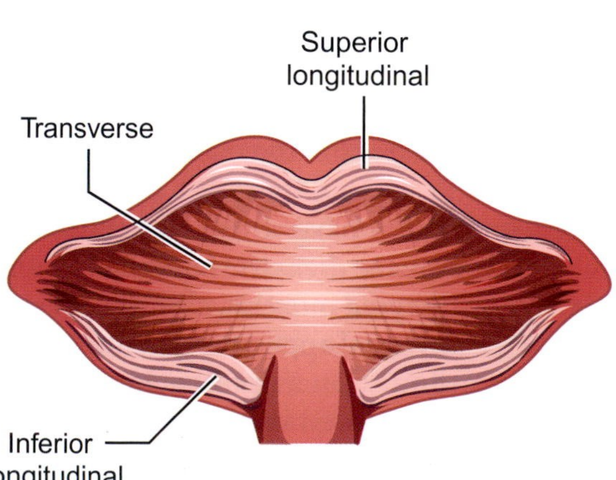

Figure 5–11. Intrinsic muscles of the tongue.

in patterns that differentially affect the regional configuration of the tongue. For example, contraction of fibers toward the front of the tongue can pull the tongue tip upward and toward the side of muscle activation. Simultaneous contractions of comparable fibers in the paired ***superior longitudinal*** muscles elevate the tongue tip without deviation to either side. For another example, contraction of fibers that insert obliquely into the edges of the tongue can pull the lateral margins of the structure upward to create a longitudinal trough down the center of the tongue toward the front.

The ***inferior longitudinal*** muscle is positioned near the undersurface of the tongue somewhat toward the side. It arises from the body of the hyoid bone at the root of the tongue and courses forward through the body of the tongue to insert near the lower surface of the tongue tip. Fibers of the ***inferior longitudinal*** muscle blend with the fibers of different extrinsic muscles of the tongue (discussed below) within the body of the tongue. Contraction of the ***inferior longitudinal*** muscle shortens the tongue and pulls the tip of the structure downward and toward the same side. Simultaneous contraction of comparable fibers in the paired ***inferior longitudinal*** muscles pulls the tongue tip downward symmetrically.

The ***vertical*** muscle originates from just beneath the dorsum of the tongue and courses downward vertically and toward the side through the body of the tongue. Fibers of the ***vertical*** muscle terminate near the sides of the tongue along its lower surface. There is some suggestion that not all fibers follow a course through the entire body of the tongue, but rather are found only in the upper half of the tongue (Miyawaki, 1974), or that there is a mixture of short and long fibers, some of which course only through the upper half of the tongue and some of which course all the way to the lower part of the tongue (Abd-El-Malek, 1939). Contraction of the ***vertical*** muscle results in a flattening of the tongue on the side of action, especially toward its lateral margins. More midline parts of the upper tongue surface may also be lowered on the side of action as a result of pull exerted during the contraction of this muscle.

The ***transverse*** muscle, as its name implies, courses side to side within the tongue. Fibers of the muscle arise mainly from the median fibrous skeleton of the tongue and course laterally, where they terminate in fibrous tissue along the side of the tongue. Upper fibers fan out in an upward direction, whereas lower fibers fan out in a downward direction. The intermingling of ***transverse*** muscle fibers with those of other intrinsic and extrinsic tongue muscles is extensive and makes it hard to determine their precise course and location within different parts of the tongue. Some fibers may not extend all the way to the sides of the tongue (Miyawaki, 1974) and the extent to which fibers are located at the back of the tongue is in question (Abd-El-Malek, 1939). The

Early X-Games

This isn't about sports, but about x-rays. Early uses of x-rays to study structures of the upper airway during speech production were quite interesting. A few tidbits should give you an appreciation. A narrow gold chain was often placed down the midline of the tongue to make its longitudinal configuration easy to visualize on single shot lateral head x-rays. Some of the first findings from different laboratories were not in agreement concerning tongue positions during vowel productions. Despite public arguments about linguistic bases for the differences, it turned out that the head had not been fixed in position and variation was related to its rotation from one exposure to another. Then, there were dangers. A pioneer in the use of x-rays for speech research entered old age unable to grow a beard on one side of his face, the side he had frequently bombarded with x-rays to get the view of the speech production apparatus he wanted to study.

transverse muscle is, however, a major constituent in the mass of interwoven muscle fibers that constitute the bulk of the tongue. Contraction of the ***transverse*** muscle results in a narrowing of the tongue from side to side and an elongation of the tongue.

The extrinsic muscles of the tongue include the ***styloglossus***, ***palatoglossus***, ***hyoglossus***, and ***genioglossus*** muscles. These are depicted in Figure 5–12.

The ***styloglossus*** muscle originates from the front and side of the styloid process of the temporal bone and the stylomandibular ligament. Fibers of the muscle course forward, downward, and toward the midline to insert into the sides of the root of the tongue. From there, they run in various directions, but primarily toward the midline and forward within the body of the tongue. Some fibers of the ***styloglossus*** muscle interdigitate with fibers of the ***inferior longitudinal*** muscle, whereas others interdigitate with fibers of the ***hyoglossus*** muscle (discussed below and in Chapter 3). Ultimate blending of different fibers makes it difficult to distinguish those of one muscle from another. Contraction of the ***styloglossus*** muscle can have multiple consequences. These include that (a) the body of the tongue can be drawn upward and backward, (b) the side of the tongue can be pulled upward to influence the structure's concavity, (c) the tongue can be shortened, and (d) the tongue tip can be pulled toward the side.

The ***palatoglossus*** muscle is discussed in Chapter 4 as a part of the velopharyngeal-nasal apparatus. There it is referred to as the ***glossopalatine*** muscle (its origin and insertion being reversed in that context). For present purposes, the ***palatoglossus*** muscle can be thought of as originating from the lower surface of the palatal aponeurosis. Fibers from the muscle course downward, forward, and toward the side (forming the anterior faucial pillar) and insert into the side of the root of the tongue. There the fibers of the ***palatoglossus*** muscle blend with those of the ***transverse***, ***styloglossus***, and ***hyoglossus*** muscles of the tongue. When the ***palatoglossus*** muscle contracts, it pulls upward, backward, and inward on the root of the tongue. Through its action, the muscle can displace the tongue mass backward in the oral cavity and increase the concavity of its upper surface. When the left and right ***palatoglossus*** muscles contract simultaneously, the result is a lengthwise grooving of the upper surface of the tongue.

The ***hyoglossus*** muscle (see also Chapter 3) is a quadrilateral structure that originates from the upper border of the body and greater cornu of

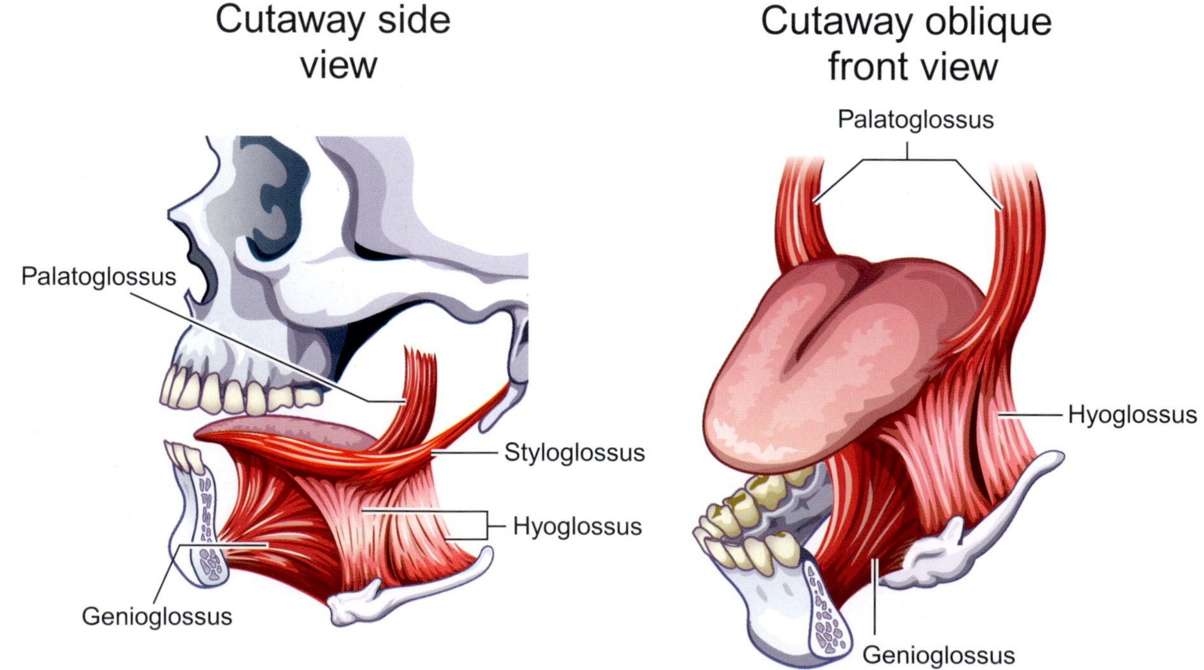

Figure 5–12. Extrinsic muscles of the tongue.

the hyoid bone and extends upward and forward to insert into the side of the tongue toward the rear. Fibers of the ***hyoglossus*** muscle intermingle with those of the ***styloglossus*** and ***palatoglossus*** muscles. Some authors consider one particular bundle of fibers within the ***hyoglossus*** muscle to be a separate muscle (Zemlin, 1998). This bundle is identified as the ***chondroglossus*** muscle and has fibers that extend from the hyoid bone farther forward into the tip of the tongue where they intermingle with fibers from intrinsic tongue muscles such as the ***inferior longitudinal*** muscle. Contraction of the ***hyoglossus*** (and ***chondroglossus***) muscle results in a lowering of the body of the tongue and a backward displacement of its mass. The lowering effect is most pronounced along the sides of the tongue (Dickson & Maue-Dickson, 1982).

The ***genioglossus*** muscle is a complex muscle that makes up a large portion of the tongue. This muscle is fan-shaped and originates as three groups of fibers from the inner surface of the body of the mandible near the midline. The lower fibers course backward to insert into the root of the tongue. The middle fibers course backward and extend upward into the tongue in the region of the juncture between the dorsum and blade of the structure. The upper fibers run vertically and forward to insert into the tip of the tongue (Langdon, Klueber, & Barnwell, 1978), although some authors report that fibers stop short of the tongue tip itself (Doran & Baggett, 1972; Miyawaki, 1974). Collectively, fibers of the ***genioglossus*** muscle travel through the body of the tongue between layers of muscle fibers formed by the ***vertical***, ***transverse***, and ***superior longitudinal*** muscles of the structure (Dickson & Maue-Dickson, 1982). Contraction of the ***genioglossus*** muscle can have a diverse set of consequences, depending on which particular fibers of the muscle are activated and in what patterns. Possible outcomes are that (a) the root of the tongue can be moved forward so as to force the tip of the tongue against the teeth or out of the mouth, (b) the front of the tongue can be pulled backward, and (c) the center line of the tongue can be pulled downward so as to form a trough-like depression along the length of the upper surface of the structure.

Figure 5–13 graphically illustrates the general force vectors associated with actions of the eight

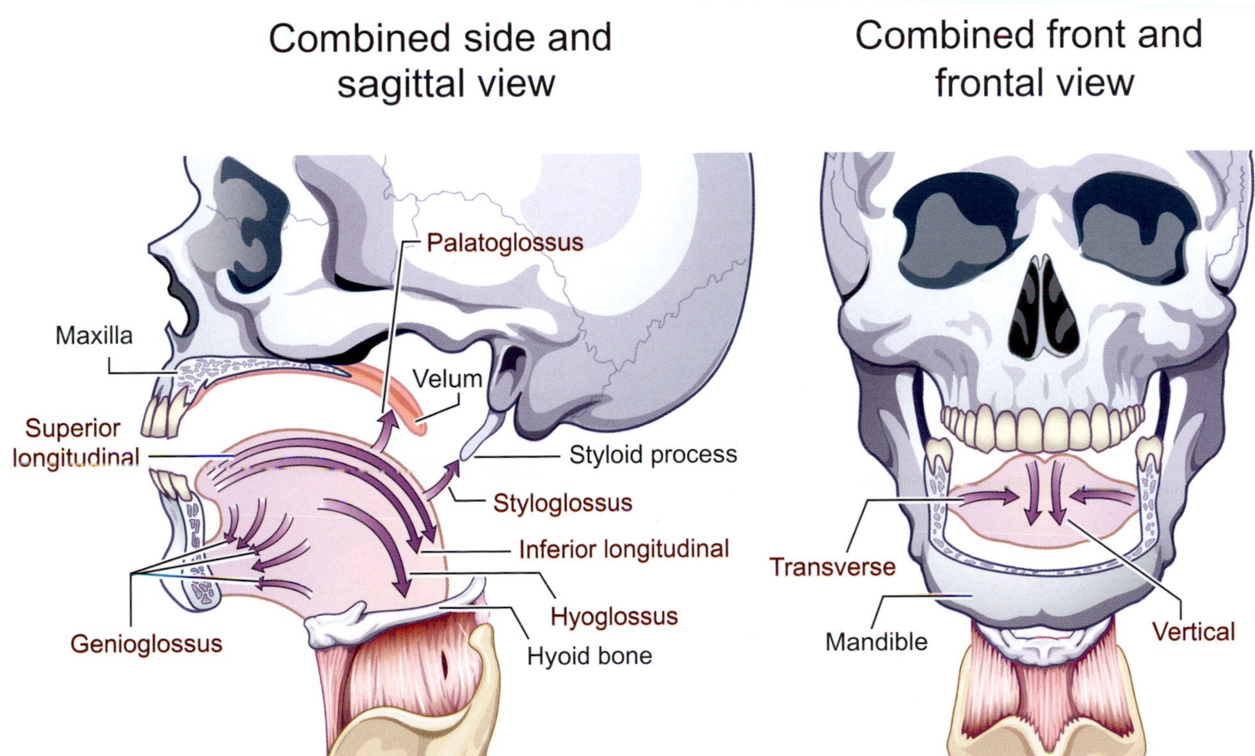

Figure 5–13. Actions of the muscles of the tongue.

muscles of the tongue. This illustration summarizes the potential active forces operating on the tongue and shows combinations of forces that could be in play at any moment to change the configuration of the tongue and its positioning within the pharyngeal-oral apparatus.

The discussion to this juncture about the individual capabilities of intrinsic and extrinsic tongue muscles is linear in nature and, although instructive, does not do justice to the intricate and interacting forces that can operate on and within the tongue to move it in different ways. Much of this has to do with special properties of the tongue that qualify it as a muscular hydrostat. These properties and the remarkable range of tongue movements are discussed below in the context of adjustment capabilities of the pharyngeal-oral apparatus.

Muscles of the Lips. The muscles of the lips are a subset of the muscles of the face. These muscles are more than a dozen in number and are portrayed in Figure 5–14 from different perspectives. The muscles of the lips include both intrinsic (contained within) and extrinsic (one attachment within) components. These muscles include the ***orbicularis oris, buccinator, risorius, levator labii superioris, levator labii superioris aleque nasi, zygomatic major, zygomatic minor, depressor labii inferioris, mentalis, levator anguli oris, depressor anguli oris, incisivus labii superioris, incisivus labii inferioris,*** and ***platysma***.

The ***orbicularis oris*** muscle is a ring of muscle within the lips that forms a sphincter at the oral end (mouth opening) of the pharyngeal-oral apparatus. The ring of muscle is complex and is constituted of fibers from both intrinsic and extrinsic sources that intertwine to form an airway valve and the most mobile part of the face. Fibers of the ***orbicularis oris*** muscle that are exclusive to the lips (intrinsic) are arranged in concentric rings around the border of the sphincter. These rings follow the outer contour of the upper and lower lips. The course of the intrinsic fibers of the ***orbicularis oris*** muscle changes with changes in the angular circumference of the

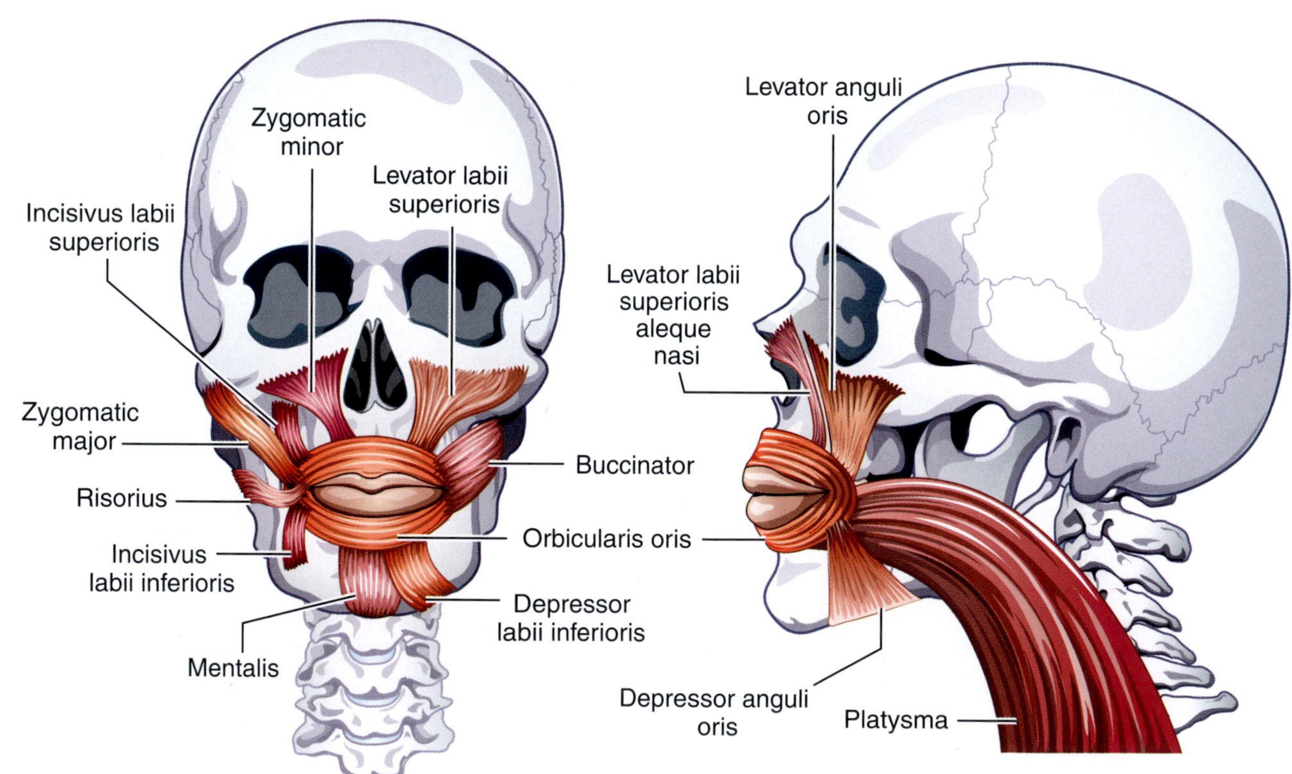

Figure 5–14. Muscles of the lips.

mouth opening. Contraction of the ***orbicularis oris*** muscle can result in several positional changes of the lips. These include movements of the lips toward one another and forward, which, if extensive enough, can result in closure of the mouth and a forcing together of the lips. The corners of the mouth may also move as a result of activation of the ***orbicularis oris*** muscle. Such movement can be upward, downward, toward the side, or toward the midline. Action of the muscle may also force the lips and/or corners of the mouth against the teeth.

Those lip muscles that are extrinsic are sometimes subgrouped into sets that follow fiber courses that are transverse (horizontal), angular (oblique to the corners of the mouth), vertical (from above or below), and parallel (adjacent to and alongside the lips). These subsets are considered, in turn, below. An additional muscle is also discussed at the end of this section. This muscle, the ***platysma***, is classified as a cervical (neck) muscle, but is included as a special case because it has extrinsic influences on the lower lip.

The transverse facial muscles that influence the lips are the ***buccinator*** muscle and the ***risorius*** muscle. The former is sometimes called the bugler's muscle and the latter is often referred to as the laughter muscle.

The ***buccinator*** muscle is a broad muscle that forms part of the cheek. It originates from the pterygomandibular ligament, the outer surface of the alveolar process of the maxilla, and the mandible from the region of the last molars. Fibers course horizontally forward and toward the midline to insert into the upper and lower lips near the corner of the mouth. Uppermost fibers of the muscle enter the upper lip, whereas lowermost fibers enter the lower lip. Fibers of the central part of the muscle converge near the corner of the mouth and cross such that the lower fibers of that part of the muscle insert into the upper lip and the upper fibers insert into the lower lip. Contraction of the ***buccinator*** muscle can pull the corner of the mouth backward and toward the side. It can also force the lips and cheek against adjacent teeth.

The ***risorius*** muscle is a small muscle located within the cheek, but closer to the surface than the ***buccinator*** muscle. It arises from fascia of the ***masseter*** muscle and courses horizontally forward and toward the midline to insert into the corner of the mouth and the lower lip. Contraction of the ***risorius*** muscle draws the corner of the mouth backward and toward the side. Contraction of the muscle may also force the lips against adjacent teeth.

The angular muscle group includes five muscles. These are the ***levator labii superioris*** muscle, ***levator labii superioris aleque nasi*** muscle, ***zygomatic major*** muscle, ***zygomatic minor*** muscle, and the ***depressor labii inferioris*** muscle.

The ***levator labii superioris*** muscle has a broad origin from below the orbit of the eye, the front of the maxillary bone, and the zygomatic bone. Its fibers

Street Talk About Talking

The folk language is filled with indications that the person on the street knows something about pharyngeal-oral function in speech production. Below is a baker's dozen of expressions that we generated off the tops of our heads. Look at these and then try to add to the list from your own knowledge of the folk language. Our favorite from the list below is the last one, used during World War II to mean be careful to whom you are talking. Here goes. "That's a real tongue twister." "We were just jawing it." "He's bumping his gums." "They were flapping their cheeks." "She's lying through her teeth." "Don't give me any of your lip." "He has a great set of pipes." "I don't chew my cabbage twice." "He's running off at the mouth again." "Hold your tongue, young man." "She's a big loudmouth." "His father told him to cork it." And our favorite, "Loose lips sink ships."

course downward and slightly inward and insert into the upper lip. Contraction of the ***levator labii superioris*** muscle results in elevation of the upper lip. Contraction may also cause an outward turning (eversion) of the upper lip.

The ***levator labii superioris aleque nasi*** muscle originates as a slender slip from the front of the maxilla and courses vertically downward and slightly toward the side. The muscle divides into a nasal segment and a lip segment. Fibers from the lip segment of the muscle insert into the upper lip where they intermingle with fibers of the ***orbicularis oris*** muscle. Contraction of the lip segment of the ***levator labii superioris aleque nasi*** muscle causes elevation of the upper lip. Contraction of the nasal segment of the muscle dilates the anterior naris on the corresponding side, as described in Chapter 4.

The ***zygomatic major*** muscle has its origin on the side of the zygomatic bone and runs down and toward the midline where it inserts into the corner of the mouth. Fibers associated with its insertion intermingle with those of the ***orbicularis oris*** muscle. Contraction of the ***zygomatic major*** muscle pulls backward on the corner of the mouth. At the same time, action of the muscle lifts the corner of the mouth upward and toward the side.

The ***zygomatic minor*** muscle originates from the inner surface of the zygomatic bone. Its fibers course downward and toward the midline where they insert into the upper lip and interweave with fibers of the ***orbicularis oris*** muscle. Contraction of the ***zygomatic minor*** muscle results in elevation of the upper lip. It also pulls the corner of the mouth upward.

The ***depressor labii inferioris*** muscle is a small, flat muscle located off the midline of the lower lip. Fibers of the muscle originate from the front surface of the mandible and course upward and inward to insert into the lower lip from near the midline to the corner of the mouth. Contraction of the ***depressor labii inferioris*** muscle pulls the lower lip downward and toward the side. It may also cause the lower lip to turn outward.

The vertical facial muscles are three in number. They include the ***mentalis*** muscle, ***levator anguli oris*** muscle, and the ***depressor anguli oris*** muscle.

The ***mentalis*** muscle lies on the front of the chin. It is a small muscle that arises from the front and side of the mandible near the midline and inserts into the ***orbicularis oris*** muscle and the skin overlying the chin. Contraction of the ***mentalis*** muscle results in upward displacement of the soft tissue of the chin, a forcing of the lower part of the lower lip against the alveolar process of the mandible, and an outward curling of the lower lip. The lower lip may also elevate somewhat during contraction of the ***mentalis*** muscle. The functional potentials described are consistent with the familiar signs of pouting and, indeed, the ***mentalis*** muscle is sometimes called the "pouting muscle."

The ***levator anguli oris*** muscle (also referred to as the ***caninus*** muscle) originates from the front of the maxilla and courses downward and forward to insert into both the upper lip and the lower lip near the corner of the mouth. There, its fibers intermingle with those of the ***orbicularis oris*** muscle. Contraction of the ***levator anguli oris*** muscle draws the corner of the mouth upward and toward the side. Activation of the muscle can also elevate the lower lip against the upper lip and force the lips together.

The ***depressor anguli oris*** muscle is also sometimes referred to as the ***triangularis*** muscle. As its alternate name implies, the muscle is roughly triangular in form. This muscle has a broad origin from the outer surface of the mandible. Its fibers course upward and converge before inserting into the ***orbicularis oris*** muscle at the corner of the mouth and into the upper lip. Contraction of the ***depressor anguli oris*** muscle pulls the corner of the mouth downward. It also forces the lips together by drawing the upper lip downward against the lower lip.

There are two parallel facial muscles. These are the ***incisivus labii superioris*** muscle and the ***incisivus labii inferioris*** muscle.

The ***incisivus labii superioris*** muscle is a small, narrow muscle that lies beneath the ***levator labii superioris*** muscle. Fibers of the ***incisivus labii superioris*** muscle originate from the maxilla in the region of the canine tooth and course parallel to the transverse fibers of the ***orbicularis oris*** muscle of the upper lip. Insertion of the muscle is in the region of the corner of the mouth where its fibers intermingle with the fibers of other muscles. Contraction of the ***incisivus labii superioris*** muscle pulls the corner of the mouth upward and toward the midline.

The ***incisivus labii inferioris*** muscle constitutes the lower lip counterpart of the ***incisivus labii superioris*** muscle. The ***incisivus labii inferioris*** muscle lies below the corner of the mouth and underneath the ***depressor labii superioris*** muscle. The muscle originates on the mandible in the region of the lateral incisor tooth and courses parallel to the transverse fibers of the ***orbicularis oris*** muscle of the lower lip. The insertion of the ***incisivus labii inferioris*** muscle is into the region of the corner of the mouth. Contraction of the muscle results in a downward and inward pull on the corner of the mouth. The downward component of this action is antagonistic to the upward pull provided by the ***incisivus labii superioris*** muscle.

The ***platysma*** muscle is a very broad muscle that covers most of the front and side of the neck and much of the side of the face. The muscle has an extensive origin from a sheet of connective tissue within the neck above the clavicle and may even extend from as far below as the front of the chest wall and regions of the back of the torso. Fibers of the ***platysma*** muscle run upward and forward to attach to the lower edge of the mandible along the side and interweave with fibers of the opposite side at the front of the mandible. Its fibers have a broad distribution about the face, which includes a blending of fibers associated with different muscles of the lower lip and the corner of the mouth. Contraction of the ***platysma*** muscle draws the skin of the neck toward the mandible. It may also pull the lower lip and corner of the mouth to the side and downward and/or force the lower lip against the lower teeth and the alveolar process of the mandible.

Figure 5–15 graphically portrays the general force vectors for the 14 muscles of the lips. These

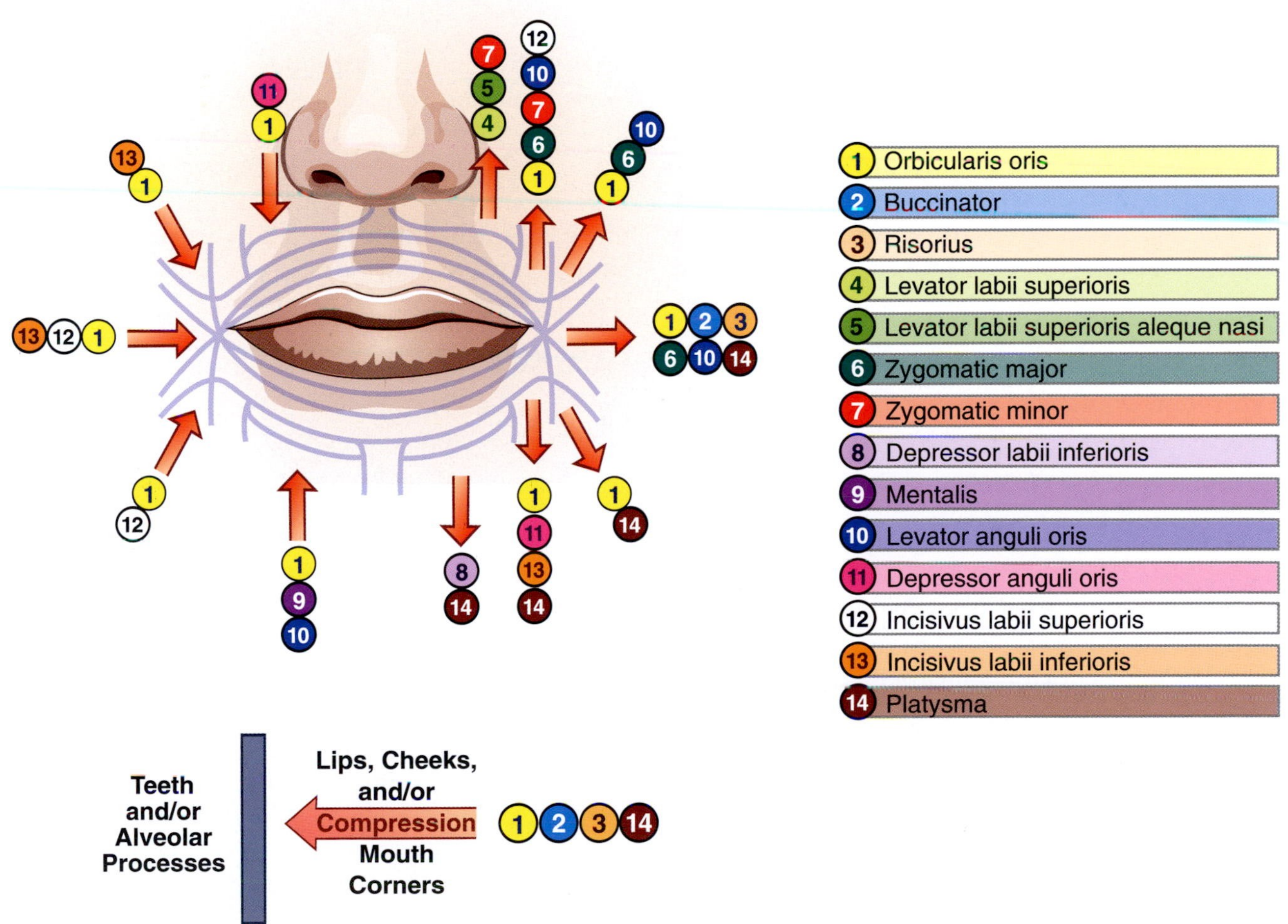

Figure 5–15. Actions of the muscles of the lips.

The Cold War

With prolonged exposure to very cold weather, your face tightens up and your speech slows down. Certain parts of your speech production apparatus actually get stiffer as you chill down. You can live with this because your body, although coping with change at the periphery, is still winning the cold war. Should things get worse, however, such that hypothermia sets in, you'll be in trouble. Hypothermia occurs when your body can't replace heat lost to its surroundings and your core temperature begins to drop. From the usual 98.6°F down to 95°F, your speech will continue to sound normal. Below 95°F down to 90°F, your speech will become "slurred" and progressively more so as temperature decreases. Once your core temperature passes below 90°F, your speech will be unintelligible. The cooling of the body is simply too much for the nervous system to handle and all remaining resources are devoted to preserving the organism.

general vectors summarize the active forces operating on the lips and their consequences on the positioning of the lips and corners of the mouth up and down, side to side, and with regard to compression against the teeth and/or alveolar processes of the maxilla and mandible. Figure 5–15 evokes images about the seeming infinite variety of lips adjustments that are possible and how those adjustments are intricately involved in human expression. Figure 5–16 offers a humorous view of how the lips can be involved in expression.

Movements of the Pharyngeal-Oral Apparatus

Movements are important to many functions of the pharyngeal-oral apparatus. Potential movements are considered below apart from the forces that cause them. The relation of forces to movements is discussed in the section on adjustments.

Movements of the Pharynx. The potential movements of the overall pharynx are discussed in detail in Chapter 4 and illustrated there (see Figure 4–13). Focus here is on potential movements of the laryngopharynx and oropharynx. These portions of the pharyngeal tube are relatively mobile and present three movement capabilities. These include (a) inward and outward movement of their sidewalls, (b) forward and backward movement of their back wall, and (c) forward and backward movement of their front wall (tongue and/or epiglottis). These movement capabilities enable the lumen of the laryngopharynx and oropharynx to be changed in size and shape.

Movements of the Mandible. The mandible is capable of a wide range of movements in three-dimensional space. Complex movements of the structure derive from its potential to move upward and downward, forward and backward, and side to side through the different hinge-like and gliding actions of the temporomandibular joints described above (see Figure 5–6).

Upward and downward and forward and backward movements of the mandible often include both rotational and translational components (Zemlin, 1998). Rotational movements are hinge-like and resemble the swinging of a two-hinged trap door about an axis that extends through the center pins of its hinges. Such movements of the mandible take place about a lateral axis that passes through the condylar processes on the left and right sides of

Say "NO" To Tax Increases!
KEN BLARRABY FOR SENATE ~2008~
CHANGE IN
Yeah, but how do we know if he's lying?
Well... his lips are moving, aren't they?

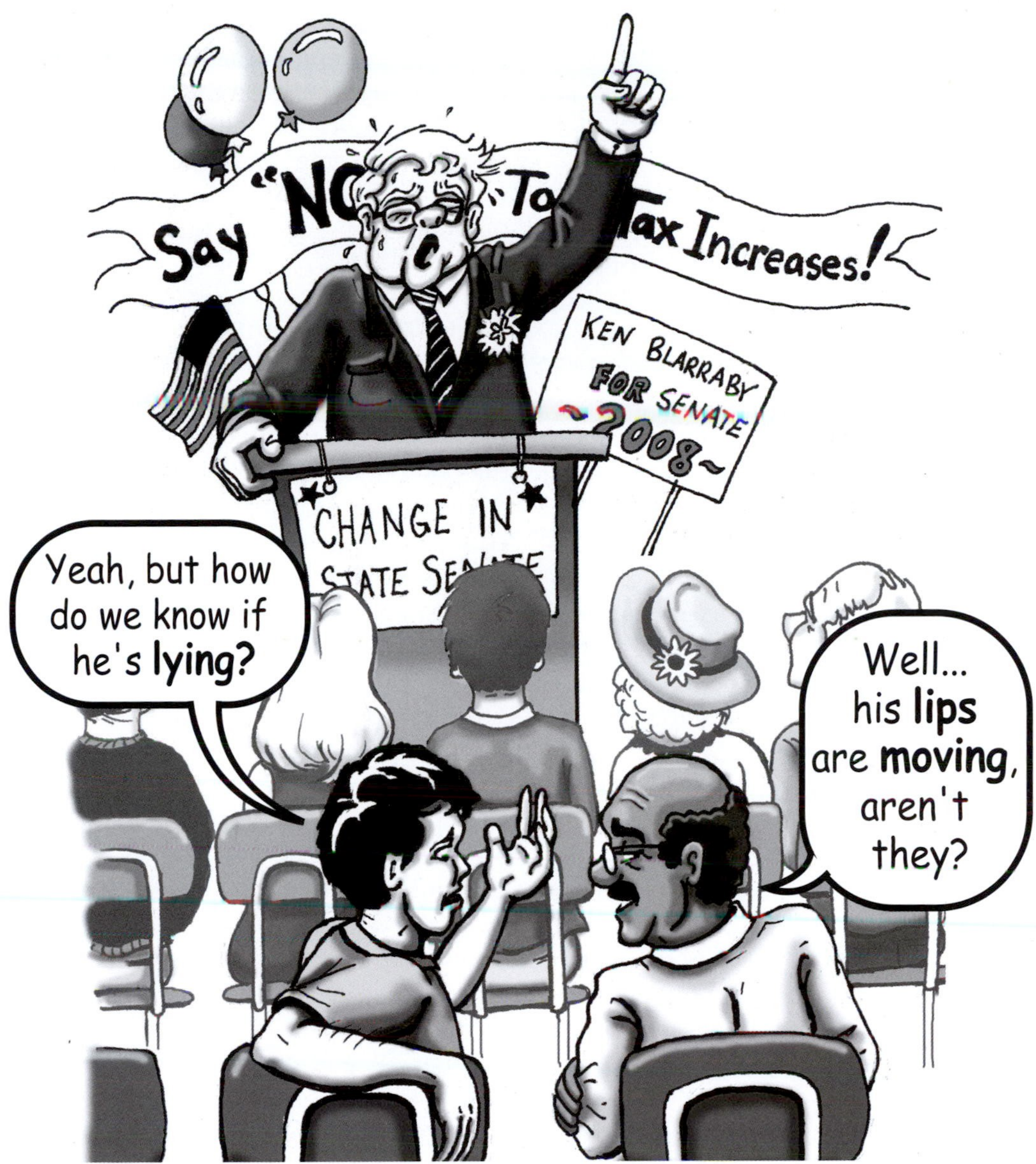

Figure 5–16. Cartoon showing a discerning potential voter.

the skull. Translational movements, in contrast, involve downward and forward or upward and backward displacements of the mandible along the rear slopes of the articular facets of the temporomandibular joints. These movements are of the nature observed when the mandible is moved forward or backward without an accompanying hinge-like rotational component and are based on the forward and backward gliding potential at the temporomandibular joints. Side-to-side movements of the mandible provide for additional complexity by taking advantage of the to-and-fro gliding action at the temporomandibular joints that enable the mandible to be moved from left to right or vice versa.

The multiple movement possibilities of the mandible can combine to pitch the structure upward or downward about a lateral axis, roll it to one side or the other about a longitudinal axis, and yaw it to the left or right about a vertical axis. An example where the three movements combine is seen in the crushing and grinding associated with chewing. The movements of boats and airplanes are also good examples of how a structure can pitch, roll, and yaw all at the same time.

Movements of the Tongue. The tongue is a fleshy muscular structure that is exceedingly mobile. Its mobility derives from the fact that (a) it rides with the mandible and floor of the oral cavity and goes as a whole where they go (see section below on adjustments), (b) its position within the oral cavity can be shifted en masse as a body (akin to moving a closed fist around in space), and (c) its shape can be changed markedly and relatively independently of the first two sources of mobility.

Movements of the tongue are often segmental and differ along its major and minor axes. Thus, one part of the structure may move more or less than another or even in a different direction than another. Movements of different points on the surface of the structure can be upward and downward, forward and backward, side to side, or different combinations of these. Vertical movements can extend from the trough of the mouth to the roof of the oral cavity. Front-to-back movements can range from a maximally forward displacement of the tongue out of the mouth to a maximally rearward displacement of the structure against the back wall of the pharynx. Side-to-side movements can range from the stretchable limits of one cheek to the other.

Movements of the Lips. The mobility of the face in the region of the lips rivals that of the fine movements of the fingers. Movements of the lips can occur along vertical, side-to-side, and front-to-back dimensions. Each lip can be moved independently of the other or the two lips can be coordinated in their movements. The upper lip is fixed in spatial coordinates to the fixed position of the maxilla, whereas the lower lip rides with the mandible and the consequences of its positional changes are dictated, in part, by the prevailing position of the mandible. The juncture of the two lips at the corners of the mouth can entail movements of both the upper and lower lips and is influenced by both intrinsic and extrinsic forces imparted by the facial muscles. The wide range of possible lip movements implicates a complex array of combinations of muscle forces operating on the lips. Experimenting with lip movements in front of a mirror gives one an almost awesome appreciation for the degrees of freedom of movement in the region of the mouth opening.

Adjustments of the Pharyngeal-Oral Apparatus

Adjustments of the pharyngeal-oral apparatus reflect the potential configurations that can be assumed by the overall apparatus and its component parts. Such adjustments involve combinations of the movements discussed in sections above.

Adjustments of the Pharynx

The pharynx is capable of many adjustments. Chapter 4 includes a discussion of adjustment capabilities within the upper part of the pharynx (nasopharynx) and their roles in adjusting the degree of coupling between the oral and nasal cavities through the velopharyngeal port. Interest here is in adjustment capabilities of the lower and middle parts of the pharynx (the laryngopharynx and oropharynx, respectively) and their roles in changing the regional lumen of the pharynx and the degree of coupling between the oropharynx and the oral cavity through the palatoglossal arch (anterior faucial pillars).

Recall that the lumen of the pharynx is oval in cross section, being larger side to side than front to back. This lumen can be adjusted so as to change both its size and/or shape. Adjustments in size can range from a maximally enlarged pharyngeal airway to one that is fully obstructed. In the case of complete obstruction, the walls of the pharynx may not only come in contact, but may also undergo forceful compression against one another. When a pharyngeal lumen exists, it can be changed in both size and shape. Shape adjustments may range from elliptical to circular or otherwise.

Certain pharyngeal adjustments, or components of them, can result from the actions of other structures. For example, lowering of the mandible results in an inward pull on the sides of the pharynx that causes a reduction in its side-to-side diameter and a smaller and more circular lumen (Minific, Hixon, Kelsey, & Woodhouse, 1970). Thus, simply raising and lowering the mandible, without the activation of muscles in the pharyngeal region, results in significant changes in the size and/or shape of the pharyngeal airway.

Passive influences notwithstanding, more purposeful adjustments of the pharynx are effected by the actions of muscles that attach to and directly influence the positioning of the four walls of the structure. Inward and outward movements of the sides of the structure are effected mainly through contractions of the ***inferior*** and ***middle constrictor*** muscles and the ***stylopharyngeus*** muscles, respectively. Forward and backward movements of the back wall of the pharynx figure into certain adjustments of the airway, whereas forward and backward movements of its front wall (tongue and epiglottis) are prominent contributors to many adjustments. The velum may also be involved in actively adjusting the lumen of the oropharynx. When at rest, the velum hangs pendulously and its upper surface forms the upper front wall of the oropharynx. As the velum moves, it changes the upper front-to-back diameter of the oropharynx. This is true until its elevation is sufficient to carry it out of the oropharynx and into the nasopharynx, whereupon its lower surface then forms the approximate upper boundary of the oropharynx.

Adjustment of the degree of coupling between the pharyngeal cavity and oral cavity is influenced by (a) upward and downward movements of the tongue, (b) upward and downward movements of the velum, and (c) side-to-side movements of the pillars of the palatoglossal arch (anterior faucial pillars). Decreases in the degree of coupling through the oropharyngeal isthmus are achieved through one or any combination of upward movement of the tongue, downward movement of the velum, and inward movement of the palatoglossal arch. Conversely, increases in the degree of coupling through the oropharyngeal isthmus are accomplished through one or any combination of opposite movements of these three components. Maximum coupling is brought about by a combined maximum elevation of the velum and maximum depression of the tongue. Decoupling results when the undersurface of the velum and the upper surface of the tongue are placed in full apposition and the oropharyngeal airway is occluded. When contact between the tongue and the velum occurs, it is also possible to have left- and right-side openings through which the pharynx and oral cavity are coupled.

Adjustments of the Mandible

The mandible can be adjusted in position, but not in shape. Such adjustment is usually considered in relation to some fixed structure of the skull. Most often that structure is the maxilla because it constitutes the opposing jaw for the mandible and is critical to certain functions that the two structures carry out collaboratively, such as chewing and speech production. Adjustments of the mandible result from individual actions or combinations of actions that displace the structure downward or upward, forward or backward, and toward one side or the other. Adjustments that involve lowering of the mandible result from the action of one or more muscles that include the ***external pterygoid*** muscle, ***digastric*** (***anterior*** belly) muscle, ***mylohyoid*** muscle, and ***geniohyoid*** muscle. In contrast, adjustments that involve elevation of the mandible result from the action of one or more muscles that include the ***masseter*** muscle, ***temporalis*** muscle, and ***internal pterygoid*** muscle. Side-to-side movements are the domain of four muscles that include the ***masseter*** muscle, ***temporalis*** muscle, ***internal pterygoid*** muscle, and ***external pterygoid*** muscle. And forward and backward movements are caused by the actions of the ***external pterygoid*** muscle and the ***masseter*** muscle and/or ***temporalis*** muscle, respectively.

Using different combinations of muscular contractions, the mandible can be protruded, retracted, lateralized, or centralized. These adjustments may be made singly or in certain combinations, except where contradictory (simultaneous protrusion and retraction), and are limited only by constraints imposed by the temporomandibular joints and the forces that can be applied to the mandible through muscle activations. Combinations of adjustments of the mandible

Take It Away

The tongue rides with the mandible and goes where it goes. Thus, when trying to interpret changes in the configuration of the tongue surface, it's necessary to determine how much is attributable to adjustment of the tongue and how much is attributable to adjustment of the mandible. Suppose you had a client with a hyperkinetic disease in which both the tongue and mandible went through adventitious involuntary excursions. How could you go about parsing them in your evaluation? Not to worry! Have the client speak through clenched teeth or while biting down on a small stack of tongue depressors. Then, the abnormal movements of the tongue are on their own and not confounded by the abnormal movements of the mandible. It's called removing a degree of freedom of performance, and the principle can be applied in many ways when analyzing different structures involved in speech production.

can result in marked changes in its positioning relative to when the upper and lower teeth are in contact along their opposing surfaces. For example, a combined adjustment in which the mandible is maximally lowered and maximally protruded might entail more than a 2-inch downward excursion of the front of the structure and a 0.5–inch forward excursion.

Adjustments of the Tongue

The enormous variety of tongue adjustments is truly amazing. What seems to be a near infinite array of adjustments has to do with the special mechanical endowment of the tongue that sets it apart from other components of the pharyngeal-oral apparatus. That endowment is that the tongue is a muscular hydrostat that can perform its functions while maintaining its overall volume (Kier & Smith, 1985; Smith & Kier, 1989). This capability is somewhat akin to adjustments that can be made in a balloon filled with water, in which the balloon, like the tongue, does not have a rigid underlying skeleton against which purchase can be gained.

Nonetheless, the tongue can protrude, retract, lateralize, centralize, curl, point, lick, bulge, groove, flatten, rotate, and do many other things. Consider for a moment the range of adjustments the tongue goes through in "picking between one's teeth" one at a time from the outside, inside, and bottom, both the uppers and lowers, after eating something like corn on the cob. The series of adjustments that characterize some of the daily activities of the tongue has been described as paralleling the adjustments of the tentacles of an octopus or the trunk of an elephant (Kier & Smith, 1985; Smith & Kier, 1989).

These adjustments are made possible by the biomechanical property of the tongue that enables it to function like a liquid-filled, pliable structure that is incompressible. This special property of the structure, along with its personal soft skeleton that encapsulates it (see above), provides leverages for the eight muscles that give rise to its motive force. These leverages enable the tongue muscles to work off one another and its connective tissue to achieve its variety of adjustments (Miller, Watkin, & Chen, 2002). Because of its hydrostatic properties, inward displacement of one part of the tongue brings about outward displacement of another part (like squeezing one part of a water-filled balloon and seeing another part bulge outward). Through the selective contraction of different muscle fibers, a relatively rigid but changing support system is created in the tongue. This changing support system provides a changing base from which the contraction of different muscle fibers can accomplish adjustments of other parts of the tongue. Thus, conceptualizing the consequences of tongue muscle actions in a classical sense is limiting and problematic. Rather, it is better to conceptualize the tongue as a mechanical platform that can change in accordance with the collective activations of the muscles within and attached to it. Because this platform maintains its overall volume, its adjustments in free space (when not contacting other structures in opposition) are best conceptualized in terms of its nature as a hydrostat.

Before the properties of muscular hydrostats were understood, a question like "How do you stick out your tongue?" would evoke an answer that usually involved a complex geometric explanation about muscle force vectors. The simple answer to this question with today's knowledge is that "You squeeze it out."

Adjustments of the Lips

As mentioned above, the lips are highly mobile and can be moved independently or in a coordinated fashion. The forces that enable adjustments of the lips derive from the many facial muscles that surround the mouth opening. Adjustments of the lips can be viewed from a variety of perspectives, such as in relation to influences on (a) the position and shape of each lip, (b) the position and shape of the corners of the mouth, (c) the resultant compression between the lips and/or between one or both lips and the teeth and gums, and (d) the resultant configuration (cross section and length) of the channel that forms the airway opening.

Frequently recognized positional adjustments of the lips include puckering, protruding, retracting, spreading, pointing, curling (inward and outward), groping, rounding, and plumping (other than with supplemental collagen). Common compressions may involve forceful airtight seals between the lips, the pushing around of one lip by the other, the thinning or thickening of the contact area between the two lips, and the placement of different parts of the lips against the maxillary and/or mandibular arches and teeth. The channel that forms the airway opening is, of course, frequently adjusted such that it can be lengthened or shortened, changed in shape, and moved from side to side (consider talking out one side of the mouth, the so-called sidewinder). The lips may even be in apposition on one side and be parted on the other, as in the dying breed of the smoker who talks with a cigarette hanging from one side of the mouth.

The multitude of possible lip adjustments are effected by a large variety of muscle activations in the facial region involving different combinations of the more than dozen muscles that impart forces to the lips. These adjustments also include those associated with a host of facial expressions, such as smiling, smirking, sulking, and sneering.

Control Variables of Pharyngeal-Oral Function

Several control variables are important in pharyngeal-oral function. Their relative importance depends on the activity being performed, whether it is breathing, speech production, singing, whistling, wind instrument playing, blowing, sucking, chewing, or swallowing, among others.

For the purposes of this chapter, discussion is devoted to four control variables of pharyngeal-oral function. These are (a) pharyngeal-oral lumen size and configuration, (b) pharyngeal-oral contact pressure, (c) pharyngeal-oral airway resistance, and (d) pharyngeal-oral acoustic impedance.

Pharyngeal-Oral Lumen Size and Configuration

The lumen of the pharyngeal-oral apparatus (its inner open space) can be changed in both size and configuration. Such changes are the result of adjustments in the positions of structures that line the pharyngeal-oral airway. Adjustments can be manifested in physical dimensions such as length, longitudinal configuration (midsaggital outline), diameter, cross-sectional area, and cross-sectional configuration.

The open space that constitutes the pharyngeal-oral lumen can be either increased or decreased from the resting configuration of the pharyngeal-oral apparatus. Figure 5–17 summarizes the structures that may contribute individually or in combination

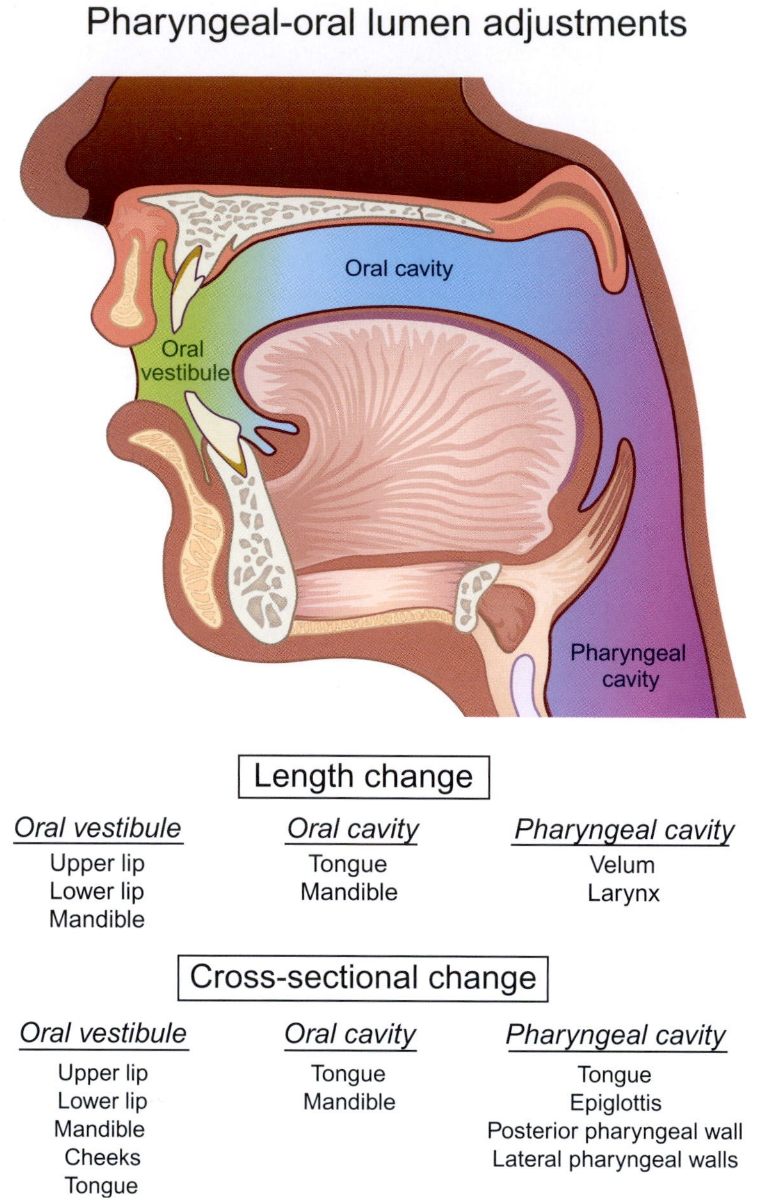

Pharyngeal-oral lumen adjustments

Oral cavity
Oral vestibule
Pharyngeal cavity

Length change

Oral vestibule	*Oral cavity*	*Pharyngeal cavity*
Upper lip	Tongue	Velum
Lower lip	Mandible	Larynx
Mandible		

Cross-sectional change

Oral vestibule	*Oral cavity*	*Pharyngeal cavity*
Upper lip	Tongue	Tongue
Lower lip	Mandible	Epiglottis
Mandible		Posterior pharyngeal wall
Cheeks		Lateral pharyngeal walls
Tongue		

Figure 5–17. Regional structures contributing to adjustments of the pharyngeal-oral lumen.

to changing the lumen of the airway in the pharyngeal cavity, the oral cavity, and the oral vestibule.

As indicated in Figure 5–17, the dimensions of the pharyngeal-oral lumen can be changed in a variety of ways. Length changes can be achieved (a) within the pharyngeal cavity, by different combinations of adjustments of the velum and larynx; (b) within the oral cavity, by different combinations of adjustments of the tongue and mandible; and (c) within the oral vestibule, by different combinations of adjustments of the upper lip, lower lip, and mandible. Cross-sectional changes can be achieved (a) within the pharynx, by different combinations of adjustments of the tongue, epiglottis, posterior pharyngeal wall, and lateral pharyngeal walls; (b) within the oral cavity, by different combinations of adjustments of the tongue and mandible; and (c) within the oral vestibule, by different combinations of adjustments of the lips, mandible, cheeks, and tongue.

Given the lengthwise and cross-sectional adjustment possibilities noted, the number of options for luminal changes in the pharyngeal-oral apparatus

Open Wide

Your mandible and maxilla are separated by only a small distance when you produce speech. Activities such as calling your dog, yelling at a football game, or singing often get you to open up more. Classical (opera) singing is one activity that gets people to open very wide. One form of classical singing teaches what is referred to as a four-finger jaw position. Try it. Place the four fingers of one hand together and then, with your thumb on that hand pointing upward, insert your fingers vertically at the midline between your upper and lower front teeth. Quite a stretch, isn't it? It comes close to maximum separation between your mandible and maxilla and gives you nearly as large a mouth opening as you can achieve (or tolerate). What a great way to get that beautiful singing voice to radiate outward from the singer to the audience.

is exceedingly large. This fact underpins the fact that the acoustic products that emanate from the pharyngeal-oral apparatus can be richly variable, as is discussed in detail in subsequent chapters.

Pharyngeal-Oral Structural Contact Pressure

Adjustments of the pharyngeal-oral apparatus can result in full obstruction of the pharyngeal-oral lumen at different locations. This is accomplished through structural contact between components that comprise the boundaries of the airway. Structures in apposition may include (a) the tongue against the pharynx, velum, hard palate, alveolar process of the maxilla, teeth, and lips, and (b) the lips against the teeth and one another. Once two structures are in apposition, the structural contact pressure between them can be adjusted to meet the needs of the situation. This is manifested as a compressive force between the two structures and can be changed in accordance with the pressure needed to maintain the contact or to increase it in magnitude. Figure 5–18 portrays structural contact and its resultant compressive force between the tongue and the alveolar process of the maxilla.

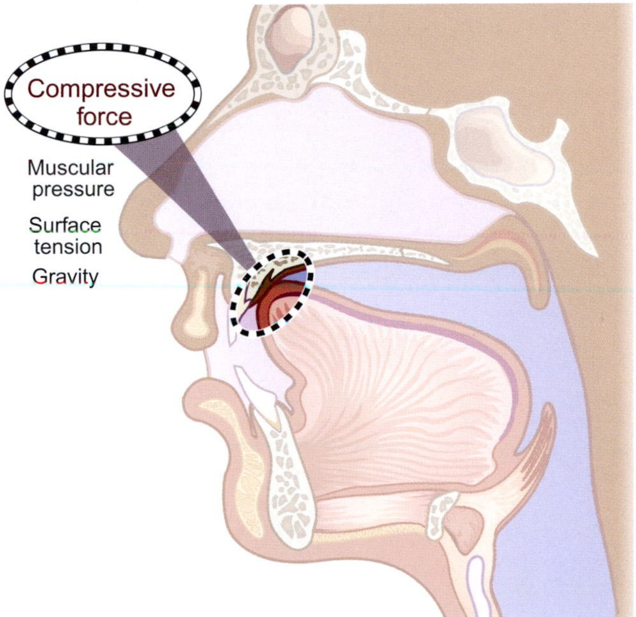

Figure 5–18. Structural contact pressure between the tongue and alveolar process of the maxilla.

Structural contact pressure can be influenced by several factors. These include (a) muscular pressure exerted by muscular components of the contacting surfaces (tongue against alveolar ridge or two lips against one another), (b) surface tension between apposed surfaces that are moist (tongue against hard palate) and hold them together, and (c) gravity that weighs down structures and acts on them differently in different body positions (or gravity fields). The most significant of these three is usually the muscular pressure exerted by one or more structures.

Surface contact pressure for an activity may require low-level muscular exertion for soft contact between structures or it may require high contact pressure when it is necessary to fortify the contact in the face of high air pressures in the vicinity. Adjustment of surface contact pressure is critical to providing the opposition needed to allow pharyngeal or oral air pressure to be raised for certain activities.

Pharyngeal-Oral Airway Resistance

Pharyngeal-oral airway resistance is a measure of the opposition provided by the pharyngeal-oral apparatus to airflow through it. As portrayed in Figure 5–19, this opposition pertains to the mass flow of air in and out of the apparatus. Pharyngeal-oral airway resistance is a property of the airway itself and is airflow dependent. This means that it increases or decreases with increases or decreases in the rate at which air moves, even without changes in the physical dimensions of the pharyngeal-oral airway. However, it is the change in the cross section of the airway that causes the greatest change in pharyngeal-oral airway resistance. Such change can occur anywhere along the length of the pharyngeal-oral apparatus, from larynx to lips, but is most prominently the result of adjustments within the oropharynx, oral cavity, and oral vestibule. By decreasing the cross-sectional area of the airway anywhere within these regions, the airway resistance will likely increase.

Airway resistance is calculated from the quotient of the pressure drop across any segment of interest and the airflow through that segment. For the entire pharyngeal-oral apparatus, airway resistance is represented by the pressure difference (in cmH_2O) between the laryngopharynx and the atmosphere divided by the airflow (in LPS) at the airway opening. The range of potential airway resistance values is from a fraction of a cmH_2O/LPS (associated with a wide open pharyngeal-oral apparatus) to infinity (associated with a closed pharyngeal-oral apparatus). The distribution of resistance along the pharyngeal-oral airway can be determined by partitioning the total resistance. All that is required is that appropriate pressure measurements be made at the two ends of each segment of interest along the airway.

Pharyngeal-Oral Acoustic Impedance

The pharyngeal-oral apparatus plays an important role in the control of acoustic impedance, which, like airway resistance, involves opposition to flow. As portrayed in Figure 5–20, this opposition is not to mass airflow, but to the movement of energy in the form of sound waves through the apparatus. In this case, however, these waves function more like an alternating current in which adjacent air molecules collide with each other and pass energy on to

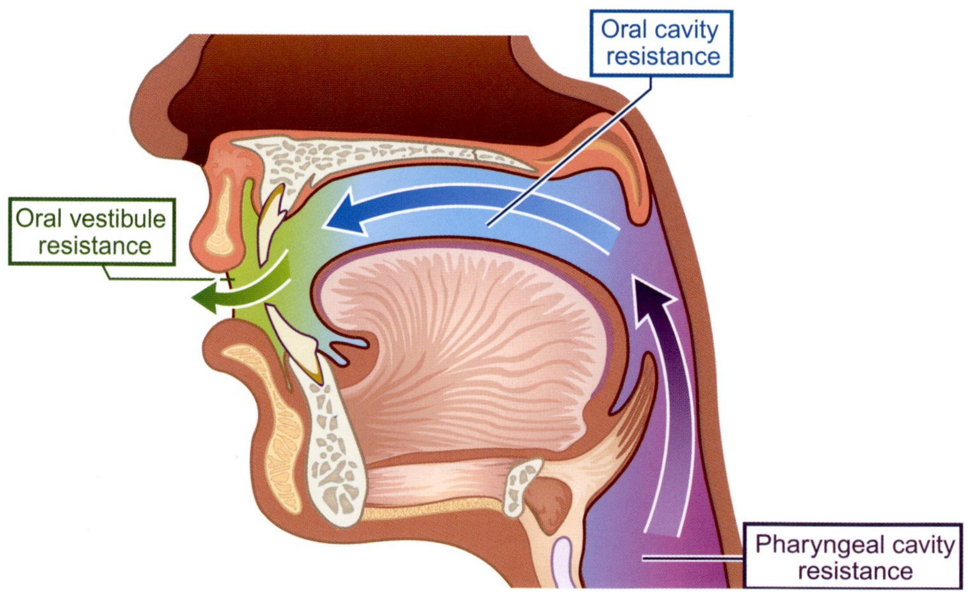

Figure 5–19. Three regional components of pharyngeal-oral airway resistance.

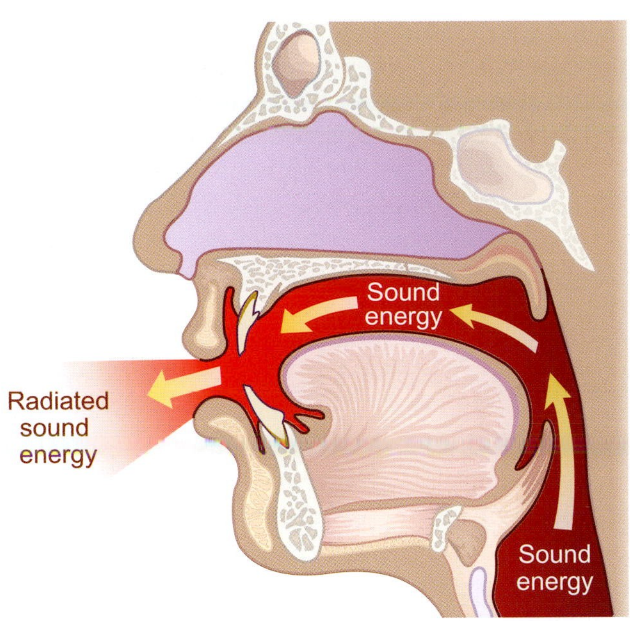

Figure 5–20. Pharyngeal-oral sound wave propagation in the presence of velopharyngeal closure.

their neighbors. Acoustic impedance influences how well sound waves propagate through the pharyngeal-oral airway.

Acoustic impedance is determined to a great extent by cross-sectional adjustments of the pharyngeal-oral airway. These adjustments influence the degree of coupling between different segments of the pharyngeal-oral apparatus. When the adjustments create a relative increase in the cross section of the lumen of the pharyngeal-oral airway, sound waves pass relatively freely along the airway. In contrast, when the adjustments create a relative decrease in the cross section of the lumen of the airway, sound energy does not pass as freely along the airway. Relative decreases in the cross section of the lumen at different locations simultaneously may also influence the degree to which different segments of the pharyngeal-oral airway interact with one another acoustically. This topic is discussed in detail in subsequent chapters.

Neural Substrates of Pharyngeal-Oral Control

Pharyngeal-oral movements are controlled by the nervous system and differ with the activity being performed. Thus, speech production and swallowing, while engaging the same structures of the pharyngeal-oral apparatus, are controlled by different neural substrates and mechanisms. Control of the pharyngeal-oral apparatus during swallowing is discussed in Chapter 12, whereas control of the apparatus during speech production is discussed here.

Although different parts of the central nervous system participate in the control of different pharyngeal-oral activities, the final forms of the control commands are sent through the same set of

Low Energy Physics

Speech is clearly an energy producing enterprise. But just how much energy is involved? One scientist has calculated that 300 to 400 ergs of energy is expended in the resultant sound wave when the sentence "Joe took father's shoe-bench out" is produced at usual loudness (Fletcher, 1953). That's not a sentence that most people run around saying and many readers might not have an appreciation for how 300 to 400 ergs relates to their everyday lives. Perhaps we can help a bit. You and 499 of your closest friends (that's a Boeing-747 aircraft with all the seats filled) would have to say "Joe took father's shoe-bench out" together at your usual loudness continuously for a year to produce enough energy to heat a cup of coffee. Holy Starbucks! That's a lot of talking. It would undoubtedly contend for a Guiness World Record, but on nature's energy scale it wouldn't amount to much.

cranial nerves. These nerves have their origins in the brainstem and course from there to provide motor innervation to the muscles of the pharynx, mandible, tongue, and lips. As shown in Table 5–1, motor innervation of the pharynx is effected through the pharyngeal plexus, which includes fibers from cranial nerves IX (glossopharyngeal), X (vagus), and possibly XI (accessory). Motor innervation to the mandible is effected through cranial nerves V (trigeminal) and XII (hypoglossal). Motor innervation of the tongue includes cranial nerves XI and XII, whereas motor innervation of the lips is effected through cranial nerves V and VII (facial).

Table 5–1. Summary of Motor and Sensory Nerve Supply to the Pharynx, Mandible, Tongue, and Lips. Cranial nerves Indicated in the table and notes are V (trigeminal), VII (facial), IX (glossopharyngeal), X (vagus), XI (accessory), and XII (hypoglossal).

	INNERVATION	
COMPONENT	MOTOR	SENSORY
Pharynx	Pharyngeal Plexus	V, VII, IX, X
Mandible	V, XII	V, XII
Tongue	XI, XII	V, VII, IX, X
Lips	V, VII	V, VII

Notes:

1. The pharyngeal plexus is a network that includes cranial nerves IX, X, and possibly XI.
2. All of the muscles of the mandible have motor and sensory nerve supply through cranial nerve V, except the ***geniohyoid*** muscle, which has motor and sensory nerve supply through cranial nerve XII.
3. All of the muscles of the tongue have motor nerve supply through cranial nerve XII, except the ***palatoglossus*** muscle, which has motor nerve supply through cranial nerve XI.
4. All of the muscles of the lips have motor nerve supply through cranial nerve VII, except the ***buccinator*** muscle, which has motor nerve supply through cranial nerve V.

Sensory innervation to the pharynx is carried by cranial nerves V, VII, IX, and X. Sensory innervation to the mandible is supplied by cranial nerves V and XII. The tongue receives sensory supply from cranial nerves V, VII, IX, and X, whereas supply to the lips is from cranial nerves V and VII. Neural information traveling along the sensory nerves supplying the pharynx, mandible, tongue, and lips results from the activation of receptors of various types within those structures. These receptors include an array of mechanoreceptors that are differentially distributed (some occurring in certain locations more than others) throughout the tissues of the pharyngeal-oral apparatus. When sound results from pharyngeal-oral activity, mechanoreceptors formed by hair cells within the cochlea (end organ of the auditory system) may be activated. Sensory information from the auditory system is effected via cranial nerve VIII (auditory).

The mechanoreceptors within the pharyngeal-oral apparatus are sensitive to a variety of stimuli

Ten Four, Good Buddy

Bell's palsy is a relatively common condition that affects cranial nerve VII, the nerve that innervates the muscles of the face. Upper and lower facial muscles can become weak or paralyzed and speech production can be impaired. Most often the cause is unknown and the problem is on one side. It may involve an autoimmune inflammatory response, a herpes viral infection, or a swelling of the nerve because of allergy. Most people who get Bell's palsy make a full recovery, especially if they're young. Exposure to cold can be a factor in Bell's palsy. Truck drivers who drive with the driver's-side window down may contract Bell's palsy from the cold. Wind chill for a prolonged period across the side of the face near the window is believed to be a contributing factor to onset of the problem. Which side depends on the country in which you're driving. What's the prevention? Close the window and turn on the air conditioner.

Gumming Things Up

Some antipsychotic drugs can have a nasty side effect called by the imposing name of tardive dyskinesia (meaning after-the-fact adventitious movement). Signs of tardive dyskinesia can include involuntary movement of the mandible, tongue, and lips and can manifest in such strange actions as lip smacking and puffing. In some individuals, these signs are permanent. Another condition may masquerade as tardive dyskinesia. Persons with poorly fitting dentures also may present with adventitious movement. The source of the problem is a changing sensory feedback from the gums caused by movement of the denture. The result is a disorganized background template of the oral cavity. This effectively gums up the control circuits for movement. Take out the denture or secure it in position and the problem will go away. When confronted with the signs of tardive dyskinesia, always check for loose-fitting dentures.

and are capable of providing the nervous system with many types of information, including information about (a) muscle length, (b) rate of change in muscle length, (c) muscle tension, (d) joint position, (e) joint movement, (f) touch, (g) surface pressure, (h) deep pressure, (i) surface deformation, (j) temperature, (k) vibration, and (l) hair deflection, among others. Mechanoreceptors within the fabric of the pharyngeal-oral apparatus and within the auditory system provide the central nervous system with information that is used to guide anticipated actions of the pharyngeal-oral apparatus and to keep track of the recent status of the pharyngeal-oral apparatus. Recent in this case means that the information conveyed is delayed by at least the amount of time it takes to transmit signals from mechanoreceptors to centers within the brain where they are processed. This processing may include the integration of various inputs coming from the periphery and the use of this collective information to execute ongoing commands from the motor side of the system.

Pharyngeal-Oral Functions

The pharyngeal-oral apparatus performs many functions. Those of interest here relate to (a) degree of coupling between the oral cavity and atmosphere, (b) chewing, (c) swallowing, and (d) sound generation and filtering.

Degree of Coupling Between the Oral Cavity and Atmosphere

Actions of the pharyngeal-oral apparatus determine the degree of coupling between the pharyngeal-oral apparatus and atmosphere. The coupling pathway in this case is through the oral vestibule. Changes in the positions of lips, cheeks, and alveolar process of the mandible influence such coupling. When breathing through the pharyngeal-oral apparatus, the oral vestibule is open, whereas when breathing through the velopharyngeal-nasal port, the oral vestibule may be closed. The lips are especially important in changing the degree of coupling between the oral cavity and atmosphere and can influence it not only in cross section but also by adjusting the length of the channel formed between the oral cavity and the airway opening.

Chewing

Chewing (mastication) is the process of grinding, mashing, gnawing, crushing, and kneading food (nutriment in solid form) with the teeth. This process is aimed at the alteration of food into smaller particle sizes that can be prepared to a swallow-ready consistency. The alignment of the maxilla, mandible, and teeth is important in this process to ensure that proper biting forces can be exerted. Chewing entails extensive movement of the mandible

Myth Conceptions

The history of speech-language pathology is rich with clinical theories and methods that don't actually involve speech production directly. These have taken many forms. One early one took the point of view that language had its beginnings in chewing and that chewing exercises had a prominent role in the evaluation and management of speech and voice disorders. The originator of this idea said that he conceived the notion when confronted with two Egyptian hieroglyphic scripts that showed a similar sign for eating and speaking. Despite using some of the same pharyngeal-oral structures, chewing and speaking are controlled differently by the nervous system and one is not a precursor or analog of the other. Other forms of nonspeech activities and devices continue to be used even today as if they were somehow beneficial to speech production. We don't subscribe to any of these misconceptions. You shouldn't either.

that may have significant vertical, side-to-side, and elliptical components. These depend, in part, on the consistency of the food being manipulated.

Swallowing

Swallowing (deglutition) is a life-sustaining function of the pharyngeal-oral apparatus. Actions of the oral cavity and oral vestibule prepare food or liquid for swallowing and then propel it backward into the oropharynx (the velopharynx being closed). Thereafter, muscles of the oropharynx and laryngopharynx act to further propel the prepared substances downward through the pharyngeal tube and into the esophagus. Chapter 12 provides a comprehensive discussion about the swallowing process that includes consideration of the role played by the pharyngeal-oral apparatus.

Sound Generation and Filtering

Much of the interest in the present chapter is with sound generation and filtering by the pharyngeal-oral apparatus. Sound generation in the apparatus can be of several types. The two of these that are most important to this book are (a) transient (popping) sounds, in which the oral airstream is momentarily interrupted and then released, and (b) turbulence (hissing) sounds, in which air is forced through a narrow constriction within the airway. Sound generated within the pharyngeal-oral apparatus or generated at the larynx and passed through the pharyngeal-oral apparatus undergoes a sound-filtering process in which its characteristics can be modified through enhancement or attenuation before becoming public at the airway opening (for details, see Chapters 7 and 8).

PHARYNGEAL-ORAL FUNCTION IN SPEECH PRODUCTION

The pharyngeal-oral apparatus is of great importance in speech production. This section and various sections of Chapters 7 and 8 emphasize this importance by stressing its role in the generation and filtering of speech sounds. Two aspects of pharyngeal-oral function are discussed here. The first is how the pharyngeal-oral apparatus makes coded adjustments that constitute the physiological bases of speech production. The second is how these coded adjustments become elaborated in real time by the pharyngeal-oral apparatus and other subsystems of the speech production apparatus.

Duck and Cover

Aeromechanical and acoustical energies come out of your mouth during speech production. Other things also make their way out. One of these is saliva. Today your salivary glands might produce up to a quart of liquid. The usually slippery oral cavity dries out when you talk, especially when the humidity is low. Tiny drops of saliva spew from your mouth when you speak. These are usually invisible and emerge as wet clouds that can hang around an hour or more and settle on nearby listeners. Each word spoken sends about 2.5 droplets of saliva into the atmosphere (Bodanis, 1995). Read this sidetrack aloud and you'll expel about 400 droplets of saliva. Do the same with the Gettysburg Address and the number will reach 700. The United States Constitution would get you about 11,000 droplets. And what would an assembly of 500 people reciting the Pledge of Allegiance get you? 40,000 droplets dispersed in 500 wet clouds.

The Speech Production Code

Previous sections have discussed the variety of adjustments that can be made by individual components of the pharyngeal-oral apparatus. Chapters 3 and 4 do likewise for the laryngeal apparatus and velopharyngeal-nasal apparatus, respectively. Adjustments across the different subsystems of the speech production apparatus comprise a phonetic code that specifies the positions and movements of structures. This code consists of groupings of adjustments that are associated with the generation of different speech sounds, each grouping being one component of an organized system of sounds in a language. Such a code contains a series of elements that differ from one another in one or more aspects that enable them to be distinguished from other elements. Coding schemes for vowels, diphthongs, and consonants of American English are considered here.

Vowel-Coding Scheme

Vowels are usually produced with voicing by the larynx (although they can be whispered) and with velopharyngeal closure (although they can be nasalized). They demonstrate different combinations of positions and movements by the pharynx, mandible, tongue, and lips. Whatever the pattern of adjustments, vowel productions involve relatively unconstricted configurations of the pharyngeal-oral airway. Laryngeal and velopharyngeal actions notwithstanding, the positions and movements of structures within the pharyngeal-oral apparatus are of foremost importance in the vowel-coding scheme. Figure 5–21 shows how vowels can be coded using the three dimensions of *place of major constriction* within the pharyngeal-oral apparatus, *degree of major constriction* within the apparatus, and *degree of lip rounding.*

Place of Major Constriction. *Place of major constriction* specifies the location at which the pharyngeal-oral airway is maximally constricted during vowel production. Three locations are coded for vowels. These include *front, central,* and *back.* The term *front* is used to designate constrictions formed between the tongue and the alveolar process of the maxilla. The term *central* is used to indicate constrictions formed between the tongue and the hard palate, or when no obvious constriction exists. And the term *back* designates constrictions formed between the tongue and the velum, or between the tongue and the posterior pharyngeal wall. Five vowels fall under the rubric *front* vowels, four are classified as *central* vowels, and five are considered *back* vowels. Changes across the *place of major constriction* dimension can

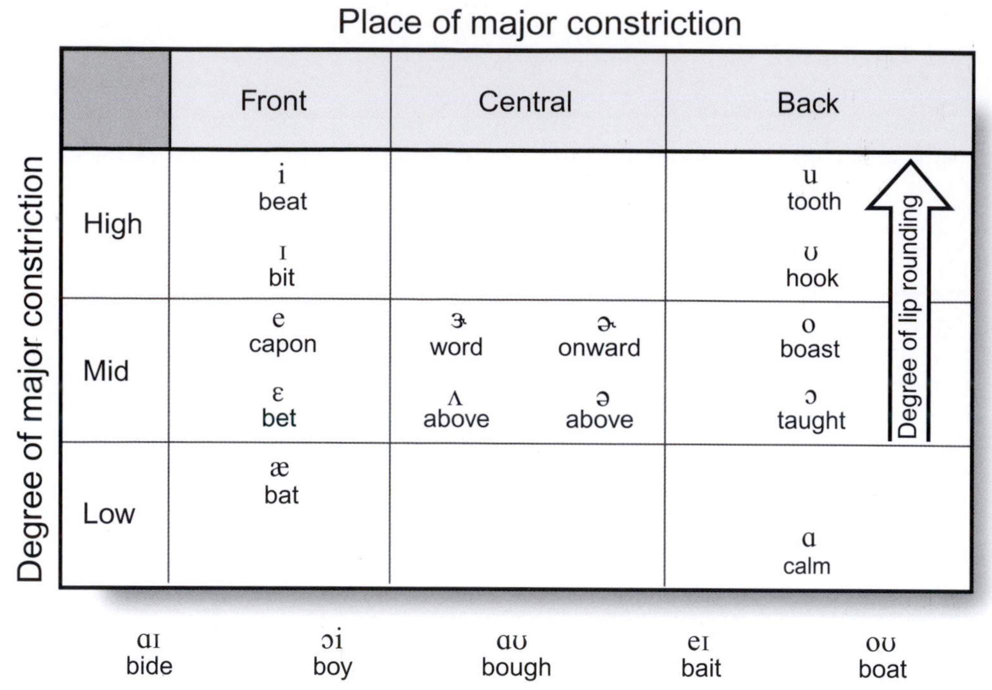

Place of major constriction

Degree of major constriction	Front	Central		Back	
High	i beat ɪ bit			u tooth ʊ hook	Degree of lip rounding ↑
Mid	e capon ɛ bet	ɝ word ʌ above	ɚ onward ə above	o boast ɔ taught	
Low	æ bat			ɑ calm	

aɪ	ɔi	aʊ	eɪ	oʊ
bide	boy	bough	bait	boat

Figure 5–21. Production coding scheme for American English vowels and diphthongs coded in terms of place of major constriction, degree of major constriction, and degree of lip rounding. Physiological clusters are based on the coding scheme advocated by Hixon and Abbs (1980). Vowel symbols are from the International Phonetic Alphabet. Word exemplars are primarily from Fairbanks (1960).

be viewed as shifts in the position of the tongue along the length coordinate of the pharyngeal-oral apparatus.

Degree of Major Constriction. *Degree of major constriction* designates the cross-sectional size of the constricted region of the airway. Coding along this dimension typically specifies a *high*, *mid*, or *low* degree of major constriction and corresponds, in most circumstances, to the location of the highest point of the tongue surface in relation to the roof of the mouth. Exceptions occur when the major constriction is formed between the back of the tongue and the posterior pharyngeal wall. *High* degrees of constriction correspond to small cross-sectional areas at the major constriction. *Mid* degrees of constriction are associated with intermediate size cross sections. And *low* degrees of constriction involve large cross-sectional areas. At times, *low* degrees of constriction may actually have larger cross-sectional areas than those associated with relaxation of the pharyngeal-oral apparatus. Four vowels are classified within the *high* degree of constriction category, eight within the *mid* constriction category, and two within the *low* constriction category. Changes across the *high* to *mid* to *low* degree of constriction categories correspond to lower and lower positioning of the highest point on the dorsal surface of the tongue.

Lip Rounding. *Lip rounding* designates the degree to which the lips are protruded. Such protrusion correlates directly with the size of the airway opening. Thus, an increase in lip rounding signifies a simultaneous lengthening and narrowing of the lip channel along the oral vestibule, whereas a decrease in lip rounding indicates a simultaneous shortening and opening up of the lip channel. In American English, lip rounding is a coding factor on only *mid*-constriction and *high*-constriction *back* vowels. For these vowels, lip rounding increases across the *mid* to *high* categories of constriction.

Diphthong-Coding Scheme

Diphthongs (pronounced DIFF-thongs) are speech sounds that are vowel-like in nature. The classic phonetic view is that they are transitional hybrids of vowels that are formed by rapidly changing from one vowel adjustment to another. Thus, they are transcribed as pairs of vowels, their being five such pairs in American English. Each diphthong is formed of a vowel pair in which the first vowel is characterized by a lesser degree of major constriction than the second vowel. Diphthongs may combine vowel pairs that transition (a) within the same place of major constriction, (b) from back to front places of constriction, and (c) from mid to high degrees of constriction that include increases in lip rounding. Given that diphthongs are transitional hybrids of vowel pairs in the classic phonetic view, their production coding may be conceptualized in terms of their vowel beginning and ending points and nearly continuous adjustments in between. This usual phonetic conceptualization of diphthongs is not without controversy. Acoustic studies of diphthong formation have suggested that they have unique features that are different from "pure" vowels and that their transitional components contain defining features that show them to be a different sound class than vowels. This topic is discussed in detail in Chapter 10.

Consonant-Coding Scheme

Consonants, unlike vowels and diphthongs, are usually produced with a substantially constricted or obstructed airway. Some are produced with voicing by the larynx and some are not. And some are produced with velopharyngeal closure and some are not. As shown in Figure 5–22, adjustments for consonant productions are coded along three dimensions. These include *manner of production* (five categories), *place of*

Manner of production

Place of production	Stop-plosive −	Stop-plosive +	Fricative −	Fricative +	Affricate −	Affricate +	Nasal −	Nasal +	Semivowel −	Semivowel +
Labial (lips)	p pole	b bowl						m sum		w watt
Labiodental (lip–teeth)			f fat	v vat						
Dental (tongue–teeth)			θ thigh	ð thy						
Alveolar (tongue–gum)	t toll	d dole	s seal	z zeal				n sun		l lot
Palatal (tongue–hard palate)			ʃ ash	ʒ azure	tʃ choke	dʒ joke				j,r yacht, rot
Velar (tongue–velum)	k coal	g goal						ŋ sung		
Glottal (vocal folds)			h hot							

Figure 5–22. Production coding scheme for American English consonants coded in terms of manner of production, place of production, and voicing. Voiceless and voiced elements are designated by – and + signs, respectively. Physiological clusters are based on the coding scheme advocated by Hixon and Abbs (1980). Consonant symbols are from the International Phonetic Alphabet. Word exemplars are from Fairbanks (1960).

production (seven categories), and *voicing* (two categories). These three dimensions yield 70 (5 × 7 × 2) unique coding possibilities. About one-third of these are used in American English.

Manner of Production. *Manner of production* specifies the way in which structures of the laryngeal apparatus, velopharyngeal-nasal apparatus, and pharyngeal-oral apparatus constrict or obstruct the airway during consonant generation. The manner of production dimension includes five adjustments, referred to as *stop-plosive*, *fricative*, *affricate*, *nasal*, and *semivowel*. Each of these adjustments is described here and considered further in Chapter 8.

Stop-plosive consonants begin with occlusion of the oral airway and a buildup of oral air pressure behind the occlusion. The airway is then abruptly opened and a burst of airflow is released. Such actions are generated in association with airtight closure of the velopharynx. Not all stop consonants demonstrate a burst of airflow following occlusion of the oral airway. Some release the pent-up air through a lowering of the velum. This allows air to escape inaudibly through the nasal cavities. Stop consonants produced in this fashion are referred to as imploded stop consonants. This type of stop consonant occurs in American English but is not phonemically distinctive.

Fricative consonants are generated when air is forced at high velocity through a narrowly constricted laryngeal or pharyngeal-oral airway. Such sounds derive their acoustic energy from turbulent airflow near their constrictions and from airflow striking nearby obstacles such as the teeth. Fricative consonants are usually produced with a closed velopharynx, although this is not obligatory if the constriction is upstream of the velopharynx, as in a fricative produced within the larynx.

Affricate consonants are usually produced with a closed velopharynx. Such consonants start out much like stop-plosive consonants in that the oral airway is occluded and air pressure builds up behind the occlusion. However, the occlusion for affricate consonants is released less abruptly than for stop-plosive consonants and the burst of airflow that follows is less vigorous. These characteristics of the release phase of affricate consonants are the main features that distinguish their productions from those of stop-plosives.

Nasal consonants are produced with an occluded oral airway and an open velopharyngeal airway. The aeromechanical and acoustical energy associated with their production is transmitted through the nasopharynx and nasal cavities and is emitted from the external nares.

Semivowel sounds are consonant sounds produced with a constricted oral airway. The constriction involved is greater than that for vowel sounds, but less than that for other consonant sounds. Semivowels are generated with the velopharynx closed

Raspberries

Raspberries (also called Bronx cheers) are sounds that resemble sustained flatulence (farting). Raspberries are made by blowing air between a protruded tongue and the lips. Adults use raspberries to indicate derision, sarcasm, or silliness. All cultures seem to have a fondness for them. Infants especially like them and use them in their early sound play. Raspberries aren't used as sounds in human languages. Thus, they fade from the repertoire of experimental noises as the infant figures out that they're not an important part of the linguistic code. Nevertheless, the skill acquired is not wasted. They return later on as full-blown Bronx cheers to be used to put someone down, sarcastically cheer a poor sports performance, or be the final gesture after a lost argument. Blow a raspberry the next time you see a primate at a zoo. Most primates make raspberries. You'll either get one back or get a weird look from a resident.

and the aeromechanical and acoustical energy associated with their production passes through the pharyngeal-oral airway.

The five manners of production just discussed are differentially represented across the consonants of American English. The fricative manner of production is a feature in more than one-third of American English consonants, whereas the stop-plosive manner of production is a feature in one-fourth of such consonants. Semivowel, nasal, and affricate manners of production are successively less prominent in proportion within the overall coding scheme.

Place of Production. *Place of production* codes for where a consonant constriction or occlusion occurs along the laryngeal and pharyngeal-oral airway. This dimension encompasses seven sites. Places of production include *labial*, *labiodental*, *dental*, *alveolar*, *palatal*, *velar*, and *glottal*. In the order listed, these constriction or occlusion sites lie progressively farther inward along the combined pharyngeal-oral and laryngeal airways.

Labial means that only the two lips participate in the primary action having to do with place of production. An exception exists for the semivowel /w/ which is also specified as requiring a high-back tongue configuration. *Labiodental* indicates that the place of production is between the lower lip and the upper teeth. *Dental*, *alveolar*, *palatal*, and *velar* places of production designate locations where the tongue contacts or comes very close to contacting the teeth, upper gum ridge (inside the teeth), hard palate, and velum (soft palate and uvula), respectively. The *glottal* place of production entails primary action of the two vocal folds.

The places of production are differentially represented across the consonants of American English. The *alveolar* and *palatal* places of production are equally prominent and one or the other of them is a feature in half of the consonants of American English. *Labial*, *labiodental*, *dental*, and *velar* places of production are less prominent than *alveolar* and *palatal* places, with the *glottal* place being a feature of only a single consonant of American English.

Voicing. The voicing dimension in the consonant-coding scheme is binary. That is, voice is either on or off for consonant productions, so consonants are categorized as either *voiced* (+) or *voiceless* (–), respectively. The majority of consonant sounds are voiced. Many of the consonants of American English form cognate pairs that differ only on the voicing dimension. Thus, two consonants in a cognate pair match one another in their manner of production and place of production, but differ from one another because one is voiced and the other is voiceless. Cognate pairs occur within the stop-plosive, fricative, and affricate manners of production and at nearly all places of production, the glottal site being the exception. The nasal and semivowel manners of production are voiced.

The Speech Production Stream

The previous section describes the nature of the phonetic code for producing the sounds of speech. This code considers each vowel, diphthong, and consonant as a discrete physiological entity that can be specified in terms of articulatory descriptions related to place-constriction-lip rounding for vowels and place-manner-voicing for consonants. This type of phonetic code is didactically convenient and serves the useful role of idealizing important aspects about the production of speech sounds. A limitation of this code, however, is that the descriptors are timeless. The speech production process is not a linear assemblage of a series of idealized physiological packets (speech sounds). That is, it is not a series of invariant positions and movement sequences strung together like beads on a string (MacNeilage, 1970).

Studies of movements of the speech production apparatus, especially of the pharyngeal-oral subsystem, reveal the limitations of a phonetic code. X-ray images, obtained from speakers of several different languages, show the mandible, tongue, velum, and lips to undergo continuous movement throughout even the simplest sequence of sounds (Munhall, Vatikiotis-Bateson, & Tohkura, 1995). Such x-ray images reveal the sequencing and coordination of articulatory events to be far more complex than a series of discrete speech sounds abutted to one another. Rather, the speech stream, as visualized at the level of articulatory movement, appears to be fluid and continuous and to show no obvious boundaries between successive sounds. Moreover, examination of x-ray images suggests that very different movements can be associated with a single

The Father Who Grew Younger

One of us had a father who had Parkinson disease. He looked younger and younger as he got older and older because increasing stiffness in his face fought off the usual wrinkling process that comes with time. Repeated muscle actions lead to the formation of the wrinkles in our faces as we age. Then there is everyday wear and tear and loss of collagen that causes sagging here and there. We wouldn't show our age so dramatically if we didn't use our facial muscles as much throughout our lives. That is, if we never smiled or frowned or puckered up we might look younger than we are. But as Kent (1997) so aptly put it, ". . . our social worlds would be much poorer for the loss of animated faces. And perhaps we would feel older while looking younger." So rather than hiding your facial expressions, cultivate them so that others will get a true sense of what you are all about. Smile.

positioned at the upper edge of the 7th cervical vertebra. This positioning lowers during adulthood until, by senescence, the lower edge of the cricoid cartilage reaches the bottom of the 7th cervical vertebra. Continuing through senescence, the cricoid cartilage descends even farther (Wind, 1970). One result of this lowering of the laryngeal framework is that the pharynx lengthens downward. At the same time the pharynx is lengthening, it is also changing in cross section. The muscles of the pharynx tend to weaken and atrophy with age and the pharyngeal lumen widens and dilates (Linville & Fisher, 1985; Zaino & Benventano, 1977).

Other features of pharyngeal structure and function also change with age. The epithelial lining of the pharynx undergoes progressive thinning (Ferreri, 1959). Sensory innervation in the pharyngeal region decreases and sensory discrimination goes through a significant decline (Aviv et al., 1994; Ferreri, 1959). The compliance (relatively floppiness) of the pharyngeal tube increases with age (Huang et al., 1998). And the capacity to voluntarily move the pharynx progressively decreases with age (Sonies, Stone, & Shawker, 1984).

The oral part of the pharyngeal-oral apparatus (defined here to include the oral cavity and the oral vestibule) also changes in several ways during adulthood. The oral airway undergoes a gradual increase in size with age, probably in both length and cross section. This is believed to occur even into senescence (Israel, 1968, 1973). It is uncertain, however, whether or not this trend applies to very old individuals (Kahane, 1990).

Other age-related changes in the oral cavity include that the oral epithelium thins, loses some of its elasticity, and becomes less firmly attached to adjacent bone and connective tissue (Squire, Johnson, & Hoops, 1976). Salivary function also changes, causing a tendency for saliva to thicken and alter in composition in older individuals (Chauncey, Borkan, Wayler, Feller, & Kapur, 1981). Reduced amounts of saliva result in dryness in the oral mucosa. Such change may result from structural changes of the salivary glands and/or from endocrine changes attendant to aging (Baum, 1981). These changes may be a factor in why elderly individuals have more oral infections, more oral lesions (sores), and more loose teeth than their younger counterparts (Sonies, 1991).

In those individuals who lose teeth with age, alveolar bone may be resorbed (dissolved), sometimes significantly so (Klein, 1980), although this is less of a problem with current high-quality dental care than in the past (Zemlin, 1998). Overall, bones of the oral cavity and oral vestibule may become more fragile, cartilages may lose some of their resiliency, ligaments may lose some of their elasticity, fat may get redistributed, and muscle bulk and power may wane with aging (Fremont & Hoyland, 2007).

Sensory and motor capabilities of the oral part of the pharyngeal-oral apparatus also decrease with age. For example, oral form, pressure, and touch discrimination are poorer in elderly adults than in young adults (Canetta, 1977). Spatial acuity on the surface of the lips also declines significantly in old age, especially in men (Wohlert, 1996c). The tongue may lose mobility with age (Amerman & Parnell, 1982) and its range of motion may decrease (Sonies, Baum, & Shawker, 1984). The ability to seal the lips may also decline with age (Hixon & Hoit, 2005). Reflex responses of lip muscles are significantly lower in amplitude and longer in latency in elderly individuals compared to young individuals (Wohlert, 1996b).

Others aspects of the nervous system go through changes with aging that affect both the pharyngeal and oral parts of the pharyngeal-oral apparatus. These include, among others, that cortical cells controlling the apparatus may atrophy, neurotransmitter production may decrease, blood flow may diminish, nerve-firing rates may decrease, and nerve conduction velocities may reduce (Kenney, 1982; Lexell, Taylor, & Sjostrom, 1988; Luschei, Ramig, Baker, & Smith, 1999; McGeer, Fibiger, McGeer, & Wiskson, 1971; Valenstein, 1981).

Some of the age-related changes discussed to this juncture may affect speech production. Three prominently discussed manifestations of aging have to do with changes in the resonance properties of the pharyngeal-oral airway, durational features of speech production, and variability of speech production. Changes in factors such as cognition, memory, and linguistic processing may also affect speech production, but they are beyond the scope of emphasis in this introductory presentation.

As discussed above, the pharyngeal and oral components of the pharyngeal-oral apparatus increase in length and cross section of their internal airways across adulthood. As considered in detail in subsequent chapters, the size of these internal airways influences the resonant properties of the pharyngeal-oral apparatus. For example, larger airways tend to have acoustic resonances that are lower in frequency. Thus, it is unsurprising that the frequencies of vowel formants (major energy concentrations, see technical definition in Chapter 7) have been reported to be lower in elderly individuals than in younger individuals (Linville & Fisher, 1985; Liss, Weismer, & Rosenbek, 1990; Watson & Munson, 2007). This age-related lowering is especially prominent in the first formant, the lowest resonance (Endres, Bambach, & Flosser, 1971; Linville, 2001; Linville & Fisher, 1985; Scukanec, Petrosino, & Squibb, 1991). The second and third formants (higher frequency resonances) are also documented to be lower in frequency in older individuals, but the effect is smaller than for the first formant (Linville & Fisher, 1985; Linville & Rens, 2001). Although there is general agreement that the age effect in vowel acoustics is related to enlargement of the pharyngeal-oral airway, there is some question concerning how the relative changes of the pharyngeal and oral parts of the apparatus contribute to the acoustic changes observed (Xue & Hao, 2003). Additional research using advanced technologies for measuring the three-dimensional configuration of the pharyngeal-oral lumen should be helpful in sorting out the details of this age effect.

Slowing is a hallmark of aging and is viewed by most experts as the most pervasive motor characteristic of getting older (Fremont & Hoyland, 2007; Welford, 1982). Slowing in the pharyngeal-oral apparatus is no exception and can be attributed to changes in the nervous system that controls the peripheral machinery of the apparatus, as well as to changes in the peripheral machinery itself (Fozard, Vercruyssen, Reynolds, Hancock, & Quilter, 1994; Kahane, 1990; Kent & Burkard, 1981; Ulatowska, 1985; Weismer & Liss, 1991). Chapters 2, 3, and 4 discuss the influences of age on breathing, laryngeal, and velopharyngeal-nasal function in speech production. Those influences combine with those of the pharyngeal-oral apparatus to produce a general slowing of speech production with advanced age. This slowing has two bases, one being that articulatory rate slows and the other being that older speakers pause more often during running speech production (Hartman & Danhauer, 1976; Hoit & Hixon, 1987; Ryan, 1972).

Measurements of the temporal characteristics of the speech of normal elderly adults shed light on how the slowing of speech is spread across the speech production stream (Liss, Weismer, & Rosenbek, 1990; Smith, Wasowicz, & Preston, 1987). Smith and colleagues, for example, studied young adults (24 to 27 years of age) and elderly adults (66 to 75 years of age) producing a variety of words and sentences at normal and fast speaking rates. They measured the durations of phonetic segments (consonants and vowels), syllables, and sentences and found that the durations for each of these measures were an average of 20 to 25% longer for elderly speakers than for young speakers at both the normal and fast speaking rates.

Liss et al. (1990) also studied a group of elderly individuals for segment durations in sentences, but in their case the participants were from among the oldest of the old (87 to 93 years of age). Liss et al. found that the segment durations they measured in these very old participants were longer than those reported in the literature for young adult speakers, but relatively similar to those produced by younger elderly speakers (65 to 82 years of age) studied by Weismer (1984).

Longer durations for speech segments in normal-speaking old and very old adults, in comparison to young adults, beg comparison to other speakers who use longer durations during speech production. One such group is young children. For all duration comparisons with such young children, the production of elderly speakers tend to be in the range of durations exhibited by 6- and 7-year-old children (Kent & Forner, 1980; Smith et al., 1983). Thus, life would appear to go full circle from young childhood to senescence, picking up speed in early life and slowing back down in later life.

The variability of movement undergoes change with age across adulthood. Such variability tends to increase with age and is often considered to be a measure of motor control integrity in general (Nelson, Soderberg, & Urbsheit, 1984; Weismer & Liss, 1991). Studies to determine whether or not such variability is also manifested in speech production with aging have included both physiological and acoustical observations.

Wohlert and Smith (1998) studied the spatiotemporal stability of lip movements in old adult and young adult speakers. Lip displacement waveforms were recorded for different rates of speech production and subjected to sophisticated analyses that captured information about variability of performance. Despite producing clear and fully intelligible speech, elderly adults spoke more slowly than their young adult counterparts and demonstrated less spatiotemporal (position and time) stability in lip movement. Findings of this nature imply that normal aging alters the fine motor control required for speech production.

Wohlert (1996a) conducted a study of the activity of muscles surrounding the lips in young and old adults during different activities, including speech production. This study was concerned with the complexity of motor patterns and whether or not they become less flexible as a consequence of aging. Patterns of muscle activation were compared among different quadrants of the lips and were found not to differ for tasks such as lip protrusion and chewing, but to differ significantly during speech production in relation to the age of the individuals studied. Specifically, patterns of muscle coupling among different quadrants of the lips (inferred from correlations of myoelectric measurements of muscle activities) showed a tendency for coupling (coactivation across quadrants) to be greater in elderly individuals than in young individuals. One interpretation of this finding is that there is a clear effect of aging on speech production and that this effect has strong implications for the motor control of speech production. Presumably, elderly individuals adopt an increased coupling strategy among quadrants of the lips as their fine motor control wanes with age and they are unable to use the lips in the variety of ways they could at younger years. Loss of fine motor control may require a reorganization of speech movements and one consequence may be an increase in their variability as the elderly adult attempts to cope with a changing nervous system.

Acoustical studies of speech also show increased variability with age (Smith et al., 1987; Weismer, 1984; Weismer & Fromm, 1983). Weismer, for example, found greater variability among normal elderly speakers than among young adult speakers for segments in sentence productions. For another example, Smith and colleagues found greater variability in elderly compared to young participants for segment durations in words and sentences produced at normal speaking rates. And in their study of the oldest of the old, Liss et al. (1990) determined that the variability in performance of the very old is even greater than the variability among younger elderly and much greater than among young adults. This is true not only for segment durations, but also for vowel formant (resonance) midpoints and formant transitions.

The process of aging imposes a slowing and reduction of precision on the pharyngeal-oral apparatus. Liss et al. (1990) noted that data on the acoustic characteristics of very old speakers show striking similarities to data obtained from speakers with Parkinson disease (Weismer, 1984). They interpreted this similarity to suggest a speech production analog to assertions that aging may involve processes similar to those seen in neural disease (Morgan & Finch, 1988). This is not to say that the very old are Parkinson-like, but that the speech motor performance of very old persons may be related, in part, to the deterioration of brain circuits that are affected in similar ways to those affected by Parkinson disease.

Sex and Pharyngeal-Oral Function in Speech Production

Everyone knows that speech usually sounds different when produced by men and women. From discussion in previous chapters, it is clear that sex-related differences in speech production and speech are strongly associated with sex-related differences in laryngeal structure and function, but that structure and function of the breathing apparatus and velopharyngeal-nasal apparatus are only minimally different between the sexes (see Chapters 2, 3, and 4). Here, attention turns to the potential contribution of pharyngeal-oral structure and function to sex-related differences in speech production and speech.

Perhaps the most obvious structural difference between men and women is size. Men tend to be larger than women overall, and this size difference is also reflected in the pharyngeal-oral apparatus. For example, the skull is larger (Zemlin, 1998) and the vocal tract (from larynx to lips) is longer in men than women (Fitch & Giedd, 1999; Vorperian et al., 2005). One of the most important sex-related differences for speech production is that the pharynx is longer by about 22% (in the resting state) in men compared to women (Fitch & Giedd, 1999). These size and length differences are not present in children. Rather, such differences emerge at puberty and continue to become more prominent until they level out around early adulthood (Fitch & Giedd, 1999; Goldstein, 1980).

Men tend to be stronger than women. This also holds true for the strength of structures within the pharyngeal-oral apparatus. For example, men produce greater maximum lip forces than women (Barlow & Rath, 1985) and the same is true for maximum tongue forces (Youmans & Stierwalt, 2006). Nevertheless, it is interesting to note that when maximum tongue force production is normalized to body muscle mass, sex-related differences disappear (Mortimore, Fiddes, Stephens, & Douglas, 1999). Finally, one study of fine force control of the lips and tongue revealed that men, when compared to women, had longer reaction times, generated higher velocities of force change, and were more accurate in holding a target force (Gentil & Tournier, 1998).

Certain features of speech production that relate to pharyngeal-oral function have been shown to differ somewhat between the sexes. For example, men produce syllable-, word-, and sentence-level utterances (Smith et al., 1987) and repetitions of speech movements (Nicholson & Kimura, 1996) at faster rates than women. Examination of a single structure, the tongue, during speech production, also shows the same sex-related pattern for speed. Specifically, during diphthong productions and productions of two consecutive vowels, the posterior tongue moves faster in men than women (Simpson, 2001, 2002). This difference in speed has been attributed to the fact that the male tongue must move a greater distance than the female tongue, particularly in the posterior region of the oral cavity where the palate is domed and the pharynx is large in men.

Sex-related differences in the size of the pharyngeal-oral apparatus influence speech in a number of ways. For example, the frequency spectrum of certain fricative consonants is lower in men than women due to size differences in the resonating cavities (Schwartz, 1968). Perhaps one of the most puzzling differences between the speech of men and women relates to the formant patterns (major energy concentrations—see Chapter 7) associated with vowel production. Although men have lower frequency vowel formants than women (as would be expected from the fact that men are larger than women), the differences in formant values are not what would be expected from size differences alone. Other factors must be also contributing.

One such factor is that men have proportionally longer pharyngeal cavities than women (Fant, 1975). Nevertheless, even this is not sufficient to explain the nonuniform differences in formants between men and women, leaving open the possibility that sex-related differences in articulatory behavior may account for at least some of the remaining variance. One suggestion is that women use smaller and longer constrictions than men in their vowel productions and these constrictions contribute to the creation of different formant patterns (Fant, 1975).

Another suggestion is that women articulate in ways that create larger acoustic differences among vowels as a means of compensating for the wider distribution of energy across frequency provided by the voice source (Ryalls & Lieberman, 1982). That is, because women have higher voice fundamental frequencies than men, their harmonics are more widely spaced and there is less acoustic energy in each formant frequency region, thereby making it more difficult to distinguish among vowels. Thus, women may compensate in ways that exaggerate the acoustical and perceptual differences among vowels. Using magnetic resonance imaging, Story, Hoffman, and Titze (1997) found the female pharynx to be about 37% shorter than the male pharynx during the production of three cardinal vowels. They concluded that the female pharyngeal-oral airway shape "contains unique qualities that cannot be explained by a simple uniform compression of the male vocal tract" (p. 36) and that the shortened pharynx in the female pharyngeal-oral apparatus may be a key factor in distinguishing between male and female voice qualities during speech production.

MEASUREMENT OF PHARYNGEAL-ORAL FUNCTION

This section considers the instrumental measurement of pharyngeal-oral function. Attention is directed to selected methods that have application to the study of normal and abnormal function. Six categories of methods are discussed, including those that take advantage of (a) x-ray, (b) strain-gauge, (c) electromagnetic, (d) ultrasonic, (e) aeromechanical, and (f) acoustical technologies.

X-ray Imaging

X-ray imaging is a powerful method for studying the positions and movements of structures of the pharyngeal-oral apparatus. Three x-ray methods for studying pharyngeal-oral function are chosen for discussion here. These include lateral still x-rays, cinefluorography (motion picture x-rays), and microbeam x-rays.

Lateral still x-rays provide images like that shown in Figure 4–26. These are most often obtained in the midsagittal plane and provide a shadow-cast "snapshot" of the pharyngeal-oral apparatus at a moment in time. Lateral still x-rays are useful for examining structures that are stationary. For example, they can be used to determine the midline positions of the lips, mandible, tongue, velum, posterior pharyngeal wall, and hyoid bone in relation to one another during sustained speech sounds where such structures are relatively fixed in position. Thus, vowels, fricative consonants, and nasal consonants are prime candidates for study.

Cinefluorography (or videofluorography) enables the x-ray study of structures in motion (McWilliams & Girdany, 1964; Moll, 1960). Fluorographic methods, and other forms of cineradiography, provide for the monitoring of the positions of different structures within the pharyngeal-oral apparatus and for determining the spatial and temporal coordination among those structures as their positions change. Thus, movement patterns can be discerned among the lips, mandible, tongue, velum, posterior pharyngeal wall, hyoid bone, and other structures. Images obtained through the use of cineflourography (or videofluorography) can be analyzed qualitatively or quantitatively. Quantitative analysis often entails a series of stop-frame observations in which the positions of structures are measured in a two-dimensional coordinate system. Such measurements are tedious and time intensive, even when semiautomated. They are, however, powerfully instructive with regard to speech production behaviors of the pharyngeal-oral apparatus in that they enable visualization of the entire apparatus in one plane. A great deal of knowledge about normal and abnormal speech production has been obtained using such methodology (Kent & Moll, 1975; Netsell & Kent, 1976).

Being able to visualize x-ray images of the outlines of stationary and moving structures of the pharyngeal-oral apparatus is enormously instructive, but there are complexities in their measurement. One approach to simplifying the quantification of the complex geometry of the pharyngeal-oral airway entails the fixing of metal markers at strategic locations on the structures being viewed and tracking these markers during x-ray observations. For example, as portrayed in Figure 5–28, small metal

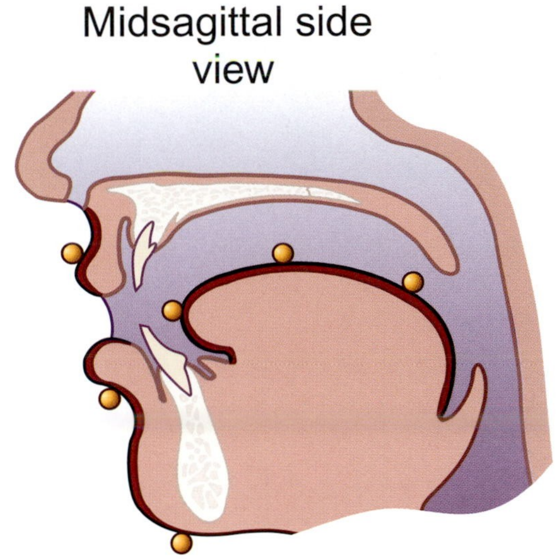

Figure 5–28. Some flesh point pellet positions used in cinefluorographic studies of speech production.

pellets can be fixed to the outside of the mandible, lips, and the dorsal surface of the tongue (at multiple locations) to make the visualization of "flesh points" on the pharyngeal-oral apparatus possible. In this way, the positions and movements of designated points on structures can be tracked and studied. All aspects of pharyngeal-oral movements are not taken into account with this procedure, but the tracking of points has been shown to be a suitable means for quantifying the nature of movement sequences during speech production. It also removes some of the ambiguities of studying complex gestures such as those involved in tongue movements (Honda, 2002; Kent, 1972; Wood, 1979).

X-ray studies of pharyngeal-oral function expose those being studied to radiation risks. For safety reasons, limits are placed on the extent to which observations can be made in both research and clinical studies. One attempt to address this problem is the x-ray microbeam system. X-ray microbeam technology was developed at the University of Tokyo (Kiritani, Itoh, & Fujimura, 1975), and in the United States is currently found at the University of Wisconsin in a facility supported as a national resource for investigators by the National Institutes of Health (Westbury, 1991).

The x-ray microbeam system is designed to track small pellets adhered to structures using an extremely thin x-ray beam. This beam focuses on the pellets specifically so that surrounding tissue receives minimal radiation. Two-dimensional positions of multiple pellets can be tracked simultaneously. Thus, in the case of the study of multiple pellets affixed to the dorsal surface of the tongue, it is possible to track the movement of different points (pellets) along the surface of the structure. Research has shown that patterns of tongue movement with and without pellets in position are not appreciably different, so that the pellet tracking protocol does not influence the usual behavior of the participant being studied (Weismer & Bunton, 1999).

Figure 5–29 shows an example of data obtained using the x-ray microbeam method during speech production. There, a pellet on the tongue blade is tracked in vertical and horizontal dimensions and the speed of movement of the pellet is also shown. The trajectories of individual pellets and groups of pellets are instructive concerning the nature of adjustments of the surface of the tongue (and mandible and lips) for speech production events and reflect on the changing midline configuration of the oral airway. Studies using the x-ray microbeam system have been exceptionally powerful in elucidating kinematic patterns within the oral apparatus in both individuals with normal speech production (Green & Wang, 2003; Nittrouer, 1991) and individuals with neuromotor-based speech disorders (Weismer, Yunosova, & Westbury, 2003).

Strain-Gauge Monitoring

Strain-gauge monitoring is often used to study pharyngeal-oral function. Strain gauges are devices that respond to the bend placed on metal beams to which they are attached. Most often they are bonded to both sides of such beams and form two arms of an electrical circuit called a Wheatstone bridge. Bending forces on the beams cause resistance changes in the strain gauges that are converted into proportional voltage changes for monitoring.

Different arrangements of deflection beams and strain gauges have been used to measure force production of various structures of the pharyngeal-oral apparatus (Hixon, 1972). Included among these are circular or straight beam configurations using strain gauges to measure the adductory force of the two lips combined (Kim, 1971), maximum and controlled

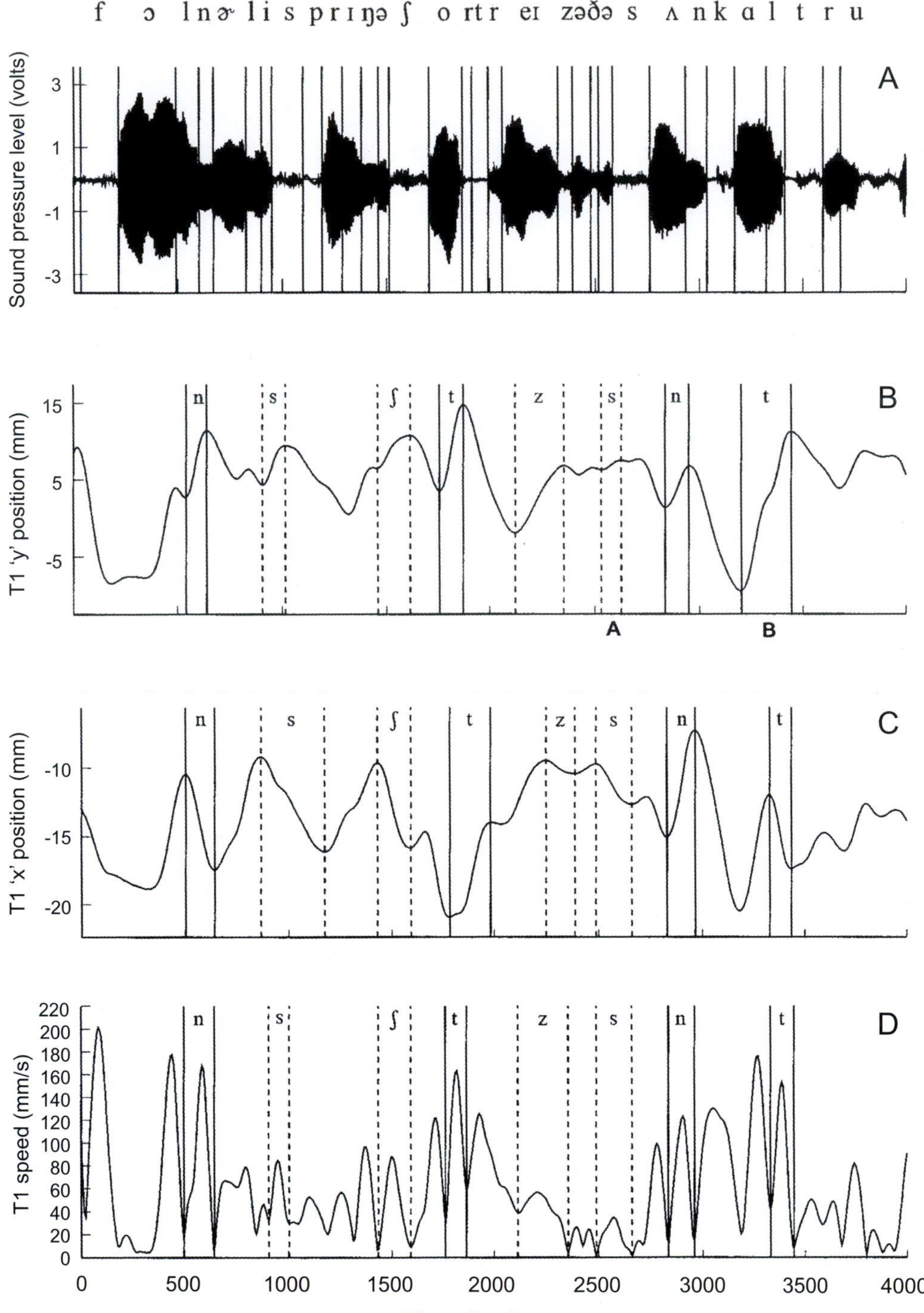

Figure 5–29. X-ray microbeam data showing the tracking of a flesh point pellet attached to the tongue blade during the production of the utterance ". . . fall and early spring, the short rays of the sun call a true . . ." Panel A shows the sound pressure level wave associated with the utterance, whereas panels B, C, and D show the pellet's vertical (upward and downward) and horizontal (forward and backward) positioning, and its speed of movement, respectively. Signals are partitioned into presumed phonetic segments. From "Defining and measuring speech movement events" (p. 129), by S. Tasko and J. Westbury, 2002, *Journal of Speech, Language, and Hearing Research, 45*, 127–142. Copyright 2002 by the American Speech-Language-Hearing Association. All rights reserved. Reproduced with permission.

sustained holding adductory forces of the upper and lower lips individually (Barlow & Burton, 1990; Barlow & Netsell, 1986; Barlow & Rath, 1985), and thrusting force of the tip of the tongue in a vector toward the alveolar process of the maxilla (Barlow & Abbs, 1983). Measurements of these types have been found to be helpful in elucidating both normal behavior and the behavior of individuals with pharyngeal-oral control problems related to cerebral palsy, Parkinson disease, and traumatic brain injury (Barlow & Abbs, 1983; Barlow & Burton, 1990).

The widest use of strain-gauge technology in the pharyngeal-oral apparatus relates to its application in the measurement of structural position and movement (Hixon, 1972). For example, strain-gauge technology has been used to measure the positions and movements of the velum (Moller, Martin, & Christiansen, 1971) and the mandible and lips (Barlow, Cole, & Abbs, 1983; Muller & Abbs, 1979; Sussman & Smith, 1971).

Figure 5–30 shows one array for recording movements of the mandible and the upper and lower lips with a strain-gauge system. The gauges are mounted on cantilever beams that yield as the mandible and lips move and deform them. Beams can be arranged to record both up and down and forward and backward displacements of the structures being monitored. As well, signals from the transducers can be processed to obtain velocity and acceleration derivatives of the displacements.

Strain-gauge systems have yielded a large amount of data on movements of the mandible and lips during speech production. Attention has focused on the nature of such movements, especially in relation to their temporal and spatial coordination (Gracco, 1994; Shaiman, Adams, & Kimelman, 1997; Smith & McClean-Muse, 1987). The simplicity and relatively low cost of strain-gauge transduction systems has fostered their continued use despite the development of other movement monitoring technologies.

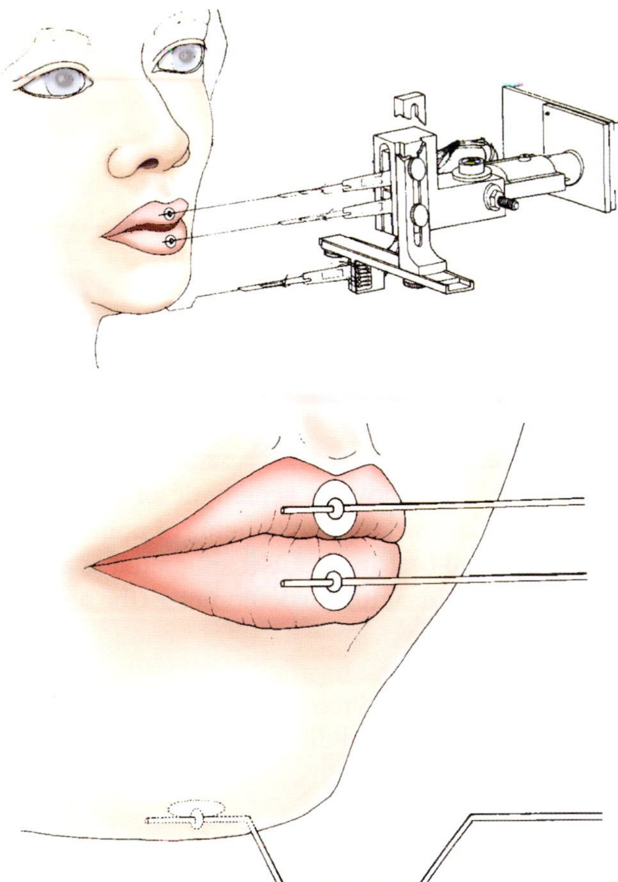

Figure 5–30. Strain-gauge array for simultaneously measuring upward and downward and forward and backward movements of the mandible and the upper and lower lips (*upper part of figure*) and cantilever attachment locations on the mandible and the upper and lower lips (*lower part of figure*). From "Strain gauge transduction of lip and jaw motion in the midsagittal plane: Refinement of a prototype system" (p. 484), by E. Muller and J. Abbs, 1979, *Journal of the Acoustical Society of America, 65*, 481–486. Copyright 1979 by the American Institute of Physics. Modified and reproduced with permission.

Electromagnetic Sensing

Electromagnetic sensing provides a means for tracking the movements of points on the inside and outside of the pharyngeal-oral apparatus. Such sensing relies on the detection and quantification of magnetic fields induced in receiving coils by generating coils. More specifically, the voltage induced in receiving coils attached to points on the pharyngeal-oral apparatus is inversely proportional to the distance between them and fixed generating coils. Suitable electronic manipulations provide a measure of the position of the receiving coils in one- or two-dimensional space, as desired.

tongue that enables it to function like a liquid-filled, incompressible, and pliable structure (a muscular hydrostat).

Movements of the lips are exceptionally versatile, with each lip being able to move independently or with the two lips coordinated in their movements, and with the range of possible adjustments including puckering, protruding, retracting, spreading, pointing, curling, groping, rounding, and plumping, among others.

The control variables of pharyngeal-oral function include pharyngeal-oral lumen size and configuration, pharyngeal-oral structural contact pressure, pharyngeal-oral airway resistance, and pharyngeal-oral acoustic impedance.

Pharyngeal-oral movements are controlled by the nervous system, with the final forms of control commands sent through cranial nerves to muscles, and with sensory innervation provided through cranial nerves to guide anticipated actions of the pharyngeal-oral apparatus and to keep track of its recent status.

Pharyngeal-oral functions of importance to this text include changing the degree of coupling between the oral cavity and atmosphere, chewing, swallowing, and sound generation and filtering.

Pharyngeal-oral function in speech production involves adjustments that physiologically code the positions and movements of structures into the formation of different speech sounds.

Vowel sounds and diphthongs are usually produced with voicing by the larynx, exclusion of nasal participation by velopharyngeal closure, and using combinations of structural positions and movements that result in relatively unconstricted configurations of the pharyngeal-oral airway that are coded along the dimensions of place of major constriction, degree of major constriction, and degree of lip rounding.

Consonant sounds are usually produced with a relatively constricted or obstructed airway, with or without voicing by the larynx, and/or with or without velopharyngeal closure, and using combinations of structural positions and movements that are coded along the dimensions of manner of production, place of production, and voicing.

The speech production stream is fluid and ongoing and structures of the pharyngeal-oral apparatus move smoothly and nearly continuously from one position to another.

Traditional theory about speech production proposes that sounds in the speech production stream influence their neighbors through processes that are anticipatory and scan ahead and processes that are a reflection of the inertial properties of the speech production apparatus.

More recent articulatory phonology or gesture theories about speech production propose that sounds in the speech production stream are assembled by the phasing of overlapping movement gestures of different structures and do not require schemes of phoneme representation to account for speech production behavior.

The development of pharyngeal-oral function in speech production involves a transition to faster speech production rates and more stable speech production movements across childhood, along with the development of muscle synergies and movement routines.

The influence of age on pharyngeal-oral function is manifested in resonances of the pharyngeal-oral airway that are lower, temporal aspects of speech production that become protracted, and variability of performance that increases in elderly individuals compared to young individuals.

Sex has certain influences on pharyngeal-oral function in speech production and speech that are related to faster utterance rates and movements in men than women and a longer pharyngeal airway in men than women that results in nonuniform differences in formants (resonances) between the sexes.

Common measurements of pharyngeal-oral function include those that take advantage of x-ray, electromagnetic, strain-gauge, ultrasonic, aeromechanical, and acoustical technologies.

Pharyngeal-oral disorders come in many forms, affect people of all ages, may be of functional and/or organic origin, and have a significant influence on the quality of life because of their behavioral, social, health, and economic consequences.

Many clinical professionals contribute to the evaluation and management of individuals with pharyngeal-oral disorders that influence speech production, including the speech-language pathologist, otorhinolaryngologist, plastic surgeon, neurologist, dentist, prosthodontist, and psychologist.

Scenario

Time has a way of healing things and it worked to his advantage. He had to learn the boundaries of a vastly altered pharyngeal-oral apparatus that was missing a tongue and some of the left side of his oral cavity. He had also lost some sensation. Chewing, swallowing, and speaking were three of his continual challenges and none of these was going well through the use of his own devices.

Once he had recovered from surgery, he was referred to a regional maxillofacial clinic that specialized in reconstructive and prosthetic treatments for people who had undergone ablative surgeries for cancer. There, a team of experts worked on his problems. When first seen at the clinic, he was struggling to meet his nutritional needs and his speech was severely wanting. Eating was difficult and largely restricted to liquids and very soft foods that he managed to move backward in his mouth by rotating his head upward. His speech was relatively unintelligible, except to his wife. His speech intelligibility for sentences was 47%, whereas intelligibility for single words was 32%. His voice was mildly hypernasal. Detailed phonetic analysis of his speech revealed that he had imprecise productions of vowels, diphthongs, semivowels, and other consonants, especially those that normally require tongue adjustments.

A prosthetic tongue was fabricated and fitted to his remaining lower teeth. This structure covered the floor of his mouth and had two prominent elevations on its upper surface, one located toward the front of his mouth and one located toward the back. A groove was included in the prosthesis that ran along the intact right side of his oral cavity so that liquid and thin, pureed foods could be channeled to the pharynx. The prosthesis was initially uncomfortable to him and created excessive saliva. These problems resolved after several days of using the device.

A speech-language pathologist worked on the design of programs to enhance drinking and eating and speech production. The prosthesis was worn during most daily activities and training was provided in its use with liquids and pureed substances. Slight upward rotation of the head was combined with slight rightward tilting of the head and elevation of the mandible. This moved substances to the right and backward within the oral cavity into the pharynx. Cheek activity on the right was also encouraged to help with rearward propulsion of substances. For meals at home, the prosthesis was sometimes removed so that semisolid substances could be handled through other mechanical compensations and propelled to the esophagus by sips of water.

An intensive speech management program was undertaken that focused on the development of compensations for a missing tongue. This program included strategies for using new places of production for certain speech sounds and capitalizing on differential actions involving the positioning of the larynx (to effect pharyngeal length changes), positioning of the lateral pharyngeal walls (to effect cross-sectional changes position, and is displaced far to the left—note at time D the wide separation of the molecules from positions 1 and 2. Clearly, the elastic recoil forces caused the molecule to move back toward the rest position at time E, position 2, but why doesn't the motion stop at the rest position? The answer is that inertial forces do not allow the molecule to "stop on a dime" at the rest position, but drive the molecule through rest and to the leftward extreme. The molecule, which has mass and opposes acceleration and deceleration, will not decelerate instantly to stop at the rest position, but rather will continue its motion through that point in space. The motion will continue leftward until the recoil forces again overcome the forces driving the molecule away from its rest position (primarily inertial). When this happens, the motion will be reversed once more, and the molecule will head back in the direction of the rest position. Once again, the motion will not stop at the rest position because of inertial forces and the molecule will continue to move back and forth around the rest position.

After the original application of the force at position 1, the back and forth motion is maintained by energy stored by the molecule itself, in the form of recoil and inertial forces. If the molecules were vibrating in a *frictionless* medium, where no energy was lost because of heat generation, the back and forth motion would continue indefinitely. Realistically, heat loss due to air molecules rubbing against each other and other surfaces will eventually cause the back and forth motion to die out if external forces are not continually reapplied to the air molecules. However, the principles of recoil and inertia forces still apply to a dying-out motion. The frictional forces simply compete with the recoil and inertial forces, and in the absence of external forces (such as another push), eventually dominate the latter two and end the motion.

The Motions of Vibrating Air Molecules Change the Local Densities of Air

The motion of air molecules and the forces that control that motion have been described. How can these ideas lead to an understanding of pressure waves? Assume that a device for measuring air pressure is placed at position 2 in Figure 6–1. *Pressure* can be defined as the force exerted over a unit area ($P = F/A$) and is proportional to the density of air. When air molecules are more densely packed, they collide with each other more frequently and generate more force and more pressure. Conversely, when air molecules are less densely packed together, the collisions are less frequent and the pressures are relatively lower. At time A in Figure 6–1, there are no external forces applied to the air molecules and the density of air is that associated with air at rest (recall the 4×10^{23} figure given above). The pressure measured at time A, position 2 (or at any other position at time A, because the density of air at rest is the same at any spatial location) is referred to as *atmospheric pressure*. The actual value of atmospheric pressure is not important to the current discussion,[2] but the *reference function* of this pressure is important. In the following discussion, atmospheric pressure (symbolized hereafter as P_{atm}) is considered as zero (0) pressure. At time B, the schematic drawing shows two molecules close together, indicating a relatively denser packing of air molecules as compared to time A. The pressure measuring device at time B, position 2 should measure a higher pressure than at time A because the denser packing of molecules will involve more frequent collisions and higher forces. Any time a pressure is above the reference pressure P_{atm}, it is referred to as *positive pressure*. The more tightly packed the molecules, the more positive the pressure.

At time D, position 2, the first and second molecules are widely separated in space. This represents the case where the density of air is less than it is at P_{atm}. The pressure-measuring device records a value below P_{atm}, which is a *negative pressure*. The less tightly packed the molecules, the more negative the pressure.

These positive and negative pressures are not positive or negative in any absolute sense. They are only positive (above) or negative (below) with respect to the reference pressure P_{atm}. Figure 6–2 shows the result of the continuous bunching up and spreading apart of the air molecules schematized in Figure 6–1.

[2]Atmospheric pressure at sea level is 14.7 pounds per square inch, or 1013 *millibars* (an alternate unit of pressure).

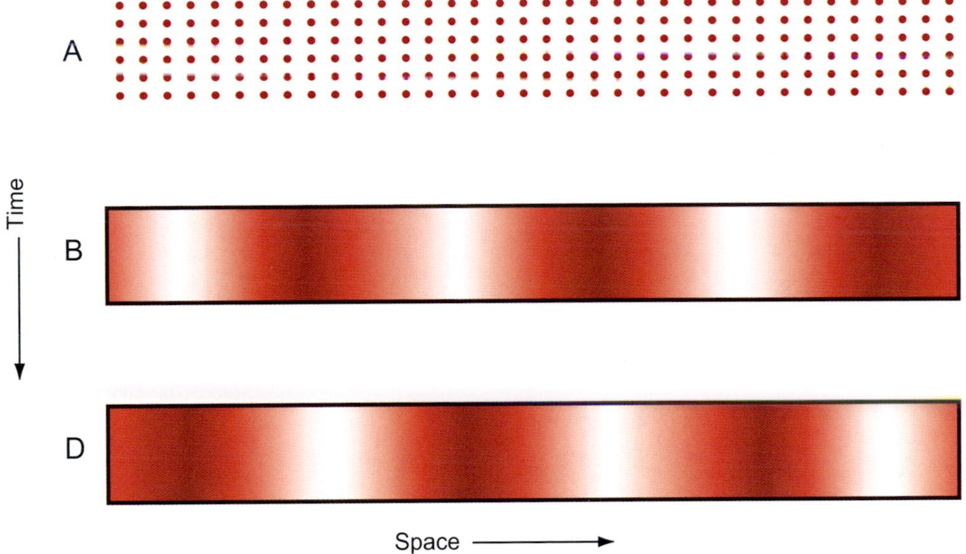

Figure 6–2. Schematic drawing of pressure waves, distributed in space and time. A, B, and D correspond to discrete times depicted in Figure 6–1. At a given point in space, pressure changes over time.

The three rows labeled A, B, D in Figure 6–2 correspond to the same rows in Figure 6–1 (rows C and E from Figure 6–1 have been omitted from Figure 6–2), indicating three different times in the evolving history of air molecule movement. At time A, the multiple dots are shown evenly distributed across space, as would be expected if the medium was not being affected by an external force. The pressure at any point throughout the distribution would be P_{atm}.

At time B, this distribution has been changed to one in which regions of low and high density alternate across space. The heavily shaded areas represent high densities (as when two molecules are immediately adjacent, as in Figure 6–1, time B, position 2), and the lightly shaded areas represent low densities (as in Figure 6–1, time D, position 2). At time D, regions of high and low densities again alternate across space, but their locations have been reversed from those at time B. In other words, for a given point in space (such as position 2), what was a high density and high pressure area at time B, is a low density and low pressure area at time D. Areas of high density and high pressure are called areas of *compression* or *condensation*[3]; areas of low density and low pressures are called areas of *rarefaction*.

A Pressure Wave, Not Individual Molecules, Propagates Through Space and Varies as a Function of Both Space and Time

Recall what was said earlier about the motion of individual air molecules. They moved around a rest position, the movement resulting from inherent elastic and inertial forces. The molecules themselves, however, do not *propagate* across space. What moves across space is the *pressure wave*, shown in Figure 6–2 from left to right as the sequence of high and low densities (pressures), or the sequence of compression (condensation) and rarefaction areas. Because these alternating regions of high and low pressures are the result of the back and forth movement of air molecules, which alternately bunches them up and spreads them apart, a given point in space will sometimes have high pressure (such as time B, position 2 in Figure 6–1), and sometimes have low pressure (time D, position 2 in both Figures 6–1 and 6–2). Thus, a pressure wave extends across space at a specific instant in time (examine Figure 6–2, across time B or D), and varies in time at a particular point in space (Figure 6–2, compare times B and D at any point in space).

[3]Condensation is the result of compression. For purposes of this text, compression and condensation are used interchangeably.

When a pressure wave moves away from the *source* of the sound waves (the origin of the forces that initiated the displacement of air molecules), the alternating regions of high and low pressures often project in a straight line, as shown from left to right in Figure 6–2. These kinds of sound waves are called *plane waves*, because the sequence of high and low pressures can be thought of as a series of pressure "slices," or planes, extending away from the source. For the present discussion, only plane waves will be considered, but other kinds of pressures waves are possible (for example, those moving sideways from a source, rather than in a straight line away from the source).

The Variation of a Pressure Wave in Time and Space Can Be Measured

There are specific measures of the temporal (time) and spatial (space) variation of pressure waves. A firm grasp of these measures is essential to understanding important aspects of the acoustic theory of speech production, covered in Chapter 7.

Temporal Measures

Figure 6–3A redraws a portion of the molecule motion shown in Figure 6–1. Of particular interest is the motion of the first molecule, shown in Figure

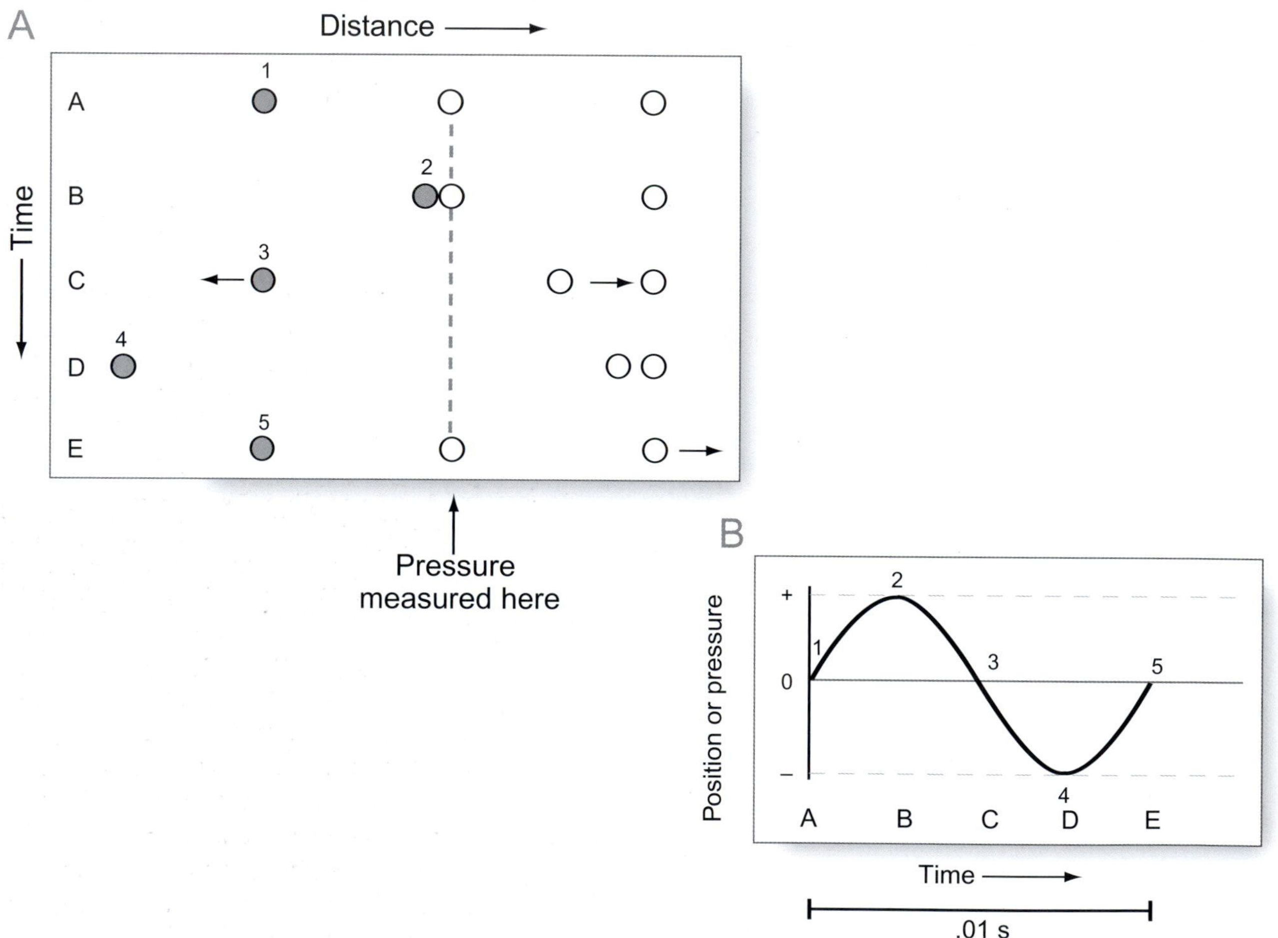

Figure 6–3. A. Schematic model of the vibration of an air molecule (*filled circle*) around its rest position. Numbers above the molecule indicate five successive points in time during its vibratory cycle. **B.** Plot of the position of the filled-circle molecule and the pressure measured at the location of the second molecule during one vibratory cycle.

6–3A as a shaded circle. As in Figure 6–1, space (distance) is shown from left to right, and time from top to bottom (times A, B, C, D, E, occurring in succession). The numbers 1, 2, 3, 4, and 5 above the filled circles show the position of the first molecule at 5 discrete points in time, starting from the molecule at the rest position "1" and ending with the molecule back at the rest position "5." At time B, the molecule is immediately adjacent to the next molecule, which will create a region of compression, or high pressure, at the point in space indicated by the upward-pointing arrow. The pressure at this point in space will become somewhat negative at time C (molecule labeled "3"), more negative yet at time D (molecule labeled "4"), and will return to P_{atm} at time E (molecule labeled "5").

The motion of the filled-circle molecule is shown as a function of time in Figure 6–3B. When any magnitude (such as displacement, pressure, speed, and so forth) is shown as a function of time, the plot is called a *waveform*. This waveform shows the position of the molecule from rest position (1), to the rightward extreme (2), the return through the rest position (3), at the leftward extreme (4), and finally back at the rest position (5). In other words, this waveform shows one complete *cycle of motion* of the molecule. If the molecule continued to move after point 5, it would repeat the 1 through 5 sequence and produce another cycle with the same motion history.

The y-axis of the waveform in Figure 6–3B is also labeled pressure because it is easy to show that air pressure (measured at position 2) and position of the first molecule change in the same way over time. The rightmost extreme of molecule movement ("2" in Figure 6–3A) is also the time when air compression is maximum at the pressure measurement point, the leftmost extreme ("4") will occur at the same time as a rarefaction at the pressure measurement point, and the rest positions ("1" and "5") will be associated with P_{atm}. Positions between these discrete times will have pressures somewhere between compressions and P_{atm} or rarefactions and P_{atm}. Thus, the waveform in Figure 6–3B also shows the temporal variation of the pressure wave.

The Period (T) Is the Time Taken to Complete One Full Cycle of Motion and Is Given by the Formula: T = 1/f, Where f = Frequency. The filled-circle molecule is plotted as *a continuous function of time* as shown in Figure 6–3B. Figure 6–3A only indicates 5 discrete points in time, but Figure 6–3B shows every possible position of the molecule from time A through E, and how those positions change over time. Time is shown on the x-axis and molecule position (or air pressure) is shown on the y-axis. The horizontal line separating the upper and lower halves of the waveform indicates the rest position of the molecule, that is, when pressure = P_{atm}. The numbers 1, 2, 3, 4, and 5 given in Figure 6–3A are indicated on the time plot in their appropriate locations. The measurement of the temporal variation of a pressure wave that repeats over time, like the one shown in Figure 6–3B, is performed by computing the time taken to complete one full cycle. This is called the *period* of vibration and is denoted by the symbol *T*. For example, according to the time scale shown on the waveform in Figure 6–3B, it takes .01 second to complete one cycle of molecule motion. Thus for this waveform

$$T = .01 \text{ second (s) or}$$

$$T = 10 \text{ milliseconds (ms).}$$

In this example, .01 s and 10 ms are the same value, but expressed in different units. In speech and hearing applications, it is typical to express time units in ms. For reference purposes, 1 s = 1000 ms, 0.1 s = 100 ms, 0.01 s = 10 ms, and 0.001 s = 1 ms.

An alternate way to express the time variation of a repeating, cyclic motion, like the one shown in Figure 6–3B, is in terms of *frequency*, symbolized with an *f*. Frequency (*f*) is simply the inverse of period (T), and can be stated in the formula

$$f = 1/T \qquad \text{Formula (1)}$$

The units for frequency are *Hertz*, abbreviated as Hz, which stands for "cycles per second." The number resulting from the formula indicates how many complete cycles of vibration occur in a 1-s period. For example, if Formula (1) is applied to the 10 ms period in Figure 6–3B, the result is

$$f = 1/10 \text{ ms or}$$

$$f = 1/.01 = 100 \text{ Hz.}$$

bridge set into vibration by the rhythmic marching of soldiers. The energy of the synchronized stepping is transferred to the bridge, which responds with large-amplitude vibrations (swayings) that can endanger its structural integrity.

The concept of resonance is introduced here by describing a simple mechanical model. Then, acoustic resonance is discussed in detail. One point of this discussion is to show how concepts from mechanical systems are directly applicable to acoustical systems.

Mechanical Resonance

Mechanical systems can be used to understand acoustical systems. This is illustrated using a spring-mass model to describe the phenomenon of resonance and how mass and elasticity determine resonant frequencies.

A Simple Spring-Mass Model Can Be Used to Explain the Concept of Resonance

Figure 6–10A shows a simple mechanism consisting of a mass (e.g., a small block of wood) labeled *M*, a spring labeled *K*, and a fixed surface to which the spring-mass assembly is attached. The spring-mass model in Figure 6–10A is not being affected by any external forces (i.e., no one is pushing or pulling it) and is, therefore, at rest. Not surprisingly, if the mass is pulled away from the fixed surface (that is, the spring is stretched) and then released (Figure 6–10B), the result is a back-and-forth movement around the original rest position (rest position indicated by the vertical dashed line at the right of the figure). As the spring-mass assembly vibrates, sometimes the spring will be stretched (Figure 6–10B) and sometimes it will be compressed (Figure 6–10C) relative to its rest length (Figure 6–10A or 6-10D). Figure 6–10D shows the spring-mass model as it passes through the rest position, either in the direction of stretching (right-pointing arrow) or compression (left-pointing arrow). The difference between Figures 6–10A and 6-10D is that Figure 6–10A shows the model at rest (no forces applied) whereas 6-10D shows a single moment in time during vibration when the spring-mass model is at a length corresponding to the length at rest.

The period of this vibration is equal to the amount of time required to complete one full cycle

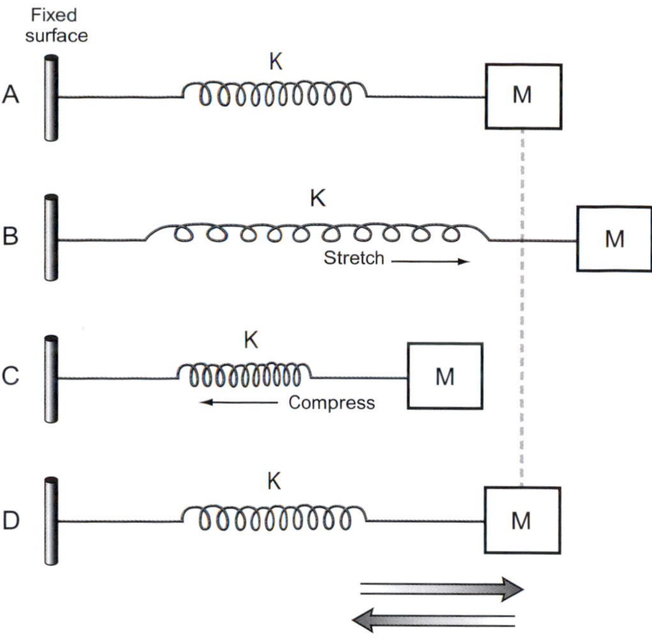

Figure 6–10. Spring-mass model that illustrates the concept of mechanical resonance. K = spring and M = Mass. **A.** Model at rest. **B.** Model stretched from its rest position. **C.** Model compressed relative to its rest position. **D.** Model passing through its rest position during vibration.

of motion (from rest, to maximum stretch of the spring, back through rest to maximum compression of the spring, and then back to rest). Alternatively, one could measure the frequency simply by counting the number of complete vibrations occurring in some unit of time and then converting to Hz, the number of complete cycles in 1 s. Notice that the motion being described—a back and forth movement around a rest position—is exactly like the one described above for the motion of air molecules (see Figures 6–1 and 6–3). The relevant question here is, "What determines the frequency of a spring-mass model after it has been set into motion by a manual stretch?"

The Relative Values of Mass (M) and Elasticity (K) Determine the Frequency of Vibration of the Simple Spring-Mass Model

As described earlier, the mass and elasticity properties of an air molecule play a critical role in maintaining the motion of the molecule. This idea is pursued here, but now with reference to the specific properties of *M* and *K* that determine vibratory frequency in the spring-mass model.

Mass. The mass of an object is defined as its weight divided by a constant, which is the value of acceleration due to gravity. Formally,

$$M = \text{weight}/g_o \qquad \text{Formula (5)}$$

where weight can be measured in pounds or grams and g_o is the symbol used to denote acceleration due to gravity, the value of which is 9.8 meters/s^2. Because g_o is a constant, mass can be considered to be directly proportional to weight for the remainder of this discussion.

Objects with mass have the property of inertia, meaning that they offer opposition to being accelerated and decelerated. This property explains why, when an air molecule recoils from a stretched or compressed position back toward the rest position, it does not stop at the rest position. The inertial forces inherent in the air molecule oppose deceleration as the molecule approaches rest position, and cause the motion to continue past rest and toward the other extreme position. Similarly, when the recoil forces overcome the inertial forces and reverse the direction of movement back toward the rest position, the molecule does not reach full speed immediately because the inertial forces oppose acceleration. These same inertial forces apply to the vibration of the spring-mass model. The foregoing explanation of mass and inertia provides the clues to how mass affects the frequency of vibration. Both recoil and inertial forces are acting at the same time during the vibration, with one or the other dominating depending on the position of the vibratory object.

Imagine that the mass in Figure 6–10 is replaced with a heavier one. Because the new mass is greater than the old one, it should demonstrate greater inertial forces. The new mass will, therefore, oppose being accelerated and decelerated to a greater degree than the old mass. How will this affect the motion of the spring-mass model? If the new spring-mass model opposes acceleration and deceleration more than the old one, it should take more time for the model to move through one complete cycle. This is the result of the greater time required to initiate movement at points in the cycle where the direction of motion is reversed (as at the end of a maximum displacement) or to slow down the movement as the spring-mass model goes through the rest position (see discussion above about air molecule motion). Thus, the effect of adding mass to the spring-mass model is to increase the period of vibration, which of course is the same as decreasing the frequency. All other things being equal, an increase in mass will decrease the resonant frequency of a vibratory object.

Stiffness. The elasticity of an object is defined by the amount of force required to displace the object some distance. Elasticity is typically measured in terms of *stiffness*, which can be expressed formally as

$$K = \text{Force}/\text{Meters} \qquad \text{Formula (6)}$$

where K is the symbol for the quantity *stiffness*, force is measured in units called *newtons*, and *meters* indicates a linear distance. Stiffness is typically schematized by a spring, as shown in Figure 6–10 and several upcoming figures. Force can be described in terms of an equivalent weight required to displace an object some distance. For example, 1 newton is roughly equivalent to the application of 0.224 pounds (or 98.7 grams; 1 pound = 439 grams) of force to an object. If there were a scale sensitive enough to register accurately fractions of a pound and enough force was applied manually to make the scale register 0.224 pounds, 1 newton of force would have been applied to the scale.

The elasticity formula shown above suggests that stiffer objects require greater force to displace them over some standard distance. This concept is illustrated in Figure 6–11, which shows two spring-mass models mounted on either side of a measuring rule marked off in centimeters. For this demonstration the two masses (M1 and M2) are assumed to be equal, but the springs, labeled K1 and K2, have some unknown difference in stiffness. The difference in the stiffness of K1 and K2 can be determined as follows. First, both spring-mass models are resting at "0" on the centimeter rule, so 1 cm can be designated as a standard displacement for both models. Next, a wire is attached to the mass of each model, and this wire is connected to a scale which registers the amount of weight applied to the spring-mass model when it is displaced 1 cm. The stiffer spring, according to the stiffness formula given above, is the one requiring more weight (greater force) to produce a displacement of 1 cm. As shown in Figure 6–11, if K2 is greater than K1, then F2 (where F = force) will be greater than F1 to produce the standard displacement of 1 cm.

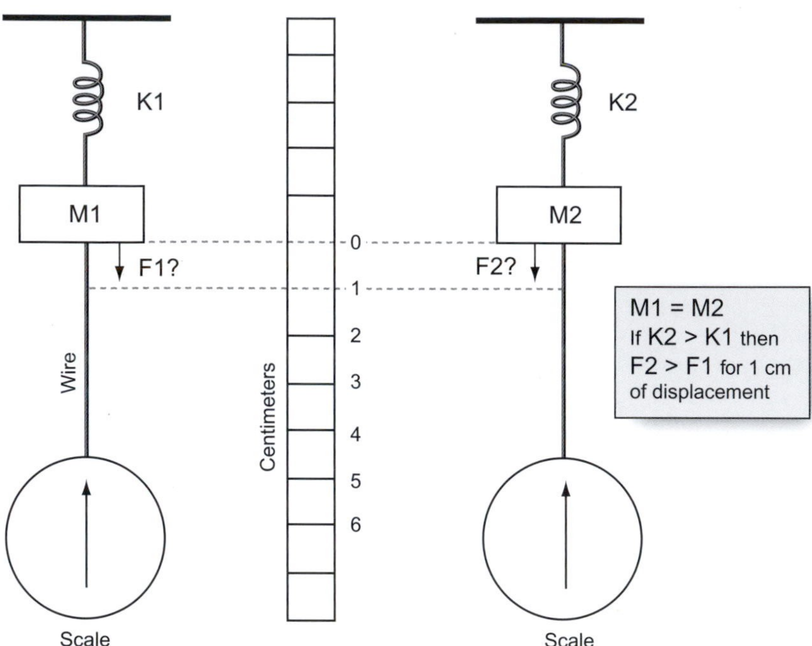

Figure 6–11. Measurement of stiffness. If the spring on the right (K2) is stiffer than the spring on the left (K1), all else being equal, it will take a greater force to displace the K2-M2 spring-mass model a 1-cm unit of length.

In the discussion of air molecule motion, it was noted that as a molecule is displaced from its rest position, a recoil force is developed which is exerted in the direction of the rest position. When any spring is stretched or compressed away from its rest position, it stores these recoil forces, which become greater with increasing displacement from the rest position. When the two springs in Figure 6–11 are stretched 1 cm away from their rest positions, it follows that the stiffer spring—K2—will generate a greater recoil force to return to the rest position because it required a greater force to displace it from the rest position. If the two springs are suddenly let go after their extension to 1 cm, they will both spring back toward the rest position, but K2's movement will be faster because its recoil forces are greater than those of K1 at equivalent displacements. In other words, greater recoil forces are associated with greater rates of movement when the forces are permitted to produce motion (as in the case of "letting the spring go").

Now assume that the original spring in Figure 6–10 is replaced with one having greater stiffness. The greater recoil forces, and thus recoil speeds, of the new spring will decrease the time required for the model to complete a full cycle of vibration. Stated in another way, if the motion of the spring-mass model is faster because of a stiffer spring, it will take less time to move back and forth. Thus, the effect of increasing stiffness is to decrease the period, which is the same as increasing the frequency. All other things being equal, an increase in stiffness will increase the resonant frequency of a vibratory object.

The Effects of Mass and Stiffness (Elasticity) on a Resonant System: A Summary

The foregoing discussion of the factors that determine the resonant frequency of a spring-mass model can be summarized by the formula

$$f_r = 1/2\pi * \sqrt{K/M} \qquad \text{Formula (7)}$$

where f_r = resonant frequency, K = stiffness and M = mass; $1/2\,\pi$ is a constant related to the circular origin of sinusoidal motion. According to the formula, increases in the numerator K will raise the resonant

Tacoma Narrows Bridge

A spectacular episode of apparent wind-induced resonance occurred in 1940, when the half-mile long Tacoma Narrows Bridge in Washington State responded to high winds with vibrations of increasingly large amplitude and eventually collapsed into the Puget Sound (see Petroski, 1992, for an interesting account of bridge structures and the potential dangers of resonance). There has been some controversy over the years about the exact cause of the bridge's collapse, but one factor seems to be that the wind "forced" the bridge to resonate and twist rhythmically until it collapsed. If you enter "Tacoma Narrows Bridge" into a search engine on the Internet, you can see photographs and even a brief movie of the bridge as it responded to the winds.

frequency f_r, whereas increases in the denominator M will lower f_r. The formula and preceding discussion also show that a decrease in f_r could be accomplished either by a decrease in stiffness or an increase in mass. Similarly, an increase in f_r could be accomplished either by an increase in stiffness or a decrease in mass. In more complicated resonant systems, both stiffness and mass will vary independently and at the same time, and their combination will determine the resonant, or natural frequency of the system.

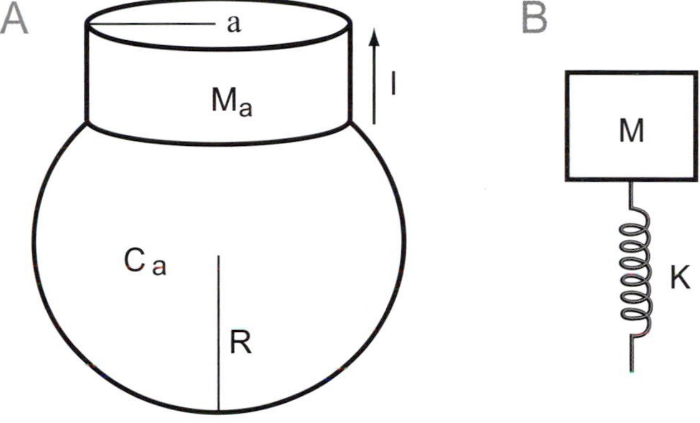

l = length of neck
a = radius of circular neck opening
R = radius of circular bowl
M_a = acoustic mass (inertance)
C_a = acoustic compliance

Figure 6–12. A. Helmholtz resonator and dimensions that determine its resonant frequency. **B.** Spring-mass model that is analogous to the Helmholtz resonator in A.

Acoustic Resonance: Helmholtz Resonators

The concepts just developed in the discussion of mechanical resonance are directly applicable to a model of acoustic resonance called *Helmholtz resonance*. Helmholtz resonance is so named because Hermann von Helmholtz, a German scientist who lived in the late 19th century, constructed acoustic resonators and studied the laws governing their vibratory behaviors. A discussion of Helmholtz resonance will not only show how concepts of mechanical resonance are equally valid in an acoustical system, but is also directly applicable to certain aspects of vowel production, as discussed in Chapter 7.

Figure 6–12A shows a drawing of a Helmholtz resonator. The resonator consists of a neck having some length l, a circular opening with radius a, and a bowl having radius R. The air contained within this resonator can be separated into two functional components corresponding to the resonator neck and bowl, respectively.

The Neck of the Helmholtz Resonator Contains a Column, or Plug of Air, That Behaves Like a Mass When a Force Is Applied to It

The air within the neck can be thought of as a plug of air having some mass. When a force is applied to

The damping factors could be increased for the second experiment by (for example) placing more of the resonator bowl in contact with some absorptive material or decreasing the ease with which air molecules move along the edges of the resonator by increasing the roughness of the interior surface (thus increasing friction). For both experiments, the brief input energy—the tap—must be identical so that differences in the acoustic measurements between the two resonator conditions can be attributed to the differences in damping, and not differences in the characteristics of the input.

Figure 6–17A shows a waveform (left) and a spectrum (right) of the acoustic energy associated with the resonator response in the condition of light damping. Two notable observations can be made about the waveform: (a) the amplitude is relatively large immediately following the input, and then decreases over time until it is zero; and (b) the waveform is periodic, but does not appear to be strictly sinusoidal, which suggests that the acoustic event is characterized by more than one frequency component.

The precise nature of the frequency components in the resonator response can be seen in the spectrum to the right of the waveform, which shows frequency on the *x*-axis and relative amplitude on the *y*-axis. The relative amplitude scale has been arbitrarily marked 0 dB at the point of maximum energy in the resonator response, and the negative numbers simply indicate sound levels (in dB) less than this maximum energy point. The function shown in the spectrum is called a *resonance curve*, which displays the computer-generated measurements of sound levels at all frequencies of interest. Because resonance is defined as the frequency at which an object (in this case the air within the resonator) vibrates with maximum energy, this resonance curve shows that this Helmholtz resonator has a natural or resonant frequency of 500 Hz. The frequency at which peak sound energy occurs along the resonance curve defines the resonant frequency.

The other frequencies along the resonance curve—those not associated with peak energy, but clearly showing some vibratory energy—reflect energy loss factors affecting this vibration. If there were no energy loss factors in this Helmholtz resonator the spectrum would show a single line at 500 Hz, indicating vibratory energy at a single frequency. Such a resonator would be said to be *perfectly tuned*. Damping factors in a resonator change this tuning, and produce energy at frequencies other than the natural frequency. The frequency-domain index of this tuning, and thus of damping, is called the *bandwidth* of the resonator. Bandwidth is defined as the range of frequencies between the two *3-dB-down points* on either side of the peak energy. In Figure 6–17A, a horizontal dashed line has been extended from the –3-dB level on the *y*-axis to intersect the resonance curve on either side of the peak (500 Hz), and from each of these intersecting points a vertical line has been dropped to the *x*-axis (frequency). The vertical lines show the frequencies where the energy is 3 dB less than the energy at the resonant frequency of 500 Hz, namely 450 Hz to the left and 550 Hz to the right. The bandwidth of this resonance, shown on the spectrum by the horizontal line terminated in arrows, is 100 Hz.

In Figure 6–17B, the time-and-frequency domain results are shown for the same resonator with greater damping. Here the waveform clearly decays faster and the bandwidth is wider than in Figure 6–17A. The spectrum in Figure 6–17B has been drawn to show an important feature of the effect of increased damping on the resonance curve: The single dot in the middle of the spectrum (arrow in Figure 6–17B) is the location of peak energy for the lightly damped resonator in 6-17A, and the peak of the more heavily damped resonance is shown at 0 dB, as in Figure 6–17A. The more heavily damped resonance of Figure 6–17B clearly does not produce the same amount of energy at the resonant frequency as the more lightly damped resonance of 6-17A, but the resonant frequency is the same for both resonators. In other words, the peak energy in Figure 6–17B is still at 500 Hz, even though it is weaker than the peak energy in 6-17A. The difference between parts A and B is clearly the bandwidth, which is wider in B (200 Hz, indicated by horizontal line ending in arrows). Changes in damping do not affect the resonant frequency(ies) of an acoustic system.

Why is bandwidth defined in terms of the 3-dB-down points on the resonance curve? The energy in a sound wave is capable of doing some *work* (such as causing an effective displacement of the human ear drum, and thus having an important effect in the perception of some sound), and there is a range of sound levels below the peak that is still effective in doing this work. The term *power* is typically used

Organic Music-Making: Hats Off to Tube Resonators

Everyone is familiar with pipe organs, the massive array of different-length tubes rising above a keyboard, the heart-thumping sound a truly great instrument is capable of generating. Obviously, a pipe organ has the ability to generate tones of a wide range of pitches by having all those pipes of different length. But it also achieves pitch variation with *individual* pipes by providing the organist with controls for "capping" one end of the tube, or leaving both ends open. Really, pipe organs are simply tube resonators in disguise as ear candy.

by scientists to designate the work capability of energy, and it can be shown that half of the peak sound power is equivalent to 3 dB below the peak sound level. The concept of the *half-power points* designating the lower limit of effective sound energy is thus the origin of the use of 3-dB-down points to determine the bandwidth. The reader should understand that the half-power (3-dB-down) points are used by agreement of the community of individuals interested in sound, and do not necessarily reflect any inherent truths about the effective nature of sound energy. This kind of *operational definition* is very common in all sciences, and serves the purpose of allowing scientists to communicate with one another and share research experiences within a common measurement framework.

AN EXTENSION OF THE RESONANCE CURVE CONCEPT: THE SHAPING OF A SOURCE BY THE ACOUSTIC CHARACTERISTICS OF A RESONATOR

In Figure 6–17 a brief input (the hammer tap) was used to show the relationship between the speed of decay of the resonant waveform and the bandwidth of the resulting spectrum (resonance curve). This impulse approach to the excitation of the resonator was useful in showing that damping can be defined in the time or frequency domains. Greater damping is indicated by faster speeds of waveform decay (time domain) and wider bandwidths (frequency domain). This idea is now extended by demonstrating how a resonator shapes the energy in an input signal.

Figure 6–18 shows an experimental arrangement similar to that in Figure 6–17, except now a continuous white noise is serving as the input signal to a Helmholtz resonator (Figure 6–18A), and a tube resonator (Figure 6–18B). A continuous, perfect white noise is an excellent input signal for evaluating the characteristics of a resonator, because the average sound level at any frequency is equivalent to the average sound level at any other frequency. This is shown in Figure 6–18 by the flatline spectrum for the input signals. Because the average sound level in the input signal is equivalent at all frequencies, any modification of the spectrum at the output of the resonator must be due to the characteristics of the resonator. Stated otherwise, any difference between the input and output spectra must be due to the resonator only, because the energy in the input spectrum is constant as a function of frequency.

Figure 6–18A shows how the Helmholtz resonator *shapes the input spectrum*. The air in the resonator vibrates with maximum energy at one frequency—the resonant frequency—and with less energy at other frequencies. The resonance curve is similar to the one shown in Figure 6–17, its shape being the result of both the physical dimensions of the resonator (which determine the resonant frequency) and the energy loss factors. The difference between the input and output spectra in Figure 6–18A is solely a result of the resonator characteristics.

Figure 6–18B shows the *input-output function* for a tube closed at one end. The tube shaped the flat input spectrum by resonating at multiple frequencies (only three are shown in Figure 6–18). Each peak in this output spectrum is a resonant frequency, and the bandwidth around each peak is

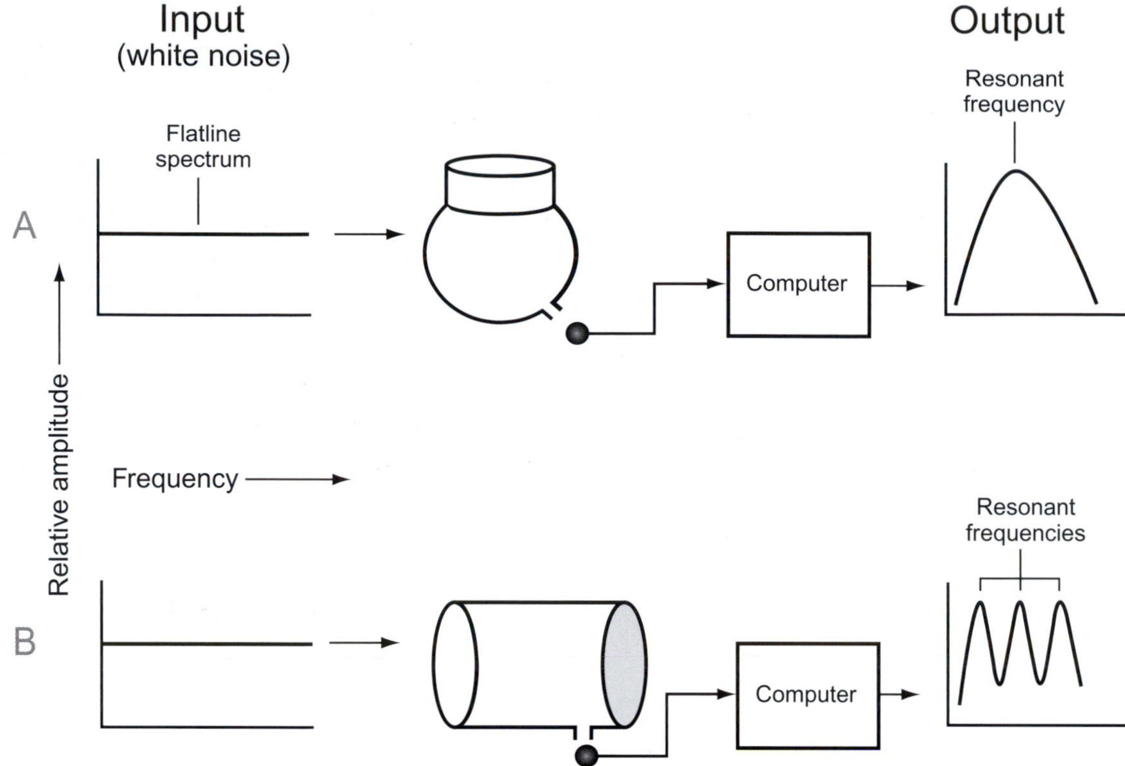

Figure 6–18. Input-output relations for a Helmholtz resonator (A) and a tube resonator (B), using white noise with a perfectly flat spectrum as the input signal. In both cases, the resonator "shapes" the input signal, as shown by the output spectra to the far right in the two panels.

determined by energy loss factors which may differ as a function of frequency (see Chapter 7).

The concept of resonators shaping an input to produce an output is a crucial one for understanding the acoustic theory of speech production. A flat input spectrum has been used to illustrate this concept, but the shaping idea applies to any situation where an input is applied to a resonator. Another way to think about the effect of a resonator on a sound source is to consider the former a *filter*. A filter is any device that passes certain inputs (i.e., allows those inputs to get through) and rejects others (i.e., stops them from getting through). Acoustic filters such as Helmholtz or tube resonators pass certain frequencies (especially the resonant frequencies) and reject others. In the case of speech production, the vocal tract can be considered as a filter that passes or rejects frequencies generated by different sources (such as the source energy generated by the vibrating vocal folds).

Resonance, Damping, and Bandwidth: A Summary

The vibratory patterns of air in resonators are not only characterized by the resonant frequency (the frequency with maximum vibratory energy), but by energy loss factors that determine the shape of the curve around the peak. The energy loss factors, or damping of a resonance, can be described in either the time or frequency domain. Greater energy loss is associated with more rapid decay of vibratory amplitude over time and with wider bandwidths. For a given resonator, variations in damping have no effect on the resonant frequencies (i.e., the locations of peaks in the spectrum). A simple way to determine the acoustic characteristics of a resonator is to perform an input-output experiment, wherein the input is a signal having the same energy at all frequencies. When this input signal is used to excite the resonator, any differences between the input and output spectra must reflect the characteristics of the resonator. Resonators are said to shape, or filter, inputs, and in so doing produce an output that reflects the combination of the input and resonator characteristics.

REVIEW

Pressure waves can be understood by examining the motions of air molecules during vibration.

These motions are governed by various forces, including those due to the elasticity and inertial properties of air molecules.

Factors that contribute to energy loss also determine how long the vibrations continue.

Sinusoids are the simplest type of acoustic vibration and can be considered as the elementary components of more complex vibrations.

A mathematical technique, Fourier analysis, allows a decomposition of a complex acoustic event into its component sinusoids.

When a computer program is used to construct a spectrum for a portion of a waveform, the program applies the Fourier technique to decompose the complexities in the time domain (the waveform) into the component sinusoids, and then displays the components in the frequency domain (a spectrum).

Fourier analysis is valid for acoustic events that repeat in time (complex periodic sounds) and for those that do not repeat in time (complex aperiodic sounds).

Resonance is the phenomenon where an object vibrates at a single frequency, or multiple frequencies, with maximal amplitude.

Two types of resonators—Helmholtz and tubes—were considered in detail.

The frequencies at which Helmholtz and tube resonators vibrate are governed by specific laws.

Resonators shape, or filter, the acoustic energy in a source of sound.

The shaping of a source by a resonator is critical to the understanding of the acoustic theory of speech production.

REFERENCES

Beranek, L. (1986). *Acoustics*. New York: American Institute of Physics.

Beyer, R. (1999). *Sounds of our times*. New York: Springer-Verlag.

Hunt, F. (1978). *Origins in acoustics*. New Haven, CT: Yale University Press.

Milenkovic, P. (2001). *TF32. User's manual*. Madison: University of Wisconsin.

Petroski, R. (1992). *To engineer is human: The role of failure in successful design*. New York: Vintage.

7

Acoustic Theory of Vowel Production

INTRODUCTION

Speech scientists and speech-language pathologists are indebted to Gunnar Fant, a Swedish speech scientist, for the development of the theoretical basis of speech acoustics. Fant performed much of the work on the theory in the 1940s and 1950s, and published his classic book, titled *Acoustic Theory of Speech Production*, in 1960. Previously, two Japanese scientists (Chiba & Kajiyama, 1941) had developed a similar mathematical theory of vocal tract acoustics, but this work was essentially unknown in western hemisphere countries until well after World War II. Fant, as well as a small group of scientists whose names are encountered throughout this text (Kenneth Stevens, Osamu Fujimura, Arthur House, James Flanagan), continued to develop and refine the theory in the 1950s, 1960s, and 1970s. Indeed, the theoretical development continues today. In particular, the texts of Flanagan (1972) and more recently Stevens (1998) showcase developments in speech acoustic theory since the original work of Fant, and Chiba and Kajiyama (see also Story, 2005). Much of the information in this and the following chapter is drawn from these sources.

The acoustic theory of vowel production can be stated in very broad terms, as follows: for vowel production, the vocal tract resonates like a tube closed at one end, and shapes an input signal generated by the vibrating vocal folds. The two major concepts suggested in this broad statement of the

Father of Speech Acoustics

Professor Gunnar Fant is a famous speech acoustician and widely regarded as the father of speech acoustics. Fant was born in Sweden in 1919 and is currently Professor Emeritus in the Department of Speech, Hearing, and Music at the Royal Institute of Technology (KTH) in Stockholm. Fant founded this department in 1951 as the Speech Transmission Laboratory, after spending 1949 and 1950 at the Massachusetts Institute of Technology working with another giant in the field, Professor Kenneth Stevens. Over the years, Fant's department has generated a wealth of valuable research in the area of speech acoustics, all of which was reported in a famous, recurring publication called the *KTH Speech Transmission Laboratory Quarterly Progress Report*. Fant's 1960 book, *Acoustic Theory of Speech Production*, is the speech scientist's bible.

theory—(a) the resonance patterns of a tube closed at one end, and (b) the shaping of an input by a resonator—are covered in Chapter 6. At this point, the broad statement of the theory refers only to vowel production. The theory is most precise for the case of vowels, primarily because its mathematical basis works best for the resonant frequencies of vowels (as compared to many consonants). The theory also addresses consonant acoustics, which is covered in Chapter 8. To explore the acoustic theory of vowel production in greater depth, this chapter addresses the following set of questions:

1. What is the precise nature of the input signal generated by the vibrating vocal folds?
2. Why should the vocal tract be conceptualized as a tube *closed* at one end (as compared to open at both ends)?
3. How are the acoustic properties of the vocal tract determined?
4. How does the vocal tract shape the input signal?
5. What happens to the resonant frequencies of the vocal tract when the tube is constricted at a given location?
6. How is the acoustic theory of vowel production confirmed?

WHAT IS THE PRECISE NATURE OF THE INPUT SIGNAL GENERATED BY THE VIBRATING VOCAL FOLDS?

The periodic vibration of the vocal folds provides the input signal to the vocal tract resonator. This periodic vibration is referred to as the *source* for vowel acoustics. As discussed in Chapter 6, any signal can be studied in both the time and frequency domains. Much of what follows is a condensation of work done by Fant (1979, 1982, 1986) as refinement of the theory first published in 1960.

The Time Domain

The identification of the precise time-domain characteristics of the signal produced by vocal fold vibration is fairly complicated. The larynx, a structure of cartilage, membrane, ligament, and muscle, is not easily accessible for direct measurement of vocal fold behavior. If a microphone is placed directly in front of a speaker's lips while he or she phonates a vowel, the recorded acoustic event will reflect the *combination* of source (vocal fold) and resonator (vocal tract) acoustics. There is no simple way to look at the waveform (time domain) of a vowel recorded in this way (such as that shown in Figure 6–8B) and identify the components due only to vocal fold vibration. Some other approach must be found to "split" the waveform of a recorded vowel into the parts contributed by (a) the vibrating vocal folds and (b) the resonating vocal tract.

One of the earliest attempts to understand the details of vocal fold vibration was described by Farnsworth (1940), who took high-speed motion pictures of the vibrating vocal folds by filming the image of the glottis as reflected in a laryngeal mirror. When played back in slow motion, these films allowed Farnsworth to view, on a frame-by-frame basis, movements of the vocal folds and the changing configuration of the glottis (the space between the vocal folds) throughout individual cycles of vocal fold vibration. A sequence of images of one vocal fold cycle, qualitatively similar to those examined by Farnsworth but collected with a contemporary device, is shown in Figure 7–1. The cycle begins with the vocal folds fully approximated (image 1). The folds separate gradually to a maximum width of the glottis (image 5), then begin to move back to the midline until they are once again fully approximated and there is no glottis (images 6–10). Scientists examined images such as these and for each one measured the width and length of the glottis, allowing them to derive the glottal area on an image-by-image basis. They then plotted *glottal area as a function of time* for a complete cycle of vocal fold vibration. A typical *glottal area function*, commonly symbolized as A_g, is shown for two cycles of vocal fold vibration in Figure 7–2A. The baseline in this plot represents full approximation of the vocal folds (i.e., $A_g = 0$), and upward movement of the function indicates increasingly larger separation of the vocal folds (i.e., increasing A_g). One cycle of vocal fold vibration is defined as the interval between successive separations of the vocal folds, as marked in Figure 7–2. Note that the vocal folds are fully approximated for a substantial portion of each cycle (nearly 40% of each cycle). The moment immedi-

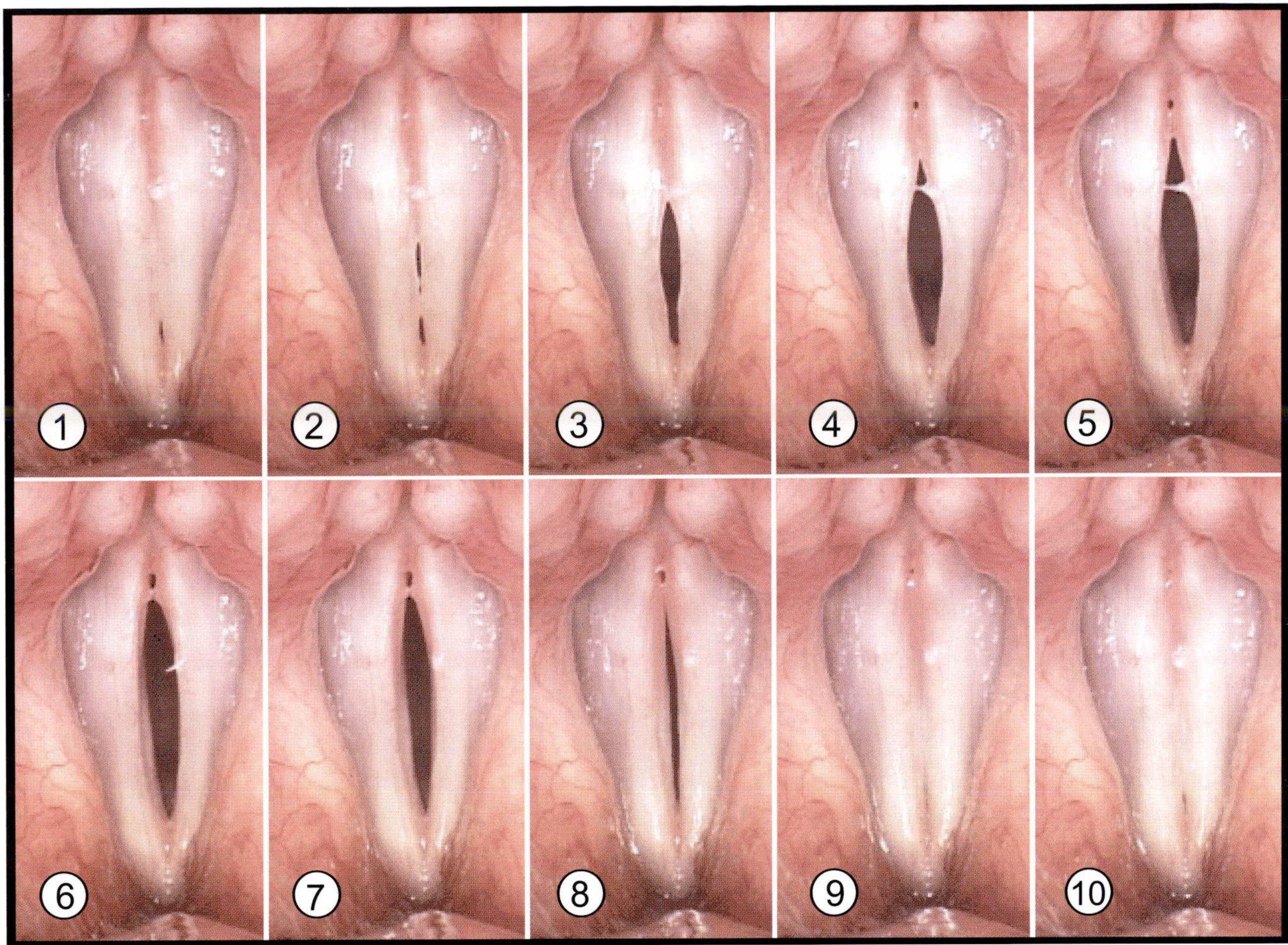

Figure 7–1. Successive images from one complete cycle of vocal fold vibration recorded via digital videostroboscopy. In these frames anterior is toward the bottom of the image, posterior toward the top. The cycle begins in the upper left frame (image 1) with the vocal folds approximated. The folds begin to separate in image 2 and reach maximum separation in image 5. Closing of the vocal folds takes place in images 6 through 10. Images provided courtesy of KayPENTAX, Lincoln Park, NJ. Reproduced with permission.

ately before the vocal folds separate has been chosen arbitrarily as the initiation of each cycle. The duration of these cycles of vocal fold vibration may range from as little as 1 ms or less (for some opera or pop singers who can produce extremely high-pitched notes) to the more typical 5 ms (adult women, as shown in Figure 7–2) or 8 ms (adult men).

The A_g function shown in Figure 7–2 is not an acoustic signal, but rather reflects a pattern of vibration that produces an acoustic signal. How does one obtain the acoustic signal associated with vocal fold vibration—separate from the influence of the cavities in the vocal tract—and how is this signal related to the A_g function just described? Imagine that it was possible to suspend, immediately above the vocal folds, a device that measures the magnitude of airflow coming through the glottis as a function of time. When the vocal folds separate during a vibratory cycle (e.g., during phonation of a vowel) airflow through the glottis is expected because speech is produced with tracheal pressures greater than those in front of the lips (i.e., P_{atm}), and air always flows from regions of higher pressure to regions of lower pressure. Intuitively, the magnitude of this airflow should be zero when the vocal folds are fully approximated (when there is no glottis to allow the passage of air), and maximum when the vocal folds are maximally apart (when A_g is the largest). In other words, the airflow coming through the glottis should increase as A_g increases, and decrease

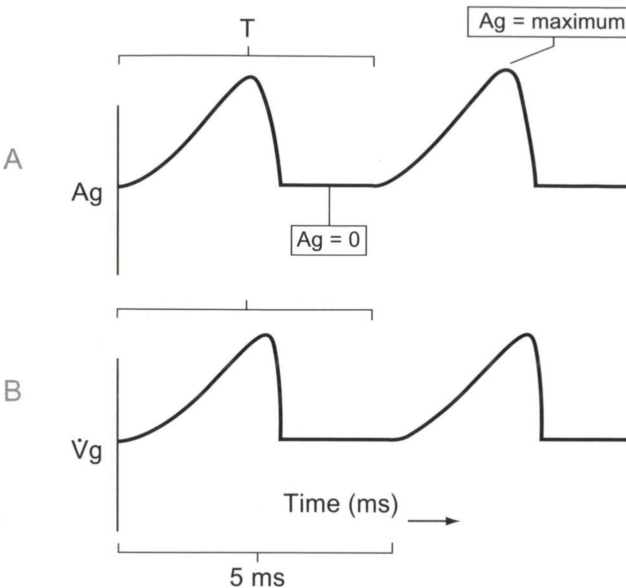

Figure 7–2. A. Glottal area function (A_g) for two cycles of vocal fold vibration. Upward displacements represent increasingly larger glottal areas, which are proportional to glottal widths measured from images like those in Figure 7–1. **B.** Glottal airflow function ($\dot{V}_g$) obtained by inverse filtering (see text). Upward displacement indicates increasing magnitudes of airflow passing through the glottis.

as A_g decreases. A plot of the magnitude of airflow coming through the glottis as a function of time should look a lot like the A_g function shown in Figure 7–2A. The time domain plot of airflow through the glottis is a *glottal flow* function, symbolized as $\dot{V}_g$. Because the $\dot{V}_g$ reflects movement of air molecules, this movement being responsible for the production of pressure waves (see Chapter 6), $\dot{V}_g$ is the proper signal to study as the source in vowel acoustics.

A $\dot{V}_g$ function is shown in Figure 7–2B. As expected, it looks very much like the A_g function (the detailed differences between the two types of waveforms will not be discussed in this text). Nevertheless, as noted above, actual measurement of the flow coming through the glottis in a phonating human is extremely difficult, if not impossible. Instead, scientists obtain $\dot{V}_g$ signals like the one shown in Figure 7–2B using an indirect approach.

Imagine a situation in which the input signal is the vibration of the vocal folds and the filter is a resonance curve associated with a specific shape of the vocal tract. From the discussion of tube resonators in Chapter 6 and introductory comments made above concerning the vocal tract resonating like a tube closed at one end, multiple peaks are expected in the resonance curve. The input signal, plus a resonance curve (filter) for this hypothetical shape of the vocal tract, are shown in the upper part of Figure 7–3. When the input signal—here labeled "glottal source signal"—is applied to the vocal tract filter, the result is the output labeled "speech signal" (Figure 7–3, upper right panel). That speech signal represents the blending of the input and filter characteristics. Because of this blending, the output signal cannot reveal the exact characteristics of the input signal unless something is done to it. What is done to it, to "recover" the input signal, is a process called "inverse filtering" as demonstrated in the lower part of Figure 7–3. On the left is the speech signal, the same one as in the upper right-hand panel of the figure. This is the "blended" signal reflecting the influence of both the source and vocal tract filter. This blended signal serves as input to a resonance curve that is a "flipped" or mirror image of the one shown in the top of the figure. In this "flipped," or "inverse filter," there are valleys at the precise locations of the peaks in the upper filter function. If the inverse filter is constructed correctly, when the "blended" input signal is run through it, the resonances will be taken away from the signal and what remains at the output of the filter is the glottal source signal. This is shown in the lower right panel as "recovered glottal source signal." In essence, the sequence of the bottom panel reverses that of the top panels, with the special adjustment of "flipping" or inverting the filter function. This is a time-honored approach to studying the glottal input signal independent of the filter function.

The technical details of inverse filtering are not important here, and the technique is more complicated (and often trickier) than implied by the straightforward logic of Figure 7–3. For current purposes, the ability to recover a glottal source signal—such as the $\dot{V}_g$ signal—is the central issue. There are three important features of the $\dot{V}_g$ signal shown in Figure 7–2B.

First, as noted above for the A_g signal, the $\dot{V}_g$ signal is periodic, meaning that its characteristic shape repeats over time. The rate at which it repeats over time is the fundamental frequency (F0) of vocal fold vibration, or how many times per second the vocal folds go through complete cycles of vibration. In adult women, a typical F0 is around 190 to 200 Hz,

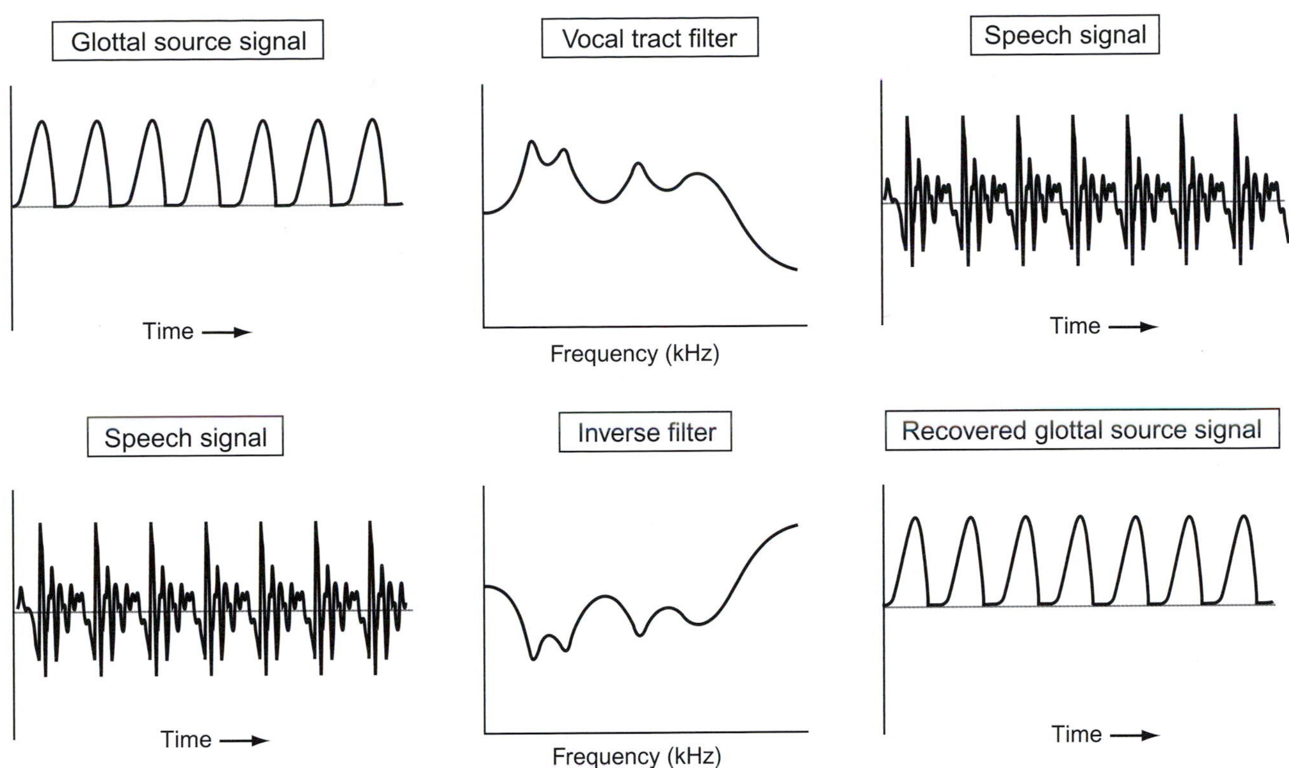

Figure 7–3. Schematic representation of steps in the inverse filtering process. *Top row of panels:* Glottal source signal serves as input to a multipeaked filter function associated with a vocal tract configuration and results in an output which is the speech signal recorded at the lips. The three-panel sequence summarizes the source-filter theory of vowel acoustics. *Bottom row of panels:* The output signal shown in the top right waveform now serves as the input to an "inverse filter," which is the "flipped" or mirror image of the filter function in the middle of the top row of panels. The inverse filter inverts the peaks shown in the top filter function and takes away the resonances from the input signal. The result of the process is the recovered glottal source signal shown in the bottom right panel. Figure provided courtesy of James Hillenbrand, Ph.D., Western Michigan University, Kalamazoo, Michigan. Reproduced with permission.

in men around 115 to 125 Hz, and in 5-year-old children around 250 to 300 Hz (Kent, 1997; Lee, Potamianos, & Narayanan, 1999). As shown in Figure 7–2 the period (T) of this time-domain signal can be measured easily, and the inverse of the period is the F0 (see Chapter 6 for discussion of $f = 1/T$).

The second important feature of the $\dot{V}_g$ signal for the kind of phonation used by most people in ordinary conversation is the shape of the opening and closing portions of each cycle. The slope of the opening phase is shallower than the slope of the closing phase, making each cycle appear as if it is "leaning to the right." This shape feature is seen clearly in the $\dot{V}_g$ signal of Figure 7–2B. The steepness of the closing phase is important because it reflects how rapidly the vocal folds come together as each cycle ends. The more rapidly the vocal folds come together, the steeper the closing part of the $\dot{V}_g$ signal. This has great importance to the frequency domain characteristics of the source, as discussed in the next section.

The third important feature is that the $\dot{V}_g$ signal shows some portions where the vocal folds are apart (i.e., where airflow is coming through the glottis), and some portions where the vocal folds are approximated. The ratio of open time to closed time for each cycle, which in normal voices is typically around 1.2:2 (i.e., the vocal folds open approximately 60% of each cycle), may be an important determinant of how much of the source signal is periodic and how much is aperiodic. This is important when considering the physiological and acoustical basis of pathological voice quality.

Figure 7–2 shows clearly that the $\dot{V}_g$ signal does not have a sinusoidal shape, but it is periodic.

Material covered in Chapter 6 suggests, then, that the signal should be described as a complex periodic waveform. Determination of the frequency components of a complex periodic waveform requires analysis in the frequency domain, and, therefore, discussion of the spectral characteristics of the source waveform.

The Frequency Domain

Imagine that the $\dot{V}_g$ signal shown in Figure 7–4A was submitted to Fourier analysis to identify the frequency components contributing to this waveform. A typical spectrum resulting from this Fourier analysis would be like the one shown in 7–4B. The important features of this spectrum are: (a) there is a series of frequency components, at consecutive-integer multiples of the lowest-frequency component; and (b) the relative amplitudes of the frequency components decrease systematically as frequency increases. This is the *glottal source spectrum*.

The lowest frequency of the glottal source spectrum is the fundamental frequency (F0), which corresponds to the rate of vibration of the vocal folds. The F0 is also called the *first harmonic* (H1) of the source spectrum. The other frequency components in the glottal source spectrum are whole number multiples of the F0. There is a component at two times the F0 (the second harmonic, H2), three times the F0 (the third harmonic, H3), four times the F0 (the fourth harmonic, H4), and so on. In theory the number of harmonics in the glottal source spectrum is infinite, but the progressive reduction in relative amplitude with increasing frequency greatly limits the significance of very high-frequency harmonics.

The reduction of energy (relative amplitude) in the harmonic components of the glottal source spectrum as frequency increases is clearly seen in Figure 7–4B. Moving from left (lower frequency) to right

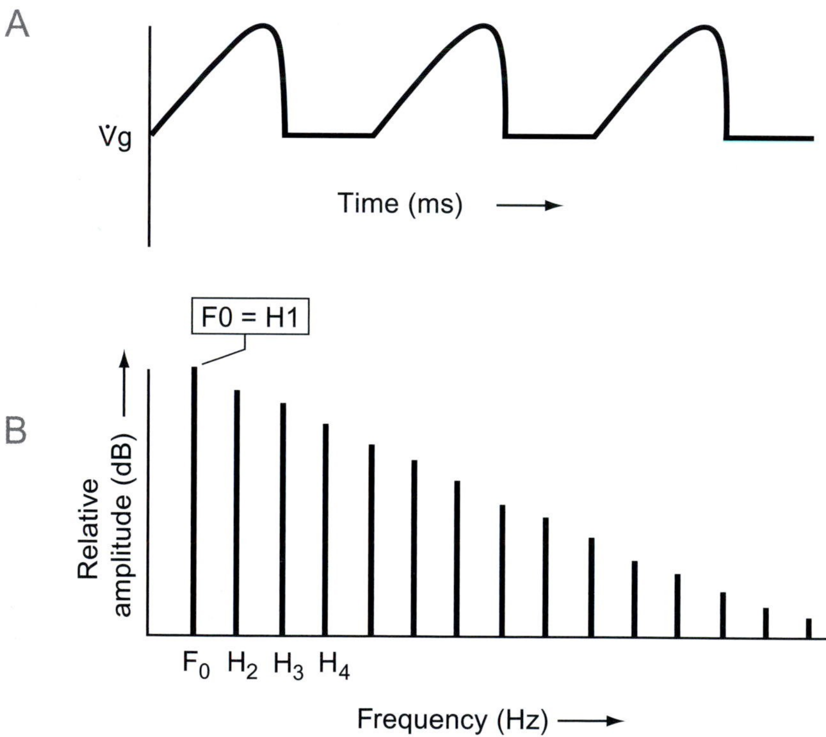

Figure 7–4. A. Time-domain and **B.** frequency-domain representations of vocal fold acoustics. The time domain is represented by the glottal airflow waveform ($\dot{V}_g$) and shows the acoustic result of vocal fold vibration. The frequency domain is represented by the glottal spectrum that results from vocal fold vibration and indicates F0, the fundamental frequency (first harmonic), and H2, H3, and H4 (the second, third, and fourth harmonics, respectively).

(higher frequency) on the x-axis, the vertical lines showing the amplitude of the components become progressively shorter. This energy reduction is systematic, with the relative amplitude decreasing approximately 12 dB for each octave increase in frequency. This gives the typical glottal spectrum a distinctly "tilted" appearance. As discussed below, changes in the nature of vocal fold vibration affect the extent to which the glottal spectrum is "tilted."

In the summary of the time domain characteristics of the glottal source, three major characteristics were identified, including (a) the periodic nature of the waveform, (b) the shape of the waveform, and (c) the ratio of open to closed time. Discussion turns now to how each of these features affects the glottal source spectrum.

The Periodic Nature of the Waveform

The $\dot{V}_g$ waveform repeats over time, is not sinusoidal, and is, therefore, a complex periodic event. The repetition of the $\dot{V}_g$ waveform is not perfectly periodic, but rather has very small variations in the periods of successive glottal cycles. This is why vocal fold vibration is referred to as *quasiperiodic*. Throughout this discussion, the term "period" refers to the average period—the small, period-to-period variations are not considered further here. The period of the glottal waveform depends on the rate of vibration of the vocal folds, which varies according to a number of factors including sex and age (see Chapter 3). Figure 7–5 shows two $\dot{V}_g$ waveforms (left part of figure) having different periods, and

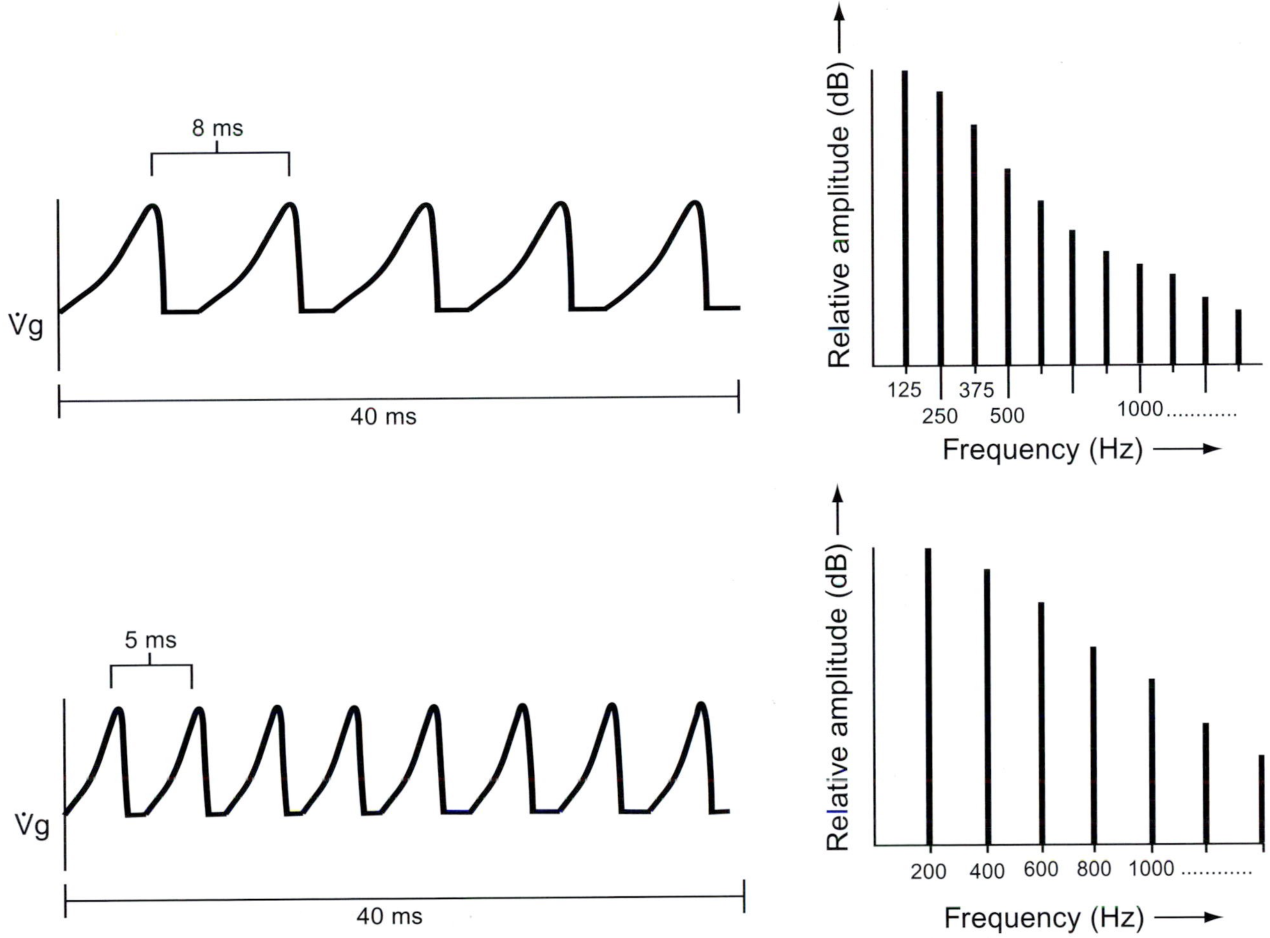

Figure 7–5. Two $\dot{V}_g$ waveforms having different periods, and their associated glottal spectra. Top: period = 8 ms, F0 = 125 Hz. Bottom: period = 5 ms, F0 = 200 Hz. Both waveforms show vibration of the vocal folds over a 40-ms interval. Note the greater number of cycles within this interval for F0 = 200-Hz waveform, as compared to the F0 = 125-Hz waveform. Note also in the glottal spectra the wider spacing of harmonics for F0 = 200 Hz (*bottom*), as compared to F0 = 125 Hz (*top*).

their associated glottal spectra (right part of figure). Note that both waveforms show the $\dot{V}_g$ over a 40-ms interval. The top waveform has a period of 8 ms (typical of many adult males), the inverse of which is an F0 of 125 Hz. This 125 Hz F0 is shown as the lowest-frequency component in the glottal spectrum to the right of the waveform. The bottom waveform has a period of 5 ms (typical of many adult females), the inverse of which is an F0 of 200 Hz. This F0 is shown as the lowest-frequency component in the corresponding glottal spectrum. The harmonics of the female glottal spectrum (bottom) are clearly more widely separated than the harmonics of the male glottal spectrum (top). This follows from the fact that the glottal spectrum consists of a consecutive integer series of harmonics: Higher F0s will yield greater spacing between successive harmonics as compared to lower F0s. The glottal spectra of speakers with low F0s, therefore, are more densely packed with harmonics when compared to the glottal spectra of speakers with high F0s. This difference between the glottal spectra of low versus high F0s explains, in part, why spectrographic analysis of vowels produced by adult males tends to be easier than spectrographic analysis of vowels produced by adult females and children.

The Shape of the Waveform

The opening and closing parts of the $\dot{V}_g$ waveform create a shape that appears to be "leaning to the right," and the steepness of the closing slope is related to how rapidly the vocal folds return to the midline for each cycle. There is a systematic relationship between this closing slope and the "tilt" of the glottal spectrum: the steeper the closing slope in the $\dot{V}_g$ waveform (the faster the vocal folds return to the midline on each cycle), the less tilted is the glottal spectrum. This relationship is exemplified in Figure 7–6, where the $\dot{V}_g$ waveform on the left has a clearly steeper closing slope than the $\dot{V}_g$ waveform on the right (see arrows indicating slopes on the closing part of the waveforms). *CP* in Figure 7–6 is the closed phase of the glottal cycle, or the portion of each cycle when the vocal folds are fully approximated, whereas *OP* stands for open phase. Note the spectra associated with these two waveforms. The glottal spectrum for the waveform with the relatively steep closing slope shows reduction in relative amplitude with increasing frequency, but not nearly as dramatically as the glottal spectrum for the waveform with the shallower closing slope. The dashed line connecting the tops of the vertical lines in the two spectra shows the rapid reduction in energy across frequency when the closing slope in the time-domain is shallow (right-hand part of figure), as compared to when it is steep (left-hand part of figure). The spectrum with the dramatic reduction in harmonic energy is said be more tilted than the spectrum with the more gradual reduction in energy. In theory, a glottal spectrum with "no tilt" would be one in which the relative amplitudes of all

Imperfect Perfection

The quasiperiodic nature of vocal fold vibration is largely a result of subtle aeromechanical imperfections. Vocal fold vibration is driven by aerodynamic forces and sustained by mechanical ones. These forces can hardly be expected to repeat themselves, across successive cycles, with perfect precision. If the forces do not repeat themselves exactly, the thing they are forcing—vibration of the vocal folds—will not either. In early versions of talking computers (speech synthesizers) scientists used a perfectly periodic, complex tone to simulate the source for vowels. Listeners didn't like it. It sounded mechanical, robotic, unfriendly. The solution was to take this complex periodic waveform and introduce into it a small amount of "jitter," or very minimal variation in the cycle-to-cycle period. Listeners found this much more pleasing. More human, you could say.

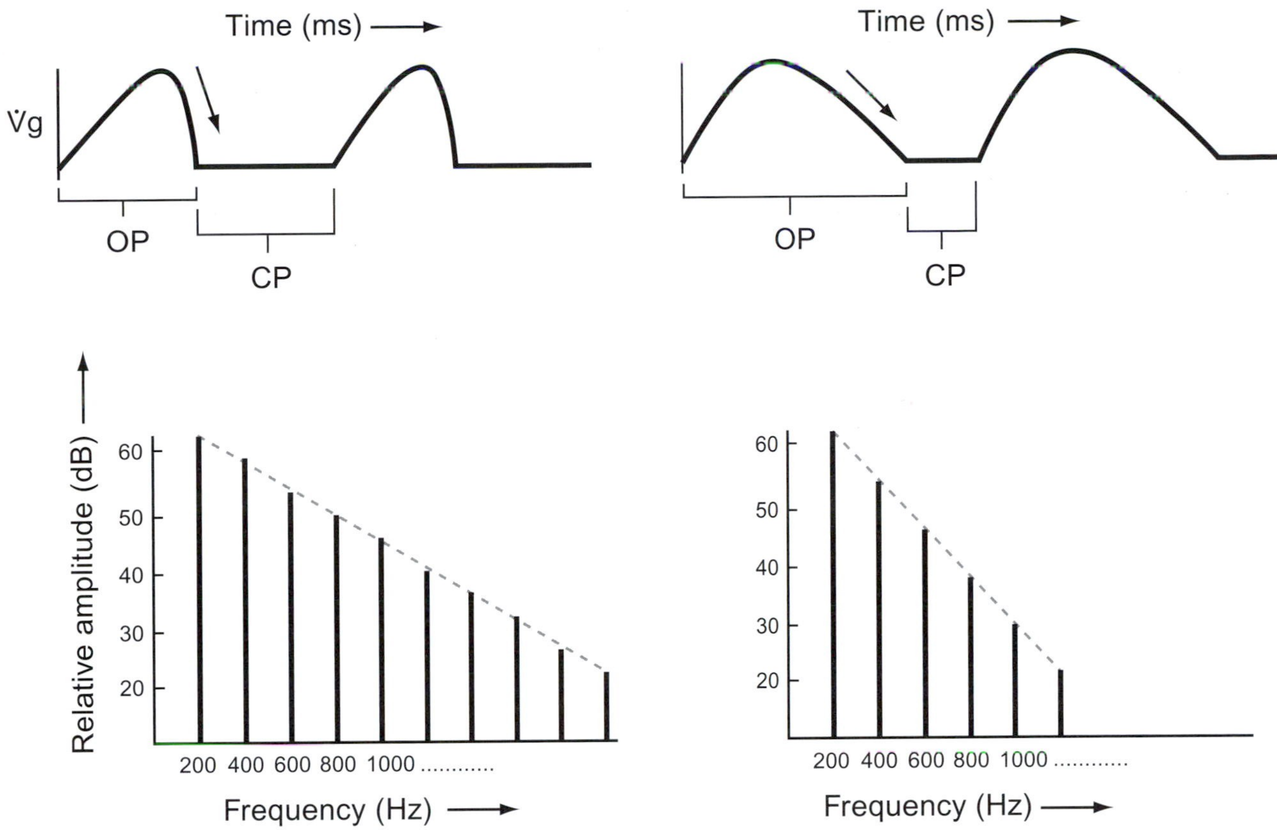

Figure 7–6. Schematic illustration of the speed of vocal fold closing and tilt of the glottal spectrum. The two upper panels show $\dot{V}_g$ waveforms, one with relatively rapid closure of the vocal folds (*left*), and one with relatively slow closure of the vocal folds (*right*). Relative speeds of closure are portrayed by the slope of the arrows alongside the closing phase of the functions. The glottal spectra immediately below the two waveforms demonstrate how speed of closure affects the tilt of the spectrum. OP = open phase (time). CP = closed phase (time).

harmonic components were equal (the dashed line connecting the tops of the vertical lines would be strictly horizontal), and a glottal spectrum with "infinite tilt" would be one in which there was energy at the first harmonic (F0), but at no other frequencies.

Another way to express the concept of tilt of the glottal spectrum is to use the 12-dB-per-octave figure given above for the typical reduction in harmonic amplitude across frequency as a reference value. $\dot{V}_g$ waveforms with very steep closing slopes (e.g., Figure 7–6, left panel) should, therefore, have a smaller dB change per octave (<12 dB per octave), and those with very shallow closing slopes should have a larger dB change per octave (>12 dB per octave).

These concepts are important in understanding the physiological and acoustical bases of so-called *hyperfunctional* and *hypofunctional* voice disorders. In hyperfunctional voice disorders, the vocal folds move together too rapidly and forcefully on each closing phase of vocal fold vibration, resulting in a glottal spectrum with less-than-normal tilt, or too much energy in the higher-frequency harmonics. Listeners interpret this kind of voice quality as abnormal, sometimes using the term *pressed voice* to describe what they hear. A pressed voice sounds overly effortful or strained. In hypofunctional voice disorders, the vocal folds move together more slowly and less forcefully, the result being a highly tilted glottal spectrum because there is so little energy in the higher-frequency harmonics. This kind of voice is often heard by listeners as weak, breathy, and thin.

The Ratio of Open Time to Closed Time

For each cycle in a typical $\dot{V}_g$ waveform, the vocal folds are apart about 60% of the time, and approximated about 40% of the time. If the two waveforms in Figure 7–6 are examined, it is fairly obvious that a waveform with a shallower (slower) closing phase is also likely to have more open time throughout a complete cycle. Similarly, a waveform with a steeper (faster) closing phase is likely to have a waveform with less open time and, therefore, a longer closed phase throughout a complete cycle. Because the speed of closing and the open time (and, therefore, the closed time) are in most cases correlated (greater speed, less open time; lesser speed, more open time), less open time will generally be associated with a less tilted glottal spectrum, and more open time with a more tilted glottal spectrum. The closing speed and ratio of open time to closed times (OP/CP) are, therefore, somewhat redundant descriptions of $\dot{V}_g$ waveforms (and spectral characteristics). However, in certain cases, they may provide independent information.

Nature of the Input Signal: A Summary

To answer the first question posed at the outset of this chapter, the precise nature of the input signal generated by the vibrating vocal folds is a complex periodic waveform whose spectrum consists of a consecutive-integer series of harmonics, at whole number multiples of the F0. The harmonics in the glottal spectrum systematically decrease in relative amplitude with increasing frequency. These harmonics serve as input to the vocal tract resonator, which shapes that input according to its resonant characteristics. Consideration turns now to the vocal tract resonator.

WHY SHOULD THE VOCAL TRACT BE CONCEPTUALIZED AS A TUBE CLOSED AT ONE END?

The vocal tract is an acoustic resonator. In Chapter 6, two general classes of acoustic resonators—Helmholtz and tube—are described. For the present discussion, accept on faith that the vocal tract is a tube resonator. It is easy to provide the proof of the tube-resonance characteristics of the vocal tract, as shown in a later section of this chapter.

If the vocal tract is regarded as a tube resonator, the question must be asked, "Does it resonate as a tube open at both ends, or closed at one end?" The answer to this question requires a brief reconsideration of the vibrating vocal folds, and how this vibration influences the acoustic output of the vocal tract.

Figure 7–7 shows two signals in the time domain, collected synchronously during phonation of a vowel. The upper signal displayed is $\dot{V}_g$, discussed above at some length. Note the upward pointing arrows at the end of the cycles in the $\dot{V}_g$ signal. These arrows mark the instant in time at which the vocal folds snap together during each cycle of vibration. At these instants, when the airflow through the glottis is suddenly blocked by closure of the airway, the air immediately above the vocal folds becomes compressed and sends a pressure wave through the vocal tract. Now, consider the situation just described. At the glottal boundary of the vocal tract, there is, for an instant, no airflow and the air molecules become compressed, whereas at the open, oral boundary of the vocal tract air molecules move freely between the lips. This appears very much like the aeromechanical conditions found in a resonating tube closed at one end, where pressure is maximum at the closed end and flow is maximum at the open end (see Chapter 6). In fact, each time the vocal folds snap together, a pressure wave is set up in the vocal tract, and this wave obeys the rules of resonance in a tube closed at one end. Another way to say this is that the vocal tract resonances are excited each time the vibrating vocal folds snap together. Because the excitation occurs when the folds approximate and the oral end of the vocal tract is open for vowel production, the vocal tract resonates like a tube closed at one end.

In Chapter 6, a model of resonance was described in which a hammer was used to tap a resonator, thus exciting the resonant frequency (Helmholtz resonator) or frequencies (tube resonator). Imagine the hammer being controlled by a periodic motor, rotating it toward the resonator and striking it, then pulling back away, rotating it back toward the resonator and striking it again, and so forth. The continuous motion of the hammer back and forth, toward and away from the resonator, is obviously important to producing the excitation of the resonator, but the actual *instant* of excitation of the resonator

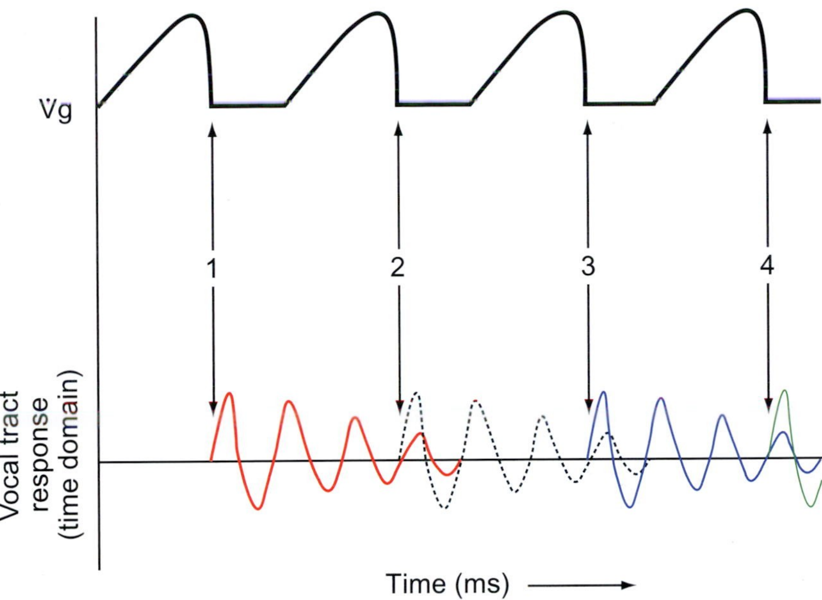

Figure 7–7. Schematic waveforms showing excitation of a vocal tract resonance (*bottom waveform*) by the vibrating vocal folds (*top waveform*). The top waveform, $\dot{V}_g$, shows four periods, with the instant of closing for each cycle marked by an upward-pointing arrow. The waveform of the vocal tract response shows a damped vibration at a resonant frequency of 500 Hz. This vibration is initiated each time the vocal folds snap shut, indicated by the downward-pointing arrows. The amplitude of the damped vocal tract resonance decays over time. Each new excitation of the resonance may overlap with the previous one, resulting in overlap (and summation) of the two damped response waveforms. All of the vocal tract resonances are excited by the closing of the vocal folds, but only a single resonance waveform (for 500 Hz) is shown for the sake of clarity.

corresponds only to the point in time when the hammer strikes the resonator. The analogy to excitation of the vocal tract resonances is direct. The motion of the vibrating vocal folds (the swing of the hammer) is important to the resonance of the vocal tract, but the actual excitation of the resonances occurs only at the instant in time of vocal fold approximation (the tap of the hammer on the resonator).

The Response of the Vocal Tract to Excitation

What does it mean to say that the vocal tract resonances are *excited* each time the vibrating vocal folds snap together? The answer is found in the bottom trace of Figure 7–7, where a waveform is initiated each time the vocal folds snap together. For purposes of simplification, a waveform for only a single resonant frequency is shown in the bottom signal of Figure 7–7, but waveforms are initiated for each resonant frequency of the tube. Think of the vocal tract response waveform shown in Figure 7–7 as corresponding to the first resonance of the tube, with a frequency of 500 Hz. The period of that waveform is 2 ms (500 = 1/T, T = .002 s or 2 ms). Note how the resonance waveform at the first excitation is initiated with relatively great amplitude, which then declines over each successive cycle until the vibration dies out completely (red waveform). In the example of Figure 7–7 note also that the resonance may be *re*-excited before the previous waveform has completely died out (compare the amplitude of the vocal tract response from excitation 1 (red waveform) and excitation 2

Of Beer Bottles and Vocal Tracts

When the vocal tract is excited by the sudden "snapping shut" of the vocal folds, the excitation has the form of a glottal spectrum. A series of such excitations, such as the 190 or so per second expected for an adult female, gives the excitation spectrum its "nice" form of discrete harmonics. This harmonic spectrum is shaped by the vocal tract filter. A historical footnote in speech acoustics was the idea that the excitation of the vocal tract was like the edge tones described in the Chapter 6 sidetrack titled, "Beer and Flutes." In this view, the resonant chambers of the vocal tract are excited by the individual puffs of air coming through the vocal folds during each cycle of vibration. The air puffs "force" air in the vocal tract into resonance, much like blowing across a beer bottle opening forces the air inside the bottle to produce a tone. This footnote view was called the "inharmonic theory" of vocal tract acoustics; it is not correct. The correct view is called the "harmonic theory," for obvious reasons. The vocal tract shapes an acoustic spectrum according to its resonant properties, rather than having its resonant frequencies "forced" into vibration by an aerodynamic event such as the air puff.

(black, dashed-line waveform). The large, 500-Hz vocal tract vibration at excitation 2 overlaps the small (decaying) vibration from excitation 1. Similar "re-excitations" are shown at excitations 3 (blue waveform) and 4 (green waveform). If Figure 7–7 showed the waveforms of all the excited and re-excited resonances, the vocal tract response signal would be visually too "busy" to illustrate the main point of this discussion. The main point is that the vocal tract responds to excitation with damped oscillations at each of its resonant frequencies. The oscillations are damped, meaning they die out over time because there is energy loss in the vocal tract due to the factors discussed in Chapter 6 (friction, absorption, and radiation).

To this point, emphasis has been placed on the time-domain characteristics of the source signal and the response of the vocal tract. The focus now turns to the question of how the vocal tract resonances shape the input signal to produce an acoustic output. Stated more simply: "What is the acoustic basis of the events known as vowel sounds?" The best approach to this problem is to consider the source signal and vocal tract resonances in frequency-domain terms.

HOW ARE THE ACOUSTIC PROPERTIES OF THE VOCAL TRACT DETERMINED?

As discussed in Chapter 6, acoustic resonators can be described in the frequency domain by a resonance curve (see Figure 6–18). The peak of the resonance curve defines the resonant frequency of the resonator, and the width of the curve between the 3-dB-down points—the bandwidth—provides an index of the amount of energy loss in the vibration. Assume, for this discussion, a vocal tract shape associated with the schwa (/ə/), a shape very much like a tube having uniform cross-sectional area from the glottis to the lips. This shape is like that of the straight tubes considered in Chapter 6, for which there are no constrictions, or narrowings, along the entire length of the tube. With such a tube, one should be able to simply apply the quarter-wavelength rule to obtain the multiple peaks of the resonance curve, provided the tube length is known. The shapes of the resonance curves (determined by the bandwidths) are also important, so some additional calculations would be necessary to arrive at a full resonance curve for the vocal tract tube.

If the mathematical tools were available to determine the bandwidths of the multiple resonances, the resonance curve for a vocal tract tube 15 cm in length and shaped for the vowel schwa would look something like the one shown in Figure 7–8. As expected, the lowest (first) resonant frequency is at c/4l = 560 Hz (where c = 33,600 cm/s and l = 15 cm), the second at 1680 Hz (3 × 560) and the third at 2800 Hz (5 × 560). Although the vocal tract tube has, like any other tube, an infinite number of resonances, only the first three are shown for the sake of clarity (as well as for other reasons that will become apparent as this discussion proceeds). The bandwidths are indicated for each peak of the resonance curve by the range of frequencies between the 3-dB-down points. For the present discussion, the bandwidths for each of the three resonances have been set to 60 Hz.

The example in Figure 7–8 was generated using simple principles established in Chapter 6 (the quarter-wavelength rule), as well as an "on faith" assumption about bandwidths. Fant (1960) needed a more comprehensive theory, however, because for most vowels the vocal tract tube does not have a uniform cross-sectional area from the glottis to the lips. Rather, *vocal tract configurations* typically involve

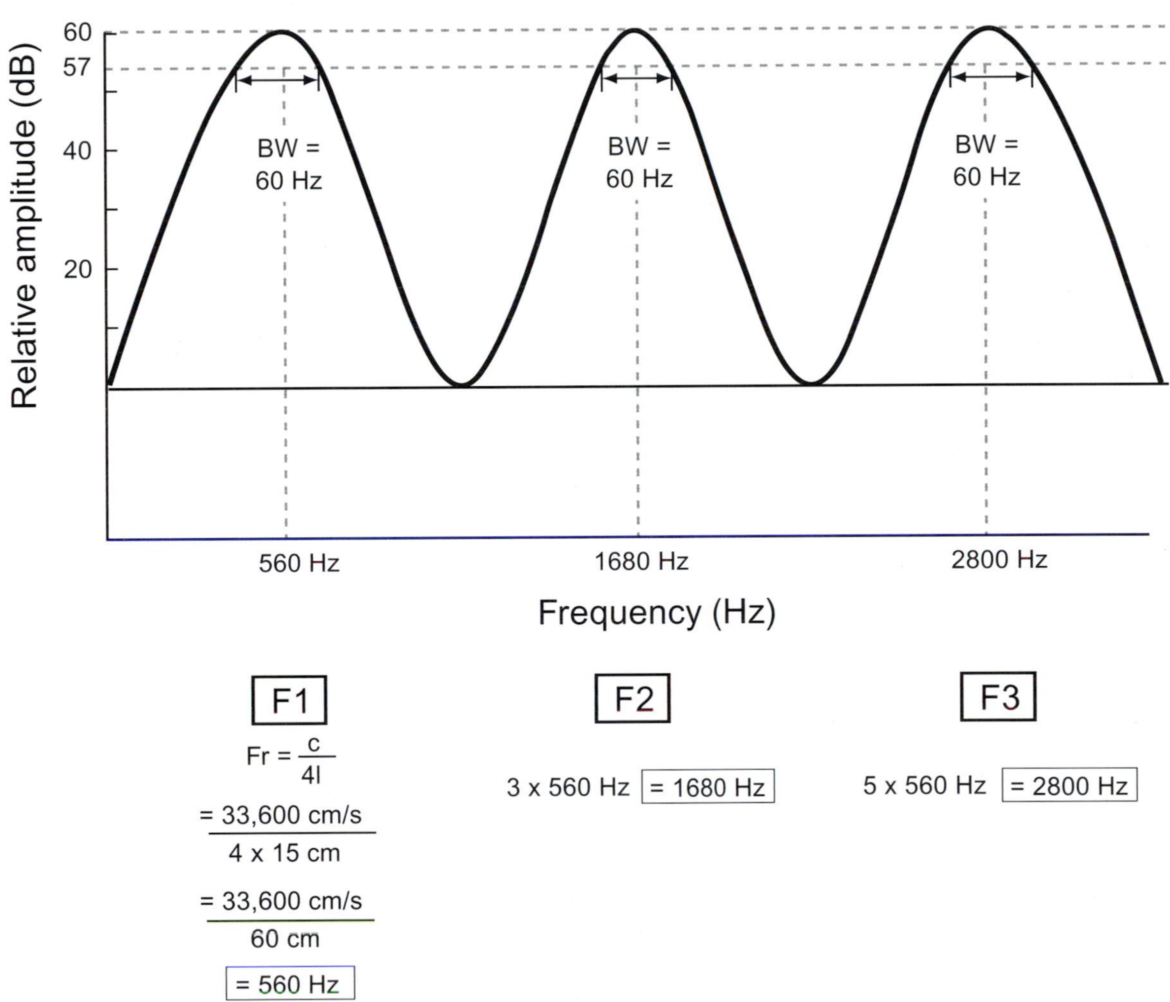

Figure 7–8. Resonance curve for a vocal tract tube in the shape of the schwa /ə/ and having a length of 15 cm. The resonant frequencies along the curve were computed by the quarter-wavelength rule, and the bandwidth of each resonance was assumed to be 60 Hz. Only the first three resonances of the tube are shown.

constrictions along the path from glottis to lips, some of which are extremely small (often referred to as "tight" constrictions). Fant approached the problem of drawing the resonance curves for different vocal tract shapes in the following way. He took sagittal x-ray pictures of an adult male speaker's productions of a variety of Russian and Swedish vowels. The soft and hard tissues of the speaker's vocal tract (tongue, lips, hard palate, velum, part of the pharynx) were coated with barium paste, which allowed easier identification of the outlines of structures in the developed film. Figure 7–9 shows a magnetic resonance image (MRI) of a speaker producing a high back vowel, with the boundaries of the air tube outlined and the air tube itself slightly shaded. The outlined and shaded tube, therefore, includes boundaries defined by the walls of the larynx superior to the vocal folds, the pharynx, hard palate, velum, tongue, lips, and other surfaces. Although Figure 7–9, is an image type much more advanced than the standard x-ray images used by Fant, his approach can be explained just as effectively using the MRI example. Fant used the x-rays he obtained of many different vowels to outline the varied vocal tract shapes. When the structures are outlined in this way, the column of air extending from the glottis to the lips can be conceptualized as a tube of varying cross-sectional area.

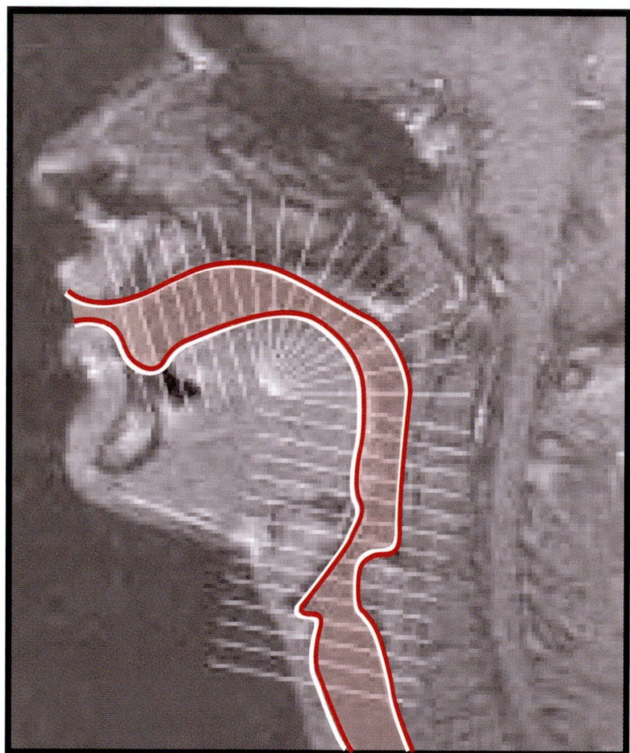

Figure 7–9. Sagittal magnetic resonance image (MRI) of a male speaker producing a vocal tract configuration for the vowel /u/. Boundaries of the vocal tract (tongue surface, hard and soft palates, pharynx, and so forth) are outlined to show the shape of the vocal tract tube and how its dimensions vary from glottis to lips. Background image obtained from Audiovisual-to-Articulatory Speech Inversion (ASPI) Web site http://aspi.loria.fr (Figure 1). Accessed August 30, 2007. Reproduced with permission.

The vocal tract length of the speaker studied by Fant (1960) was approximately 17.5 cm. Fant plotted the varying cross-sectional area of the vocal tract by estimating the area of the air tube at 0.5-cm increments from glottis to lips. This kind of "sectioning off" of the vocal tract is shown in Figure 7–9 by the sequence of straight lines drawn through the vocal tract tube which is outlined in red. If a line is imagined running straight forward from the glottis to the lips, along the long axis of the vocal tract, each of the straight lines seen in Figure 7–9 can be thought of as intersecting this long axis line at a right angle. The part of the intersecting line within the vocal tract—between the red outline in Figure 7–9—defines the "size" of the vocal tract tube at that location. The distance between adjacent lines defines a small section, or "tubelette" within the vocal tract (Story, 2005), for which width measurements can be made. For example, the tubelettes are quite narrow toward the back of the oral cavity, where the tongue is raised toward the boundary of the hard and soft palates. However, the tubelettes are much wider toward the front of the vocal tract. Fant sectioned his vocal tract images into 35 "pieces" (2 measurements per cm of vocal tract, $2 \times 17.5 = 35$). The width of each one of these section lines was measured and entered into a simple formula used to compute the area for that slice of the vocal tract. What emerged from this exercise was an *area function of the vocal tract*.

Area Function of the Vocal Tract

An area function of the vocal tract is a plot of cross-sectional area as a function of distance along the vocal tract from glottis to lips. This distance is described by the succession of the measurement "slices" shown in Figure 7–9. Figure 7–10 shows an area function for the vowel /i/. Here area, in cm^2, is plotted on the y-axis and section (slice) number (i.e., distance) is plotted on the x-axis. The low section numbers are near the glottis (i.e., section 1 is immediately above the glottis), and the measurement moves toward the lips from left to right. Each section number has an area value, so the function is actually a string of discrete points. For illustration purposes, the discrete points have been connected and the area function is represented in Figure 7–10 as a continuous line. This is justified because the measurements of successive slices were made sufficiently close together (in 0.5-cm increments) to minimize the likelihood of major changes in cross-sectional vocal tract area between the measurement steps along the vocal tract length.

The area function in Figure 7–10 shows relatively large cross-sectional areas in the lower and upper pharyngeal regions (the left side of the x-axis), with relatively smaller areas toward the front of the vocal tract. A very tight constriction—that is, small cross-sectional areas—is present between sections 22 and 27. This function is intuitively consistent with phonetic descriptions of the vowel /i/ as a high-front vowel, where the major constriction is in the front of the vocal tract.[1]

The area functions supplied the link between the configuration of the vocal tract tube, as shaped by the oral and pharyngeal structures, and the resonant frequencies of that tube. Fant (1960) developed a mathematical technique for estimating the tube resonances from the area function. The specifics of the mathematical technique are not covered here,

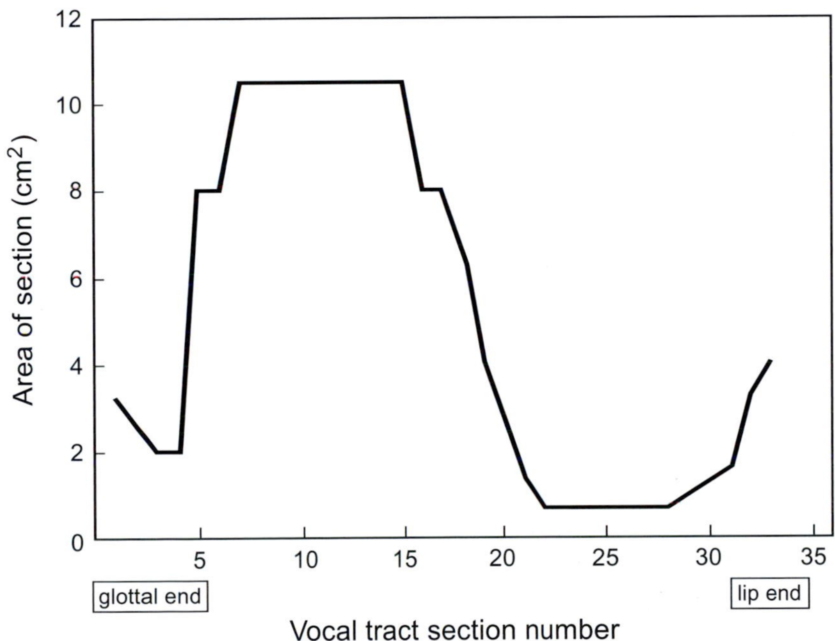

Figure 7–10. Area function for the vowel /i/ plotted from data reported by Fant (1960, p.115). Vocal tract section number (from 1–35, with sections extending from the glottis to the lips) is plotted on the x-axis. Cross-sectional area (in cm^2) is plotted on the y-axis. Even though the cross-sectional area is measured in discrete steps (for each section), individual points are connected by a straight line to give the impression of a continuous area function.

[1]The relatively large areas in the back portion of the vocal tract may not be intuitive from a standard phonetic perspective, which typically classifies vowels according to (a) the degree of tongue advancement and (b) the height of the tongue. Neither of these classificatory dimensions implies anything about the size of the pharyngeal airway.

but the conceptual link between the area function and estimation of vocal tract resonant frequencies is straightforward, and makes use of information developed in Chapter 6. Chapter 6 described the role of mass and compliance in determining the resonant frequency of an acoustical resonator. Imagine that the air contained within the boundaries of any two adjacent measurement points (that is, within a tubelette corresponding to the small air column between two measurement lines) has certain mass and compliance properties. If these properties are specified for each of the 35 sections of air, all of the information relevant to the resonant frequencies of the vocal tract should be available. Fant's mathematical theory allowed him to estimate mass and compliance properties from the area measurement for each section, or tubelette. Based on the mass and compliance estimates from *all* 35 sections, the theory produced an estimate of the resonant pattern for the entire vocal tract. When mathematical information concerning energy loss factors was included, Fant was able to draw the complete resonant curve (resonant frequencies and bandwidths as in Figure 7–8) for a given vocal tract configuration.

The conceptual basis of Fant's (1960) theory is, therefore, fairly simple. If the mass and compliance characteristics of the vocal tract tube can be determined, the resonance curve for the tube can be constructed. Because the vocal tract resonates like a tube, there are multiple peaks (i.e., resonances) along the resonance curve, each with its own bandwidth.

At this point in the development of Fant's (1960) theory, it is important to recognize that the vocal tract resonance curve is computed from the measured area function. The resonant peaks are determined mathematically, rather than being measured by analyzing the spectrum of a produced vowel. For this reason the computed resonance curve is called a *theoretical spectrum*, or a *filter function*. This theoretical spectrum, or filter function, shows where the resonances for this particular vocal tract configuration should be. The term *filter function* is particularly interesting, because it implies that the vocal tract acts like a filter, allowing energy to pass through only at certain frequencies. The regions of the spectrum where energy passes through, of course, are those regions at and in the immediate vicinity of the resonant peaks. The next section discusses the way in which the source spectrum and filter function (theoretical spectrum) are combined to produce an output spectrum—a measured spectrum, as for a phonated vowel. This discussion will show why the theoretical spectrum (the filter function) is not always exactly the same as the output spectrum (the spectrum of a produced vowel).

HOW DOES THE VOCAL TRACT SHAPE THE INPUT SIGNAL? (HOW IS THE SOURCE SPECTRUM COMBINED WITH THE THEORETICAL VOCAL TRACT SPECTRUM TO PRODUCE A VOCAL TRACT OUTPUT?)

The two questions heading this section are merely variants of the same problem, which is to determine how the acoustic characteristics of the source and vocal tract combine to produce a vocal tract output, which in this case is a vowel sound. The frequency-domain representation of the vocal tract output is called an *output spectrum*. This is the spectrum measured, with appropriate instruments, from an actual vowel produced by a talker.

Figure 7–11 presents a simple graphic answer to the question posed above. The input (source) spectrum, as described in a preceding section, is shown at the left of the figure. The filter function is shown in the middle of the figure as a resonance curve with three peaks, corresponding to the first three resonances of a vocal tract tube in an /i/ shape. Note the multiplication sign between the input spectrum and filter function. To determine the output of the vocal tract (the right panel in Figure 7–11), the energy in the input spectrum is multiplied by the energy in the filter function.[2] To be a little more explicit about what this process of multiplication means, the axes of both the input (source) spectrum and the filter function are the same—frequency on the *x*-axis, relative amplitude on the *y*-axis (i.e., they are both spectra). The input spectrum shows the relative

[2]The idea of the source being multiplied by the energy in the filter function is somewhat of a simplification, but one that does not violate the essentials of the theory. In precise mathematical terms, the output of the vocal tract is determined by the convolution of source and filter energy. It is like a "blending" of the source and filter functions.

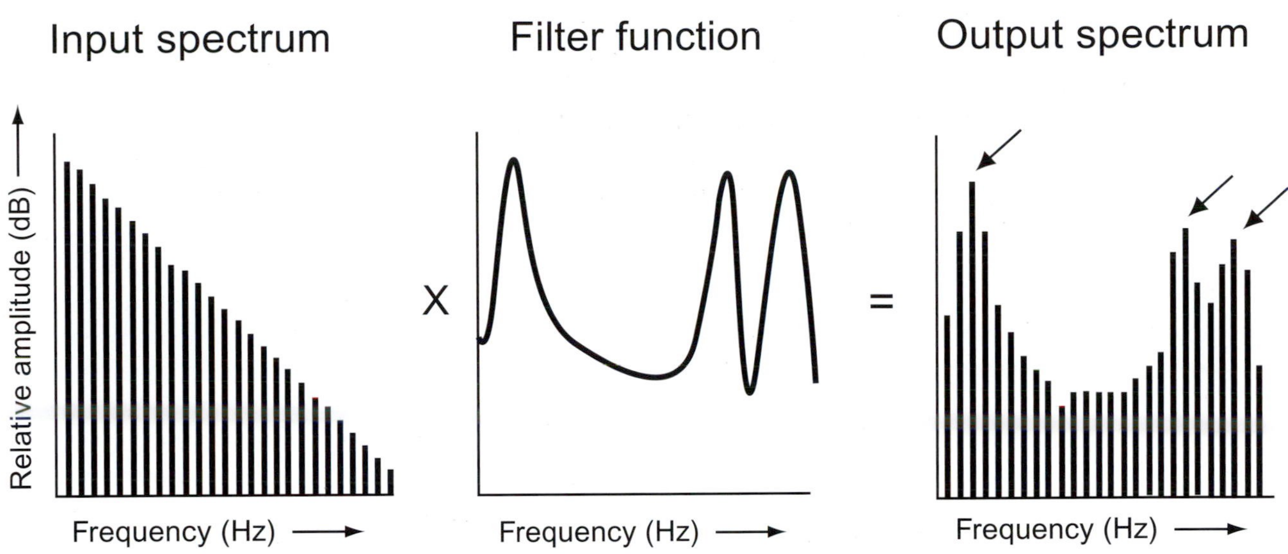

Figure 7–11. Schematic representation of how the source or input spectrum and filter function are combined to produce a vocal tract output. The left panel depicts the input spectrum, the middle panel the filter function for a vocal tract in an /i/ configuration, and the right panel the output spectrum. The output spectrum shows which harmonics are and are not emphasized by combining the input and filter functions. The peaks in the output spectrum are formants (F1, F2, F3) representing the first three resonant frequencies of the vocal tract.

amplitude of discrete frequency components, and the filter function shows the frequencies at which energy applied to it will be "amplified" (the resonances) or "de-emphasized" (the valleys of the resonance curve, between the resonances). Thus the multiplication being described here is simply another way to understand the shaping of the input (source) spectrum by the filter function. The harmonics in the input (source) spectrum will be shaped by the form of the filter function. At resonant frequencies of the filter function, energy in the input (source) spectrum will be multiplied strongly, and will appear in the output spectrum as prominent energy components. At valleys in the filter function, energy in the input (source) spectrum will be multiplied weakly or not at all, and will not appear (or appear only weakly) in the output spectrum.

The result of the multiplication of the input (source) spectrum by the filter function (equivalently, the shaping of the input [source] spectrum by the filter function) is indicated by the "=" sign and shown in the output spectrum of Figure 7–11. This spectrum shows the harmonics, now reshaped from their form in the input (source) spectrum. An important feature of the glottal source spectrum is the systematic decrease in harmonic amplitude as frequency increases, but in this output spectrum some of the higher frequency harmonics actually have greater relative amplitude than some of the lower frequency harmonics. This is because of the shaping of the input (source) spectrum by the filter function, which emphasizes some higher frequency harmonics while de-emphasizing some lower frequency harmonics. The rise and fall of the harmonics in the output spectrum of Figure 7–11, it will be noted, follow pretty closely the locations of the resonances in the filter function. However, all of the peaks in the filter function were computed as having roughly equal amplitudes, but in the output spectrum the higher-frequency "peaks" (see arrows) have less amplitude than the lower-frequency peaks (note the decline in peak amplitude across the three peaks in the output spectrum). This is because the energy available in the input (source) spectrum decreases with increasing frequency, meaning there is less energy to multiply by the roughly equivalent peaks in the filter function. So, an output spectrum may show a general decrease in harmonic energy with increasing frequency, but in some cases higher frequency harmonics will have greater amplitudes than lower-frequency harmonics.

The distinctions between harmonics in the source (input) spectrum and peaks in the output spectrum can be confusing, so it is useful to pursue this description a little further. In the output spectrum of Figure 7–11, there is a series of harmonics whose amplitudes rise and fall according to peaks and valleys of the filter function. But there is no systematic relationship between the frequency locations of the harmonics in the source (input) spectrum and the frequencies of the peaks in the filter function. The frequencies in the source (input) spectrum are determined by the rate of vibration of the vocal folds (the F0), and the frequencies of the peaks in the filter function are determined by the configuration of the vocal tract. In the acoustic theory of vowel production, then, the source and filter are independent.[3] Two simple examples of the independence of the source and filter in the theory are as follows: (a) for a given speaker, the same vowel (produced by a single filter function) can be produced with many different F0s and, therefore, many different source spectra; and (b) for a given speaker, many different vowels can be produced with the same F0. Thus, either the source or the filter can be adjusted without affecting characteristics of the other component.

A graphic example (Figure 7–12) illustrates the independence of the source and filter in the acoustic theory of vowel production. The example also highlights a distinction in the theory between *computed and measured* resonances. Figure 7–12 shows two graphs, both of which have a computed (theoretical) filter function with resonances at 300 Hz, 2300 Hz, and 3000 Hz. This filter function would be a reasonable set of formant frequencies for an adult male's production of /i/. Because the source spectrum and filter function are shown as spectra, one can superimpose two different source spectra on these identical filter functions. Source spectra with F0s of 100 Hz and 120 Hz are shown in Figures 7–12A and 7–12B, respectively. Because the F0s of these two source spectra are slightly different (by 20 Hz), so are the frequencies of the consecutive-integer series of harmonics. For example, for the F0 of 100 Hz there is a 3rd harmonic at 300 Hz, a 23rd harmonic at 2300 Hz, and a 30th harmonic at 3000 Hz. In this case, there is harmonic energy *exactly* at the location of the computed resonances of the filter function, as well as harmonic energy 100 Hz above and below these frequencies. The harmonic energy around the peaks in this filter function, but especially exactly at the peaks, will contribute to emphasizing energy in the output spectrum in the immediate region of the computed peaks.

Hardheaded Speech Acoustics

First (Chapter 6) we used a hammer analogy for the excitation of resonators, then in the previous sidetrack we said that wasn't exactly the way the vocal tract was excited for speech, now we're going to say that the vocal tract *can* be excited "inharmonically," if you care to do so. Vowel-like vocal tract sounds can be produced by banging the skull (usually toward the front of the head, in the middle, with your knuckles) with the vocal tract open (flicking the neck with your fingers can produce roughly the same effect). Try this with your vocal tract in the shape of the vowel in "oh" and then "ee." You'll probably hear the difference, and most certainly a listener will. This is simply the case of the vocal tract being excited by a source different from the harmonic glottal spectrum. The vocal tract will respond with damped oscillation of the resonant frequencies, "ringing" in response to the skull bangs.

[3]This statement is true for the purposes of this textbook; it can be shown that there are some effects of the filter on the source under certain conditions, but these are beyond the scope of this text.

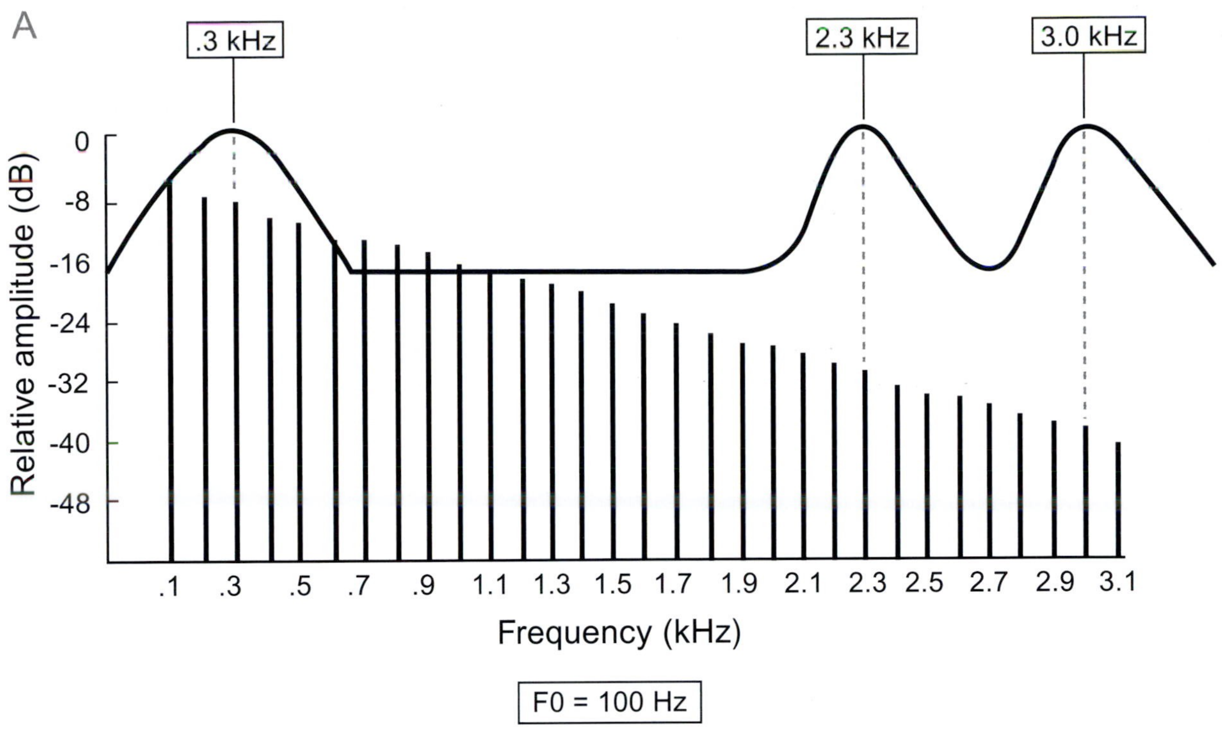

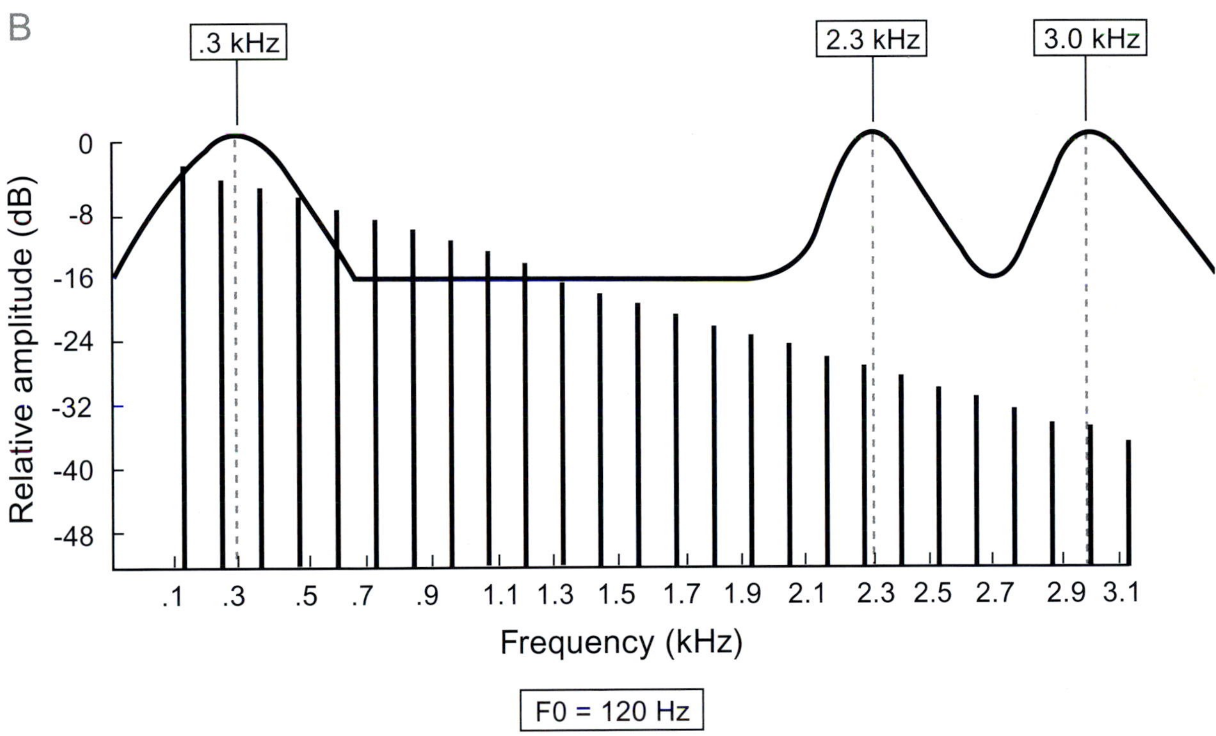

Figure 7–12. A single filter function (appropriate for the vowel /i/) superimposed on two source spectra having different fundamental frequencies and, therefore, different spacing between harmonics. In panels A and B, the filter function is superimposed on a source spectrum having an F0 = 100 Hz and 120 Hz, respectively. When F0 = 100 Hz, frequencies of the harmonics match the frequencies of the computed resonances of 300 Hz, 2300 Hz, and 3000 Hz. When F0 = 120 Hz, frequencies of the harmonics do not match the first and second resonances, but do match the third resonance ($120 \times 25 = 3000$ Hz).

In fact, when the energy in this source spectrum is multiplied by the values along the filter functions, the peaks in the output spectrum are likely to coincide exactly with the computed (theoretical) peaks because there is harmonic energy precisely at the location of the computed peaks. This is the case for the superimposed source and filter characteristics in Figure 7–12A.

Now consider the case of the source spectrum and filter function in Figure 7–12B. Here the F0 of 120 Hz will *not* produce harmonics coinciding exactly with the computed peaks at 300 Hz and 2300 Hz, but the 25th harmonic matches the resonance at 3000 Hz. For example, the second and third harmonics in this source spectrum will be located at 240 and 360 Hz, values only in the general neighborhood of the computed first resonance at 300 Hz. Similarly, the 19th and 20th harmonics of 120 Hz will be located at 2280 and 2400 Hz, values that do not coincide exactly with the computed second resonance of 2300 Hz. When the energy at these harmonic frequencies is multiplied by the values along the filter function, the general region around the first and second computed resonances will be emphasized in the output spectrum, but the location of these peaks in the output spectrum may not coincide exactly with the theoretical peaks in the filter function.

The harmonics in the source spectrum are not *purposely* matched up with the locations of the computed (theoretical) peaks of the filter function. They do not have to be matched up in this manner, because the general region of resonance given by a computed peak will be emphasized in either case (i.e., whether or not a harmonic is exactly located at a peak in the filter function). But this discussion explains why the output peaks in the measured spectrum may not coincide exactly with the computed (theoretical) peaks in the filter function. Only when a harmonic in the source spectrum has exactly the same frequency as a computed resonance will a computed (filter function) and measured (output spectrum) peak be precisely the same.

The general regions of resonance in the output spectrum have been emphasized in this discussion, rather than specific values of harmonics. In the output spectra—the kinds of spectra typically measured in the laboratory, these regions of high energy are called *formants*. Because the individual harmonics are not of great importance, output spectra are typically shown as smooth curves that can be described as tracing an *envelope* along the varying harmonic amplitudes resulting from the shaping of the source spectrum by the filter function. Figure 7–13 presents output spectra for the isolated vowels /i/ (top spectrum), /ɑ/ (middle spectrum), and /u/ (bottom spectrum), spoken by an adult male. These spectra show how a *spectral envelope* can be drawn by connecting the tops of the harmonic lines with a smooth curve. The harmonic spectra in Figure 7–13 were generated with Fourier analysis, whereas the smooth, spectral envelopes superimposed on the tops of the harmonics were generated by linear predictive code (LPC) analysis, a special computer algorithm for locating formant frequencies (discussed more fully in Chapter 9). Each spectral envelope shows three peaks, labeled *F1, F2,* and *F3* (F1 = first formant, F2 = second formant, F3 = third formant). The higher frequency peaks typically have somewhat lower amplitude than the lower frequency peaks, primarily because the energy in the source spectrum decreases as frequency increases (see above). The relative amplitudes of peaks in the output spectrum do not seem to be particularly important for either the acoustic or perceptual specification of vowels, so the frequency locations of the measured peaks—the formant frequencies—will dominate the discussion of vowels.

A great deal of research, some of which is reviewed in Chapter 10, has shown that the first three peaks in a vowel spectrum have great importance for the acoustic and perceptual specification of vowel identity. The frequency locations of these first three peaks is sometimes referred to as the *F-pattern* of a vowel, and this terminology will be used throughout this text. For example, the F-patterns of the vowels shown in Figure 7–13 are F1 = 237, F2 = 2283, and F3 = 3058 Hz for /i/, F1 = 775, F2 = 1012, F3 = 2713 Hz for /ɑ/, and F1 = 280, F2 = 732, and F3 = 2218 Hz for /u/ (measurements made by author GW). Although the F-pattern of a vowel is always stated in terms of these three frequencies, the exact frequency value attached to each of the formants does not mean that other frequencies in the vowel spectrum are unimportant in the acoustic and perceptual specification of vowels. It is better to think of these numbers as *center frequencies* denoting a region of *spectral prominence*. In the region of spectral prominence for

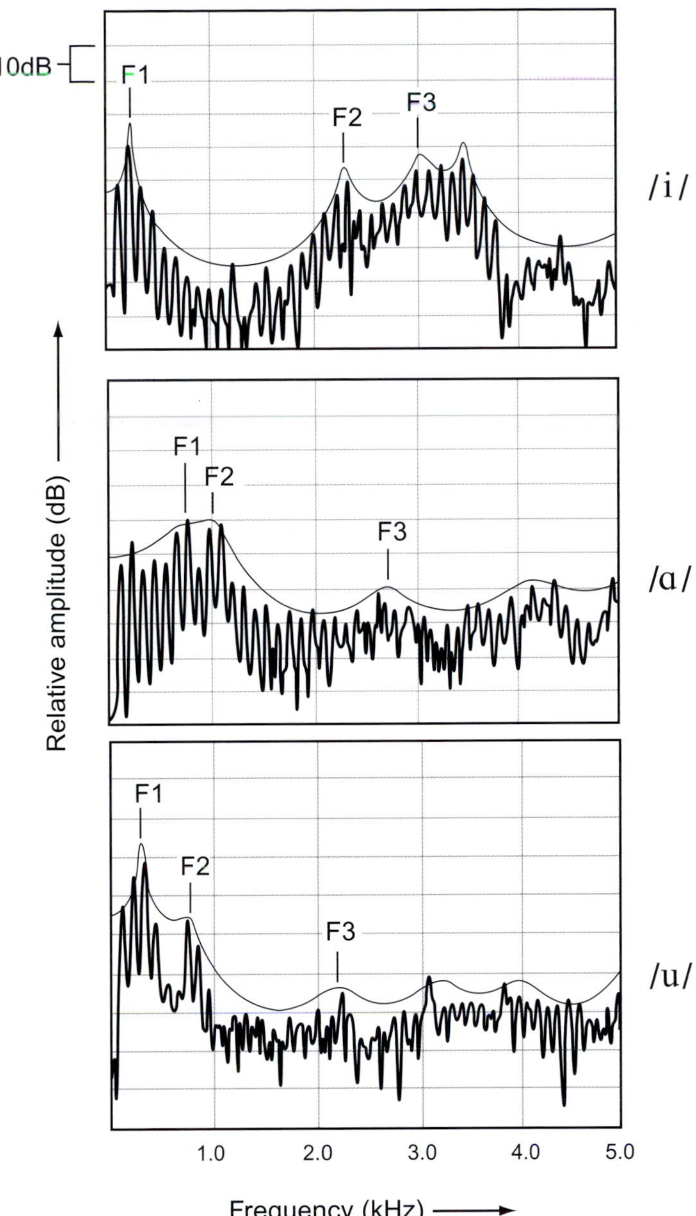

Figure 7–13. Output spectra for the vowels /i/ (*top panel*), /ɑ/ (*middle panel*), and /u/ (*bottom panel*), showing how the tops of the harmonics computed by Fourier analysis can be connected to draw a smooth curve, or spectral envelope, computed by linear predictive code (LPC) analysis. The peaks in the envelope are the formant frequencies, marked F1, F2, and F3 in each spectrum. Spectra are shown for the 0- to 5-kHz range. Each vertical division (*y*-axis, relative amplitude) is equal to 10 dB.

each formant, there is a small range of frequencies that reflects the resonance characteristics of the vocal tract (recall the discussion of bandwidth in Chapter 6). The F-pattern is always stated with respect to the frequencies measured at the highest peaks in the output spectrum.

All /i/s Are Not Created Equal

Formant frequencies do, as Fant proposed, completely specify vowels, but the more you look into the relationship between formant values and vowel identity, the more you realize this statement requires some qualification. One such qualification has emerged from the recent trend in speech acoustics research comparing acoustic phonetic data between different languages. Although many different languages "share" certain vowels, such as /i/, the formant frequencies often differ across the languages. How is it that the same vowel—at least, one transcribed with the same phonetic symbol—has a different F-pattern in different languages? Think about it. We'll tell you more in Chapter 10.

Formant Bandwidths

Chapter 6 presented a brief discussion of the factors responsible for energy loss in acoustic systems. These factors, which include friction, absorption, and radiation, are all operative in the vocal tract and contribute to the shape of the resonances (formants) in the output spectrum.

When air molecules vibrate within the vocal tract they rub against each other and also against soft and hard tissues. This friction generates heat, which dissipates a small amount of the vibratory energy. The vibration of the air molecules may also be taken up by nearby structures whose own resonant frequencies are close to the frequencies propagated through the vocal tract. For example, the cheeks and possibly the tongue appear to have resonant frequencies in the neighborhood of 200 Hz, close to the typical first formant frequencies of several vowels (Fujimura & Lindquist, 1971). When a formant frequency is close to the resonant frequency of a structure such as the cheek, the tissue will absorb some of the energy and transform it into its own vibratory event. This absorption of acoustic energy by vocal tract structures is another form of energy loss and contributes to the damping of vocal tract resonances. Under certain conditions, such as when the nasal cavities are connected to the oral cavity or the oral cavity is connected to the subglottal cavities (e.g., the trachea) because the vocal folds are abducted, the amount of energy loss may be greatly increased partly because there is more tissue to absorb sound energy. Thus, nasalized vowels tend to have greater formant bandwidths than non-nasalized vowels, and the bandwidth of the first formant is greater when a vowel is produced with breathy, as compared to regular, phonation. Finally, the radiation of sound from the mouth results in some loss of energy as the sound changes environment from an enclosed tube (the vocal tract) to the open atmosphere. Megaphones are effective in transmitting sound over a relatively great distance partly because their gradually flared design decreases the radiation loss from the vocal tract to the atmosphere. The flare of the megaphone provides a gradual transition from the vocal tract shape to the "shape" of the atmosphere, thus reducing the amount of energy loss in the propagation of sound from the vocal tract to the atmosphere.

Table 7–1 (data from Fujimura & Lindqvist, 1971) contains some estimates of formant bandwidths, and provides a rough range of the formant values associated with the bandwidths. The formant val-

Table 7–1. Approximate Bandwidths of the First (F1), Second (F2), and Third (F3) Formants of Vowels, and Frequency Ranges for Those Formants*

	F1	F2	F3
Bandwidth	45–90	40–90	40–150
Formant Freq. Ranges	250–800	500–2500	2400–3300

*These data were taken from graphs published by Fujimura and Lindqvist (1971). All values are in Hz, and include data for men and women.

ues are provided to support the statement that vowel resonances are relatively *sharply tuned*. In other words, the resonances in the spectrum have rather narrow bandwidths compared to the actual frequencies of those resonances. For example, bandwidths of 45 to 90 Hz are relatively narrow compared to typical F1 values which range between 250 and 800 Hz, depending on the vowel. These bandwidths are very definitely narrow compared to the higher formant frequency values for F2 and F3.

How does bandwidth affect the acoustic categorization and perception of vowel sounds? Earlier it was noted that the F-pattern (the first three formant frequencies) seemed to be sufficient as an acoustic index of vowels. Information on formant amplitudes and bandwidths does not seem to be particularly useful for the acoustic categorization of vowels. When speech synthesizers are used to systematically increase the bandwidth of vowel formants while maintaining constant formant frequencies, listeners do not hear a change in vowel category. Rather, vowels are perceived as increasingly "muffled" as bandwidths are increased. This "muffling" effect is sometimes heard in the speech of children and adults with craniofacial deficits and associated velopharyngeal incompetence. The perception of muffled vowels in these speakers may be explained, in part, by the increased bandwidths resulting from the undesired coupling of the oral and nasal cavities. Even though the increased "muffling" of vowel quality may not have an effect on the perception of vowel categories, there may be an effect on general speech intelligibility and naturalness.

Acoustic Theory of Vowel Production: A Summary

Information presented to this point can be summarized as follows. First, the input, or source, for vowel production is the acoustic result of vocal fold vibration. This acoustic event can be described in the frequency domain as a series of consecutive integer harmonics whose energy systematically decreases with increasing frequency. The exact shape of this glottal spectrum depends on how fast the vocal folds snap together on each cycle of vibration. When the vocal folds snap together very quickly, the harmonic energy decreases relatively slowly with increasing frequency (less tilted spectrum). When the vocal folds move together slowly, the harmonic energy decreases relatively rapidly with frequency (more tilted spectrum).

The resonator in vowel acoustics is the vocal tract, which extends from the top margin of the vocal folds to the lips. The vocal tract resonates like a tube closed at one end, the closed end being the vocal folds, the open end being the lips. The vocal tract resonances are excited at the instant of closure for each cycle of vocal fold vibration. This excitation causes the vocal tract to respond with an infinite series of damped resonances.

A mathematical theory developed by Fant (1960) relates the area function of the vocal tract to the specific resonant frequencies of the tube. The area function is a plot of the cross-sectional area of the vocal tract from glottis to lips, and can be thought of as a description of the shape of the air column formed by the articulators and the more or less fixed structures of the vocal tract (such as the hard palate). By using this shape to estimate the mass and compliance of consecutive sections of the air column, Fant was able to calculate the resonant frequencies of differently shaped tubes (i.e., air columns). For current purposes, calculation of only the lowest three resonances is important. The resonance curve that results from these calculations shows the peaks at resonant frequencies, the bandwidths of those peaks, and the valleys between the peaks. This curve is called the filter function. At any frequency, the filter function shows how the energy at the corresponding frequency in the glottal spectrum will be transferred by the vocal tract. At frequencies where there are peaks in the filter function, energy transfer will be maximum, meaning that the energy will appear prominently in the output spectrum. At frequencies where there are valleys in the filter function, the energy at corresponding frequencies in the glottal spectrum will not appear prominently in the output spectrum.

The actual acoustic event that emerges from the lips—a vowel sound—is the product of the acoustic characteristics of the glottal spectrum (the amplitudes of the harmonic frequencies) and the varying amplitudes along the filter function. The output spectrum shows which frequencies are prominent, and which are not. Peaks in the output spectrum, where energy transfer is maximal, are called formants. The first three formant frequencies of a vowel are referred to as the F-pattern of that vowel. The F-pattern is vitally important in the understanding of speech acoustics and perception.

The acoustic model of the vocal tract as a tube closed at one end is a central concept in the development of this theory. The tubes studied in Chapter 6, however, were all of uniform cross-sectional area, like a straight pipe having no constrictions along its length. As mentioned above, the articulation of the schwa may be performed with a vocal tract shape somewhat like a straight tube or pipe, but other vowels clearly require tube shapes of varying cross-sectional area from glottis to lips. Is there a straightforward way to understand how constrictions along the vocal tract tube cause changes in the resonant frequencies known to occur in a straight tube with one end closed? With no constrictions in a tube closed at one end, the quarter-wavelength rule accounts for the resonant frequencies, provided the length of the tube is known. What happens to these resonant frequencies when a constriction is introduced somewhere in the tube? Fortunately, the mathematical details of Fant's (1960) theory do not need to be studied to understand when and how the resonances change with constrictions in a tube. There is a simple conceptual basis for these changes, and the background for the concepts has already been established in Chapter 6. Discussion now turns to constrictions in the vocal tract tube, and their effect on formant frequencies.

WHAT HAPPENS TO THE RESONANT FREQUENCIES OF THE VOCAL TRACT WHEN THE TUBE IS CONSTRICTED AT A GIVEN LOCATION?

At the end of the discussion of tube resonances in Chapter 6, a graph (Figure 6–16) of the pressure distributions for the first three tube resonances is shown. This graph is reproduced in Figure 7–14A. The pressure distributions for the first three resonances correspond to one-quarter of the wavelength for the first resonance (solid blue curve), three-quarters for the second resonance (short-dashed red curve), and five-fourths for the third resonance (long-dashed green curve). (In these graphs "maximum pressure" can mean either maximum positive or maximum negative pressure. The sign of maximum pressure is not important for the discussion that follows.) As stated in Chapter 6, there are many other pressure distributions in this tube corresponding to

The Unknown Vocal Tract

Type in the words "voice disguise acoustics" on a search engine and you will be directed to all sorts of sites for electronic devices that guarantee to change your voice so people can't recognize it. With so many millions of voices in the world, it is remarkable that people can make fantastically accurate identifications based on a relatively brief voice sample. No wonder, then, that voice disguise is big business (we won't dwell on why you would want to disguise your voice). In the old days, some would-be voice disguisers spoke through the cardboard tube inside a roll of toilet paper, effectively lengthening their vocal tracts and lowering all the formants. Others (this one turns up in old movies) put a handkerchief over the telephone receiver to "muffle" their voices, increasing sound absorption and, therefore, widening formant bandwidths. Both of these antique maneuvers are easily reversed by signal processing tricks that "take away" the suspected cover-up. Modern electronic devices make it much harder to undo the disguise and recover the real voice behind the deception.

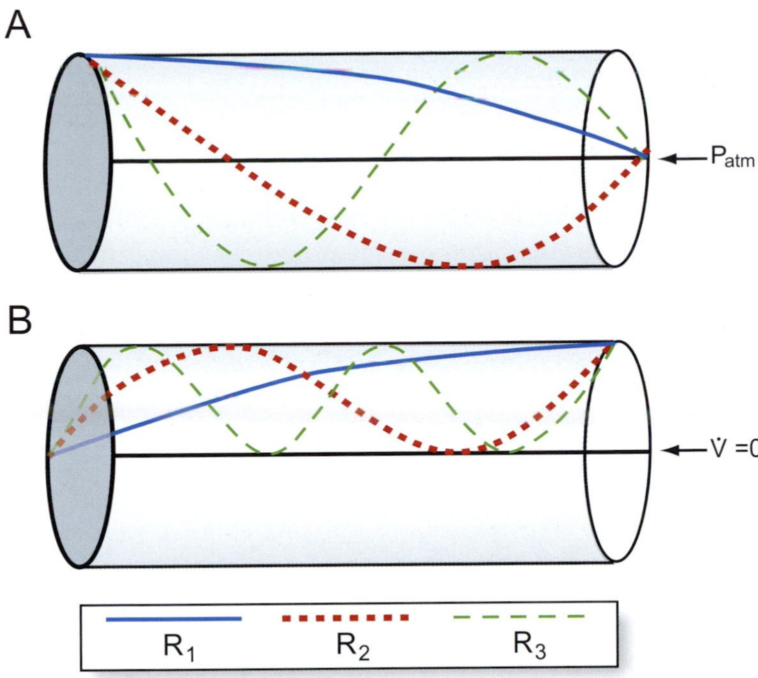

Figure 7–14. A. Modificattion of Figure 6–16 showing the pressure distributions corresponding to the first three resonances of a tube closed at one end. Pressure distributions follow the quarter-wavelength rule. **B.** Velocity distributions for the first three resonances of the tube shown in A. Velocities at any point in the tube are the exact mirror image of the pressure distributions. Thus, when pressure is maximum, velocity is zero, and vice versa. The center horizontal line in A represents P_{atm}, whereas the center horizontal line in B represents zero velocity. Maximum pressure in A can mean either maximum positive or maximum negative pressure.

the higher resonances. They are not shown here partly for reasons of clarity, but also because the first three resonances are the ones of chief concern in vowel acoustics.

As introduced in Chapter 6, Figure 7–14A shows the three pressure distributions superimposed on one another in the tube. The expected maximum pressures at the closed end of the tube can be seen for all three distributions, as well as other locations of maximum and zero (atmospheric) pressure that are specific to a particular wavelength. For example, the first resonance has maximum pressure at the closed end which falls to P_{atm} at the open end. The second resonance has maximum pressure at the closed end, which decreases to P_{atm} about one-third of the way toward the open end, decreases to maximum (negative) pressure about two-thirds of the way toward the open end, and then returns to P_{atm} at the opening. Examination of the pressure pattern for the third resonance reveals two regions of maximum pressure in addition to the maximum pressure at the closed end. Thus, along the length of this tube there are a number of regions of maximum pressure associated with each of the three lowest resonances.

Regions of high pressure result when molecules are packed together and in a relatively motionless state (i.e., at one of the extremes of the simple harmonic motion). It follows that if a measurement were made of the velocity of air molecules at the regions of high pressure in the tube, the value would be zero (i.e., no displacement as a function of time = zero velocity). P_{atm} is indicated in Figure 7–14A by a horizontal, solid black line running through the center of the tube. When the wavelengths associated with the different resonances cross this line, meaning that their pressure value is equal to P_{atm}, the air molecules are minimally packed together and move at their maximum velocity. Note the inverse relationship between pressure and velocity in the tube. When pressure is maximum, velocity of air molecules is zero, and when pressure is zero (= P_{atm}), velocity is maximum. In fact, when the distributions for air molecule velocity are drawn for the first three resonances, they are exact mirror images of the distributions of pressure shown in Figure 7–14A. Those velocity distributions are shown in Figure 7–14B. The velocity pattern for the first resonance is shown by the solid blue line, for the second resonance by the short-dashed red line, and for the third resonance by the long-dashed green line. The information in either the pressure or velocity distributions is redundant with respect to the other distribution. If the value of pressure at a given point within the tube is known, it implies the value of air molecule velocity at that same point (and vice versa). For current purposes, the important point is that, at regions of high pressure, the velocity is low and at regions of low pressure the velocity is high. This can be confirmed in Figure 7–14 by matching the regions of maximum pressure for a given resonance with regions of zero velocity. This relatively straightforward concept is critical to understanding why and how resonances of the tube change when a constriction occurs at a specific location.

Imagine a constriction placed in the tube, exactly at a location of maximum pressure (and, therefore, zero velocity of air molecule movement). This situation is schematized in Figure 7–15A, which shows the three-quarters wavelength distribution of pressure associated with the second resonance. There is a maximum pressure at the closed end of the tube, and one about two-thirds of the way toward the open end (the maximum pressures are shown here on both the positive and negative sides, emphasizing the importance of the *absolute* maximum, rather than the sign of the pressure). The tube has been constricted at this latter pressure maximum (arrow, Figure 7–15A). What is the effect, if any, of this con-

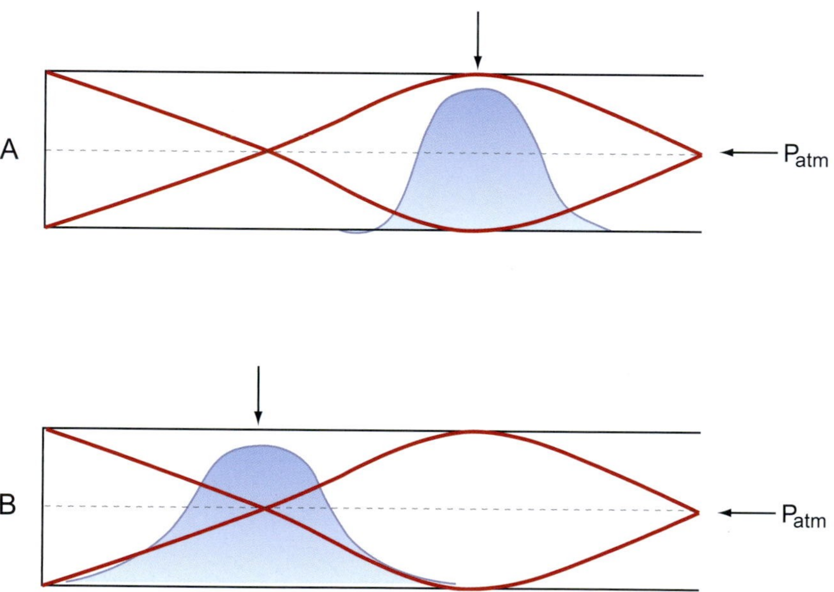

Figure 7–15. A. Tube closed at one end showing the three-quarter-wavelength distribution of pressure associated with the second resonance. A constriction is placed in the tube at the pressure maximum (*arrow*), about two-thirds of the way toward the open end. **B.** Same tube and pressure distribution as in A, but with the constriction positioned farther back in the tube, at a location where pressure = 0 and velocity, therefore, is maximum. Pressure distributions are shown as both positive and negative, emphasizing the maximum pressure locations regardless of sign.

striction on the air vibrating within the tube? The constriction in the region of maximum pressure compresses the air molecules even more, forcing them farther from their rest positions. As air molecules (or any elastic object) are displaced farther from their rest positions, they become stiffer. Thus, a constriction in a region of maximum pressure increases the stiffness of the air molecules. Increased stiffness in a vibratory system results in a higher resonant frequency, which is exactly what happens in this example. The second resonance of the tube in Figure 7–15A, with a constriction placed at a maximum pressure region along its wavelength, increases in frequency relative to the case when the tube has no constrictions. Stated otherwise, if the length of an unconstricted tube is known, the second resonance (symbolized here as f_{r2}) can be computed as $f_{r2} = (3) * c/4l$. When a constriction is placed at a region of maximum pressure, the second resonance increases relative to the value computed for the unconstricted tube. In this sense, the resonances of the unconstricted tube are reference frequencies, and the frequencies of constricted tubes can be regarded as deviations from these reference values.

What happens if the constriction is moved back in the tube to where the pressure is zero (P_{atm}) and velocity is maximum (Figure 7–15B)? In the region of the tube where velocity is maximum, the air molecules are moving at top speed. To attain that top speed, the molecules will have to undergo substantial acceleration. As described in Chapter 6, objects with mass (like air) demonstrate inertia, which is an opposition to acceleration and deceleration. When air molecules are flowing through a tube and encounter a constriction they speed up, increasing their effective mass at the point of constriction. The effective mass is increased because the maximum velocities are increased at the constriction, and the inertia of the molecules becomes greater with the requirement to accelerate to higher velocities. The narrower the constriction, the higher the velocities of the air molecules and hence the greater the inertial effects. This is the explanation for the increased acoustic mass of Helmholtz resonators with narrower necks. Logic would suggest, then, that when a constriction is placed at a point of velocity maximum (pressure minimum) the tube resonance in question decreases relative to the case when the tube is unconstricted. This is because a constriction in the region of a velocity maximum has the effect of increasing the acoustic mass, which will lower the resonant frequency of a vibratory system. Thus, the second resonance of the tube in Figure 7–15B shows a decreased frequency when the constriction is placed at a velocity maximum.

The examples given in Figure 7–15 make use of the pressure (or its mirror image, velocity) distribution only for the second resonance of a tube closed at one end, but the principles can be generalized to the pressure (or velocity) distributions of all tube resonances. The principles, and some subprinciples, are as follows:

1. A constriction located at a pressure maximum raises the frequency of the resonance whose wavelength "carries" the pressure maximum. This is because the constriction increases the stiffness of the air along that wavelength.
   a. The greater the degree of the constriction at a pressure maximum, the stiffer the air molecules become and, therefore, the greater the increase in the resonant frequency (tighter constrictions at pressure maxima will result in greater increases in the resonant frequency).
2. A constriction located at a velocity maximum lowers the frequency of the resonance whose wavelength "carries" the velocity maximum. This is because the constriction increases the acoustic mass of the air along that wavelength.
   a. The greater the degree of the constriction at a velocity maximum, the more inertive are the moving air molecules and, therefore, the greater the decrease in the resonant frequency (tighter constrictions at velocity maxima will result in greater decreases in the resonant frequency).
3. A constriction between a pressure or velocity maximum changes the frequency of the relevant resonance according to the relative magnitudes of the pressure and velocity at the point of constriction. Thus, a constriction at a point where the pressure is above P_{atm}, but not maximum, may increase or decrease the resonant frequency, depending on the actual magnitudes of the pressures and velocities at that point in the tube. In other words, the effects of constrictions on resonant frequencies are continuous (i.e., they do not apply only at pressure or velocity maxima).

In principles 1 and 2, the phrase "whose wavelength *carries* the pressure (velocity) maximum . . . " is important, because the constrictions shown in Figure 7–15 affect only the second resonance (because it is that resonance's pressure and/or velocity maximums that are being constricted). The effects of the constrictions are always specific to the pressure (or velocity) regions of a specific resonance. But the point has been made that the pressure (or velocity) distributions for *all* of the resonances are "superimposed" on each other as the tube vibrates. A reasonable question is: "What happens when a constriction occurs on these superimposed distributions?"

Figure 7–16 displays a midsagittal-view drawing of a vocal tract, below which are three tubes closed at one end. The vocal tract drawing is lined up with the tubes such that the glottal end matches the closed end of the tubes, and the lip opening matches the open end of the tubes. It is useful to think of the tubes as straightened out versions of the vocal tract, in which the right-angle bend of the pharyngeal-oral airway has been eliminated. The top tube shows the pressure distribution for the first resonance, the middle tube the pressure distribution for the second resonance, and the bottom tube the distribution for the third resonance. These pressure distributions are superimposed on each other in the vocal tract tube, but they are shown separately here for the sake of clarity. For this discussion, assume a tube length of 15 centimeters (like the length of an adult female vocal tract), which in the case of no constrictions would yield the first three resonances at c/4*15 = 560 Hz, 1680 Hz (3 × 560), and 2800 Hz (5 × 560) (where c = 33,600 cm/s).

Imagine a constriction placed toward the front of the vocal tract, roughly at the location indicated by the number "1" in Figure 7–16. This is the constriction location expected for the high-front vowel /i/. The corresponding location of this constriction along the three pressure distributions is shown by the vertical, dotted line extending down from the number "1" above the top tube. The constriction falls at a region of relatively low pressure (i.e., relatively high velocity) for the first resonance, maximum pressure for the second resonance, and between zero and maximum pressure for the third resonance, perhaps closer to maximum than zero pressure. The effect of this constriction on the first resonance is to lower its frequency somewhat relative to the resonance when the tube is unconstricted (i.e., 560 Hz), because it occurs at a region of relatively high velocity, toward the front of the tube. The constriction, therefore, increases the acoustic mass, which produces a lower resonant frequency relative to the first resonance of the unconstricted tube. The same constriction, however, occurs at a maximum pressure region for the second resonance. The constriction will, therefore, increase the second resonant frequency relative to second resonance of the unconstricted tube, because the air along this wavelength becomes stiffer as the region of high pressure is compressed. Finally, the constriction occurs between zero and maximum pressure for the third resonance, but closer to the maximum pressure. The third resonance, therefore, has a slightly higher frequency when compared to the third resonance of the unconstricted tube. This is because the constriction slightly increases the acoustic stiffness for this resonance.

In this example, it is important to recognize that a single constriction causes different effects for the different resonances, depending on the location of the constriction and the distributions of pressure (velocity) along the tube. The effects of the constriction are all simultaneous, but may cause changes in resonant frequencies in different directions. Constriction "1," for example, causes a decrease in the first resonance, but a large increase in the second resonance and a somewhat smaller increase in the third resonance.

Example 2 in Figure 7–16 shows a more posterior constriction in the vocal tract, one that might be observed for the production of the high-back vowel /u/. The dotted line extending through the tubes from the number "2" shows a constriction at a mid-pressure (mid-velocity) location for the first resonance, close to a velocity maximum for the second resonance, and close to a pressure maximum for the third resonance. Compared to constriction "1," then, constriction "2" would produce a somewhat higher first resonant frequency, a much lower second resonant frequency (because constriction "2" occurs close to a velocity maximum for the second resonance, whereas constriction "1" occurs at a pressure maximum), and perhaps a higher third resonance.

Example 3 in Figure 7–16 is like a constriction at the lip opening of the vocal tract. This is an interesting case because the constriction occurs at a

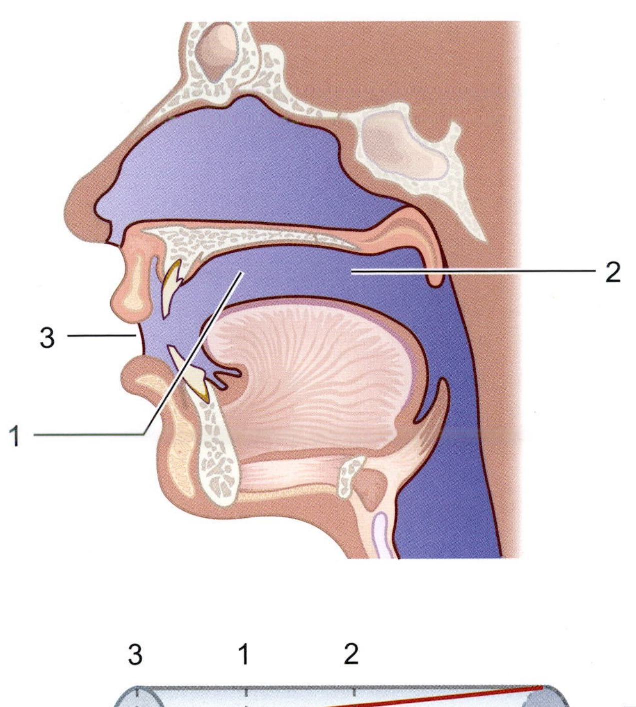

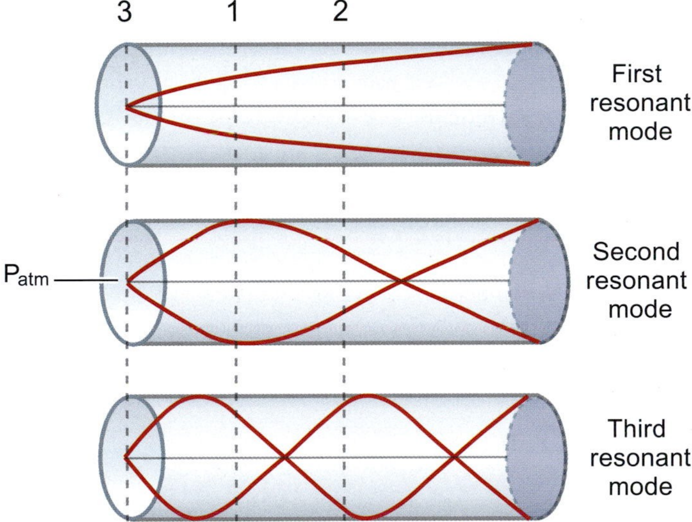

Figure 7–16. Midsagittal depiction of a vocal tract, below which are three tubes showing the pressure distributions for the first three resonances. The closed end of the tube is analogous to the glottal end of the vocal tract, whereas the open end of the tube is analogous to the lips. The numbers 1, 2, and 3 show locations of hypothetical constrictions within the vocal tract and their corresponding locations relative to the pressure distributions within the tube. High pressures within the tubes are indicated when the wavelength pressure distribution is against the edges of the tube. Sign of the pressure is not relevant. The thin horizontal line within each tube indicates atmospheric pressure.

region of zero pressure (maximum velocity) for all three resonances. This constriction should, therefore, lower all of the resonant frequencies, because the constriction increases the acoustic mass for all resonant modes. In fact lip rounding, which produces a constriction at the open end of the vocal tract tube, has the effect of lowering all of the resonant frequencies of the vocal tract. In addition, note that the tongue-constriction effects described above for constriction "2," as in the vowel /u/, may be changed if lip rounding (constriction "3") is combined with the tongue constriction. For example, the slight raising of the third resonance produced by the tongue constriction "2" (close to a pressure maximum—see Figure 7–16) may be offset by the lowering effect of lip constriction.

In summary, any constriction in the vocal tract affects all resonant frequencies of the tube. Because the pressure (or velocity) distributions for all resonances are superimposed on each other when the air in the tube vibrates, any constriction affects the pressure (or velocity) distributions for every resonance. The simple concepts of stiffness and mass explain why a constriction in the region of a pressure maximum raises a resonant frequency, and why a constriction in the region of a velocity maximum lowers a resonant frequency. A given resonance may be affected by two simultaneous constrictions, for example by the tongue and lips, but the stiffness and mass rules described here continue to explain what happens to the resonance when a previously straight tube is constricted.

Vowel articulation can be thought of as the creation of vocal tract tubes with different area functions. The area functions are modified by the kinds of constrictions described above, which result in different resonant frequencies for different vowels. Resonant frequencies in the vocal tract change according to the principles discussed here. There is a lawful connection between articulatory configuration and vocal tract resonant (formant) frequencies.

The theory of tube resonance presented above is referred to as *perturbation theory*. It is called perturbation theory because it explains how the resonances of a tube are changed when the cross-sectional dimensions of the tube are perturbed, or constricted. The theory explains why constrictions in a tube modify the resonant characteristics of the tube. Because the ultimate interest is in the relationship between articulatory configurations and vocal tract resonances, it would be convenient to have a small set of articulatory rules that account for the changes in vocal tract resonant frequency with changes in vocal tract shape. This would be much simpler than asking exactly where a constriction was located relative to the pressure (velocity) distributions of the resonant modes. Stevens and House (1955) studied this problem intensively, and developed a *three-parameter model of vowel articulation* to account for the relationships between vowel articulations and vocal tract resonances. It is useful to describe this model in some detail because it illustrates one way in which vowel acoustic theory was tested.

A Chance Encounter

Imagine being a professional speech acoustician, on vacation in the city of Odense, Denmark, and spending a July day in 2004 visiting several museums. At the end of the day you are tired, but you still have the Funen Art Museum on your list. On the second floor you discover the work of Martin Riches. Riches' art is the creation of what he calls "machines," two of which are arty speech synthesizers! Riches is not a speech acoustician, but he read Fant's book and then created a piece he calls "Talking Machine." Riches studied Fant's area functions and carved vocal tract shapes out of wood blocks, for all sounds, then fitted them with a reed as a source and powered each reed/block with an air supply. The vocal tract blocks are mounted on a "wall," and the machine talks when the operator enters a word on a keyboard. The synthesized speech is very intelligible. Not a bad demonstration of the "truth" of area functions, and pleasing art as well.

The Three-Parameter Model of Stevens and House

Fant (1960) worked on his theory by marking sagittal tracings of the vocal tract into 35 half-centimeter sections from glottis to lips. Based on the cross-sectional area of each of these sections, Fant estimated their effective acoustic mass and compliance. If the acoustic mass and compliance are known for each of the 35 vocal tract sections, then it is known for the entire vocal tract and the full set of vocal tract resonances can be computed.

Stevens and House (1955) created an analog model of Fant's theory by using their knowledge of electrical circuits. The model can be explained by describing several simple characteristics of electrical circuits and components (prior knowledge of electrical circuit theory is not necessary to follow this discussion). The term *analog model* indicates that the electrical model is studied as an analogy of the acoustic properties of the vocal tract.

A simple electrical circuit is shown in the lower right-hand part of Figure 7–17. The circle labeled "S" represents a source of energy that supplies a flow of electrons to the circuit. This flow of electrons is called *current,* and the two long curved arrows around the bottom of the circuit show it flowing both from the negative side of the source to the positive side, and vice versa. This current source generates a sinusoidal signal, depicted in the upper left-hand corner of Figure 7–17, with the speed of electron movement varying between zero (e.g., at the peaks of the sinusoid, when the direction changes from upward to downward, or vice versa) and some

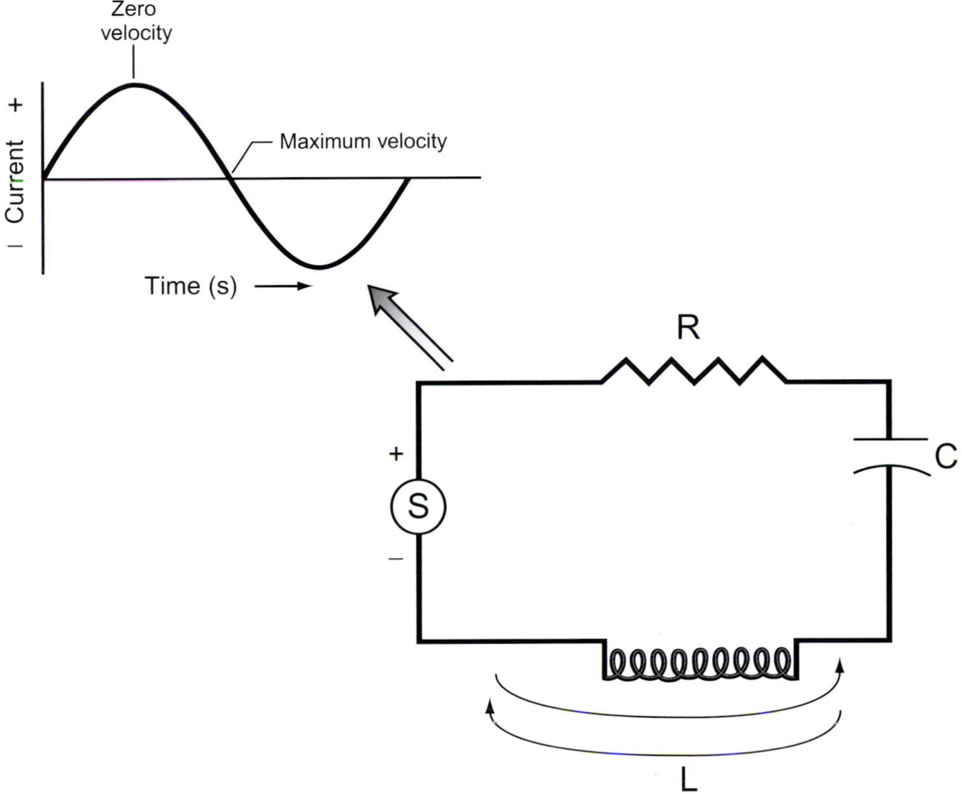

Figure 7–17. Schematic portrayal of a simple RLC electrical circuit (*bottom right*). S indicates a source of energy that produces current in the circuit. Current varies sinusoidally, as shown in the waveform inset (*top left*) of the figure. R = resistor. L = inductor. C = capacitor. When current flows through the circuit, R dissipates some of the energy in the form of heat, whereas L and C react to the current, as explained in the text. Waveform inset in the figure shows how current varies as a function of time.

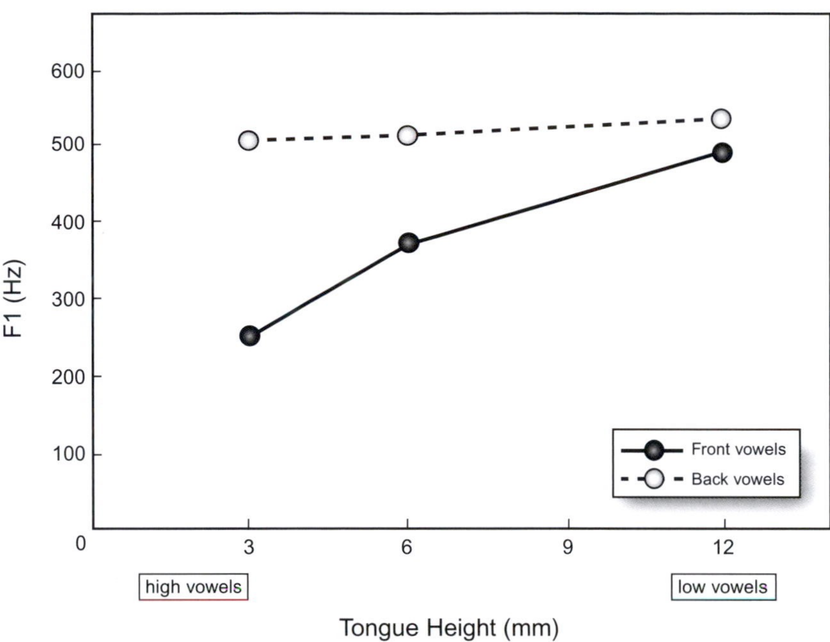

Figure 7–18. Graph illustrating the effect of changes in tongue height on the first formant frequency (F1). Tongue height is plotted on the *x*-axis as the distance between the highest point of the tongue and the palate. Higher numbers indicate lower tongue heights (that is, a more open vocal tract). Frequency of F1 is plotted on the *y*-axis. Filled circles, connected by solid lines, plot the effect for front vowels. Unfilled circles, connected by dashed lines, plot the effect for back vowels. Data extrapolated from Stevens and House (1955).

are toward the back of the vocal tract. There are also a few vowels in American English whose constrictions are in a relatively central location in the vocal tract (between front and back vowels). These would include /ɛ,ə,ɚ,ʌ/. When Stevens and House (1955) held all other factors constant as they simulated constrictions from the back to front of the vocal tract, two clear effects were observed. First, as the constriction moved from back to front, the frequency of F2 increased dramatically. This effect was more dramatic when the model was set for high tongue heights (as in moving from a /u/ to /i/ configuration) as compared to low tongue heights (as in moving from an /ɑ/ to /æ/). Second, back-to-front movements also resulted in a decrease in the frequency of F1. A summary of these findings is that increases in tongue advancement result in an increasing F2 and a decreasing F1.

The effect of tongue advancement on F2 is shown in Figure 7–19. Tongue advancement, plotted on the *x*-axis, is measured as the distance of the major vowel constriction from the glottis. Small distances (to the left of the x-axis) would represent relatively back constrictions, and large distances relatively front constrictions. To simplify the presentation, F2 values are plotted only for a constriction at 4 cm above the glottis (a back constriction) and at 13 cm above the glottis (a front constriction). Filled circles connected by solid lines plot F2 values for a relatively high tongue height (shown in Figure 7–19 by $r = 0.4$ mm indicating the radius of the constriction between the highest point on the tongue and the palate), and unfilled circles connected by dotted lines plot F2 values for a relatively low tongue height (indicated by $r = 0.8$ mm). For high tongue positions (filled circles), moving the tongue from front to back

The Three-Parameter Model of Stevens and House

Fant (1960) worked on his theory by marking sagittal tracings of the vocal tract into 35 half-centimeter sections from glottis to lips. Based on the cross-sectional area of each of these sections, Fant estimated their effective acoustic mass and compliance. If the acoustic mass and compliance are known for each of the 35 vocal tract sections, then it is known for the entire vocal tract and the full set of vocal tract resonances can be computed.

Stevens and House (1955) created an analog model of Fant's theory by using their knowledge of electrical circuits. The model can be explained by describing several simple characteristics of electrical circuits and components (prior knowledge of electrical circuit theory is not necessary to follow this discussion). The term *analog model* indicates that the electrical model is studied as an analogy of the acoustic properties of the vocal tract.

A simple electrical circuit is shown in the lower right-hand part of Figure 7–17. The circle labeled "S" represents a source of energy that supplies a flow of electrons to the circuit. This flow of electrons is called *current*, and the two long curved arrows around the bottom of the circuit show it flowing both from the negative side of the source to the positive side, and vice versa. This current source generates a sinusoidal signal, depicted in the upper left-hand corner of Figure 7–17, with the speed of electron movement varying between zero (e.g., at the peaks of the sinusoid, when the direction changes from upward to downward, or vice versa) and some

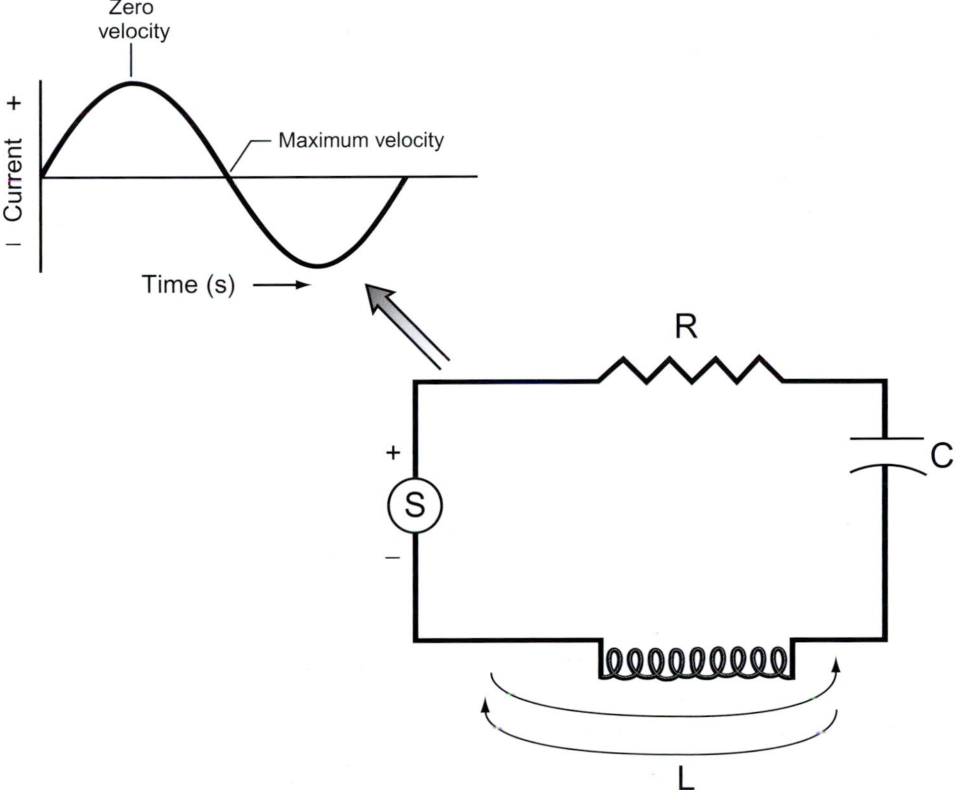

Figure 7–17. Schematic portrayal of a simple RLC electrical circuit (*bottom right*). S indicates a source of energy that produces current in the circuit. Current varies sinusoidally, as shown in the waveform inset (*top left*) of the figure. R = resistor. L = inductor. C = capacitor. When current flows through the circuit, R dissipates some of the energy in the form of heat, whereas L and C react to the current, as explained in the text. Waveform inset in the figure shows how current varies as a function of time.

maximum value (e.g., when the sinusoid is passing through the "rest" position as shown in the waveform in the upper left part of figure). The sinusoidal variation of the current also accounts for the alternating movement of the electrons (i.e., from negative to positive, and positive to negative) indicated by the two curved arrows around the bottom of the circuit.

The circuit in Figure 7–17 contains three components. The component labeled *R* is a *resistor*, whose primary characteristic is to create a certain amount of *frictional opposition* to the passage of electrons through the circuit. Friction, as discussed in Chapter 6, is a form of energy loss in which molecules rubbing against one another produce heat and, therefore, dissipate energy. Stevens and House (1955) used resistors in their model to simulate energy loss in the vocal tract and thus the bandwidth characteristics of the formants.

The resonances (formants) of the vocal tract were simulated by Stevens and House (1955) with the components labeled *L* and *C*. *L* stands for an *inductor*, an electrical component that opposes the acceleration and deceleration of moving electrons. If electrons are moving around a circuit with changing velocities, the accelerations are sometimes very high, and other times very low and even zero. Acceleration is defined as the change in velocity over time, so at those times during sinusoidal motion when the velocity is approaching zero—when velocities have to change rapidly from very high to near zero—there will be very high accelerations. One example of a high acceleration is part of the waveform in Figure 7–17 where the velocity is changing rapidly over time to reduce to zero, just before the waveform changes directions from up to down. The inductor will oppose these high accelerations, which are greater for high, as compared to low, frequencies. Not only do the changes from high to low velocities (and, therefore, high accelerations) occur more rapidly for high, as compared to low frequencies, but there are more such changes per unit time for high frequencies. Note that the discussion of the role of acoustic mass in determining resonant frequencies depended on the concept of inertia, the tendency for objects to oppose being accelerated and decelerated. The inductor opposes acceleration of electrons in the way that objects having mass oppose acceleration and deceleration. The inductor can, therefore, be used in an electrical circuit to simulate an acoustic mass in the vocal tract.

The *C* in the circuit stands for a *capacitor*, an electrical component that stores electrons and offers opposition to the flow of current in proportion to how many electrons it has stored. The capacitor can be thought of as a closed container through which electrons try to flow. As electrons enter this container they sometimes get stuck inside, and the capacitor gradually "fills up" with more and more electrons. The fuller the capacitor, the harder it is to get more electrons inside, which results in a reduction of the current in the circuit. The current is reduced because the electron flow in the overall circuit is partially blocked by the nearly-full capacitor, through which the electrons are trying to flow. Imagine a closed volume of air, such as you find in the bowl of a Helmholtz resonator (e.g., see Figure 6–13). If a plunger is placed in the neck of the resonator and moved into the bowl at an *intended* constant velocity, the air inside the bowl becomes increasingly stiff with increasing displacement of the plunger. Because the increasing stiffness develops a recoil force in proportion to the displacement of the air molecules (i.e., the displacement of the plunger), the *intended*, constant velocity of the plunger is opposed by the increasingly stiff air molecules. Thus, even though the plunger velocity was intended to be constant, the developing and increasing recoil force slows down the plunger movement. This is a fancy way to explain the fact that, with any spring (i.e., any volume of air), the more it is displaced from its rest position, the more difficult it is to move. Note the direct analogy to the electrical capacitor. The fuller the capacitor gets (the more the air molecules are compressed), the more opposition it offers to current flowing into it (like a recoil force). The capacitor is, therefore, an electrical version of an acoustical compliance (the inverse of stiffness), and can be used in an electrical circuit to simulate an acoustical compliance in the vocal tract.

Inductors and capacitors come in different sizes, much like masses and springs come in different magnitudes. As Fant (1960) did, Stevens and House (1955) estimated the cross-sectional area, and hence the acoustic mass and compliance, of each one of 35 sections of the vocal tract. They then used rules (not discussed here) to select the proper inductor and capacitor to simulate the acoustic mass and compliance of each section. They ended up with a device having 35 connected "RLC circuits" (circuits with a resistor [R], inductor [L], and capacitor [C]). The selection of the LC components was a simulation of the vocal tract area function, which, of course, depends on articulatory configuration. The LC settings of the whole, 35-section device could, therefore, be interpreted in terms of articulatory configuration.

This last point, that the model could be interpreted in terms of articulatory configuration, is especially important. Ideally, it would be useful to know the precise acoustic output for every possible vocal tract configuration (assuming a constant source spectrum). For any number of reasons, it is impossible to command a human to produce all these different configurations. But, with an electrical simulation of vocal tract (articulatory) configuration, small and precise changes in the configuration can be made (i.e., simulated) and the ensuing output observed. This is exactly what Stevens and House (1955) did. They changed the model's L and C characteristics in small steps to generate a complete "map" of the relation of vocal tract configuration to vocal tract acoustic output. By using an appropriate, electronically generated wave to simulate the source waveform, and an instrument to measure peaks in the output spectrum of the 35-section model, they measured the "formants" of the model for all possible articulatory configurations.

Based on these manipulations of the model, Stevens and House (1955) offered the following conclusions. The mapping between vocal tract configuration and vocal tract output for the first three formants did not need to be specified for each possible articulatory configuration. Instead, this mapping could be described fairly accurately with just three parameters.[4] More importantly, the three parameters made sense in terms of traditional phonetic descriptions of vowel articulation. The parameters included (a) *tongue height*, (b) *tongue advancement*, and (c) *configuration of the lips*.

Tongue Height

In traditional phonetic descriptions, vowel tongue height describes the relative height of the tongue at the location of the major vocal tract constriction. For vowels made in the front of the vocal tract, the tongue height series from lowest (most open vocal tract) to highest (most closed vocal tract) is /æ,ɛ,ɪ,i/. The corresponding series for back vowels is /ɑ,ɔ,o,ʊ,u/. When Stevens and House (1955) simulated changes in tongue height (or equivalently, mouth opening) the main acoustic effect was on the first formant frequency (F1). Specifically, F1 decreased with increases in tongue height (as vowels went from low to high). This effect was more pronounced for the front vowel series as compared to the back vowel series (see section on perturbation theory on page 394). Figure 7–18 illustrates the tongue height-F1 relationship by plotting tongue height on the *x*-axis and F1 on the *y*-axis. High tongue heights (short distances between the highest point on the tongue and the palate), as in vowels like /i/ and /u/, are indicated by low numbers on the *x*-axis ("0" represents complete closure of the vocal tract, as in a stop consonant). Moving from left to right on the *x*-axis, therefore, represents high to low tongue heights. The tongue height-F1 relationship is plotted separately for front (filled circles connected by a solid line) and back (unfilled circles connected by a dotted line) vowels. For front vowels, the graph shows clearly that F1 changes from about 250 Hz to slightly below 500 Hz as the tongue moves from a high to low position. For back vowels, there is only a small change with adjustments of tongue height, but it is in the same direction as the change for front vowels.

Tongue Advancement

Tongue advancement refers to the relative frontness or backness of the major constriction for vowels. In American English, the major constrictions for vowels such as /æ,ɛ,ɪ,i/ are toward the front of the vocal tract, whereas the major constrictions for /ɑ,ɔ,o,ʊ,u/

[4]Scientists typically deal with very complex phenomena, with many variables, but do not like to summarize their observations by describing each phenomenon and every variable. They are always looking to reduce the complexity of the real system to a few manageable parameters. If these few parameters capture the major performance characteristics of the system, this type of complexity reduction is deemed appropriate. Stevens and House's (1955) three-parameter model does not work perfectly, but it provides a good approximation to the relation of vocal tract configuration to vocal tract output.

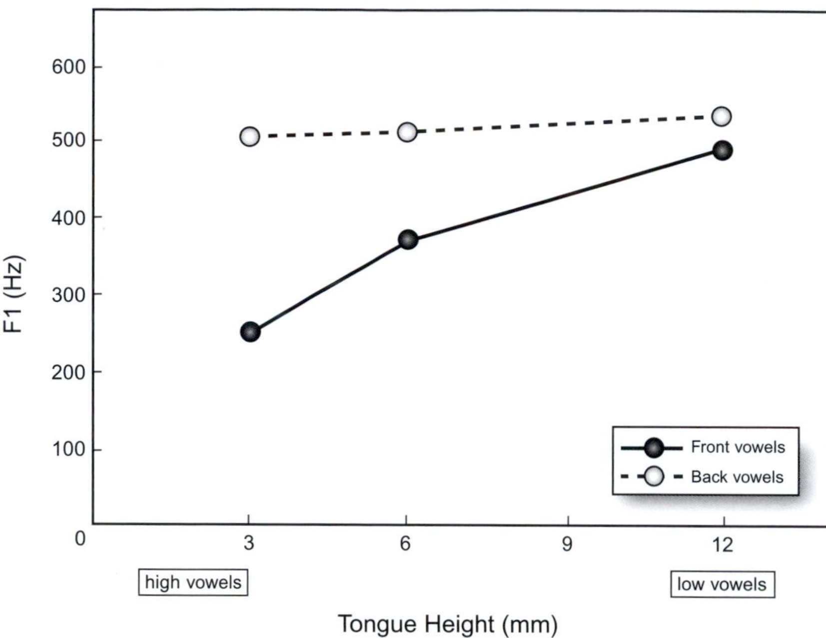

Figure 7–18. Graph illustrating the effect of changes in tongue height on the first formant frequency (F1). Tongue height is plotted on the *x*-axis as the distance between the highest point of the tongue and the palate. Higher numbers indicate lower tongue heights (that is, a more open vocal tract). Frequency of F1 is plotted on the *y*-axis. Filled circles, connected by solid lines, plot the effect for front vowels. Unfilled circles, connected by dashed lines, plot the effect for back vowels. Data extrapolated from Stevens and House (1955).

are toward the back of the vocal tract. There are also a few vowels in American English whose constrictions are in a relatively central location in the vocal tract (between front and back vowels). These would include /ɛ,ə,ɚ,ʌ/. When Stevens and House (1955) held all other factors constant as they simulated constrictions from the back to front of the vocal tract, two clear effects were observed. First, as the constriction moved from back to front, the frequency of F2 increased dramatically. This effect was more dramatic when the model was set for high tongue heights (as in moving from a /u/ to /i/ configuration) as compared to low tongue heights (as in moving from an /ɑ/ to /æ/). Second, back-to-front movements also resulted in a decrease in the frequency of F1. A summary of these findings is that increases in tongue advancement result in an increasing F2 and a decreasing F1.

The effect of tongue advancement on F2 is shown in Figure 7–19. Tongue advancement, plotted on the *x*-axis, is measured as the distance of the major vowel constriction from the glottis. Small distances (to the left of the x-axis) would represent relatively back constrictions, and large distances relatively front constrictions. To simplify the presentation, F2 values are plotted only for a constriction at 4 cm above the glottis (a back constriction) and at 13 cm above the glottis (a front constriction). Filled circles connected by solid lines plot F2 values for a relatively high tongue height (shown in Figure 7–19 by $r = 0.4$ mm indicating the radius of the constriction between the highest point on the tongue and the palate), and unfilled circles connected by dotted lines plot F2 values for a relatively low tongue height (indicated by $r = 0.8$ mm). For high tongue positions (filled circles), moving the tongue from front to back

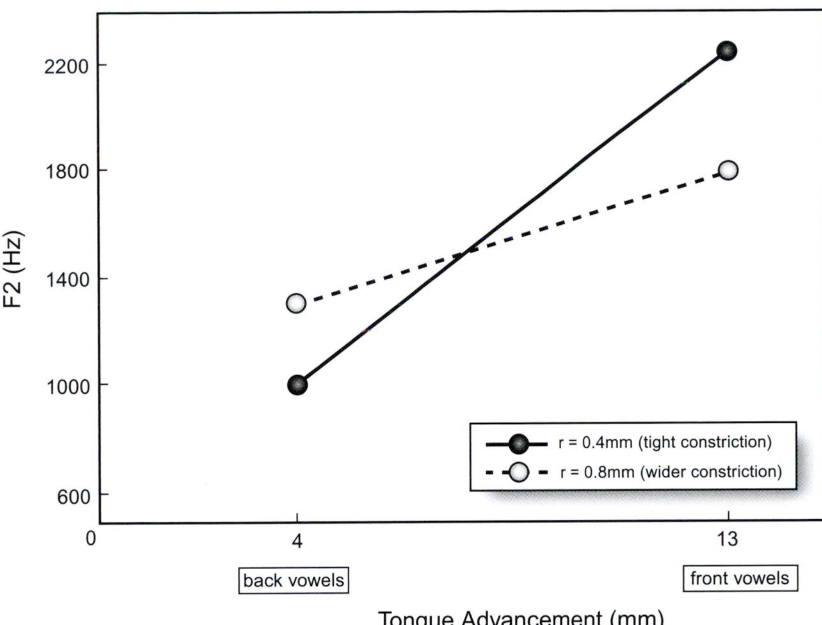

Figure 7-19. Graph illustrating the effect of changes in tongue advancement on the second formant frequency (F2). Tongue advancement is plotted on the *x*-axis as the distance of the major vocal tract constriction from the glottis. Higher numbers indicate constrictions made more forward (toward the front) of the vocal tract. Frequency of F2 is plotted on the *y*-axis. Filled circles, connected by a solid line, plot the effect for relatively small constriction radii (relatively high tongue heights). Unfilled circles, connected by a dashed line, plot the effect for relatively large constriction radii (relatively low tongue heights). Data extrapolated from Stevens and House (1955).

results in an F2 change from about 1000 Hz to 2250 Hz. For low tongue positions (unfilled circles) the same increase in tongue advancement changes the F2 from roughly 1300 Hz to 1800 Hz. For the sake of simplicity, these effects are shown as linear changes (straight lines connecting the two measurement points) but articulatory-to-acoustic transformations are, in many cases, not linear. Readers interested in more details of the complex nature of articulatory-to-acoustic transformations are encouraged to consult Stevens and House (1955) and Stevens (1989).

Configuration of the Lips

Some vowels of American English are said to be produced with rounded lips. These vowels include /u,ʊ,o,ɔ/. American English does not have a vowel opposition that depends on rounded versus unrounded lips. For example, the high-back-rounded vowel /u/ does not have a high-back unrounded counterpart. Many languages of the world, however, do have vowels distinguished by lip rounding. For example, Swedish has a rounded and unrounded high-front vowel (/i/ versus /y/), and Japanese has a rounded and unrounded high-back vowel (/u/ versus /ɯ/). Stevens and House recognized the importance of lip rounding in languages of the world by systematically varying lip configuration in their model and observing the effects on formant frequencies. They conceptualized the lip section of the vocal tract as a separate "compartment," whose dimensions could be measured by calculating (a) the area enclosed by the open lips, and (b) the length of the "compartment," measured as the distance between the front of the teeth and the most forward edge of the lips. Imagine a speaker's face when he or she is producing an exaggerated /u/, with lips rounded. If one were looking at the speaker from the front, the rounding of the lips would produce a very small mouth opening, or area. If one were looking from the side and knew roughly where the speaker's teeth were, the lips would extend well in front of the teeth and the lip "compartment" would be relatively long. When the lips were spread, as in /i/, the opposite would occur. Then, there would be a relatively large area between the spread lips, which would be pulled close to the teeth making the distance between the teeth and lips relatively small. Stevens and House used the ratio of the area of the opening enclosed by the lips (*A*) to the length of the lip compartment (*l*) as an index of lip rounding, with smaller values of the ratio *A*/*l* (smaller area, longer length) indicating more rounded lips. They applied the same principles of acoustic-to-electrical modeling used for tongue height and tongue advancement, and observed the effects of different degrees of lip rounding on formant frequencies. By varying lip rounding at different settings for tongue height and tongue advancement, Stevens and House were able to identify the entire range of acoustic effects due to lip rounding.

The general effect of lip rounding can be stated as follows: as the lips become more rounded, *all* formant frequencies decrease. Because rounding of the lips is somewhat like extending the length of the vocal tract, increased lip rounding should lower all formant frequencies of the vocal tract because a longer tube will have lower resonant frequencies than a shorter tube, all other things being equal. The vocal tract is typically not a tube with uniform cross-sectional area, however, so lip rounding does not affect all resonances equally. The greatest decreases in formant frequencies with lip rounding are seen in F2, with somewhat lesser (but roughly equal) effects on F1 and F3. Moreover, the influence of lip rounding on F2 depends substantially on tongue height: the higher the tongue, the more lip rounding will cause F2 to decrease. The general effects of lip rounding on F2 are illustrated in Figure 7–20. Two degrees of lip rounding are plotted on the *x*-axis. An *A*/*l* ratio of 0.4 represents a highly rounded condition and a ratio of 6.7 a highly spread (unrounded) condition. For each rounding condition, there are four plotted points. High-back vowels are shown by filled circles connected by a heavy solid line, low-back vowels by unfilled circles connected by a heavy dashed line, high-front vowels by lightly shaded diamonds connected by a thin solid line, and low-front vowels by unfilled diamonds connected by a thin dashed line. Consistent with Stevens and House's (1955) general findings concerning the effects of lip rounding on vowel formants, all of the points at the 0.4 *A*/*l* value have lower F2 values than corresponding points at the 6.7 value. If the amount of F2 change from the 0.4 to 6.7 value is studied for each

Dynamic Analogies

In the text, mechanical, aerodynamic, acoustic, and electrical systems have been introduced. In several cases, a single physical principle has been shown to be relevant to all systems. Take inertia, for example. Inertia is a property of things having mass, such as a block of wood. In an aerodynamic system, a plug of air has mass, called an inertance, which has relevance to acoustic resonance. Inertance, in turn, can be simulated with the electrical component called an inductor. The representation of a single physical concept in several different systems is referred to as a *dynamic analogy*. The term is used particularly for the representation of mechanical and acoustic concepts in an electrical circuit, like the Stevens and House model. Dynamic analogies have been exploited to create electrical models of the auditory system, as well.

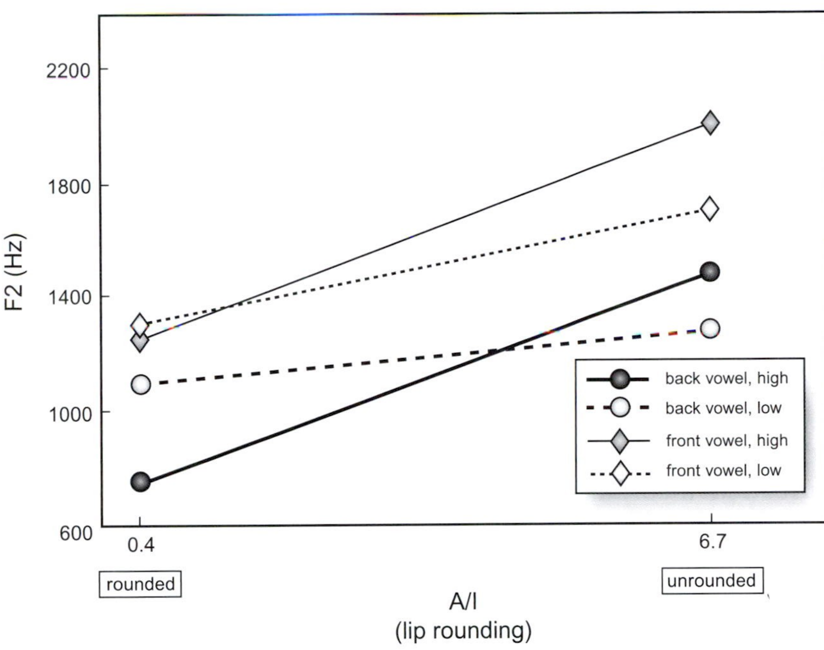

Figure 7–20. Data showing the effect of changes in lip rounding on the second formant frequency (F2). Lip rounding is plotted on the *x*-axis as the ratio of the area of the lip section to the length of the lip section (A/l). Higher numbers indicate more spread lips (less lip rounding). Frequency of F2 is plotted on the *y*-axis. Filled circles, connected by a thick solid line, show the effect for back, high vowels. Unfilled circles, connected by a thick dashed line, show the effect for back, low vowels. Filled diamonds, connected by a thin solid line, show the effect for front, high vowels. And, unfilled diamonds, connected by a thin dashed line, show the effect for front, low vowels. Data extrapolated from Stevens and House (1955).

vowel type, there are clearly greater effects of lip rounding on the F2s of high, as compared to low, vowels.

Importance of the Stevens and House Rules: A Summary

The findings of Stevens and House (1955) are often stated in the form of simple rules for relating changes in articulatory configuration to changes in formant frequencies. A clear statement of these rules is a good way to summarize the preceding discussion.

Rule 1. F1 varies inversely with tongue height. The higher the tongue, the lower the F1. The rule applies more dramatically to front, as compared to back vowels.

Rule 2. F2 increases, and F1 decreases, with increasing tongue advancement. The rule applies dramatically for high vowels, and somewhat more weakly for low vowels.

Rule 3. All formant frequencies decrease with increased rounding of the lips, but the major effect is on F2. The rule applies more dramatically to high as compared to low vowels.

An additional aspect of Stevens and House's (1955) modeling experiment is worthy of mention. The behavior of the third formant was not as easily related to changes in articulatory dimensions (tongue height, tongue advancement, configuration of the

Why Are the Stevens and House Rules Important?

The systematic study of articulatory behavior in speech production has a relatively brief history. Certainly, the interest in phonetics has a solid historical basis, but concentrated study of the physiological and acoustic behavior of the vocal tract did not occur until well after the beginning of the 20th century. The relative youth of the science of speech production can be explained on the basis of technical limitations. Before the 20th century, instruments for direct visualization of some of the "hidden" articulators (such as the tongue, velum, and larynx) were not available, nor was it possible to make acoustic recordings and spectral analyses of vocal tract output.

The seeds for the explosive growth in communication sciences as a vibrant academic discipline were sown in the 1950s and 1960s, a period during which Fant developed and elaborated his acoustic theory. This period also saw the first systematic collection and analysis of data concerning tongue behavior during speech. X-ray motion pictures, a technology originally developed for medical diagnoses of gastrointestinal function (upper and lower GI studies), were adapted to the study of speech production. A subject had the tongue and other articulators coated with barium paste to make the soft tissue more visible in the developed films. These films were analyzed by hand tracing the outlines of articulatory structures on a frame-by-frame basis. In later variations on this technique, small pellets were fixed to the tongue, lips, and velum and the movements of these points were measured by hand from the x-ray films. This approach eliminated the need to trace whole, sometimes poorly imaged vocal tract structures, but still required a fairly intensive effort on the part of an investigator or clinician. The latest development of this technology involves computerized tracking of the movements of pellets placed on the tongue and other articulators, using either x-rays or electromagnetic fields. The automated collection and storage of the moving pellets greatly reduces the amount of time spent in learning something about what an articulator is doing during an utterance.

This small digression on techniques of visualizing hidden articulators highlights the difficulty of obtaining information on the articulatory function of structures such as the tongue. Most of these techniques involve a substantial amount of subject preparation (e.g., fixing the pellets, or magnetic coils, to the tongue), and the instruments are not readily available to practitioners (see below). Moreover, any x-ray technique carries with it some health hazard (there are no currently known health hazards associated with electromagnetic techniques), and the cost of any of these techniques, plus the expertise needed to use them, make their broad application seem very unlikely.

This is where the importance of the Stevens and House rules enters the picture. The Stevens and House (1955) rules allow a practitioner to examine an acoustic record of an utterance, locate the formant frequencies from this record, and *infer* the likely vocal tract configuration(s) that produced those formants. Because of the nonuniqueness problem there may be some ambiguity in these inferences, but for the most part, the formant frequencies provide good information on articulatory positions and time histories (changes in position over time). All this can be done by making recordings of a person's speech, and then submitting the recordings to the proper analyses.

Who are the practitioners referred to above? These include researchers and clinicians, both of whom are interested in having access to techniques that allow them to draw objective, cost-effective, and *noninvasive* conclusions about a speaker's articulatory behavior. A noninvasive technique is one in which instruments do not have to be introduced into the body to obtain diagnostic and or prognostic information, or one that does not create a potential health risk to the participant or client. Obviously, x-ray procedures must be considered invasive, and the electromagnetic technologies mentioned above are not cost-effective. The use of acoustic analysis to draw reasonable inferences about articulatory behavior should be viewed as the most likely technique to upgrade the ability of speech-language clinicians to account for their diagnostic and management observations concerning speech production abnormalities. There is a high level of skill required to make these inferences, but it is the purpose of texts such as this one, and appropriate university-level coursework, to supply the framework for these skills.

The Idiomatic Toolbox: Speech Phrases

"Don't give me any lip," "Flapping your gums," "Jawboning," and "Gave him a real tongue lashing" are all well-known phrases that refer to speech acts. To make their point, these phrases refer to part of the speech production apparatus that can be seen more or less easily. It is probably not an accident that potential phrases referring to "hidden" articulators, such as "Oh, raise your velum, please!" to ask someone to stop whining or "Slow down your vocal folds!" to calm someone, are not in the idiomatic toolbox.

CONFIRMATION OF THE ACOUSTIC THEORY OF VOWEL PRODUCTION

Theories are proposed explanations of how something happens. Fant's (1960) theory is designed to explain how vowel sounds happen, but like all theories it may be false, either completely or, perhaps, just in parts. The confirmation of the acoustic theory of vowel production has taken several forms including analog experiments and human experiments.

Analog Experiments

As discussed earlier, the experiments of Stevens and House (1955) were based on an electrical model of the acoustic characteristics of the vocal tract. Stevens and House were able to get their model to sound like human vowels (albeit crudely) when they selected electrical components to simulate the area functions of the vocal tract. For example, because the model sounded like an /i/ when the components were mimicking an /i/ area function, this was fairly compelling evidence in favor of the theory. If the vocal tract did not resonate like a tube closed at one end and respond acoustically to constrictions according to the principles of perturbation theory, it is hard to see why the electrical model would have worked so well. Many scientists believed that the electrical analog experiments served as strong confirmation of Fant's (1960) theory.

Human Experiments

A powerful way to test the correctness of Fant's (1960) theory is to compare formant patterns predicted from the area functions to those actually measured when people produce vowels. The formant patterns predicted from area functions depend on the "goodness" of various aspects of the theory. If the calculated (theoretical) formants match the measured formants, the theory can be broadly confirmed. A comparison of theoretical and human formant frequencies is shown in Figure 7–22, in the form of F1-F2 (left) and F2-F3 (right) plots. These are very popular plots, where the values of two formant frequencies are plotted as coordinates in a simple scatterplot (in theory, a plot could be made of three or more simultaneous formant frequencies, as a set of coordinate points in three-space, or *n*-space for more than three formants). In the left plot, F1 is on the *x*-axis, and F2 is on the *y*-axis. In the right plot F2 is on the *x*-axis and F3 is on the *y*-axis.

In both plots, the filled circles (labeled "electrical analog") show theoretical locations of F1-F2 or F2-F3 coordinates as generated by an electrical analog of the vocal tract constructed by Fant, based on the area functions obtained from his x-rays of the vocal tract. Fant's analog was very much like the one studied by Stevens and House (1955), described above. These points are theoretical in the sense that they are based on an ability to use the area function to estimate the inertances (acoustic masses) and compliances of small sections of the vocal tract and to represent those with inductors and capacitors in

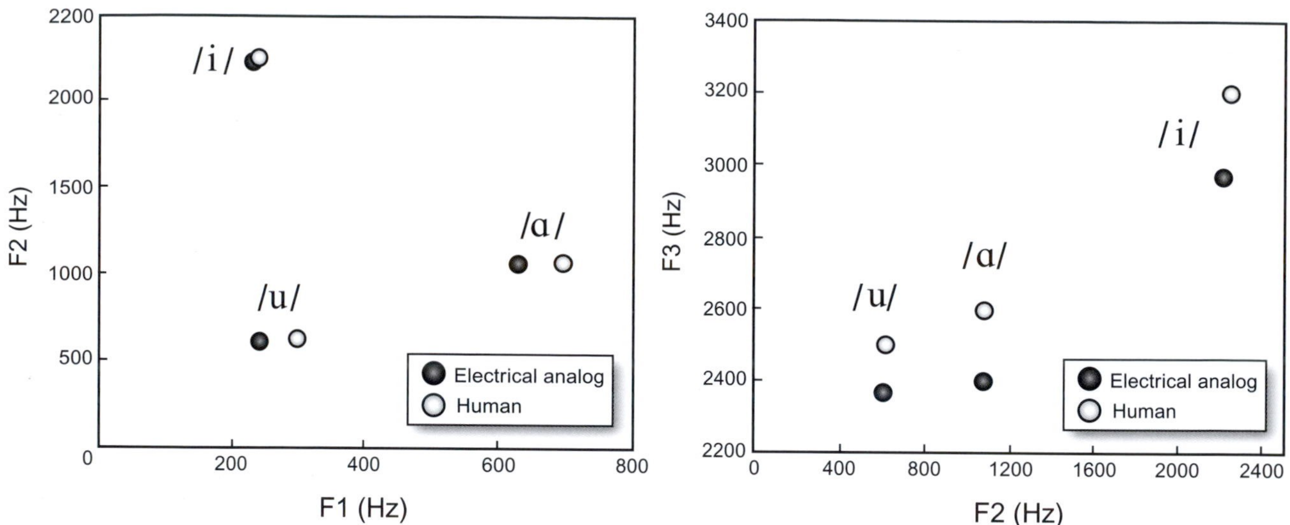

Figure 7–22. F1-F2 (*left*) and F2-F3 (*right*) plots for the vowels /i/, /u/, and /ɑ/ produced by an electrical analog based on Fant's (1960) theory (*filled circles*) and by a human producing the vowels during an x-ray filming procedure (*unfilled circles*). Agreement between the theoretical and human data suggests that the acoustic theory of vowel production is generally correct. Data plotted from Fant's Table 2.31-1 on p. 109 (1960).

an electrical model that can generate sound. The unfilled circles (labeled "human") are actual formant frequencies measured by Fant (1960, p. 109), from the sustained vowels produced by the speaker whose vocal tract was being x-rayed for the study. Data are shown for three vowels, /i/, /u/, and /ɑ/.

One test of the goodness of the theory is the extent to which the theoretical (electrical analog) points agree with the human points. Examination of the two plots in Figure 7–22 suggests that the agreement is fairly impressive, especially for F2. Even in cases where there seem to be differences between the theoretical and human measurements (as in F1 for /u/ and /ɑ/, and in F3 for all three vowels), the differences are relatively small. These data suggest that Fant's (1960) theory predicts human formant frequency data with a fairly high degree of accuracy.

It should also be noted that the electrical analog generates formant measures from the area functions for /i/, /u/, and /ɑ/ that are consistent with the Stevens and House (1955) rules listed and explained above. For example, /i/ is the highest and most front vowel in the phonetic working space and, therefore, has a very high F2 and very low F1. The opposite case is seen for the back and low vowel /ɑ/, which has a very low F2 and very high F1. This is yet another piece of evidence in favor of the theory's goodness.

Why don't the human and electrical analog formant frequencies match exactly? There are several ways to answer this question, but the general answer is, "The lack of exact matches between the theoretical and human formant frequency coordinates does not invalidate the theory." First, it is very rare for a theory to be confirmed by exact, quantitative matches to theoretical predictions. Scientists always expect some error between their predicted (theoretical) and obtained measurements. There may have been some error in estimating the area functions, perhaps deriving from certain inexact measures of the x-ray images. Alternatively, the actual measures of the formant frequencies, whether done by hand or by computer, may be subject to error. Second, and perhaps most importantly, a theory can be correct in many ways but subject to refinement in its details. This is certainly the case for the acoustic theory of vowel production. It is correct, for example, to claim that the area function predicts the locations of formant frequencies, but the precision of those predictions—how close the theoretical values come to actual values—may depend on details that have yet to be discovered, or ultimately, may be unknowable.

REVIEW

The acoustic theory of vowel production has a source, or input (the vibrating vocal folds which produce a glottal spectrum) and a filter (the vocal tract resonator), which combine to produce an acoustic output measured directly in front of the lips.

The source produces a complex periodic waveform whose spectrum consists of a consecutive-integer series of harmonics.

The vocal tract filter, or resonator, can be modeled as a tube closed at one end.

When the source and filter combine to produce an output spectrum, the peaks in this spectrum are referred to as formants.

The formants are essentially the resonances of the vocal tract, which change according to changes in the shape of the vocal tract tube.

The vocal tract configuration for a schwa is most like the case of a tube closed at one end and having uniform cross-sectional area (i.e., no constrictions) from one end to the other; this tube has a set of formant frequencies predicted from the quarter-wavelength rule.

When constrictions are introduced into the tube —when articulatory configuration changes from schwa to other vowels—the formant frequencies change according to certain rules.

These rules can be stated in terms of the location of a constriction relative to pressure and flow distributions within the tube so that constrictions near a pressure maximum will increase the formant frequency whereas constrictions near a flow maximum will decrease the formant frequency.

Alternatively, the rules can be stated in articulatory terms as described by Stevens and House (1955), which include (a) tongue height, (b) tongue advancement, and (c) configuration of the lips.

Such terms are consistent with traditional descriptions of vowel articulation.

Increases in tongue height (higher tongue heights) result in decreases in F1, increases in tongue advancement (moving the tongue from back to front) result in increases in F2 and decreases in F1, and increased lip rounding decreases all formant frequencies but most notably F2.

The lawfulness of the relations between articulatory configuration for vowels and the formant frequencies of the vocal tract acoustic output make it possible to infer articulatory behavior from just the acoustic analysis, without need for direct examination of articulators such as the tongue.

REFERENCES

Chiba, T., & Kajiyama, M. (1941). *The vowel: Its nature and structure.* Tokyo: Tokyo-Kaiseikan.

Fant, G. (1960). *Acoustic theory of speech production.* Hague, Netherlands: Mouton.

Fant, G. (1979). Glottal source and excitation analysis. *Speech Transmission Laboratory—Quarterly Progress and Status Report, 1,* 85–107.

Fant, G. (1982). Preliminaries to the analysis of the human voice source. *Speech Transmission Laboratory—Quarterly Progress and Status Report, 4,* 1–27.

Fant, G. (1986). Glottal flow: Models and interactions. *Journal of Phonetics, 14,* 393–399.

Farnsworth, D. (1940). High speed motion pictures of the human vocal cords. *Bell Laboratories Record, 18,* 203–208.

Flanagan, J. (1972). *Speech analysis, synthesis, and perception.* Berlin: Springer-Verlag.

Fujimura, O., & Lindqvist, J. (1971). Sweep-tone measurements of vocal tract characteristics. *Journal of the Acoustical Society of America, 49,* 541–558.

Kent, R. (1997). *The speech sciences.* San Diego, CA: Singular Publishing Group.

Lee, S., Potamianos, A., & Narayanan, S. (1999). Acoustics of children's speech: Developmental changes of temporal and spectral parameters. *Journal of the Acoustical Society of America, 105,* 1455–1468.

Stevens, K. (1989). On the quantal nature of speech. *Journal of Phonetics, 17,* 3–46.

Stevens, K. (1998). *Acoustic phonetics.* Cambridge, MA: MIT Press.

Stevens, K., & House, A. (1955). Development of a quantitative description of vowel articulation. *Journal of the Acoustical Society of America, 27,* 484–493.

Story, B. (2005). A parametric model of the vocal tract area function for vowel and consonant simulation. *Journal of the Acoustical Society of America, 117,* 3231–3254.

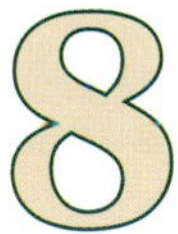

Theory of Consonant Acoustics

INTRODUCTION

Chapter 7 showed how fairly simple concepts from basic acoustics are put together to construct a theory of vowel acoustics. Essentially, the theory can be viewed as a combination of the following concepts: (a) input signals, (b) resonance and resonators, and (c) output signals. These concepts were developed in Chapter 6. As stated in Chapter 7, the basic theory was presented for the case of vowels because the theory is most precise and accurate for this class of sounds. There is, however, an acoustic theory of *speech* production, not just vowel production. The purpose of this chapter is to establish the theoretical basis for the vocal tract acoustics of nonvowel sounds. Many of the concepts developed for the vowel theory are applicable in this chapter, but some new concepts, specific to the acoustics of consonants, are introduced. The following questions are addressed in this chapter:

1. Why is the acoustic theory of speech production more accurate for vowels, as compared to consonants?
2. What are the acoustics of coupled resonators, and how do they apply to consonant acoustics?
3. What is the theory of fricative acoustics?
4. What is the theory of stop acoustics?
5. What is the theory of affricate acoustics?
6. What kinds of acoustic distinctions are associated with the voicing distinction in obstruents?

WHY IS THE ACOUSTIC THEORY OF SPEECH PRODUCTION MOST ACCURATE AND STRAIGHTFORWARD FOR VOWELS?

Table 8–1 lists several reasons why the acoustics of sound classes such as obstruents, nasals, and at least one semivowel require some theoretical elaboration over and above that provided for vowels. First, the theory of vowel acoustics is relatively simple because the resonators can be described as contained within a single tube which extends away from a source. The single tube, in this case, is the vocal tract, and the source is the vibrating vocal folds. There are sound classes, however, for which the single tube model is not adequate. For example, production of the nasal sounds /m/, /n/, and /ŋ/ involves two major tubes—the pharyngeal-oral and nasal—which communicate with each other.[1] This kind of arrangement produces certain acoustic effects different from those associated with the single tube of vowel acoustics.

Second, the important frequencies for vowels, which are below about 4000 Hz, all have wavelengths considerably longer than the cross-sectional dimensions of the vocal tract. To make this statement more concrete, consider the cross-sectional areas of the vowel /i/ along the length of the vocal tract. In measurements reported by Fant (1960, p. 115), the cross-sectional areas of the vocal tract for /i/ ranged between 0.65 cm^2 (at the site of the front constriction)

[1]Chapter 4 contains detailed discussion of the double-barreled nature of the nasal cavities and its functional significance. Nevertheless, because the double-barreled nature is relatively inconsequential to the acoustic product, it is treated as a single tube in the present context.

Table 8–1. Reasons Why the Acoustics of Obstruents, Nasals, and Some Semivowels Are Not Completely Covered by the Theory of Vowel Production Presented in Chapter 7.

1. The production of nasals, laterals, and obstruents involves *coupled* resonator tubes, rather than the single-tube resonators of vowels. The acoustics of coupled, or *shunt* resonators, are somewhat different from the acoustics of single-tube resonators.
2. The important acoustic energy in vowels is located at frequencies below 4000 Hz, for which the wavelengths exceed the cross-sectional dimensions of the vocal tract. In this case, only plane waves propagate in the vocal tract and the acoustics are easily related to the area function. Obstruents sounds have important energy at frequencies above 4000 Hz, where wavelengths are less than the cross-sectional dimensions of the vocal tract. In this case, the sound waves are more complex than planar and the area function does not completely describe the tube acoustics.
3. Vowels have a complex periodic source produced by vocal fold vibration, this source being located at one end of the single-tube resonator. Obstruents have aperiodic sources produced by air flowing through and against vocal tract structures. These sources may be located between resonant cavities of the vocal tract.

and 10.5 cm^2 (in the region of the relatively open pharynx). The F-pattern for /i/ reported by Fant (1960, p. 109) for a representative speaker is F1 = 240 Hz, F2 = 2250 Hz, and F3 = 3200 Hz. By applying the wavelength formula ($\lambda = c/f$) to these frequencies and assuming the speed of sound in air (c) to be 33,600 cm/s, then λ1 (wavelength for F1) = 140 cm, λ2 = 14.9 cm, and λ3 = 10.3 cm. Because the range of cross-sectional areas given above will be far greater than the simple distances (i.e., radii) used to compute the areas, the wavelengths computed for the first three formants are clearly greater than the cross-sectional dimensions of the vocal tract for the vowel /i/. The importance of this fact is that, in the case of vowels, *sound waves will travel through the vocal tract only as plane waves*. In other words, when the wavelengths of frequencies are greater than the cross-sectional dimensions of a tube such as the vocal tract, the pressure waves propagate along the long axis of the tube (from one end to the other), but not in other dimensions (such as from the center to the sides of the tube). When pressure waves are propagated mostly as plane waves, the area function of the tube can be used to predict the resonant frequencies of the tube, as discussed in Chapter 7.

At frequencies above 4000 Hz, many wavelengths are shorter than the cross-sectional dimensions of the vocal tract and pressure wave propagation in the vocal tract becomes more complex. The mathematics underlying the theory also are more complex, and more prone to error. Many consonants—especially obstruents, which include stops, fricatives, and affricates—have substantial amounts of energy above 4000 Hz, so the theory is not as accurate for this class of sounds, as it is for vowels.

Finally, the theory of vowel acoustics requires a complex periodic source, described in Chapter 7. The spectrum of the voicing source can be related in a straightforward way to the movements of the vocal folds. In obstruent consonants, however, many sources are aperiodic and depend on complex interactions between airflow and structures within the vocal tract. In addition, some sources for obstruents may be located *between* resonant chambers of the vocal tract, rather than at one end of the vocal tract as in the case of vowels.

In this chapter the theoretical concepts required to understand the case of coupled or "shunt" resonators are discussed. Then, vocal tract aeromechanics in obstruent production are described and related to previously discussed concepts from vowel acoustics. Sections cover points 2 and 3 in Table 8–1, and show how the acoustics of stops, fricatives, and affricates are logical consequences of the articulatory positions, configurations, and movements in obstruent production.

WHAT ARE THE ACOUSTICS OF COUPLED (SHUNT) RESONATORS, AND HOW DO THEY APPLY TO CONSONANT ACOUSTICS?

The English nasals /m/, /n/, and /ŋ/ are produced with oral airway closure and an open velopharyngeal port. Because the oral closure involves a complete obstruction to airflow through the vocal tract, /m/, /n/, and /ŋ/ are sometimes called "nasal stop consonants." In fact, the place of complete closure for the three nasals is essentially the same as the place of closure for the stops /b/, /d/, and /g/ (and cognates /p/, /t/, and /k/). Nasals are, therefore, like stop consonants produced with an open, rather than closed, velopharyngeal port. The interval during which the oral closure coincides with the open velopharyngeal port is referred to as the *nasal murmur*. This term is used to distinguish the acoustics of nasals produced with complete oral closure from the acoustics of vowels produced with a somewhat open velopharyngeal port—that is, nasalized vowels. The theory of nasal murmurs is discussed first, followed by the more complex case of *nasalization*, the term used to describe the acoustic effect of coupled resonators with an open oral tract.

Nasal Murmurs

Figure 8–1 shows a schematic tube model of the vocal and nasal tracts during production of an /m/. Several features of this model are different from the vowel tube model discussed in Chapter 7. First, the lip end of the pharyngeal-oral tube is closed, consistent with the labial closure for /m/. The rest of the pharyngeal-oral tube has been constricted roughly in the shape appropriate for the vowel /i/ (tight constriction in the front of the vocal tract, more open tube in the back). Second, the velopharyngeal port is open, also consistent with the production of /m/ or any other nasal sound. As shown in Figure 8–1, the open velopharyngeal port couples the pharyngeal-oral and nasal tracts. Tubes coupled in this way are referred to as *shunt resonators*, one of the resonators being a shunt, or diverging tube, relative to the other resonator. Third, there are additional shunt resonators coupled to the nasal tract, shown as tubelettes communicating with the nasal cavities. These tubelettes represent the sinuses, which contribute in important ways to the acoustics of nasal sounds (Dang, Honda, & Suzuki, 1994; Dang & Honda, 1996). The source is located at the glottal end of the tube and has a harmonic spectrum produced by the vibrating vocal folds, just as in the production of vowels. All English nasals are produced as voiced sounds.

As in the case of vowels, the resonators shown in Figure 8–1 shape the spectrum of the source. When shaping the source spectrum for vowels, there are frequency regions at which sound transmission through the vocal tract is maximum. Those regions appear in both the theoretical (i.e., com-

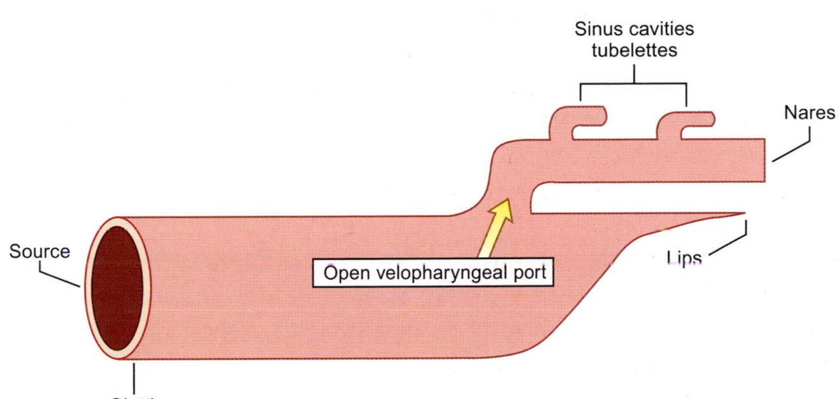

Figure 8–1. Tube model of the vocal tract with coupled resonators. The open velopharyngeal port couples the nasal and pharyngeal-oral cavities, and the sinus cavities are coupled to the nasal cavities. The front end of the tube, where the lips are located, is closed.

Of Mufflers, Heating Systems, and Nasals

The concept of shunt resonators is well known to engineers interested in noise reduction in cars, motorcycles, and heating systems. A shunt resonator traps energy at certain frequencies and reduces the amount of energy radiating (coming out) of an acoustic system. This is why car mufflers are constructed with multiple side branches off the main pipe, and heating ducts often have small, dead-end chambers off their main path. Although nasals don't "require" sound reduction, listeners seem to take advantage of it and use it as one cue that a nasal has been produced.

puted from the mathematical theory) and measured spectra as peaks, otherwise known as resonances or formants. The frequency regions between these spectral peaks, or spectral valleys, have substantially less energy than the resonances because the vocal tract shape does not emphasize energy in these regions. Although the reasoning in this last statement may sound circular, it serves to highlight the primary difference between theoretical and measured spectra of vowels and nasals. In the case of the coupled (shunt) resonators shown in Figure 8–1, there are actually frequency regions where sound energy is "trapped," thus producing *antiresonances*. For example, the closed oral tube shown in Figure 8–1 will shape a frequency region of the source spectrum, but that energy will be "trapped" in the closed resonator. Energy may also be trapped in the smaller sinus resonators shown in Figure 8–1. The sinus cavities are closed resonators. These regions of antiresonance, where energy is trapped because two or more tubes are coupled together and one or more of the tubes has a dead end, can be calculated based on resonator type and size, just as in the vowel theory. Moreover, an antiresonance affects a measured spectrum in several ways, most notably by eliminating or reducing energy in its vicinity.

Because the nose is an acoustic tube open to the atmosphere at the nares, nasal murmurs have resonances (formants) related to the shape and size of the nasal passages. Antiresonances may originate in the sinus cavities and the closed oral cavity. Nasal sounds, therefore, have spectra consisting of a mix of resonances and antiresonances. The concept of an antiresonance is illustrated in Figure 8–2, which shows theoretical speech-sound spectra from Fant (1960) for a vowel (/ɑ/) and two nasals (/m/ and /n/). The theoretical spectrum for the vowel /ɑ/ was computed, as discussed in Chapter 7: the estimated area function, based on midsagittal x-ray tracings of a single speaker producing a sustained /ɑ/, was used to compute the resonance curve for the vowel. The theoretical spectra for the nasals were also estimated from area functions of the nasal cavities, but the process was somewhat more complex than the case for vowels. Sagittal x-rays could not produce a satisfactory image for the computation of nasal area functions, so Fant used a plastic model of the nasal cavities obtained from a cadaver, and adjusted this model to fit the dimensions of the single speaker. The nasal area functions derived from this model were then submitted to the mathematical theory which generated the nasal resonances as well as the antiresonances due to the coupling of the nasal and pharyngeal-oral cavities. It should be noted that modern imaging techniques allow very accurate reconstructions of nasal and sinus cavity dimensions and, therefore, estimates of nasal cavity area functions (Dang & Honda, 1996; Dang et al, 1994).

The first three peaks in the theoretical vowel spectrum are shown clearly in Figure 8–2A. These peaks correspond to the first three formants of the vowel /ɑ/. Note how the peaks in this spectrum are *sharply tuned*, with relatively narrow bandwidths. Of special interest are the valleys of the computed resonance curve. The arrow on the vowel spectrum indicates a valley around 1800 Hz where the energy is nearly 40 dB less than the energy of the first peak. This is a substantial energy difference between the highest peak in the spectrum and the valley, but note that the valley develops between the second

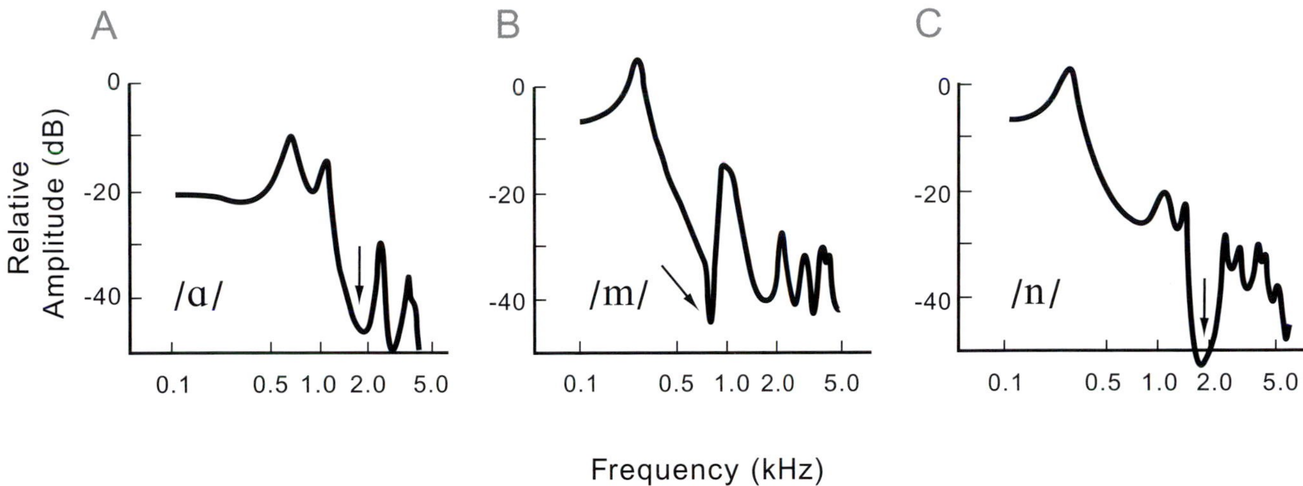

Figure 8–2. Computed spectra based on area functions, showing resonances for /ɑ/ (*panel A*) and resonances and antiresonances for two nasal murmur spectra /m/ (*panel B*) and /n/ (*panel C*). From *Acoustic theory of speech production* (pp. 144, 153), by G. Fant, 1960, The Hague: Mouton. Copyright 1960 by Mouton de Gruyter. Modified and reproduced with permission.

The Sinuses Are Helmholtz Resonators

In a beautifully done experiment, Dang and Honda (1996) used Magnetic Resonance Imaging (MRI) to measure the structural characteristics of the sphenoid, maxillary, and frontal sinuses in three participants. These characteristics included the volume of each sinus, as well as the dimensions of the small anatomical "tube" connecting the sinus cavity to the main nasal pathways. For each sinus volume Dang and Honda computed a value for compliance, and for each connecting tube a value for inertance. They entered these values into the formula for Helmholtz resonators (see Chapter 6) and obtained the theoretical location of antiresonance frequencies for each sinus (remember: the sinuses are closed cavities). Then, they compared the calculated antiresonance frequencies to actual measurements of antiresonances during the participants' production of nasals. The calculated and measured antiresonance frequencies matched within 10% of each other!

and third peaks in a relatively gradual way. Stated otherwise, there is no rapid decrease in the energy along this curve—nothing that resembles a sharply tuned, upsidedown peak in the spectrum. The valley in the vowel spectrum is partly the result of the decreasing energy in the source spectrum with higher frequency (see Chapter 7), and partly the result of the close spacing of F1 and F2 for this vowel (see Fant, 1973, Chapter 1, for information on formant frequency spacing and formant intensity).

The theoretical spectrum for /m/ shows peaks, much like the vowel spectrum, but it also shows what appears to be a reverse, or upside down peak. This sharply tuned, reverse peak, which is indicated in Figure 8–2B by an arrow, and occurs around 800 Hz, is the antiresonance which results from

closure. The sealed, oral tube will shape the source spectrum according to its resonator size, but the energy shaped by that tube will be trapped there because its outlet to the atmosphere is closed. This results in an antiresonance, or a reverse peak in the spectrum. The sinus cavities coupled to the nasal tract may also function as closed resonators and contribute antiresonances to the spectrum of a nasal murmur. Antiresonances affect a measured spectrum by reducing or eliminating energy at and around the frequency of the reversed peak. The energy in the spectrum of a nasal murmur is also reduced because of the relatively high damping of the nasal formants which results from absorption of sound by the extensive surface area in the nasal cavities. Whereas antiresonances are an important characteristic of nasal murmurs, there are also resonances of the nasal cavities, the most important of which is a low frequency formant between 250 to 300 Hz. This formant frequency is relatively constant for the three nasals of English, because the pharyngeal and nasal cavities responsible for the formant do not change shape for the different places of articulation. There are higher formants for the nasal murmurs as well, roughly at 1000-Hz intervals beginning at 1000 Hz. The specific frequencies of these upper formants vary with context and across speakers.

Nasalization

The acoustic theory of nasalization has many similarities to the theory of nasal murmurs, but is somewhat more complicated. As in nasal murmurs, the pharyngeal-oral and nasal airways are coupled, but in the case of nasalization both tracts are open to atmosphere. Thus, the overall output of the vocal tract for nasalized vowels represents a mixture of the resonant characteristics of the nasal and pharyngeal-oral cavities, as well as the effects of their coupling.

When the nasal and pharyngeal-oral airways are coupled, with both open to atmosphere, sound waves will propagate through both airways and radiate from the mouth and nares. Each of these tracts has resonant characteristics dependent on the size of the cavities (and, hence, the inertance and compliance of the air in those cavities). The oral resonances should be roughly, but not exactly (see below) the same as when the nasal cavities are not coupled to the pharyngeal-oral cavities. Thus one major effect of coupling the nasal to the pharyngeal-oral cavity during a vowel should be the addition of resonances from the nasal cavities. To a large degree, this is exactly what happens. In effect, the spectra of nasalized vowels have extra formants due to the addition of a second resonant tube.

There is another effect of coupling the oral and nasal cavities. Recall from the discussion of nasal murmurs that sound is trapped in the closed oral cavity, thus introducing an antiresonance into the spectrum. In nasalized vowels, antiresonances are also introduced to the spectrum as a result of energy trapping in the paranasal sinuses (Dang et al., 1994; Stevens, Fant, & Hawkins, 1987). The main antiresonance in nasalized vowels appears to occur at a relatively low frequency, between about 300 Hz and 1000 Hz. Interestingly, the primary *resonance* of the nasal cavities also occurs in this frequency region, as does the first formant (F1) of most non-nasal vowels. Nasalized vowels, therefore, contain a low-frequency spectrum (between about 300-1000 Hz) having a nasal resonance, an antiresonance, and a pharyngeal-oral resonance (the F1 of the oral vowel). For several writers (Hawkins & Stevens, 1985; Stevens et al., 1987), this resonance-antiresonance-resonance pattern in the region around F1 of the oral vowel is the defining acoustic feature of nasalization.

The low-frequency spectra of four nasalized and non-nasalized vowels are shown in the four panels of Figure 8–4. Each panel shows the energy level, in relative amplitude (dB), across the frequency range from 0 to 1300 Hz. The "zero" point on the dB scale is arbitrary. The blue curve in each panel shows the spectrum for the non-nasalized vowel and the red curve shows the spectrum for the nasalized version of the vowel. The only articulatory difference between these non-nasalized and nasalized vowels is found at the velopharyngeal port. For non-nasalized vowels, the port is closed, whereas for nasalized vowels, the port is open. Note for the vowel /ɑ/ the peaks in Figure 8–4 in the non-nasalized spectrum (blue curve) at roughly 680 Hz and 1100 Hz, and the absence of any sharply tuned, reversed peaks (antiresonances). The frequency location of the peaks is consistent with the typical F1 and F2 values observed in the /ɑ/ spectra of adult males. The label $F1_0$ indicates the first oral

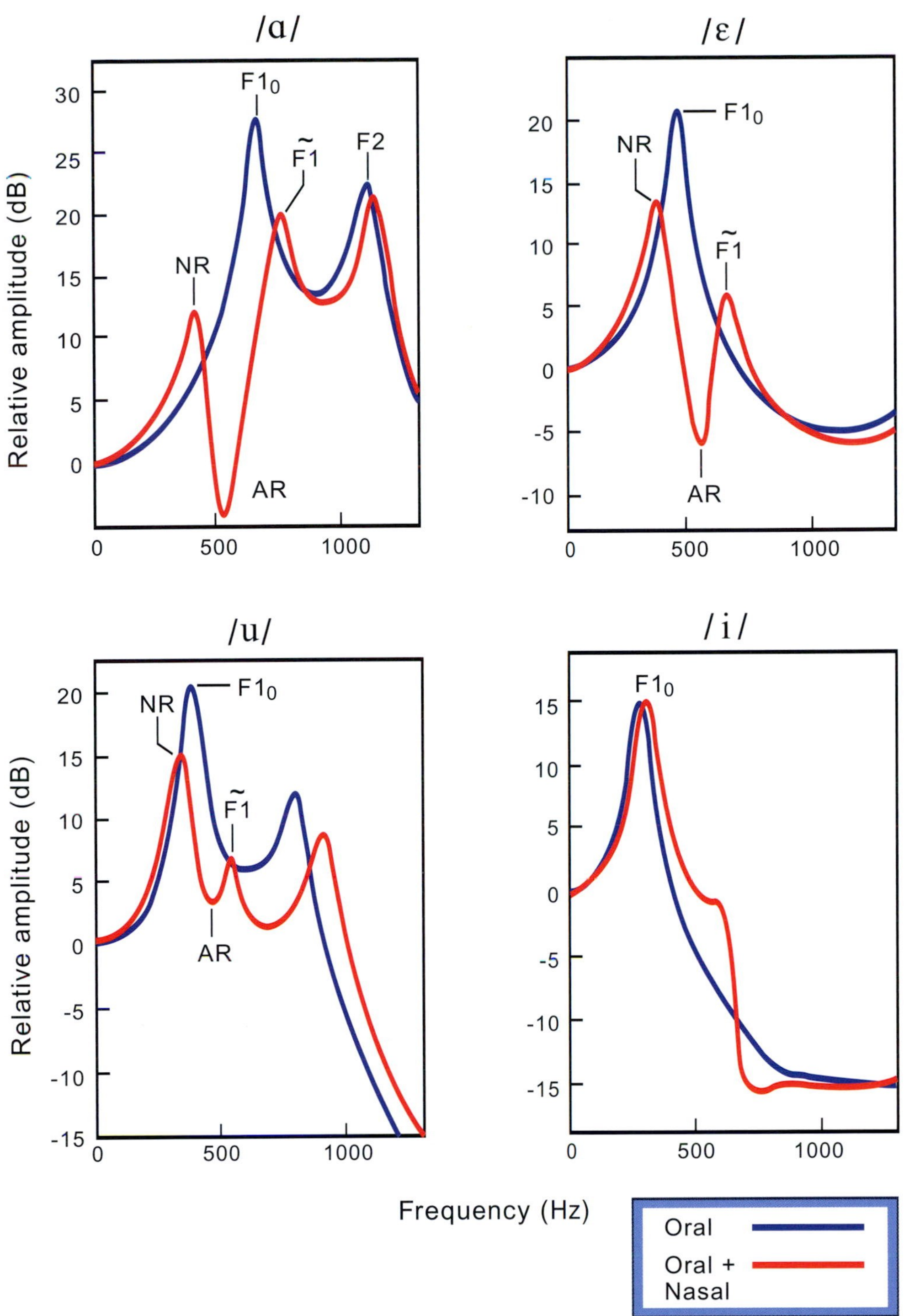

Figure 8–4. Spectra for the vowels /ɑ/, /ɛ/, /u/, and /i/ for both non-nasalized (*blue lines*) and nasalized (*red lines*) conditions. Frequency, between 0 and 1300 Hz, is plotted on the abscissa and relative amplitude, in dB, is plotted on the ordinate. NR = nasal resonance. AR = antiresonance. $F1_0$ = F1 of non-nasalized vowel. $\tilde{F}1$ = F1 of nasalized vowel (combined oral and nasal outputs). For each vowel except /i/, note the nasal resonance-antiresonance-F1 pattern in the nasalized spectra. For /i/, the nasal resonance is canceled by the antiresonance because of the small coupling (small velopharyngeal port opening) between the oral and nasal cavities. From "Some acoustical and perceptual correlates of nasal vowels," by K. Stevens, G. Fant, & S. Hawkins in *In honor of Ilse Lehiste* (p. 246), Edited by R. Channon and L. Shockey, 1987, Dordrecht, Netherlands: Foris. Copyright 1987 by Foris. Modified and reproduced with permission.

resonance (i.e., the first formant) of the non-nasalized vowel. The spectrum for the nasalized /ɑ/ (that is, /ɑ̃/: red curve) shows two peaks in roughly the same location as the peaks of the non-nasalized spectrum, but the nasalized peaks are at slightly higher frequencies than the non-nasalized peaks. Note the label $\tilde{F1}$ indicating the location of the first oral resonance for /ɑ̃/.

The /ɑ̃/ spectrum is different from the /ɑ/ (non-nasalized) spectrum in several important ways. First, $\tilde{F1}$ clearly has a lower amplitude than $F1_0$. There is a corresponding amplitude difference for the F2 peaks (around 1100 Hz), but not of the same magnitude. Second, there is a clear antiresonance, labeled AR on the graph, just above 500 Hz in the /ɑ̃/ spectrum. This antiresonance is a result of the coupling of the sinus cavities to the pharyngeal-oral and nasal cavities for the production of /ɑ̃/. The antiresonance also accounts for the relatively low amplitude of $\tilde{F1}$ as compared to $F1_0$. Recall that antiresonances tend to reduce energy at and around their frequency locations. The location of the antiresonance, just above 500 Hz is close enough to the F1 of /ɑ/ to have a major effect on its amplitude in the nasalized version of the vowel. Third, there is a low-amplitude peak in the nasalized spectrum, around 400 Hz, that is not present in the non-nasalized spectrum. This is the primary resonance of the nasal tract, labeled *NR*, which mixes with the oral resonances and is seen in the output spectrum of a nasalized vowel.

The resonance-antiresonance-resonance pattern in /ɑ̃/, therefore, consists of the nasal tract resonance (*NR*) around 400 Hz, the antiresonance (*AR*) just above 500 Hz, and the F1 in the vicinity of 700 Hz. This general pattern is seen for other nasalized vowels, with variations that depend on vowel identity. Note for the vowels /ɑ̃/, /ɛ̃/, and /ũ/ how $\tilde{F1}$ is shifted up in frequency relative to $F1_0$, as well as the lower amplitude of $\tilde{F1}$ as compared to $F1_0$. In each of these cases, the antiresonance resulting from the coupling of sinus cavities to the pharyngeal-oral and nasal cavities reduces the amplitude of the first oral resonance. Also noteworthy is the fairly consistent frequency of the nasal resonance (NR) for the vowels /ɑ̃/, /ɛ̃/, and /ũ/. This consistency has the same explanation as the consistent nasal resonance in nasal murmurs. The area function of the nasal tract does not change substantially during speech production and, therefore, neither do its resonances.

The non-nasalized and nasalized spectra shown for the vowel /i/ (Figure 8–4) seem to violate these acoustic principles of nasalization. No antiresonance (AR) is indicated, nor is there a nasal resonance (NR). The absence of the resonance-antiresonance-resonance pattern in the /ĩ/ spectrum can be attributed to the small amount of coupling between the pharyngeal-oral and nasal cavities for this vowel. It is well known that the size of the velopharyngeal port in nasalized vowels is greater for low and mid-vowels (such as /ɑ/ and /ɛ/) than it is for the high vowel /i/ (see Bell-Berti, 1993). Stated in acoustic terms, the coupling between the pharyngeal-oral and nasal cavities is greater for low and midvowels than it is for high vowels such as /i/. When the coupling between the pharyngeal-oral and nasal cavities

More to Vowels Than Meets the Ear

How are vowels distinguished in a language? Well, according to tongue height, tongue advancement, and lip configuration, right? Actually, a more precise answer is yes, but not absolutely. In their 1996 book, *The Sounds of the World's Languages*, the great phoneticians Peter Ladefoged (1925-2006) and Ian Maddieson described and discussed "minor features of vowel quality," meaning vowel differences involving contrasts of (for example) voice quality and nasalization. Among the several "minor" contrasts in vowel quality discussed by Ladefoged and Maddieson, the opposition between an oral vowel and its nasalized counterpart (/i/ vs. /ĩ/ for example, as in French or Portuguese) is said to be the most common among languages of the world.

is small, the nasal resonance (NR) and the antiresonance (AR) have essentially the same frequency. When a resonance and antiresonance associated with the same cavity have the same frequency, they cancel each other and their effects are not seen in the output spectrum. The absence of a nasal resonance and antiresonance in the /ĩ/ spectrum is a result of this cancellation. The lack of effect of an antiresonance on F1 for /ĩ/ is readily apparent in its amplitude, which is essentially the same as the amplitude of $F1_0$.

Nasalization: A Summary

Nasalization is the term used to describe the production of vowels with an open velopharyngeal port. The acoustic theory of nasalization differs somewhat from the theory of nasal murmurs because in the former the oral airway is open, whereas in the latter the oral airway is closed. The primary acoustic effects of nasalization are seen in the frequency range between 0 and 1000 Hz and include (a) the introduction of an "extra" resonance from the nasal tract, usually in the 300- to 500-Hz region; (b) an antiresonance located at a slightly higher frequency than the nasal tract resonance, probably due to trapping of energy in the paranasal sinus cavities which act as side-branch resonators to the main nasal cavities; and (c) a first oral resonance ($\tilde{F}1$) which may be slightly higher in frequency than the non-nasalized F1 ($F1_0$) and is usually of lesser amplitude than the non-nasalized F1. The reduction of F1 amplitude is due to the nearby antiresonance. Because of the reduction in $\tilde{F}1$ amplitude, nasalized vowels will typically have less overall amplitude than corresponding non-nasalized vowels.

The Importance of Understanding Nasalization

Why is nasalization important (see Stevens et al., 1987)? First, when English vowels are articulated either before or after nasals, some portion of the vowel is produced with an open velopharyngeal port. Even though the vowels of English are described as being non-nasal, and, therefore, produced with a closed velopharyngeal port, the open velopharyngeal port required for the nasal consonant will "spread" an acoustic effect to adjacent vowels. This spreading of articulatory (and, therefore, acoustic) characteristics from one type of segment to another is called *coarticulation*, as discussed in Chapter 5. For example, the open velopharyngeal port of the nasal murmur cannot be closed instantaneously for the articulation of a following vowel. Thus, a vowel following a nasal consonant will be nasalized for a brief period of time, during which the output of the vocal tract will reflect the effects of combined oral and nasal acoustics. Similarly, a vowel preceding a nasal consonant will be nasalized for a certain period of time when the velopharyngeal port is opened prior to the oral articulation of the nasal murmur. This opening of the velopharyngeal port during the vowel is often thought to reflect anticipation of the articulatory requirements of the nasal murmur. These coarticulatory effects of nasalization may serve as important cues to phonetic perception (that is, the presence of an upcoming nasal), even though there is no contrast in English between nasalized and non-nasalized vowels.

The second reason for understanding nasalization is suggested by the closing statement of the preceding paragraph. Whereas English does not have a *phonemic* opposition for nasalized and non-nasalized vowels, such contrasts are phonemic in languages such as French and Hindi (a language spoken in northern India). A comprehensive theory of speech acoustics should be able to explain the acoustic basis of sound systems for many (if not all) languages of the world, not just English.

A third reason for considering an acoustic theory of nasalization is the more practical one of children and adults with structural or neurological disorders that prevent the decoupling of the pharyngeal-oral and nasal cavities in speech production. Craniofacial anomalies, seen in many different syndromes, often involve structural deficits in the velopharyngeal port area which make velopharyngeal closure impossible or inadequate. Many different neurological diseases cause *dysarthria*, which affects the ability of the muscles of the speech production apparatus to function properly. A typical sign in many cases of dysarthria is chronic or intermittent hypernasality, sometimes similar to that seen in craniofacial anomalies. Regardless of the cause of inadequate or absent velopharyngeal closure, the effect will be the same, the chronic or intermittent nasalization of vowels (as well as additional effects on consonant production and acoustics). Speech-language pathologists should know the theory of nasalization as part of their basic scientific knowledge and as a foundation for diagnostic, prognostic, and management plans and statements. A speech-language pathologist who understands the acoustics of nasalization will be able to provide a coherent account to other health care professionals, such as physicians, as to why the speech of a child with a repaired cleft palate, but lingering velopharyngeal inadequacy, produces "muffled" and soft speech. The extra absorption of sound energy in the nasal cavities and the presence of antiresonances from the sinus cavities widen the bandwidths and reduce the overall amplitude of the sound, respectively, producing the muffled, soft speech quality referred to above.

Coupled (Shunt) Resonators in the Production of Lateral Sounds

Figure 8–5A shows a tracing from a midsagittal x-ray of a speaker producing an /l/. Note the con-

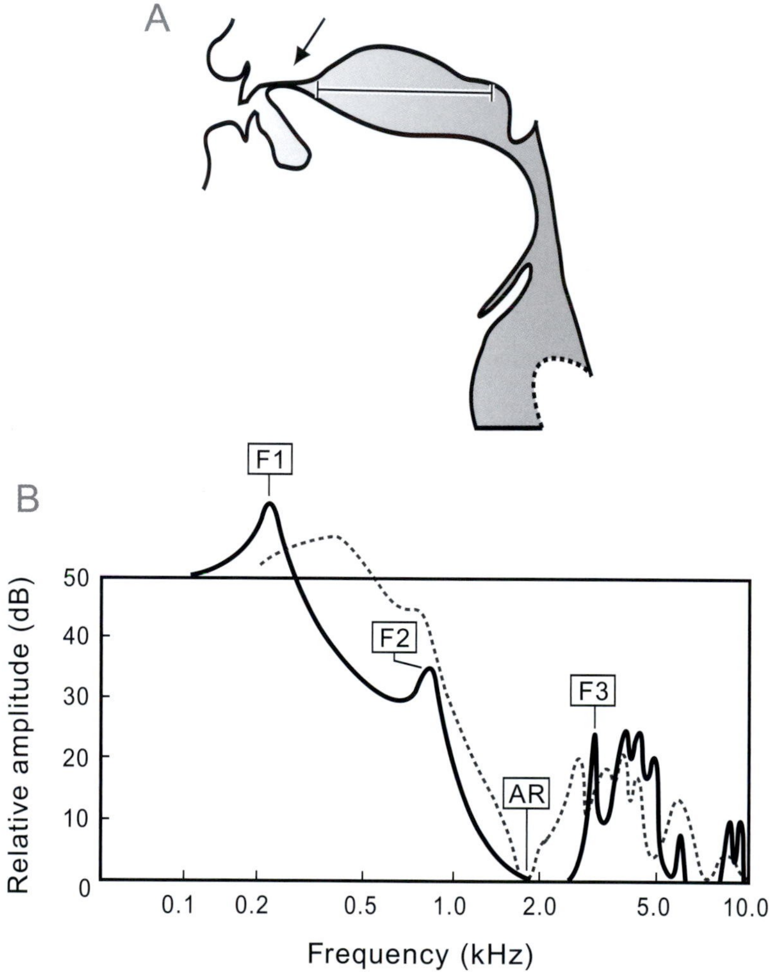

Figure 8–5. A. Midsagittal x-ray tracing of a lateral /l/ production. The contact of the tongue apex to the alveolar ridge is indicated by an arrow. The cavity where energy is trapped, thus introducing an antiresonance into the /l/ spectrum, is indicated by the horizontal line ending in short vertical bars. **B.** Theoretical (*solid line*) and measured (*dotted line*) spectra for lateralized /l/. Note the antiresonance (AR) in both the theoretical and measured spectra around 1800 to 2000 Hz. F1, F2, and F3 are indicated on the theoretical spectrum. From *Acoustic theory of speech production* (pp. 163, 165), by G. Fant, The Hague: Mouton. Copyright 1960 by Mouton de Gruyter. Modified and reproduced with permission.

tact of the tongue apex at the alveolar ridge (arrow). This contact is often accompanied by a lowering of the sides of the tongue, which creates two parallel chambers, one on either side of the midline of the vocal tract. This style of /l/ production is commonly referred to as a *lateral* manner of articulation, to denote the articulatory configuration just described and hence the propagation of sound waves through the lateral passageways.[3] The cavity immediately behind the apical closure, however, will trap sound energy at frequencies determined by the size of the closed resonator, and will, therefore, introduce an antiresonance into the /l/ spectrum. Thus, the cavity behind the apical closure can be considered a shunt resonator, in much the same way as described above for nasals.

The antiresonance in lateralized /l/ spectra derives from the cavity extending from the apical closure to the uvula, as indicated in the x-ray tracing of Figure 8–5A by the horizontal line ending in short vertical bars. Figure 8–5B shows the computed (theoretical) and measured spectra for an articulatory configuration like that shown in Figure 8–5A. If the spectra shown by the solid (theoretical) and dashed (measured) lines are compared, both show roughly the same frequency location of the antiresonance, or reverse peak (labeled AR in Figure 8–5B). This antiresonance occurs around 1800 to 2000 Hz and produces a substantial "dip" in the spectrum between the second and third formants. The antiresonance probably has the greatest effect on the amplitude of F3, which is quite low in both the theoretical and measured /l/ spectra in Figure 8–5B.

Coupled (Shunt) Resonators in the Production of Obstruent Sounds

Shunt resonators also occur in obstruent production. For all sounds considered so far (vowels, nasals, laterals), the theory involves a voicing source located at the back end of the vocal tract tube. The production of obstruents, however, involves a source of sound located *between* two resonating cavities. For example, in the production of /ʃ/ there is a noise (aperiodic) source generated in the vicinity of the supraglottal constriction. A magnetic resonance image (MRI) of a speaker producing an /ʃ/ is shown in Figure 8–6. The lips are to the right of the image and the air-filled cavities are shown as illuminated passageways. The /ʃ/ constriction is indicated by an arrow, and in and near this constriction a source of frication energy is generated (see below for more details on frication sources). Just as the vibrating vocal folds produce a spectrum shaped by the vocal

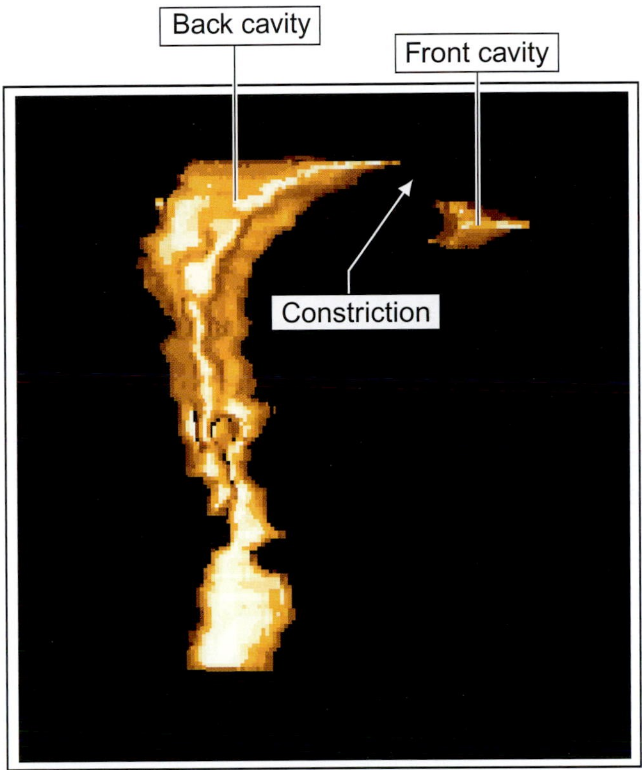

Figure 8–6. Midsagittal magnetic resonance image (MRI) of a speaker's vocal tract in the articulatory configuration for /ʃ/. The arrow indicates the /ʃ/ constriction, which is one location of the noise source whose spectrum is shaped by the front and back cavities shown. The back cavity is effectively a closed resonator and can be considered as a coupled, or shunt, resonator. It, therefore, contributes an antiresonance to the /ʃ/ spectrum. Image provided courtesy of Brad Story, Ph.D., University of Arizona, Tucson, Arizona. Reproduced with permission.

[3]The articulatory configurations for /l/ may not always conform to the lateral description given here. For example, word-final /l/ (as in the words *bowl* and *heel*) is often produced with a retracted tongue and no contact with the alveolar ridge (the so-called "dark /l/" discussed in many phonetics textbooks). Some dialects use the lateralized version of /l/ more often than other dialects.

tract resonators, the /ʃ/ noise source has its spectrum shaped by the vocal tract. Even though the /ʃ/ noise source sits roughly between two resonators—the cavity in front of the constriction (Figure 8–6, "front cavity"), and the cavity in back of the constriction (Figure 8–6, "back cavity")—both cavities contribute to the vocal tract output because sound waves are propagated away from the source in both directions (forward and backward). Because the back cavity is effectively closed, it traps energy at frequencies determined by its size and, therefore, generates an antiresonance. In this sense, the back cavity acts as a coupled or shunt resonator in the production of /ʃ/, and the antiresonance has an influence on the shape of the output spectrum. These kinds of coupled or shunt resonators are seen in the production of fricatives, stops, and affricates, as discussed more fully in the next section.

WHAT IS THE THEORY OF FRICATIVE ACOUSTICS?

Special features of fricatives make the theory of fricative acoustics different from those of the other sounds discussed thus far. These features can be understood by considering the general nature of fluid flow in pipes, and how different conditions within a pipe may change the nature of the flow and, therefore, its acoustic results.

Fluid Flow in Pipes and Source Types

As mentioned above, obstruents are typically produced with a noise source, usually located in the vicinity of the major constriction or at the point where an obstacle (e.g., the teeth) interrupts airflow within the vocal tract. These noise sources are aperiodic (unlike the periodic voicing source), and can be related to patterns of airflow in the vicinity of the major constrictions or obstacles. In cases where the obstruent is voiced (such as a /b/, /z/, or /dʒ/), the voicing source may be superimposed on the vocal tract noise source. This case of *mixed sources* is discussed more fully in a later section of this chapter.

An understanding of aperiodic noise sources requires some background information on how patterns of airflow in tubes are modified at constrictions along the path of flow. Figure 8–7 shows a tube in which air molecules are flowing, as indicated by the parallel arrows. The arrowheads show the direc-

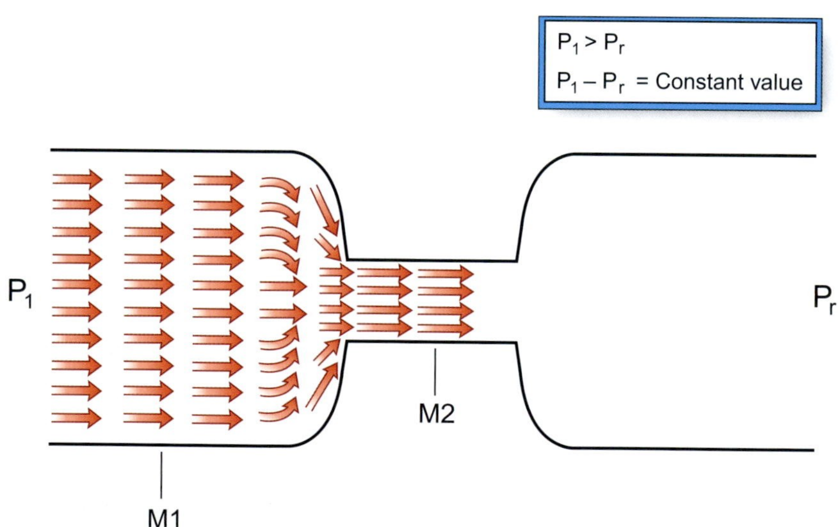

Figure 8–7. Laminar airflow within a tube. Laminar airflow is indicated by the parallel lines ending in arrowheads. Pressure at the left of the tube (P_1) is greater than pressure at the right of the tube (P_r), so that air flows from left to right, toward the lower pressure. M1 indicates a measuring device placed at a relatively wide part of the tube and M2 indicates a measuring device placed at a relatively constricted part of the tube.

tion of the flow. Air is flowing through this tube because there is a *pressure differential* between the two ends of the tube. Air flows from regions of higher pressure to regions of lower pressure, so the movement of air molecules from left to right implies that P_1 is greater than P_r (where "r" means "reference"). The pressure differential $P_1 - P_r$ is assumed to be constant for the remainder of this discussion.

When air molecules flow through a tube in parallel streams, as shown in Figure 8–7, the flow is referred to as *laminar*. If the air flowing within the tube is not compressed as if moves from one end of the tube to the other, the air volume flowing past any one point in the tube per unit of time must be equivalent to the air volume flowing past any other point in the tube in the same unit of time. "Volume" can be interpreted as an amount, such as one might place in a container. It is typically measured in liters (L) (like milk, soda, or any other fluid, air being a fluid) or milliliters (ml).

Consider the tube shown in Figure 8–7 and imagine two volume-measuring instruments, one placed at a wide section of the tube (M1) and the other at a narrow section (M2). According to the law stated above, the volume of air moving past M1 in 1 s must equal the volume moving past M2 in the same time interval. The only way to get the same volume per unit time through a narrow section of the tube (at M2) as through a wide section of the tube (at M1) is for the speed of the air molecules to be greater through M2, as compared to M1. Thus, air molecules flowing through a tube speed up as they go through a constriction.

Figure 8–8 reproduces the essential features of Figure 8–7 and adds two new conditions that have direct relevance to obstruent production, including the immediate case of fricatives. First, the flowing air molecules are shown both entering and exiting the constriction. Second, the flowing air molecules are shown striking a small rectangular obstacle, near the right-hand end of the tube.

As the air molecules enter the constriction they increase their speed, as discussed above. These fast-moving molecules are then "shot out" of the constriction exit in the form of a narrow stream or *jet* which expands as it moves downstream, toward the end of the tube. This jet of air is shown emerging from the constriction exit as a group of narrowly focused parallel lines. Note also in Figure 8–8 the circular motions of air molecules indicated along the edges of the jet. This circular flow pattern, which is clearly different from the parallel streaming of laminar flow, is called *turbulent flow*, or *turbulence*. When a constriction is narrow enough and the flow through it is sufficiently rapid, turbulent flow is produced in the manner shown in Figure 8–8. Because the temporal and spatial characteristics of these rotating air molecules are random (i.e., they are not periodic), their acoustic correlate is an aperiodic sound. The complex aperiodic acoustic event resulting from turbulent flow provides a sound source for fricatives, which have the kinds of narrow constrictions

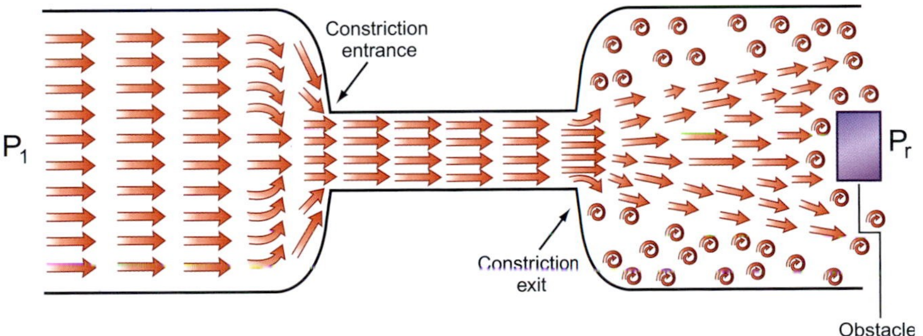

Figure 8–8. Air flowing in a tube, as in Figure 8–7, except that this tube has a very narrow constriction through which air is forced by a pressure differential across the two ends of the tube. Parallel lines indicate laminar airflow. Laminar airflow emerges from the constriction as a narrow jet, at the edges of which are erratic and rotational motions of air molecules called turbulent flow. An obstacle is in front of the constriction and in the path of the airflow. When the laminar jet strikes the obstacle, air molecules move erratically and create additional turbulent airflow.

and high flows discussed in conjunction with Figure 8–8. Just as in the tube shown in Figure 8–8, air molecules speed up as they go through fricative constrictions and emerge from the constrictions as jets surrounded by regions of rotating and erratically-moving air molecules, or turbulent flow. In fricative production, the turbulence generated at the exit of the supralaryngeal constrictions is called a *frication source.* This frication source is shaped by the resonant characteristics of the vocal tract, just as the vocal tract shapes the glottal source spectrum in vowel production.

The obstacle shown in Figure 8–8 produces a similar effect on the moving air molecules. When molecules strike the obstacle, they rotate and move erratically if certain conditions are met,[4] producing a significant amount of turbulent flow. The turbulence in the region of the obstacle functions as a frication source, just like the turbulence in the region of the constriction exit. When there is a sufficiently narrow constriction and a great enough flow (the conditions necessary for turbulence to be produced), plus an obstacle in the path of the expanding air jet "shooting out" from the constriction, there may be multiple frication sound sources. For example, one source might be located near the constriction exit with the other at the "downstream" obstacle.

What is the difference in the acoustic characteristics of a frication sound source with and without an obstacle like the one shown in Figure 8–8? Imagine an experiment in which the frication source characteristics generated by air rushing through a constriction is first measured without the obstacle in place, followed by an experiment in which the obstacle is placed in the path of the air jet. The primary difference in the source spectrum would be a greater amount of overall energy in the "constriction + obstacle" case as compared to the "constriction only" case. The presence of the obstacle results in an acoustic event of greater amplitude (see below). In fact, if the linear distance between a constriction and a downstream obstacle is not too great, the frication source at the obstacle will be powerful enough to dominate the amplitude of the acoustic event.

The tube model shown in Figure 8–8 is a fairly good representation of the aeromechanic and acoustic conditions generated in real fricative productions. Fricatives are associated with narrow constrictions and relatively high airflows, as mentioned above, and some fricatives (certainly /s/, /z/, /ʃ/, /ʒ/) have obstacles, in the form of teeth, located downstream from the constriction, in the path of the air jet.

An estimate of the source spectrum for fricatives is presented in Figure 8–9. Just as in the case of the voicing source for vowels, the spectral characteristics of frication sources are nearly impossible to measure directly, but must be inferred from the study of mechanical models and acoustical theory (Shadle, 1985, 1990). The spectrum shown in Figure 8–9 is not exactly correct, but is likely to be a very close approximation to the aperiodic source spectrum for fricatives. Stevens (1998), based on his own work and that of Shadle (1985, 1990), has argued that a source spectrum such as the one shown in Figure 8–9 is generally applicable to *all* fricatives. This "prototype" fricative source spectrum has slowly declining energy over the 0- to 10-kHz frequency range, with a roughly 20-dB difference between the highest-amplitude, low-frequency energy and the lowest-amplitude, high-frequency energy. In the 0- to 5-kHz range, the spectral energy changes only a little, and can be described as more or less flat. There are fricative-specific modifications of this general spectrum, the most prominent one being the relative amplitude of the whole spectrum. As suggested by Stevens (1998), fricatives with greater source energy—those with obstacles (teeth) relatively close to the constriction—move the spectrum up the relative amplitude scale but leave the basic spectral shape unchanged. Those fricatives with lesser source energy—the ones made in the front of the vocal tract, near its exit to the atmosphere—have the source spectrum moved down on the relative amplitude scale. These fricative-specific changes in the overall level of the "prototype" source spectrum are indicated in Figure 8–9 by the arrows pointing up for /sʃzʒ/ and down for /fθvð/. In addition, because voiceless fricatives have greater oral pressure (P_o, see below) and hence greater air flow through the constriction as compared to their voiced cognates, the "prototype" fricative source

[4]The conditions include the speed of the flow, the sharpness of the obstacle's edges, and the angle at which the flow strikes the obstacle.

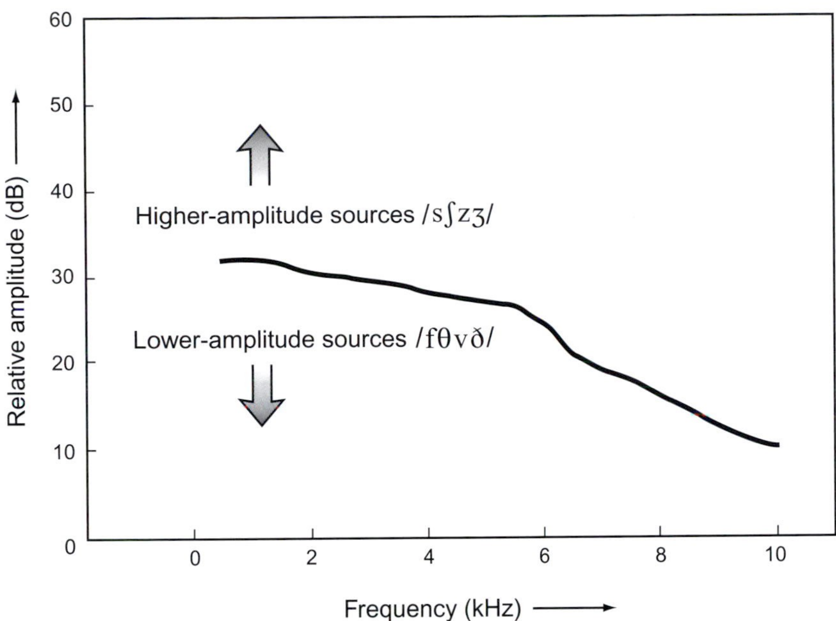

Figure 8–9. "Prototype" source spectrum for fricatives, modeled after data described by Stevens (1998) and work of Shadle (1985, 1990). The entire prototype spectrum is moved up the relative amplitude scale for fricatives in which an obstacle in the path of airflow contributes heavily to the source of energy (/sʃzʒ/) and down the scale for fricatives in which obstacles play only a minor role or no role at all (/fθvð/).

Good Dental Health = Nice Fricatives

Even before Shadle's (1985) experiments on how obstacles influence the aperiodic source for fricatives such as /s/ and /ʃ/, the University of Michigan phonetician J. C. Catford had described a relevant little experiment in his 1977 text, *Fundamental Problems in Phonetics*. He located two people with full dentures and asked them to produce /s/ and /ʃ/ with their dentures in, and with them out. Catford compared the teeth-in to teeth-out fricative spectra and found a dramatic difference in spectral intensity. The more intense fricative spectra occurred for the teeth-in productions, of course.

spectrum is of higher amplitude for voiceless as compared to voiced fricatives.

Actual fricative source spectra may deviate from the prototype shown in Figure 8–9 for several reasons. As demonstrated by Shadle (1985, 1990), the shape and degree of the fricative constriction, the magnitude of airflow through the constriction, the angle at which air flow strikes an obstacle, and the distance of the constriction from an obstacle are all factors that adjust details of the fricative source spectrum shape. These modifications, however, do not change the general description of an aperiodic source spectrum that gradually declines in energy from low to high frequency, and is more or less flat from 0 to 5 kHz.

Mixed Sources in Fricative Production

The production of the English fricatives /v/, /ð/, /z/, and /ʒ/ involves the turbulent airflow events discussed above, but also may be accompanied by vibration of the vocal folds. These voiced fricatives are, therefore, produced with two types of sources —one associated with the aperiodic, turbulent flow generated in the vocal tract and the other with the periodic vibration of the vocal folds. Fant (1960) used the term, "mixed source" to describe the case in which two sources were active in the production of a sound. When a mixed source occurs, as in the case of voiced fricatives, both source spectra will be shaped by the resonant characteristics of the vocal tract. It is as if the two sources are superimposed on each other, and the vocal tract resonators act on them (i.e., shape their spectra) simultaneously.

Shaping of Fricative Sources by Vocal Tract Resonators

The foundation for the understanding of resonances in fricative production has been prepared by (a) the discussion of resonator size and resonant frequency (Chapter 7), and (b) the discussion of antiresonances in cases where sources are located between two resonant cavities.

The narrow vocal tract constriction required for fricatives can be thought of as dividing the vocal tract into a front and back cavity. The source is located in the vicinity of the constriction, or in front of the constriction (e.g., at the teeth), and its energy is propagated in both directions along the long axis of the vocal tract. Both the front and back cavities shape the source spectrum. However, the back cavity behaves as if it is "closed" and will trap energy at frequencies determined by its size (i.e., just as open cavities—cavities that can radiate their sound to the atmosphere—amplify energy at frequencies determined by their size). Thus, the back cavity shapes the source spectrum by introducing antiresonances into the fricative output spectrum. The front cavity, however, shapes the source spectrum by emphasizing a region of the spectrum. These emphasized frequencies appear in the output spectrum as high-amplitude regions, or peaks, at particular frequencies. A general, simplified rule for the way in which these cavities shape fricative spectra is as follows. As the cavity in front of the constriction gets smaller, the resonances of the frication spectra move to higher frequencies, consistent with the idea that the air in smaller resonating cavities is stiffer than the air in larger cavities. As the cavity behind the constriction gets smaller, the frequency of the antiresonances increases for the same reason.

Fricative spectra contain peaks, but they are not nearly as easy to identify as they are in vowel spectra. The peaks in fricative spectra are often broad, extending over a fairly large frequency region (perhaps 300–700 Hz). This is unlike vowel spectra in which the peaks are relatively narrow, with bandwidths in the 40- to 70-Hz range. Figure 8–11 presents

Sound Change

Speech sounds are subject to evolutionary selection pressures. One selection pressure is for a sound to be sufficiently distinct from other sounds so that it can function phonemically. When two phonemes in a language have very similar acoustic characteristics, their effectiveness as separate phonemes may be compromised. The two sounds may begin to merge into a single sound class and function more or less as allophones of one phoneme. Some believe this is happening to /f/ and /θ/ in African-American English, where the two sounds appear to be interchangeable in certain word positions. The weak, very similar spectra for these two fricatives make them ideal candidates for this kind of sound change—well known in the history of many languages.

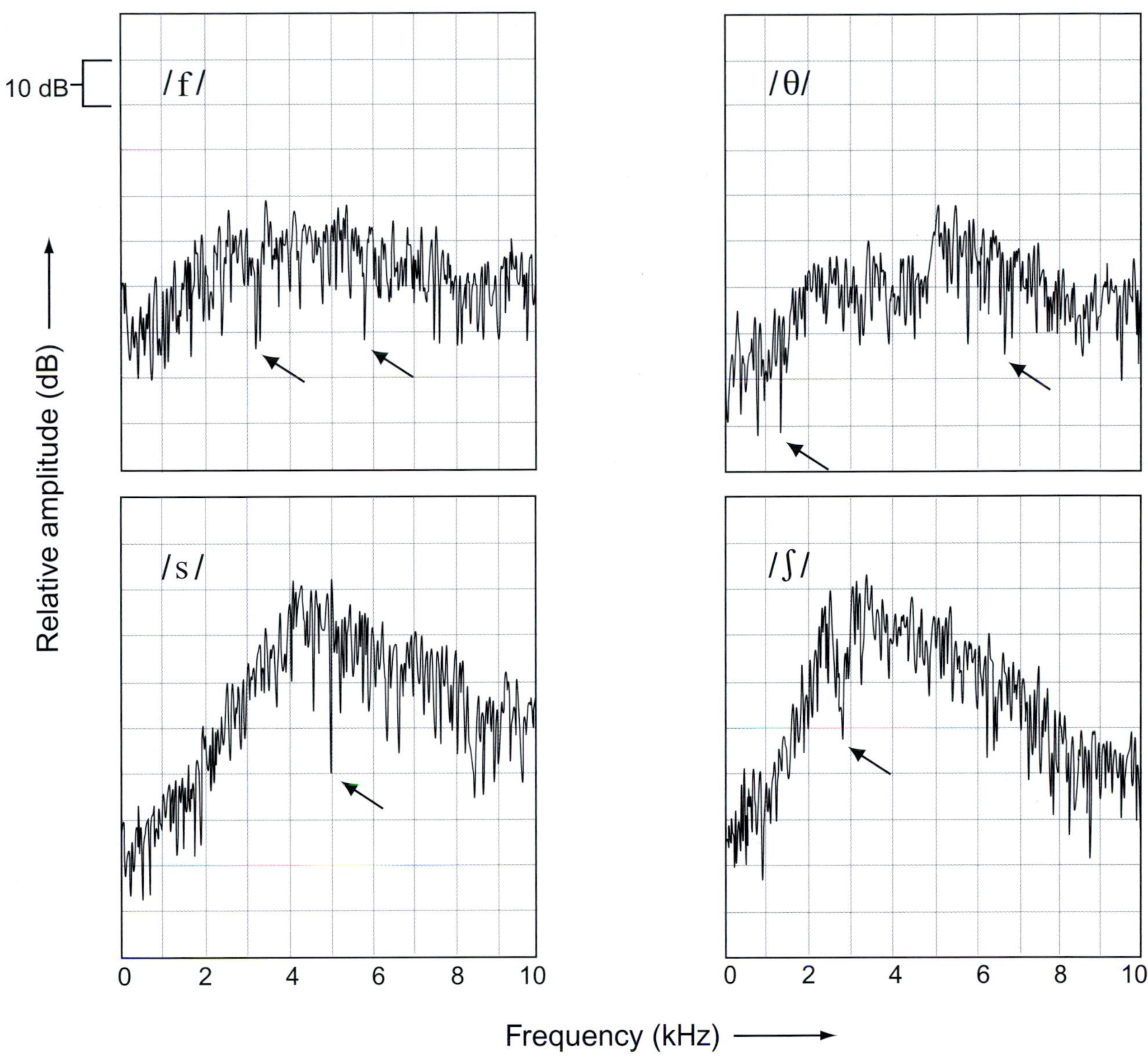

Figure 8–11. Output spectra for /f/ (*upper left*), /θ/ (*upper right*), /s/ (*lower left*), and /ʃ/ (*lower right*), produced by a 57-year-old adult male. The fricative spectra were computed from 50-ms intervals extracted from the middle of the frication noises in an /æCæ/ frame, where C = fricative. Arrows indicate probable antiresonances.

examples of fricative spectra for /f/, /θ/, /s/, and /ʃ/. The fricatives were spoken in an /æCæ/ frame, where C = fricative, and the spectra were computed from the middle 50 ms of the frication noises. These spectra have a frequency range of 0 to10 kHz on the *x*-axis and relative amplitude, in 10-dB steps, on the *y*-axis. The fricatives were all recorded under exactly the same conditions, so relative amplitudes can be compared directly across the four spectra. Both the /f/ and /θ/ spectra are relatively weak compared to the /s/ and /ʃ/ spectra. The peak amplitudes in the latter spectra are roughly 20 dB greater than the peak amplitudes of the former spectra. The /f/ spectrum is relatively flat, whereas the /θ/ spectrum has increasing amplitude up to 5.0 kHz and is relatively flat or slightly decreasing in energy thereafter. There is either a very small or nonexistent cavity in front of the constrictions for

/f/ and /θ/, so the spectra of these fricatives might be expected to have an extremely high resonance frequency, or perhaps no clear region of resonance. In the case of an extremely small resonating cavity, the resonant frequency may be above the frequency limit of the spectra in Figure 8–11 (10 kHz) and, therefore, not visible. If the constriction is sufficiently anterior in the vocal tract and there is no effective front resonating cavity, the spectra may look like unfiltered versions of the source spectrum. Compare, for example, the shape of the prototype fricative source spectrum shown in Figure 8–9 to the /f/ output spectrum shown in Figure 8–11. With the exception of the low frequencies, the two spectra are quite similar. The /f/ and /θ/ spectra of Figure 8–11 also reflect the influence of antiresonances, as indicated by the upward-pointing arrows aimed at sharp "dips" in the spectra. As noted above, these result from energy trapping in the large back cavity.

A comparison of the /s/ and /ʃ/ spectra in Figure 8–11 illustrates nicely the principle of cavity size and resonant frequency. The constriction location for /s/ is more forward than it is for /ʃ/, resulting in a smaller front cavity for /s/. Higher frequency peaks should, therefore, be observed for /s/, as compared to /ʃ/. Examination of the /s/ and /ʃ/ spectra in Figure 8–11 confirms this, showing a prominent, broad peak between 4.0 and 5.0 kHz for /s/ as compared to the peak in the /ʃ/ spectrum located between 2.5 and 3.5 kHz. The probable locations of antiresonances in the /s/ and /ʃ/ spectra have been indicated by upward-pointing arrows.

Figure 8–12 summarizes the relation of constriction location to the frequency location of major resonances by showing a sequence of spectra from a vocal tract maneuver in which one of the authors moved his tongue continuously from an /x/ to an /s/ position, sliding it forward from the back position while generating frication noise. The /x/ sound is a fricative heard in languages such as German and Yiddish (as in German "ach" /ɑx/ and Yiddish "chutzpah" /ˈxʊtspɑ/). The three spectra shown are "slices" in time from the beginning (top spectrum), middle (middle spectrum), and end (bottom spectrum) of the back-to-front gesture. Note how the major concentration of spectral energy moves from a lower to a higher frequency region as the constriction is moved forward. The peak energy in the /x/, /ʃ/, and /s/-like positions of the tongue are indicated by arrows, and are located roughly at 1.5, 2.4, and 5.3 kHz, respectively. This is consistent with the increasingly small front cavity as the constriction is moved from back-to-front in the vocal tract.

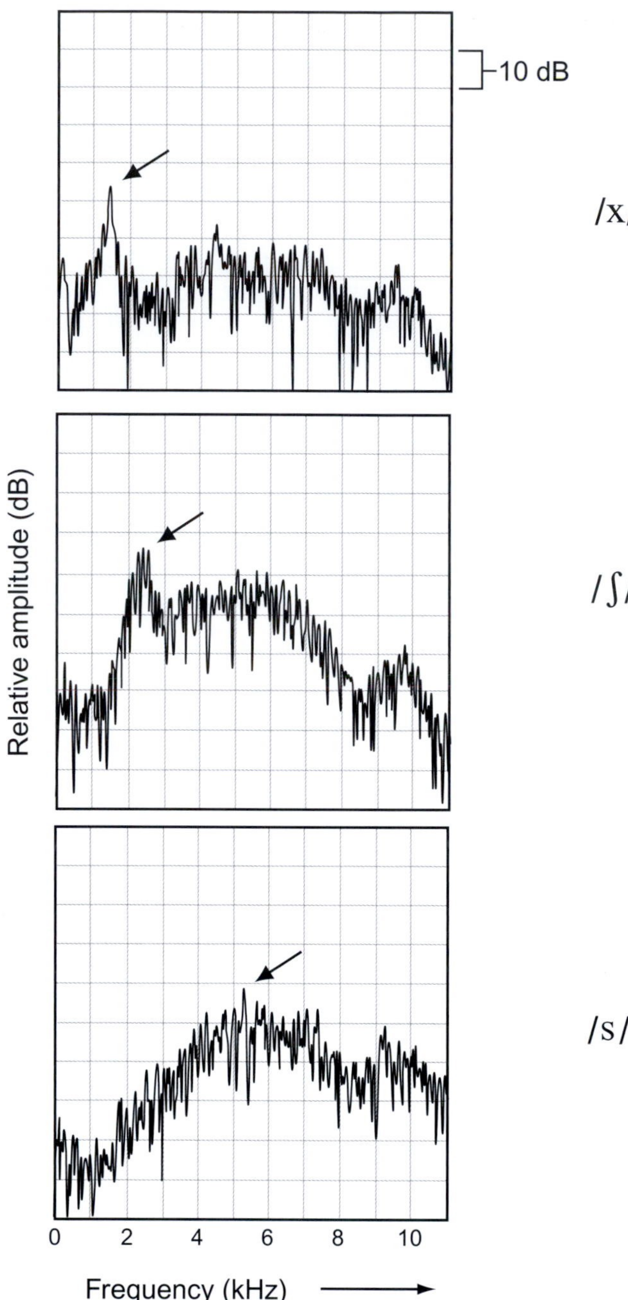

Figure 8–12. Sequence of spectra as one of the authors moved his tongue continuously forward from an /x/ to /s/ position while generating frication noise. Each spectrum is a "slice in time" from the continuous back-to-front gesture. The change in frequency emphasis as the tongue moves forward is related to the increasingly smaller front cavity. Arrows indicate peaks in the spectra.

Measurement of Fricative Acoustics

Both spectral and temporal measures are important in the description of fricative acoustics. The measures reviewed below are used frequently in scientific and clinical applications, but do not exhaust the possible measures that could be used to describe fricative acoustics.

Spectral Measurements

In the acoustic theory of vowel production, the measurement of formant frequencies is highlighted as an important way to capture the essential acoustic characteristics of vowels. The F-pattern (the frequencies of the first three formants) is an accepted way to represent the acoustic characteristics of vowels. Unfortunately, there is no standard way to measure fricative spectra. The goal of a measurement strategy for fricative spectra is to obtain a number, or small set of numbers, that reliably distinguishes between fricatives having different places of articulation, and possibly even between fricatives having the same place of articulation but different voicing characteristics.

Figure 8–13 shows two different approaches to the measurement of fricative spectra, using /f/ (top) and /s/ (bottom) spectra as examples. These fricative spectra are smoothed versions of the ones shown in Figure 8–11. "Smoothed" means that the general shape of the spectrum is shown as a smooth line connecting the peaks of the Fourier spectrum. For present discussion, the spectra are shown in this simplified way to facilitate the explanation of fricative spectrum measurement. The smoothing technique is discussed further in Chapter 9. The arrows in each spectrum point to the primary peak, or the frequency associated with the greatest amplitude. This measurement is called the *peak frequency* of a fricative spectrum. This is a simple and straightforward approach to the measurement of fricative spectra, and is conceptually similar to the measurement of peaks (formants) in vowel spectra. In particular, because the primary resonance of fricatives depends on the size of the front cavity (the cavity in front of the constriction) the peak frequency is, in many cases, correlated with the place of articulation. Higher peak frequencies are expected for fricatives with smaller front cavities (such as /s/), and lower peak frequencies for fricatives with larger front cavities (such as /x/ or /ʃ/). In Figure 8–13 the /f/ peak frequency of 3.5 kHz is clearly different from the /s/ peak at 4.6 kHz.

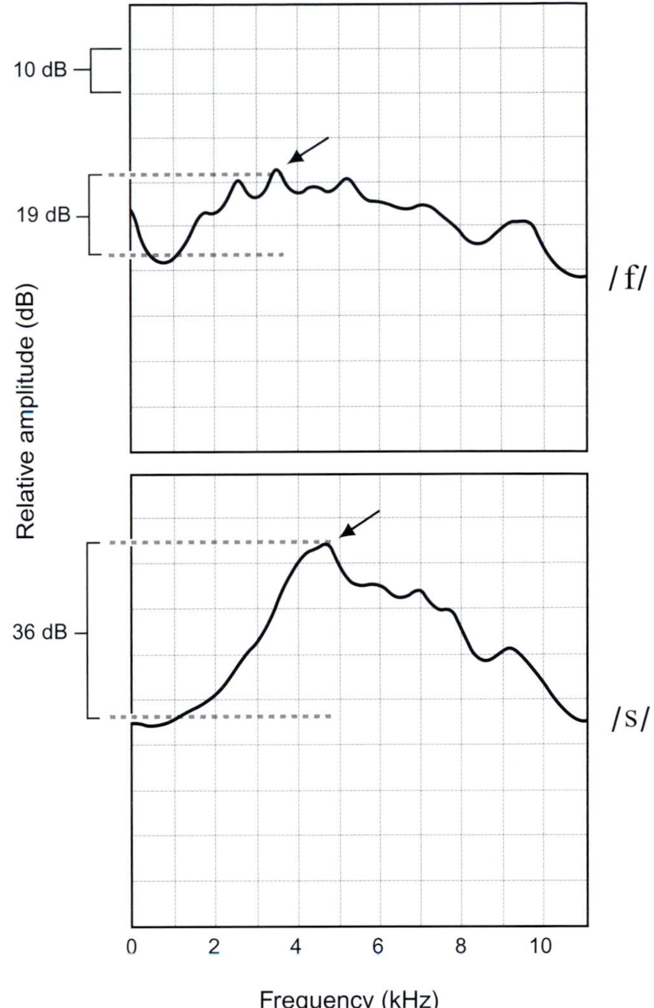

Figure 8–13. An /f/ (*upper panel*) and /s/ (*lower panel*) spectrum, showing two different ways to quantify spectral characteristics. Peak frequencies in both spectra are shown by downward-pointing arrows. Dynamic range of the spectra is indicated by the distance between the upper and lower dashed lines in each panel.

Although there has been some success classifying fricative place of articulation with peak frequency measurements (Jongman, Wayland, & Wong, 2000), the measures are not as reliable in separating fricatives as formant frequency measures are in separating vowels. Many fricative spectra have multiple peaks of relatively similar amplitude, making the use of a single peak frequency relatively unreliable in distinguishing among different places of fricative articulation. This is illustrated in Figure 8–13 by the

/f/ spectrum which has three peaks—at 2.6, 3.5 (highest peak), and 5.2 kHz—of very similar relative amplitude. What if measurements were made of the frequencies of the two or three highest peaks in a fricative spectrum? This increases the *dimensionality* of the measurement (as in vowels, where three peaks are used) and may, therefore, lead to better acoustic discrimination of fricative place of articulation. Unfortunately, the peaks in fricative spectra are often not as well defined (sharply tuned) as in vowel spectra and can be difficult to identify. It would seem as if other types of measurements should be explored, possibly in combination with the measurement of peak frequency(ies).

One such measurement is the *dynamic range* of the fricative spectrum. Figure 8–13 shows for the two spectra, the range of amplitudes between the highest and lowest energies along the smoothed curves. This range is indicated on each spectrum by the two horizontal, dashed lines, and the range value in decibels is shown to the left of each spectrum. In this example, the dynamic range measurement has been limited to the frequency range 1.0 to 10.0 kHz to avoid low energies at the extremes of the spectrum that are likely to have more to do with the way the fricatives were recorded and analyzed than with their actual acoustic characteristics. The substantially larger dynamic range of 36 dB for /s/ as compared to 19 dB for /f/ is a quantitative approach to capture the subjective impression of the relative flatness of the /f/ spectrum as compared to the /s/ spectrum. Although dynamic range measurements have not been explored in great detail for fricative spectra (see Shadle, 1985), the combination of such a measure with peak frequencies could result in better ability to distinguish between the acoustic characteristics of fricatives like /s/ and /ʃ/, or /f/ and /θ/ (or their voiced cognates).

Finally, fricative spectra can be quantified by treating the spectrum as a distribution of numbers and computing parameters that describe the central tendency, dispersion, tilt, and "peakiness" of the set of numbers. One of the first lessons of basic statistics concerns the existence and characteristics of a *normal distribution*. Using the normal distribution as a reference, any distribution can be described by (a) an average, or *mean* of all the numbers (i.e., the central tendency); (b) a *variance*, which is the tendency of the numbers to spread more or less around the mean (dispersion); (c) a *skewness*, an index of how much the distribution curve deviates from strict symmetricality and leans left or right (tilt); and (d) a *kurtosis*, an index of how much the distribution deviates from the "normal" peakiness (either more "peaky" or more flat). These are called the first four *moments* of a distribution, and when they are applied to acoustic spectra they are called *spectral moments*. It is easy to see how the spectra in Figures 8–11, 8–12, and 8–13 look like distributions of numbers that deviate from the typical "bell-shape" of the normal distribution. Computer programs are available to compute spectral moments. These pro-

Parsing Parsimony

The term "reducing the dimensionality" of measurement is well known in many branches of science, including speech acoustics. How many numbers does it take to represent the fricative /ʃ/ so that it is completely distinguishable from other fricatives? Is the peak frequency measured at the halfway point of a fricative waveform sufficient, or do you need additional numbers (such as secondary and tertiary peak frequencies, fricative amplitude, and so forth). Scientists typically prefer the simplest measurement possible, so they spend a lot of time trying to determine the smallest set of numbers required to capture the essence of a physical phenomenon. The concept of *parsimony*—achieving adequate description or explanation using the simplest devices—is deeply entrenched in the souls of scientists.

grams provide a four-number index (mean, variance, skewness, and kurtosis) of a fricative spectrum, or of any speech sound spectrum for that matter. These measures can be obtained automatically and rapidly, and it is known that certain fricatives can be distinguished from each other quite well using this approach (Forrest, Weismer, Milenkovic, & Dougall, 1988. The articulatory interpretation of spectral moments, however, is sometimes not straightforward, which may limit their application in clinical settings. Spectral moments are discussed in greater detail in Chapter 10.

Temporal Measurements

The waveform in Figure 8–10 illustrates clearly the different appearance of the vowel (periodic) and fricative (aperiodic) energies. Even in the case of voiced fricatives, where some vocal fold vibration may be mixed with frication noise, vowels and fricatives look quite different in a waveform display. These different appearances of vowels and fricatives permit *segmentation* of the waveform into pieces that correspond to vowels, and pieces that correspond to fricatives. The "pieces" will correspond to *segment durations*, where "segment" refers to a sound category (vowel or fricative). The "pieces" are equivalent to durations, because they are defined along the *x*-axis of the waveform, which is time. Specific rules for the temporal segmentation of a speech waveform or *spectrogram* are given in Chapter 9. There is an extensive literature on segment durations (see Chapter 10), which have been used more than any other measure to describe and sometimes classify different types of speech disorders.

The Acoustic Theory of Fricatives: A Summary

The acoustic theory of fricatives shares with the acoustic theory of vowels the concepts of source and filter. In fricative production there is a source generated supralaryngeally, as a result of turbulent airflow (a) in the vicinity of the constriction, (b) at an obstacle in the path of airflow, or (c) along the walls of the vocal tract. A particular fricative may have turbulent noise sources at any combination of these three sites. This turbulent source is aperiodic and produces a spectrum that is nearly flat, or in some cases slightly falling, as a function of frequency. When airflow strikes an obstacle directly, as in the case of /s/ and /ʃ/, where the flow hits the teeth, the frication source has relatively great amplitude. When airflow strikes other surfaces in a more indirect manner, as in the case of /f/ and /θ/ where airflow may glance off the teeth and/or lips, or when the airflow encounters no obstacles in its pathway, the frication source is relatively weak. These differences in source amplitude are largely responsible for the pronounced, overall amplitude differences between fricatives with constrictions within the vocal tract (/s/, /ʃ/, /z/, /ʒ/) and those with constrictions at the outlet of the vocal tract (/f/, /θ/, /v/, /ð/).

The filter in fricative production is the vocal tract, as it is for vowels. Because the source propagates in both directions along the long axis of the vocal tract, all cavities contribute to the shaping of the source spectrum, even though the source location may be well in front of the cavity behind the constriction. The primary resonances in fricative spectra are due to the cavity in front of the constriction. As this cavity decreases in size, as when a fricative constriction is moved from the back to front of the vocal tract, the primary resonances will increase in frequency. Fricative spectra also contain antiresonances, which are due primarily to the back cavity and its behavior as a closed resonator that traps acoustic energy.

There is no standard approach to the measurement of fricative spectra, as there is in the case of vowels. However, three candidate measurements—peak frequencies, dynamic range, and spectral moments—appear to be useful. Future research should show which of these (or other) measures does the best job of distinguishing between the fricatives, and which can be most easily interpreted in articulatory terms.

WHAT IS THE THEORY OF STOP ACOUSTICS?

Figure 8–14 shows a tube model similar to the one shown for fricative aeromechanics (see Figure 8–8). Unlike the tube in Figure 8–8, which contains a narrow constriction through which air flows, the tube

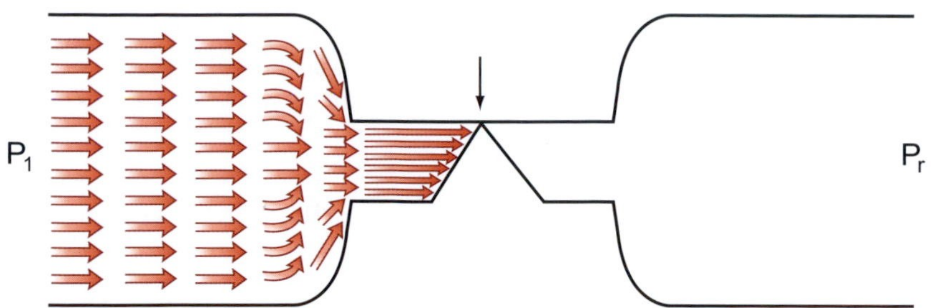

Figure 8–14. Airflow in a tube like that in Figures 8–7 and 8–8, except that a complete constriction in the tube (*arrow*) prevents air from passing through to the right side. Pressure builds up behind the constriction, as is the case for stop consonants. P_1 is the pressure behind the constriction and P_r is the reference pressure (atmospheric pressure).

in Figure 8–14 has a complete constriction (at the downward-pointing arrow) that can be conceptualized as a closed valve blocking the flow of air. When a pressure differential exists between the two ends of the tube, with P_1 greater than P_r, air flows from the left end of the tube to the right end, as shown by the arrows in Figure 8–14. The airflow is blocked by the complete constriction, causing compression of the air molecules behind the constriction. Compression of air molecules results in increasing pressure and the pressure continues to rise until the constriction is broken or the air volume becomes maximally stiff and cannot be compressed further.

During speech production, completely closed tubes such as the one shown in Figure 8–14 occur for the articulation of stop consonants. The complete blockage of airflow for stops may be formed at several places throughout the vocal tract (at the lips, between the tongue and various locations along the hard and soft palates, and at the glottis), and generally lasts for no longer than about 100 ms (1/10 of a second). When the air flowing through the vocal tract is blocked by a stop constriction, the molecules within the volume behind the constriction are compressed uniformly and simultaneously. For example, in the production of a voiceless stop consonant, the vocal folds are separated and the volume in back of a vocal tract constriction includes the air spaces of the trachea and lungs (as well as those of the vocal tract). The nasal cavities are excluded from this volume because the velopharyngeal port is closed for the production of stops, as for all obstruents. The complete blockage of airflow at the stop constriction results in compression of air molecules throughout the volume behind the constriction. This compression is uniform and occurs fairly rapidly throughout the enclosed volume, so the pressure should be the same—especially when it reaches its peak value—at all points in back of the constriction.

This condition is illustrated in the schematic speech production apparatus of Figure 8–15A, where a complete lingua-alveolar constriction is shown for the voiceless stop /t/, and the volume in back of the constriction is indicated by the shaded area. Three pressures are indicated within this volume. *Oral air pressure* is symbolized by P_o, which as reviewed above in the section on fricatives is the pressure measured within the vocal tract. P_t is *tracheal air pressure*, measured immediately below the vocal folds. P_{alv} is *alveolar air pressure*, or the pressure inside the lungs. When air is compressed behind a complete vocal tract constriction for a voiceless stop, the peak (highest) value of P_o is roughly equivalent to the peak values of P_t and P_{alv} because the vocal folds are separated during the stop closure, creating the condition for the volume of air behind the constriction to be continuous from articulatory constriction to trachea and lungs. In an utterance such as /ɑtɑ/, P_o is nearly zero (P_{atm}) during the first vowel, begins to rise when the complete constriction is made for the /t/ until a magnitude of 5 to 10 cmH_2O is reached, and then drops rapidly back to nearly zero when the constriction is released into the following vowel. During vowel production, of course, P_t and P_{alv} will be above zero (around 5–10 cmH_2O) so that air can flow from the

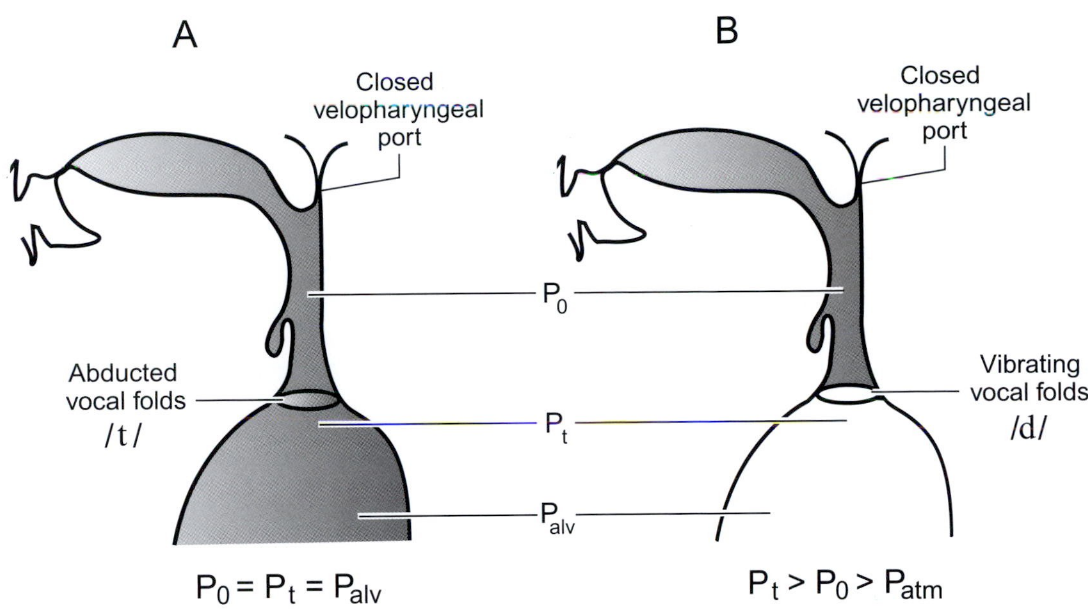

Figure 8–15. A. Schematic drawing of the speech production apparatus, showing a complete constriction at the alveolar ridge for the voiceless stop /t/. The volume of air that is compressed during the stop closure interval is indicated by the shaded parts of the drawing and includes the vocal tract spaces behind the constriction as well as the spaces within the trachea and lungs. Oral, tracheal, and alveolar air pressures are all equal. **B.** Schematic drawing of the speech production apparatus, showing a complete constriction at the lingua-alveolar ridge for the voiced stop /d/. The volume of air that is compressed during the stop closure interval is indicated by the shaded parts of the drawing and includes only the spaces between the constriction and the larynx. Tracheal air pressure is greater than oral air pressure and both are greater than atmospheric air pressure. The unshaded oval at the level of the glottis indicates that the larynx is closed during the closed phase of the vibratory cycle.

trachea and through the vocal folds, setting them into vibration. As mentioned above, the complete constriction for voiceless stops is generally maintained for no longer than 100 ms. It is during this closure interval that air is compressed and P_o rises above zero.

In the case of voiced stop consonants, the aeromechanical situation is somewhat different because the vibrating vocal folds separate the tracheal and pulmonary air volumes from the vocal tract air volume. In this case, the peak value of P_o typically does not equal P_t and P_{alv} because as air flows through the vibrating vocal folds there is some loss of pressure, resulting in P_o values that are generally lower than the pressures in the trachea and lungs. In Figure 8–15B the shaded area behind the lingua-alveolar constriction shows the compressible volume associated with P_o for voiced stops. This volume extends only between the constriction and the vocal folds, the latter shown as an unshaded oval to indicate the closed phases during each vibratory cycle. As long as P_t is greater than P_o by a critical amount (typically 1 or 2 cmH_2O) the vocal folds continue to vibrate during the voiced stop closure interval, because air flows from the higher to lower pressure region.[7] Values of P_o for voiced stops are typically about

[7]There are cases in which P_o rises to the same magnitude as P_t during the closure interval of a voiced stop. When this occurs, there is no pressure differential across the glottis, and hence no airflow and vocal fold vibration. This set of conditions might even be more common if it were not for an articulatory gesture that seems to be specific to voiced stops. In several studies (Bell-Berti, 1975; Kent & Moll, 1969), it has been shown that the volume of the cavity behind the vocal tract constriction and above the glottis actually *enlarges* during the closure interval of voiced stops. The enlargement is accomplished by muscular

1.5 cmH_2O less than values for voiceless stops, ranging between about 3.5 to 8.0 cmH_2O. The duration of the closure interval for voiced stops is about the same as that for voiceless stops, usually not exceeding 100 ms.

Both voiceless and voiced stops, therefore, have a buildup of P_o during their closure intervals. The vocal tract is "sealed" by the stop articulation (e.g., between the lips, or between the tongue and palate) as well as by the closure of the velopharyngeal port. The seal briefly prevents air from escaping the vocal tract to the atmosphere and results in the P_o buildup. From here, the next step is to link these aeromechanical events with the acoustic characteristics of stop consonants.

Intervals of Stop Consonant Articulation: Aeromechanics and Acoustics

Stop consonant articulation is often said to have several successive components. These include the closure, release (burst), frication, and aspiration intervals (the latter only occurring for voiceless stops). Voice-onset time (VOT) includes the burst, frication, and aspiration intervals in the case of voiceless stops, and the burst and frication intervals for voiced stops.

Closure (Silent) Interval

In an articulatory sequence such as /ɑtɑ/ the vocal tract is open for the first vowel and then closed for the /t/ by contact of the tongue tip with the alveolar ridge. The closure interval of the stop is also called the *silent interval*, because during this interval the vocal tract generates little or no acoustic energy. In other words, if the vocal tract is completely sealed, there is no orifice from which acoustic energy can be radiated. The closure intervals of voiceless stops are typically completely silent, but the closure intervals of voiced stops may show evidence of weak periodic energy from vibration of the vocal folds. This weak periodic energy during the closure interval is not the result of a pressure wave emerging from the mouth or nose, because the vocal tract is completely sealed. Rather, vocal fold vibration during a closure interval causes the walls of the vocal tract to vibrate, thus generating a pressure wave in the outside air which may be sensed by the ear or by a microphone.

Figure 8–16 shows two speech waveforms to illustrate the closure interval for /ɑtɑ/ (left) and /ɑdɑ/ (right) utterances. P_o and $\dot{V}_o$ (oral air pressure and airflow) traces are shown below and synchronized in time with each acoustic waveform. The vowels surrounding the closure intervals are easily identified by their large amplitude, periodic energy. For the /ɑtɑ/ traces, a pointer marked "onset of /t/ closure" indicates the final glottal pulse of the first vowel, after which there is minimal or no acoustic energy for a period of about 70 ms. This is the closure interval of the voiceless stop consonant. The onset of the /d/ closure is also indicated by a pointer, but in this case the following closure interval contains some weak, periodic energy, as shown by the low-amplitude glottal pulses that terminate shortly before the burst. This is the energy from vocal fold vibration, transmitted to the microphone via vibration of orofacial tissue such as the neck and cheeks.

The airflow coming through the mouth ($\dot{V}_o$) is approximately 130 cc/sec during the first vowel, and decreases rapidly to zero at the onset of the closure interval. For both voiceless and voiced stops, P_o is nearly zero (P_{atm}) during the vowels and begins to rise at the onset of the closure interval. The P_o continues to rise until it is released at the point on the acoustic waveforms marked "burst" (see next section). Note the very brief, high airflow (peak $\dot{V}_o$) at the instant of release of the stop. This results when the stop constriction is opened suddenly and the high P_o developed during the closure interval decreases to nearly P_{atm} over an interval of just a few

---

mechanisms that widen the pharynx, lower the larynx, and raise the velum. In a closed volume, the product of pressure and volume is a constant; this aeromechanical characteristic of closed volumes is known as *Boyle's law*. Thus, if the volume behind the constriction and above the vocal folds is enlarged during the closure interval, the pressure within that volume should be reduced to meet the constancy described by Boyle's law. The reduced pressure tends to keep P_o below P_t, and allows vocal fold vibration to be maintained throughout much or all of the closure interval. This enlargement of the vocal tract volume behind the constriction does not occur for voiceless stops because there is no need to maintain a pressure difference across the glottis (i.e., there is no need to maintain vocal fold vibration, which requires a pressure difference across the glottis).

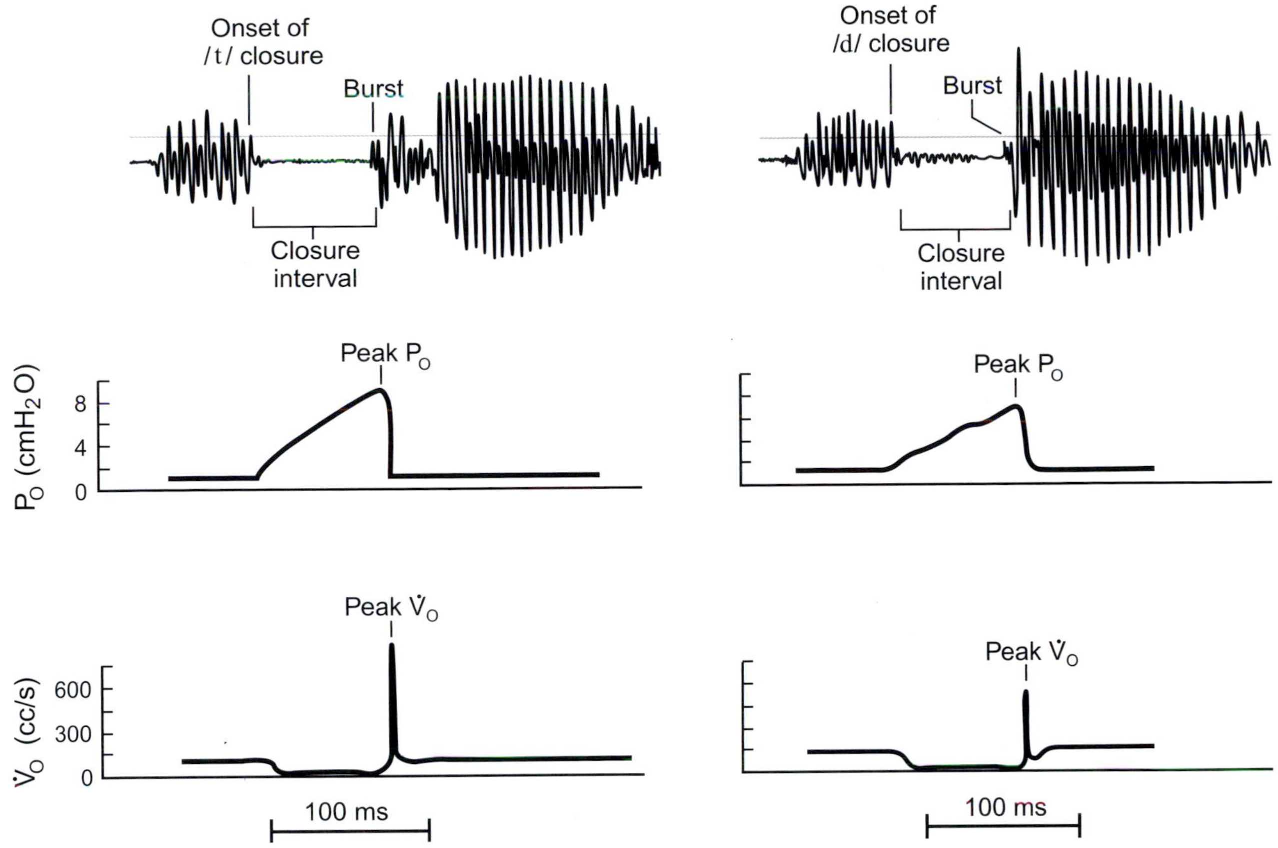

Figure 8-16. Acoustic waveforms for /ɑtɑ/ (*left*) and /ɑdɑ/ (*right*). Below each acoustic waveform are synchronized oral pressure, P_o, and oral airflow, $\dot{V}_o$, signals. See text for details.

milliseconds or less. The relationship between the aeromechanical and acoustical events shown in Figures 8–16 for /ɑtɑ/ and /ɑdɑ/ is elaborated in the following descriptions of the burst, frication, and aspiration intervals.

Release (Burst) Interval

The sudden drop of P_o at the instant of stop closure release creates an acoustic source of energy, originally referred to by Fant (1960) as *shock excitation.* Shock excitation sources typically have very brief durations (perhaps no longer than 2 ms) and relatively flat spectra. As in the case of turbulent noise sources for fricatives, shock excitation sources for stops are located in the vicinity of the constriction and their spectra are shaped mainly by the cavity in front of the constriction. In Figure 8–16, the acoustic result of the sudden release of P_o is shown as the sudden "spike" at the end of the closure interval, labeled as the *burst*. Bursts are distinctive acoustic characteristics of both voiceless and voiced stops, although they are not always present for stop production (see Byrd, 1993, and Chapter 10). The typically greater P_o for voiceless, as compared to voiced stops (compare peak P_o for voiceless and voiced stops in Figure 8–16) generally results in bursts having somewhat greater amplitude in the voiceless case (Stevens, 1998).

Frication and Aspiration Intervals

When the constriction is released, the pressure differential between the cavity behind the constriction (P_o) and the cavity in front of the constriction (P_{atm}) generates an airflow of relatively great magnitude. This event is shown in Figure 8–16 by the sudden "spikes" of airflow—the peak $\dot{V}_o$—marking the end of the closure intervals during which airflow is zero. The passage of this flow through narrow constrictions

stops are produced with a *succession* of changing sources. In the silent interval there is no source, followed by the shock excitation source of the burst, which then gives way to two turbulent noise sources in the case of voiceless stops (frication and aspiration) or a single turbulent noise source in voiced stops (frication).

Earlier it was noted that it is very difficult to state the precise spectral characteristics of fricative noise sources. This comment also applies to sources associated with stop consonant production. Reasonable estimates of stop source spectra are available in the acoustic phonetics literature, however, and can be offered here. No description is required for the silent interval, of course, because there is no source.

The shock excitation source of the burst is a very brief event, lasting only as long as the time required for the peak P_o reached during the closure interval to decline to near P_{atm}, following release of the stop (see Figure 8–16). This interval lasts only a few milliseconds, and may be as brief as 0.5 ms (Stevens, 1998). Shock excitation, therefore, qualifies as an *impulse-like event*, or one that is characterized by a large change in amplitude (in this case, pressure) over a very brief interval. Impulse-like events are known to "spread acoustic energy" across a wide range of frequencies, producing a spectrum having roughly equal energy at all frequencies. The source spectrum of shock excitation is roughly consistent with that of an impulse-like event, but like the frication source spectrum decreases in energy as frequency increases. For the purposes of this text it can be assumed that the source spectrum of shock excitation is roughly like that shown for fricatives in Figure 8–9. The different places of articulation for stop consonants have only a slight effect on the shock excitation source spectrum. Fant (1960) suggested that the source spectrum for /t/ shock excitation is flatter (shows a shallower decrease in energy across frequency) than for /p/ and /k/. This description of shock excitation source spectra also applies to the voiced cognates (/b,d,g/).

The source spectra for the stop frication interval are also essentially the same as the source spectra for fricatives shown in Figure 8–9. The aeromechanical phenomena that produce sources for fricatives, and sources for the stop frication intervals, are identical. Figure 8–9 showed some place-of-articulation differences in the source spectra for fricatives, and these apply to the frication intervals of /p,b/ versus /t,d/ and /k,g/. The frication source for bilabials typically has weaker energy than the frication sources for lingua-alveolar and dorsal stop consonants, consistent with the place-related differences in frication source energy shown in Figure 8–9.

The source spectrum for the aspiration interval of voiceless stops has energy concentrated in the mid-frequencies (1.0–4.0 kHz), with less energy in the lower and higher frequencies. A single aspiration source spectrum should apply to all three places of articulation of stops, because variation in place of articulation should not affect the acoustic result of turbulence at the glottis. This source spectrum is, therefore, somewhat different from the relatively flat source spectra of the shock excitation and frication intervals.

The Shaping of Stop Sources

The acoustic shaping of the shock excitation and frication sources in stop articulation is consistent with the shaping of fricative sources, described above. Shock excitation and frication sources are typically located within the vocal tract, between two resonators. As in the case of fricatives, the cavity in front of the source provides the primary emphasis of energy (resonance) in the output spectrum and the cavity behind the source contributes one or more antiresonances to the output spectrum.

Figure 8–18 presents fairly typical spectra for the three stop places-of-articulation, measured over a 10-ms interval beginning at the burst. The spectra have been smoothed in the same way as the fricative spectra in Figure 8–13. These spectra were derived from the voiceless stops, but the description provided here can be applied to the voiced cognates, as well. The shapes of these three burst spectra are consistent with the ideas developed above in the section on fricative spectra. For example, for the bilabial stop /p/ there is no vocal tract cavity in front of the constriction. A relatively flat output spectrum for the /p/ burst might be expected because there is no front cavity to emphasize a particular region of the shock excitation source spectrum. The /p/ burst spectrum shown in Figure 8–18 (left spectrum) is, in fact, relatively flat between roughly 0 Hz and 7000 Hz (compare this to the description of the /f/ output spectrum, and Figure 8–11). Note the slight, right-

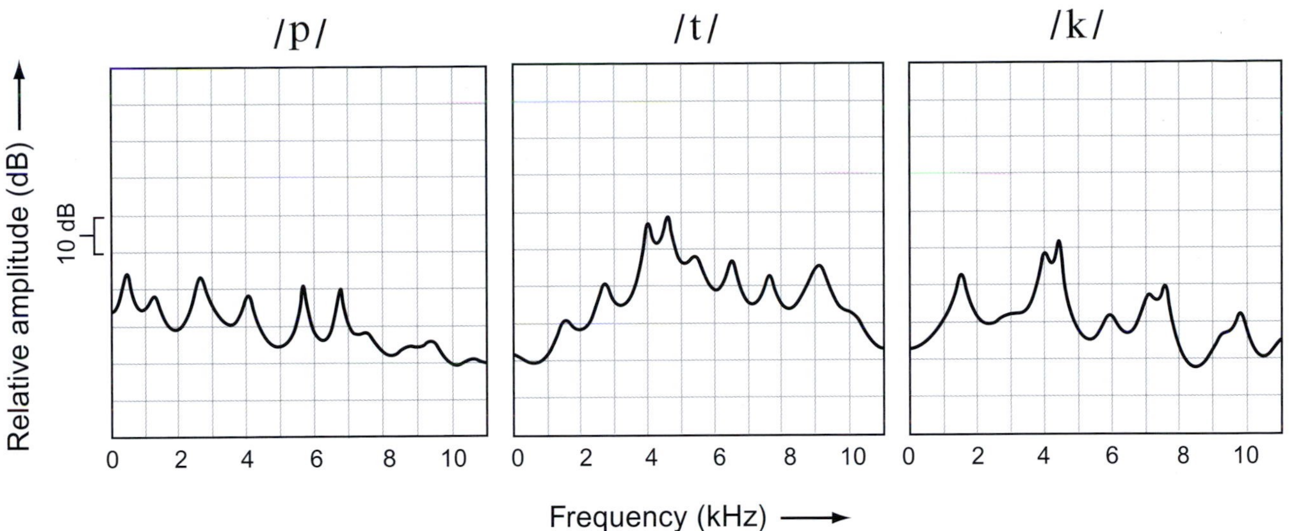

Figure 8–18. Sample output spectra (smoothed) for the burst interval of voiceless stop consonants. Each spectrum is computed from a 10-ms interval starting at the burst. The spectra for voiced stop consonants are similar to these, but may show somewhat less overall energy and some additional low-frequency energy.

> **Counteracting Pop**
>
> Rock vocalists are famous for appearing to chew the microphones they are singing into. This is one way to control variations in voice intensity that result from changing the distance between the mouth and the microphone. If the singer is always lip-to-foam, the only variations in voice intensity heard by the adoring crowd will be those with artistic intent—that is, changed by the singer as she or he delivers the song. The "foam" to which the singer's lips are applied is called a wind or pop screen. Pop screens are designed specifically to disperse the bursts produced for /p/s and /b/s. When the oral pressure is released for bilabial stops, the sudden spike of airflow has the potential to overdrive the microphone, producing acoustic distortion. Pop screens scatter bilabial airflow spikes and prevent them from creating aural unpleasantries.

ward tilt of the /p/ burst spectrum, indicating a relatively gradual decrease in energy with increasing frequency. This flat or gradually declining spectrum for the /p/ burst is considered a classic characteristic of bilabial stops. As in fricatives, the cavity behind the shock excitation source contributes antiresonances to the spectrum.

The effect of the size of the cavity in front of the constriction is illustrated by comparing the burst spectra for /t/ (Figure 8–18, middle spectrum) to that for /k/ (Figure 8–18, right spectrum). The energy in the /t/ burst spectrum seems to rise sharply from 0 Hz to roughly 4.5 kHz, with a clear spectral emphasis (the location of greatest energy) between 4.0 and 5.0 kHz. The /k/ burst spectrum, on the other hand, shows a very prominent peak at 1.5 kHz, in addition to peaks in the vicinity of 4.0 kHz. The emphasis at higher frequencies in the /t/ burst spectrum makes sense because the cavity in front of the constriction is smaller than in the case of /k/

(or, stated otherwise, the large peak at 1.5 kHz in the /k/ burst spectrum, in contrast to the weak energy at this frequency in the /t/ spectrum, makes sense because the cavity in front of the /k/ constriction is larger than in the case of /t/). As the cavity in front of the stop constriction becomes smaller, the emphasis in the spectrum moves to higher frequencies. In this sense, the general *spectral shapes* of stop bursts are related to articulatory configurations in the same way as discussed above for fricatives. Chapter 10 contains a detailed discussion of spectral shapes for stop bursts.

Stop burst spectra contain antiresonances. The same rules relating cavity size to location of frequency peaks (or reverse peaks) apply to the locations of antiresonances as well as to resonances: Large cavities yield low-frequency resonances or antiresonances, and small cavities yield high-frequency resonances or antiresonances. The spectra in Figure 8–18 do not show antiresonances because the smoothing of the spectra ignores the locations where large "dips" occur.

Measurement of Stop Acoustics

Both spectral and temporal measurements have been used to quantify the acoustic characteristics of stops. As in the case for fricatives, the discussion below is not exhaustive but rather describes frequently made measurements.

Spectral Measurements

Surprisingly, even though stop burst spectra have played a prominent role in theories of speech production and perception, there has not been much agreement concerning their measurement. Earlier in this chapter it was pointed out that there is much discussion (and not much agreement) concerning the proper way to measure fricative spectra. The issues are similar for the measurement of stop burst spectra, with one important difference as reviewed below.

As in the case of fricative spectra, the goal of a measurement strategy for stop burst spectra is to obtain a small set of numbers that distinguishes among the three places of articulation. Stop burst spectra have numerous peaks and valleys, as is evident in the three spectra shown in Figure 8–18. In fact, these spectra are quite similar to fricative spectra (compare spectra in Figure 8–18 to those in Figure 8–11). Thus, peak frequencies could be measured for stop burst spectra but have the same problems as those discussed for fricatives. Similarly, dynamic range could be measured for burst spectra, but laboratory experience suggests that this would not provide a useful way to distinguish stop place of articulation.

Many researchers have focused their attention on the shape of the stop burst spectrum. Earlier, spectral moments were described as one means to obtain a numerical index of the shape of fricative spectra. When spectral moments are applied to stop burst spectra, they do a very good job of distinguishing place of articulation (Forrest et al., 1988; see additional discussion in Chapter 10). A nonnumerical, *prototype* approach to the classification of place of articulation for stop consonants involves the use of *spectral shape templates*. These templates, developed originally by Blumstein and Stevens (1979), provide a prototype burst spectrum for the frequency range 0 to 5000 Hz for each place of articulation and an allowable range of variability for that prototype. For example, if a stop burst spectrum fits within an allowable range of variability for the bilabial template, or prototype, it is classified as a bilabial stop.

Blumstein and Stevens (1979) constructed the templates based on their careful examination of many burst spectra, and then quantified the number of spectra that could be correctly classified using the templates. They had relatively good success in this exercise, classifying the place of articulation correctly about 85% of the time. This success makes the template approach attractive because it offers a relatively simple procedure for classifying acoustic events (burst spectra) according to phoneme category (i.e., place contrasts). For example, a computer could store the kinds of templates developed by Blumstein and Stevens (1979) and measure real burst spectra (for example, produced by clients with speech disorders) for comparison to the templates. In a clinical setting, this may serve as a simple approach to an objective evaluation of a client's articulatory capabilities for stop consonants. The procedure has certain limitations, however, which would have to be worked out prior to widespread clinical or research use. For example, the classification accuracy of the original templates was evaluated by Blumstein and Stevens using a small number of speakers (3) who articulated simple syllables in a very careful way. It is not known if the same template approach would work for child speakers, older speakers, or any speaker using a more casual form of articulation. Also, it is not clear how an "unclassifiable" burst spectrum is to be interpreted. In Blumstein and Stevens' study, there were some spectra that did not fit any of the templates. Persons with speech disorders often produce stops that sound as if they are "in between" the normal places of articulation. The template system would have to be expanded to capture these important articulatory events. These are areas in need of careful research if these objective measures are to have an impact in the clinic (see Chapter 10 for more material on spectral templates for stop consonant place of articulation).

Spectral measures can also be made of the frication and aspiration intervals following the stop release. The measurement issues for these spectra are the same as discussed above for the burst. The details of frication interval spectra for the different places of articulation are very similar to the details of burst spectra. In other words, the shape of the burst spectrum for an apical stop is very much like the shape of the frication interval spectrum for that stop. Spectra of aspiration intervals of voiceless stops have not been studied extensively, but they generally show a pattern similar to the formant pattern of the following vowel. This is because the aspiration source, which is located at the glottis, excites the resonances of the vocal tract as it opens following the stop release to the position for the following vowel. Unlike burst and frication interval spectra, spectra of aspiration intervals do not show significant variation across stop place of articulation.

Temporal Measurements

As in the case of fricatives, temporal segmentation of stop consonant waveforms is relatively straightforward. The waveforms in Figures 8–16 and 8–17 show the closure interval and VOT segments quite clearly. In real speech waveforms, it is often more difficult to find the dividing lines between the burst, frication, and aspiration intervals. Many measurements of closure intervals and VOTs have been reported in the literature and applied to clinical populations.

Stop Consonants: A Summary

Stops are produced when there is a constriction in the vocal tract that completely blocks the airstream for a brief interval. During this closure interval the pressure behind the constriction (P_o) builds up and is suddenly released when the articulators break the constriction. The sudden drop in pressure serves as an acoustic source called shock excitation, the spectrum of which is shaped by the vocal tract cavities. Typically, the cavity in front of the stop constriction provides the major resonance that shapes the shock excitation source, whereas the cavity in back of the constriction contributes antiresonances to the output spectrum.

Following the closure interval, there is a sequence of acoustic events associated with stops. For voiceless stops, the sequence is the burst, frication interval, and aspiration interval. The burst is associated with the release of P_o, the frication interval with high airflow rushing past the narrow vocal tract constriction immediately following the release, and aspiration interval with high airflow rushing past the vocal folds as they move together. The aeromechanical basis of the frication and aspiration intervals is turbulent airflow, the acoustic counterpart of which is aperiodic energy (i.e., noise). Voiced stops have burst and frication intervals, but lack an aspiration interval because the vocal folds are not separated from the midline during the closure interval, as they are for voiceless stops.

The spectra of the burst and frication intervals are unique for each of the three stop places of articulation. The uniqueness of these spectra can be traced largely to the size of the cavity in front of the constriction. In bilabial stops, the cavity is infinitely large (i.e., there is no vocal tract cavity), so the output spectrum tends to be flat. In lingua-alveolar stops, the cavity is very small, which results in a high-frequency emphasis in the output spectrum. In dorsal stops, the cavity is relatively large, resulting in a concentration of energy in the mid-frequencies of the output spectrum.

The output spectra of voiced and voiceless stops at the same place of articulation are essentially the same, with greater overall amplitude for the voiceless stop spectra. Voiced and voiceless stops may be distinguished from each other by (a) the appearance of glottal pulses during the closure interval of voiced, but not voiceless stops; and (b) longer VOTs for voiceless, as compared to voiced stops.

WHAT IS THE THEORY OF AFFRICATE ACOUSTICS?

Affricates combine features of stop consonants and fricatives. Like stops, affricates have a closure interval during which P_o rises and is released when the articulatory constriction is broken. When the constriction is broken, there is a fairly long interval of frication energy generated by turbulent airflow in the vicinity of the expanding constriction. What seems to distinguish affricates from stops is the fairly long interval of this frication noise. In stops, the frication may last for about 30 to 50 ms, whereas in affricates this interval may be as long as 60 to 80 ms. As described above, frication noise results when the conditions for turbulent airflow exist, these conditions being (a) a flow of sufficient magnitude (i.e., "high enough" flow) and (b) a sufficiently narrow constriction. The longer frication interval in affricates, as compared to stops, suggests that following the release of an affricate, the conditions for turbulence exist for a greater amount of time than they do following the release of a stop. This is why affricates are sometimes referred to as "slowly released stops." The affricates of American English, which include /tʃ/ and /dʒ/, may also have a place of articulation that is different from the lingua-alveolar place of /t/ and /d/. Affricates are discussed more fully in Chapter 10.

WHAT KINDS OF ACOUSTIC DISTINCTIONS ARE ASSOCIATED WITH THE VOICING DISTINCTION IN OBSTRUENTS?

Four intervals for stop consonants have been defined and discussed above. The first three of these (closure interval, burst, and frication interval) apply to both voiceless and voiced stops, whereas the aspiration interval is only found for voiceless stops.

Slowly Released Slops

Affricates combine stop (closure and burst) and fricative features (a relatively long period of frication noise). This phonetic double-identity is represented in the transcription symbols for English affricates, /tʃ/ and /dʒ/. But are affricates really two sound classes—stops and fricatives—in rapid succession, or should they be accorded their own unique sound class? The famous linguist/phonetician Leigh Lisker (1918–2006) called affricates "slowly released stops," by which he meant to say they were neither stops nor fricatives, but something different. Another form of evidence for the unique status of affricates is what happens when the sound class is involved in a spoonerism. "Flipping the channel" becomes "chipping the flannel"; the /tʃ/ in "channel" does not separate into a stop and fricative component, with either one moving independently (nor does the /fl/ cluster separate for this switch—that's another story). Here is another one that makes the same point for /dʒ/, spoken by the actor Peter Sellers in the Pink Panther classic, *A Shot in the Dark* (1964): "killed him in a rit of fealous jage."

VOTs of voiceless stops are typically longer than those of voiced stops, partly because of the aspiration interval in the former case. Typical VOTs for voiced stops are between 0 and 20 ms, whereas VOTs for voiceless stops are typically between 40 to 80 ms. A VOT of zero means that glottal pulsing begins at the same time as the release of the stop (i.e., the burst). The difference in VOTs for voiceless and voiced stops is illustrated by comparing the left and right waveforms in Figure 8–16.

The relatively short VOTs of voiced stops are not only due to the absence of the aspiration interval, but also reflect burst and frication intervals that are somewhat shorter than those found in voiceless stops. The shorter burst and frication intervals are probably the result of the lower P_o in voiced, as compared to voiceless, stops. In addition, the vocal folds begin vibrating almost immediately after the vocal tract closure for voiced stops has been released. This follows because, during the stop closure, the vocal folds are held near or at the midline, and may actually vibrate to produce voicing, as shown in the closure interval of Figure 8–16 (right). At the release of a voiced stop, the vocal folds are, therefore, immediately (or nearly so) ready to begin vibration for the following vowel.

The activity at the level of the larynx for voiceless stops (and for any voiceless obstruent), however, is substantially different than in the case of voiced stops. This activity receives detailed consideration in Chapter 10, where acoustic data and physiological interpretations are presented on the voicing distinction for stops, fricatives, and affricates.

REVIEW

In this chapter, the theory of consonant acoustics is presented, with special emphasis on the acoustic basis of antiresonances and the aeromechanical basis of noise sources.

Antiresonances occur when two resonators are coupled, as in the case of nasals and laterals, or when a source sits in between two vocal tract resonators, as in the case of stops, fricatives, and affricates.

Turbulent airflow is generated when a great enough airflow is forced through a sufficiently narrow constriction.

The acoustic correlate of turbulence is noise, which accounts for frication and aspiration sources in the speech production apparatus.

The measurement of consonant spectra is fairly complicated, but several alternative approaches are discussed.

Data from several studies in which stop, fricative, and nasal spectra have been measured are presented in Chapter 10.

REFERENCES

Bell-Berti, F. (1975). Control of pharyngeal cavity size for voiced and voiceless stops. *Journal of the Acoustical Society of America, 57*, 456–461.

Bell-Berti, F. (1993). Understanding velic motor control: Studies of segmental context. In M. Huffman & R. Krakow (Eds.), *Phonetics and phonology: Nasals, nasalization, and the velum* (pp. 63–85). New York: Academic Press.

Blumstein, S., & Steven, K. (1979). Acoustic invariance in speech production: Evidence from measurements of the spectral characteristics of stop consonants. *Journal of the Acoustical Society of America, 66*, 1001–1017.

Byrd, D. (1993). American stops. *UCLA Working Papers in Phonetics, 83*, 97–116.

Catford, J. (1977). *Fundamental problems in phonetics.* Bloomington: Indiana University Press.

Dang, J., & Honda, K. (1996). Acoustic characteristics of the paranasal sinuses derived from transmission characteristic measurement and morphological observation. *Journal of the Acoustical Society of America, 100*, 3374–3383.

Dang, J., Honda, K., & Suzuki, H. (1994). Morphological and acoustical analysis of the nasal and paranasal cavities. *Journal of the Acoustical Society of America, 96*, 2088–2100.

Fant, G. (1960). *Acoustic theory of speech production.* The Hague, Netherlands: Mouton.

Fant, G. (1973). *Speech sounds and features.* Cambridge, MA: MIT Press.

Forrest, K., Weismer, G., Milenkovic, P., & Dougall, R. (1988). Statistical analysis of word-initial voiceless obstruents: Preliminary data. *Journal of the Acoustical Society of America, 84*, 115–124.

Fujimura, O. (1962). Analysis of nasal consonants. *Journal of the Acoustical Society of America, 34*, 1865–1875.

Hawkins, S., & Stevens, K. (1985). Acoustic and perceptual correlates of the non-nasal-nasal distinction for vowels. *Journal of the Acoustical Society of America, 77*, 1560–1575.

Jongman, A., Wayland, R., & Wong, S. (2000). Acoustic characteristics of English fricatives. *Journal of the Acoustical Society of America, 108*, 1252–1263.

Kent, R., & Moll, K. (1969). Vocal tract characteristics of the stop cognates. *Journal of the Acoustical Society of America, 46*, 1555–1559.

Klatt, D., Stevens, K., & Mead, J. (1968). Studies of articulatory activity and airflow during speech. *Annals of the New York Academy of Sciences, 155*, 42–55.

Ladefoged, P., & Maddieson, I. (1996). *The sounds of the world's languages*. Oxford, UK: Blackwell.

Pruthi, T., & Espy-Wilson, C. (2004). Acoustic parameters for automatic detection of nasal manner. *Speech Communication, 43*, 225–239.

Sellers, P. (1964). *A shot in the dark* [Motion picture]. B. Edwards (Director). United States: MGM Entertainment.

Shadle, C. (1985). *The acoustics of fricative consonants*. Doctoral Dissertation, Massachusetts Institute of Technology, Cambridge.

Shadle, C. (1990). Articulatory-acoustic relationships in fricative consonants. In W. Hardcastle & A. Marchal (Eds.), *Speech production and speech modeling* (pp. 187–209). Dordrecht, Netherlands: Kluwer Academic.

Stevens, K. (1998). *Acoustic phonetics*. Cambridge, MA: MIT Press.

Stevens, K., Fant, G., & Hawkins, S. (1987). Some acoustical and perceptual correlates of nasal vowels. In R. Channon & L. Shockey (Eds.), *In honor of Ilse Lehiste* (pp. 241–254). Dordrecht, Netherlands: Foris.

9

Speech Acoustic Analysis

INTRODUCTION

Chapters 7 and 8 are devoted to the theoretical bases of speech acoustics, with acoustic patterns of various speech sounds presented to illustrate the theory. There are a variety of techniques for generating the speech acoustic displays shown in Chapters 7 and 8, and for using the displays to obtain speech acoustic measurements. These displays and measurements are the subject matter of the current chapter.

The current use of the term "techniques" goes beyond consideration of the instruments used to store, analyze, and represent (i.e., graph) the speech acoustic signal. In this chapter, the term includes the *conceptual* tools that have been developed to make sense of vocal tract output. When a speech signal—the acoustic output of the vocal tract—is displayed in the several ways discussed below, a large amount of information is available, not all of which may be relevant to each of the many reasons for studying speech acoustics. For example, some individuals study the speech signal to make inferences about the articulatory behavior that produced the signal (as discussed in Chapters 7 and 8). Others may be interested in the characteristics of the signal used by listeners to understand speech. Still others may be interested in which parts of the speech signal are the best candidates for computer recognition of speech (i.e., machines that understand speech). And, of course, many scientists have studied the speech acoustic signal to develop computer programs for high-quality speech synthesis. Sometimes what is important about the speech signal is relevant to all four of these

> **Computers Are Not Smarter Than Humans**
>
> Speech recognizers are computer programs that analyze a speech signal to figure out what was said. The programs use acoustic analysis and other data (such as stored information on the probability of one sound following another) and produce a set of words that represents a best "guess" about the true nature of the input signal. These programs learn the patterns of a single talker's speech, and in doing so improve their recognition performance over time for that talker. Unfortunately, the improved performance does not transfer to a new talker, whose acoustic-phonetic patterns are just different enough from the original talker's to confuse the speech recognition program. Humans, it should be noted, typically have no trouble transferring their speech recognition skills from one talker to another.

stylus was applied to this paper and heated in proportion to the voltage output from the analysis. As the analysis band was swept slowly across the frequency range, the stylus was synchronously transported up the vertical dimension of the spectrogram (see frequency dimension along the drum in Figure 9–6). The varying voltages from the analysis band were burned onto the special paper, with darker regions representing areas of relatively greater acoustic energy, and lighter regions representing areas of relatively lower acoustic energy. The entire process of recording a speech signal onto the tape loop, to mounting the paper around the drum and burning a complete frequency-by-time pattern onto the paper, took about 100 seconds to complete. All this to obtain acoustic knowledge of no more than 2.5 seconds of speech!

The Original Sound Spectrograph: Summary

There are several reasons why a fair amount of discussion has been devoted to the origins and function of the sound spectrograph. Most importantly, the invention of this instrument initiated a scientific revolution in the study of speech production, because for the first time, and with relative ease, the *time-varying* characteristics of articulatory processes could be studied. These time-varying characteristics were revealed most prominently by the always changing formant frequencies. The discovery of these changes led to new ideas and insights about the behavior of the articulators in speech production.

The discussion of the spectrograph should demystify, at least in part, the general engineering concepts of speech acoustic analysis. An engineering degree is not necessary to understand the conceptual basis of producing a spectrogram. The amplitude and frequency characteristics of a speech signal are stored as a function of time on magnetic tape. The time-varying patterns of electromagnetic strength are submitted to a spectrum analyzer in the form of time-varying voltages (corresponding to the time-varying intensity of the magnetic fields on the tape), where voltage is proportional to sound intensity (greater voltage = greater intensity) and the speed with which the voltage changes is proportional to frequency (faster voltage changes [shorter periods] = higher frequencies). The energy in the spectrum is sampled using an analysis band, or filter, that covers a 300-Hz range and is swept continuously across the entire frequency range of interest. Because the voltage output from the analysis band is available for all frequencies and at every point in time, it can be used to create a total picture of the speech spectrum as a function of time. This picture is created by burning the energy patterns onto a piece of heat-sensitive paper, which results in a picture called a spectrogram. This process is summarized in Figure 9–6, by following the arrow from the turntable (the magnetic tape) all the way around to the stylus at the spectrograph drum.

Today, when scientists or clinicians make spectrograms to study speech they do so digitally, using a desktop or laptop computer. These *digital spectrograms* are displayed on computer monitors and look very much like the one shown in Figure 9–5, but can

Speech Acoustics as a Health Hazard?

Those of us of a certain age, who were making spectrograms before digital spectrograms became a reality, may read the title of this sidetrack and find themselves smiling nostalgically. As the pattern was burned onto the special paper, carbon smoke would float away from the spinning drum and fill the room with the smell of speech acoustics. That smell was something like the exhaust of a car with a corroded, burned-out muffler. The wearing of light-colored clothes to the lab was discouraged—one would find fine black specks on a nice white sweater after a few hours of spectrogram-making. Some people—especially graduate students assigned to prepare spectrograms—took to wearing surgical masks in the lab.

be produced almost instantaneously after an utterance has been recorded onto the computer (some instruments actually display the spectrogram in *real time*, as the utterance is being produced). The computer allows a spectrogram to be generated in just a fraction of the time required to produce the burned records described above, but the analysis technique is essentially the same as that used in the original spectrograph. The rapid development of computer-based analysis of speech has also resulted in a host of new analyses for speech acoustics, but the spectrogram remains the gold standard because it is such an immediate and rich source of information about speech production and perception. Especially in clinical settings, the spectrogram has great, but unfortunately unrealized, potential for providing both qualitative and quantitative data concerning a client's speech production deficit.

A detailed presentation of spectrograms and their interpretation is now provided. Selected information on the application of spectrographic analysis to the understanding of speech disorders is presented in Chapter 10.

Interpretation of Spectrograms: Specific Features

Figure 9–8 shows a spectrogram of the utterance, *Peter shouldn't speak about the mugs*. A broad phonetic transcription of the sounds in the utterance is provided at the bottom of the display. Immediately above the spectrogram, on the same time scale, is the waveform of the utterance. The utterance was produced by an adult male aged 52 years, at a normal rate of speech and without any special emphasis

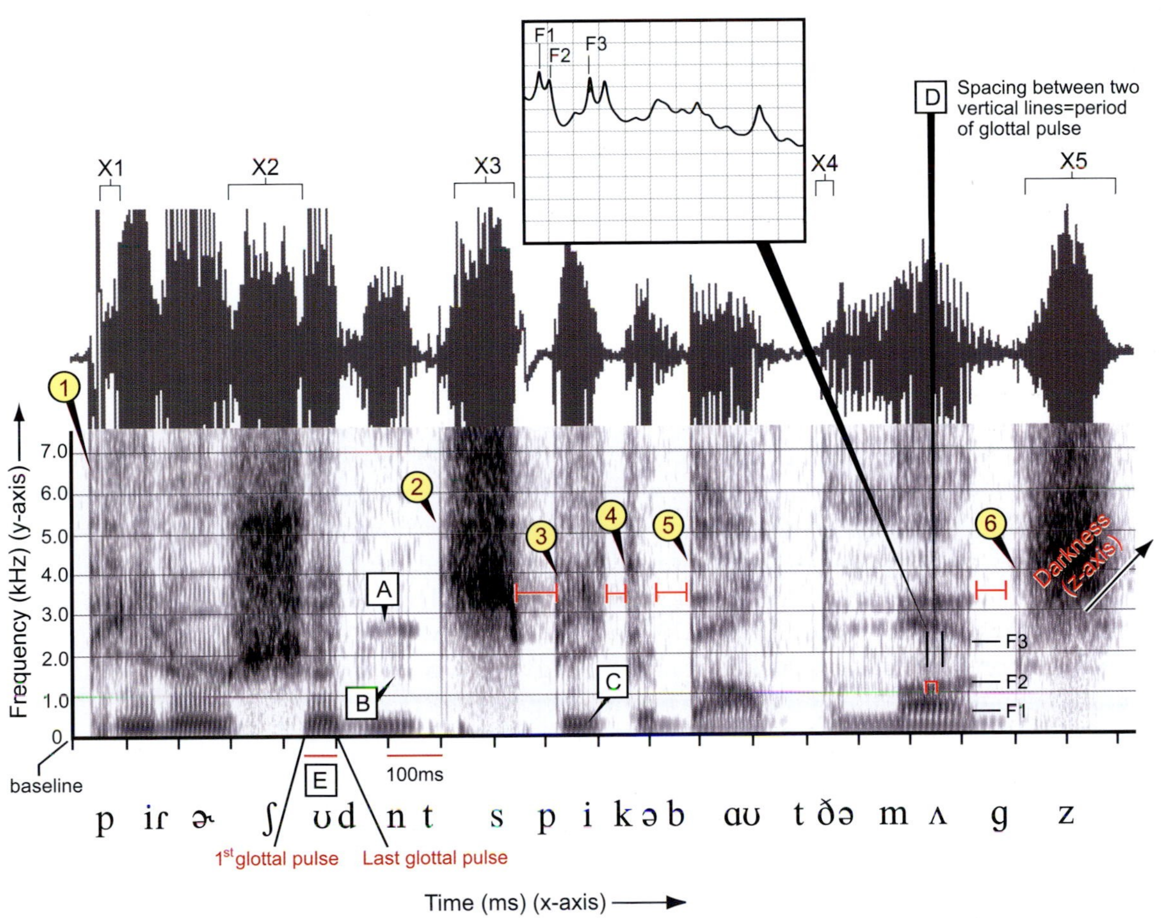

Figure 9–8. Spectrogram showing important features of a spectrographic display. Follow text description for information on axes, glottal pulses, formant frequencies, silent intervals, stop bursts, and aperiodic intervals.

on a particular word. The utterance was chosen for its ability to showcase certain spectrographic patterns, not because it has special meaning (as far as we know, Peter does not plan on ruining a surprise birthday present of really nice coffee mugs by telling the intended gift-receiver about them before the package is opened). This spectrogram was produced with the computer program *TF32*, written by Professor Paul Milenkovic of the Department of Electrical and Computer Engineering at the University of Wisconsin-Madison. *TF32* is a complete speech analysis program that includes algorithms for recording, editing, and analyzing speech waveforms, as well as displaying the speech signal as a spectrogram. Most of the speech analysis displays shown in this text were produced with *TF32*.

The important features of the spectrographic display in Figure 9–8 include the *x*-, *y*-, and *z*-axes; *glottal pulses; formant frequencies; silent intervals; stop bursts*; and *aperiodic intervals*. Each of these features is discussed below, but it is important to point out here that a casual glance at the spectrogram suggests a series of chunks, or *segments*, as the pattern is inspected from left to right. If an individual with no training in speech acoustics was shown this spectrogram and asked to find natural "breaks" in the pattern along the time axis, he or she could probably do this quite easily (try it!). The chunks, or segments, are important because they often correspond roughly to speech sounds. Chapter 10 presents detailed information on the specific acoustic characteristics of the sound segments of English.

Axes

A general orientation to the axes of a spectrographic display has been given above (see Major Roitman's explanation of what he called a *voice print*). The *x*-axis is time, and is marked off in successive 100-ms intervals by the short vertical lines occurring at regular intervals along the baseline of the spectrogram. These 100-ms *calibration intervals* are similar in length to many of the segments in this spectrogram, suggesting a relatively short time span for many of the important events of speech production. Using these calibration intervals, it is possible to estimate the entire duration of the utterance at just under 2000 ms, or a little less than 2 s. This does not seem like a particularly long time, but it is fairly typical for an utterance duration, and even such a relatively brief interval contains many distinct segments.

The *y*-axis is frequency, which in the current spectrogram extends from 0 kHz to about 7.5 kHz. Calibration of the frequency axis is shown as the series of horizontal lines marked off in 1.0-kHz increments. The 0- to 8.0-kHz range is often considered as a standard for spectrographic displays because most of the important acoustic energy for understanding articulatory events, as well as how the speech signal is used in the perception of speech, is thought to be contained within this range. This is true for the most part, but spectrograms can be generated for any frequency range. In the current text, a variety of spectrographic frequency ranges is used, depending on the purpose of the illustration. It is always important to check the frequency calibration along the *y*-axis of a particular spectrogram.

The *z*-axis (indicated on the right side of the spectrogram in red print), or third dimension of the spectrogram, is intensity. Unlike time (*x*-axis) and frequency (*y*-axis), in this type of spectrographic display intensity cannot be measured directly. Rather, intensity is coded by the darkness of the pattern at any time-frequency coordinate (that is, at any point on the spectrographic display). The darkness at any time-frequency coordinate can be compared to the darkness at any other time-frequency coordinate *only in relative terms*. This kind of coding is called a *gray scale*, which allows only *ordinal* comparisons between event magnitudes. For example, the intensity of the formant indicated by arrow A, roughly at the time-frequency coordinate of 600 ms (*x*-axis) and 2.7 kHz (*y*-axis) where the segment is marked phonetically as [n], is clearly greater (i.e., darker) than the formant above arrow B at the same segment (time-frequency coordinates of roughly 600 ms and 1.5 kHz). Similarly, the formant marked by arrow C, which occurs at a time-frequency coordinate of roughly 950 ms and 0.3 kHz where the segment is marked as [i], is slightly darker (more intense) than A. These comparisons are not stated in terms of numbers, but only as "greater than" or "less than" relations. This is what is meant by the gray scale allowing only ordinal comparisons. Time and frequency, on the other hand, can be measured directly from the spectrogram and actual numerical differences between points can be determined. There are other ways to determine numerical intensity differences (e.g., difference in decibels) between two different regions of a spectrogram, but not in the type of display shown in Figure 9–8.

Glottal Pulses

Certain segments in Figure 9–8 have a characteristic appearance of a series of dark, vertical lines. These same segments are also the ones containing the dark bands identified above as the vowel formants. In fact, the vertical lines appear to be running throughout the segments containing the most obvious formants, such as the /i/ in /pi/ and the /ʊ/ in /ʃʊd/. The vertical lines are the acoustic result of vocal fold vibration, with each individual line reflecting a single glottal pulse. More precisely, in Chapter 7 the vocal tract resonances are said to be excited each time the vocal folds snap shut during a series of glottal cycles. Each of the vertical lines in the spectrogram represents this point of excitation, where the vocal folds close quickly at the end of a glottal cycle and create a pressure wave whose spectrum is shaped by the vocal tract filter. The shaping of the source spectrum by the vocal tract filter is shown on the spectrogram as darkened areas—that is, the dark bands—at the frequencies of the vocal tract resonances. Thus, the vertical lines and the formants are not really different characteristics of the spectrogram. Rather, the formants are darkened areas along the vertical lines, showing where energy in the glottal source spectrum is emphasized (i.e., resonated) by the vocal tract filter.

Within any segment having the series of glottal pulses represented by vertical lines, the spacing of the lines appears to be very consistent. As described in Chapter 7, vocal fold vibration is quasiperiodic, with consecutive periods of nearly the same duration. The consistent spacing of the vertical lines along the time dimension (x-axis) of the spectrogram, therefore, reflects the quasiperiodic nature of vocal fold vibration, and the spacing between any two vertical lines is equal to the period of the glottal cycle (see example D, incomplete red box in Figure 9–8 showing the distance between two glottal pulses). Although this kind of spectrogram does not provide a direct display of the F0 of vocal fold vibration, segments can be compared visually for the relative spacing of the glottal pulses and, thus, their relative F0s. For example, compare the spacing of the glottal pulses in the two segments marked as /i/ (in /spik/) and /ʌ/ (in /mʌgz/). The vertical lines, or glottal pulses, are closer together in /i/, as compared to /ʌ/. Another way to make this comparison is to say that the number of vertical lines *per unit time* is greater for /i/ than for /ʌ/. A greater number of glottal pulses per unit time means a shorter period and a higher F0. Thus, /i/ has a higher F0 than /ʌ/.

Formant Frequencies

The dark bands seen in the patterns with regularly spaced glottal pulses have already been identified as the formants. This pattern is seen for any speech sound requiring a relatively open vocal tract and voicing, including vowels, diphthongs, and semivowels (/l/, /w/, /ɹ/, /j/). In addition, nasals are voiced and radiate sound through the open nares, thus producing a similar kind of pattern. The spectrographic patterns seen above the phonetic symbols for these kinds of segments (in Figure 9–8, /i/, /ɚ/, /ʊ/, /n/, /i/, /ə/, /aʊ/, /ə/, /m/, /ʌ/, from left to right) confirm this distinctive appearance.

In most cases, it is relatively easy to look at a spectrogram and determine which dark band is F1, which is F2, and so forth. The general rule is to start at the baseline (where frequency = 0 Hz) and move up the frequency scale, or y-axis, until the first dark band is encountered. This is the first formant, or F1. Continue up the frequency axis until the next dark band is found, which is F2. The next dark band above F2 will be F3, and so forth. In Figure 9–8, the first three formants for the terminal part of the vowel /ʌ/ in the word /mʌgz/ have been identified in this way. This is exactly the same approach used to identify formants in the spectrum plots presented in Chapter 7 (e.g., Figure 7-13), where frequency is on the x-axis and relative amplitude is on the y-axis. Starting from zero frequency on these plots, the first peak is labeled as F1, the next peak as F2, and the next as F3 (see spectrum inset, Figure 9–8, where the formant peaks are shown from the middle of the vowel). When the formants are labeled as F1, F2, F3, . . . Fn in a spectrographic display, the peaks in the spectrum are identified exactly as in the spectrum plots, except that the spectrogram displays frequency on the y-axis and the spectral peaks are shown as the darkened bands.

interval preceding the burst-like feature, suggesting the articulation of a stop consonant. Second, this spike has substantial energy at frequencies other than those associated with the formants of the adjacent vowel. Note, for example, the spike energy from 1.5 to 2.0 kHz, 3.5 to 4.0 kHz, and 7.0 to 7.5 kHz. The following vowel does not contain formant peaks at these frequencies. However, the next two criteria for identifying stop bursts are more ambiguous. This burst does seem to have a formant structure, with darker marks in the vicinity of F1, F2, and F3 of the adjacent vowel. And the interval between the burst and the following glottal pulse is not so different from the intervals between any of the glottal pulses in the /aʊ/ diphthong. Does the failure to meet clearly the third and fourth criteria for distinguishing a stop burst from a glottal pulse cast doubt on the identification of this acoustic event as a stop burst? Probably not, in this case, because the evidence for the closure interval is very clear, as is the evidence for voicing (glottal pulses) during the closure interval. This reasoning is consistent, of course, with knowledge that a /b/ was intended by the speaker. Thus, a voiced closure interval would be expected, and it would follow that a /b/ burst would be superimposed on the continuous series of glottal pulses extending through the closure interval and into the diphthong.

There are many cases, however, in which this kind of simple reasoning—which includes expectations about what has been spoken, who has spoken it, and how it has been spoken—cannot be applied. For example, acoustic analysis of disordered speech must often proceed with very imperfect knowledge of what has been spoken. In this case, the *who has spoken the utterance* (for example, a client with a neurologically based speech disorder) and the *what has been spoken* are very much intertwined. If the client has reduced speech intelligibility and the examiner has difficulty generating a reliable gloss of the utterance, a decision about the spike-like event labeled as 5 in Figure 9–8 (is it, or is it not a burst?) becomes more problematic. This may even be a problem in the speech of persons with no speech disorder, depending on *how* an utterance is produced. The utterance displayed in Figure 9–8 was spoken by one of the authors in a somewhat formal way, very unlike his speech patterns in more casual speech. In casual speaking styles, speakers often produce much blurrier acoustic landmarks than those seen in Figure 9–8, and in the case of stop consonants may even omit bursts all together. This goes against textbook descriptions of stop consonant production. Crystal and House (1988) and Byrd (1993) concluded from their acoustic analyses of connected speech that as many as 50% of stop consonants have no identifiable burst!

How does one distinguish between a pause and a closure interval for a voiceless stop consonant? As described above, voiceless stop closures are identifiable on a spectrogram by an interval of no energy—a silent interval—but would not the same thing be expected of a pause, for which no energy is being generated by the vocal tract?[3] Obviously, if an interval of no energy is terminated by a burst, there is a good chance it is the acoustic result of a voiceless stop closure. Not all stops, however, have bursts (see above) and in some speech disorders bursts may be present but extremely weak. The potential for confusion between pauses and voiceless stop closures, therefore, must be recognized. In the speech of individuals who are free from speech disorders, there is a general criterion for distinguishing voiceless stop closure intervals from pauses, based on the duration of the silent interval. Actual pauses in speech are typically no less than about 150 ms in duration, whereas voiceless stop closure intervals are typically no more than about 120 ms. To be on the conservative side, many scientists have adopted a criterion of 200 ms for the identification of a pause. Silent intervals 200 ms or greater are identified as pauses, those less than 200 ms are subject to further evaluation (using information such as the presence of a burst). This criterion is somewhat less reliable in certain speech disorders, for which very long stop closure intervals may be one result of a very slow speaking rate, quite common in many cases of motor speech disorders. Clearly, in these cases, the 200-ms criterion may not be effective, and the potential for confusion between stops and pauses is increased.

[3]Reference is made here only to the kind of pause that is silent, typically called an *unfilled* pause. Obviously, in the case of *filled* pauses, such as the many "um's" found in everyday spoken discourse, there would be no confusion with a voiceless stop consonant.

Aperiodic Intervals

As described in Chapter 8, aperiodic energy is produced within the vocal tract in several different ways and is an important component of the acoustic characteristics of fricatives, stops, and affricates. Aperiodic energy is shown in a spectrogram as an interval of energy having no repeating pattern. These aperiodic intervals are most commonly associated with fricatives and the release phase of stops and affricates. Aperiodic energy may also be mixed with periodic energy for certain sound segments (such as voiced fricatives) or phonation types (such as breathy voice).

In Figure 9–8, five intervals of aperiodic energy, labeled X1, X2, X3, X4, and X5, are marked at the top of the spectrogram by horizontal bars terminated by short, downward vertical lines. These five intervals vary in their duration (i.e., their extent along the *x*-axis), the range of frequencies over which energy is distributed, and the intensity of the energy. The duration of each interval can be estimated by comparing the length of each horizontal bar to the length of the time calibration ticks (at 100-ms increments) at the base of the spectrogram. The short, vertical lines extending downward from the ends of each horizontal bar show the location of the operationally defined onset and offset of each interval. The range of frequencies is indicated by the locations along the *y*-axis where there are light, medium, or dark tracings, and the relative intensity of that energy is indicated by the darkness of those tracings. Based on these characteristics, intervals X2, X3, and X5 appear fairly similar to one another, each having relatively long duration and fairly intense energy distributed across a wide range of frequencies. In general, aperiodic intervals of relatively long duration and intense energy are the result of voiceless fricative articulations, especially those produced with a lingua-alveolar or linguapalatal constriction (i.e., /s/ and /ʃ/, see Chapter 8). There are subtle, but important differences in the distribution and intensity of energy for intervals X2, X3, and X5. For example, very dark tracings indicating relatively intense energy extend down to about 1 kHz for segment X2, but not much lower than 2.5 kHz for segments X3 and X5. These differences are discussed in Chapter 8, where the relations of place of articulation to fricative intensity are considered.

Segments X1 and X4 differ from X2, X3, and X5 by virtue of their extremely brief durations. At its outset, segment X1 shows aperiodic energy in the form of a very brief "spike," the darkness of which is fairly constant between 0 and 7.0 kHz. This is, of course, a stop burst, and its distribution of energy across frequency is related to the place of articulation of the stop, as discussed in Chapter 8. Immediately following the burst is an interval of roughly 40 ms during which aperiodic energy is distributed broadly across frequency, but is relatively more intense in the 2.0- to 5.0-kHz range. This is the frication interval of the stop (see Chapter 8), and its distribution of energy should also be related to the place of articulation. Segment X4 is very brief, showing a spike-like event that, in this case, is not associated with a stop articulation, but rather with the voiced fricative /ð/. Some fricatives, especially those produced at the front of the vocal tract (e.g., /θ,ð,f,v/), may show little, if any, energy on a spectrogram, and in some cases the energy that is visible will be very brief as in segment X4.

Segmentation of Spectrograms

The process of segmenting a spectrogram involves the identification of pieces of the display that correspond roughly to phonemic or phonetic units. The distinction between "phonemic" and "phonetic" is important, because typically there are more phonetic units per spectrogram than phonemic units.

Glottal pulses play an important role in the measurement of various attributes of the spectrogram. The term *segment* has been introduced above as a temporal chunk or piece of the spectrogram that is somehow distinguishable from an adjacent chunk. These chunks also have some rough correspondence with sound categories, as indicated by the phonetic symbols at the bottom of the spectrogram. When scientists and clinicians want to know something about these chunks, however, they usually want to go past the very coarse observation of matching a given chunk with a sound type. Specifically, they are interested in making measurements to provide *quantitative information* about a segment. For example, a clinician might be interested in measuring the duration of the vowel /ʊ/ in the word /ʃʊd/, but cannot do so unless there are some rules for defining the onset and offset of the vowel. The rules for the boundaries, or onsets and offsets of many segments, often depend on the first and last glottal pulses of voiced segments. The glottal pulses shown as vertical lines in the spectrogram, therefore, play an important role in segmentation of spectrograms. Segmentation of the vowel /ʊ/ in /ʃʊd/ is shown in Figure 9–8 as example E, where the upward-pointing lines indicate the first and last glottal pulses of the vocalic segment. The first glottal pulse is considered to be the onset, or beginning of the vowel, and the last glottal pulse the offset or end of the vowel. The distance between the first and last glottal pulses along the *x*-, or time axis—the interval "E"—can be converted to time to determine the duration of /ʊ/.

The use of glottal pulses to identify onsets and offsets of segments in a spectrogram is a well-accepted practice, but must be recognized as a form of *operational definition,* and not as the *truth*. Investigators, whether they are in the laboratory or clinic, use such definitions to describe measurements precisely and to allow other investigators to make exactly the same measurements using the same criteria. When an investigator identifies the first glottal pulse of a vowel as the onset of the vocalic event, it does not necessarily imply a belief that this point in time is where the brain initiates a vowel, or even that the brain represents onsets and offsets of speech segments.

Segmentation of vowels is relatively straightforward when vowels are located between two obstruents. The beginning of the vowel is taken as the first "full" glottal pulse, and the end of the vowel is the last full glottal pulse. A full glottal pulse is one that extends from the baseline at least through F2 of the display. The requirement that the glottal pulse go at least as high in frequency as F2 distinguishes it from the glottal pulses seen in voiced stops, affricates, and fricatives, as well as some low-intensity pulses that extend only through F1. According to this reasoning, a glottal pulse that extends through at least F2 is visible only if the vocal tract is still open. If the vocal tract were closed, the sound energy generated within the vocal tract would not be visible at such high frequencies because these frequencies are filtered out by the vocal tract walls. Clearly, when trying to find the acoustic boundaries of a vowel, a clinician or scientist would like to identify the first and last instants in time when the vocal tract is open. When vowels are located before or after nasals, the "full glottal pulse" criterion cannot be used to segment a vowel from a nasal, but the change from an oral to nasal filter function, discussed in Chapter 8, can be used to find a vowel-nasal or nasal-vowel boundary. A sudden change in intensity at the boundary between a nasal and a vowel, and the sudden appearance of the low-frequency F1 characteristic of nasal cavity resonance, are good criteria for this segmentation problem. When vowels are located before or after semivowels (/l,w,ɹ,j/) or diphthongs (/ɑɪ, ɔɪ, ɑʊ, eɪ, oʊ/) the segmentation problem is very difficult because there are no natural boundaries. In general, the conservative approach in sequences such as "yellow" (/jɛloʊ/ or "I honor" (/ɑɪjɑnɚ/) is not to attempt a segmentation for phonetic or phonemic "chunks."

Segmentation of obstruents is also fairly simple in many cases. When an obstruent follows a vocalic segment (vowels, diphthongs, semivowels), the last full glottal pulse of the preceding vocalic is taken as the instant before closure of the vocal tract, and, thus, as the beginning of the closure interval. The same criterion can often be applied to nasal + obstruent sequences because nasals are voiced and have an obvious formant pattern. In the case of stops, the offset (or end) of the stop is taken as the burst (same for the closure offset of affricates). In the case of fricatives, the offset is taken as the end of the frication noise, or the first full glottal pulse of the following vowel. Even though this latter measurement point (the glottal pulse following the frication noise) produces a fricative interval that may be slightly longer than the actual frication, it is more reliable than trying to locate the precise ending of the frication noise. When fricatives and stops are abutted, as in an /s/ + stop sequence, separation of the frication from the closure interval must rely on the termination of frication noise and the onset of silence (i.e., no energy in the closure interval). When two fricatives follow each other, the changing spectrum must be used to identify the end of one and beginning of the other. When two stops follow each other, the only way to distinguish the closure intervals is if the first stop is released, and produces a burst.

Returning briefly to the issue of phonemic versus phonetic segmentation, the case of voiceless stops provides a good example of this problem because the stop includes a closure interval, a burst, a frication interval, and an aspiration interval. These are all intervals that could potentially be identified as segments on the spectrogram, but they are all associated with a single stop. If all these intervals were identified by segmentation, the segmentation is labeled "phonetic" because the different segments all relate to the same phoneme (i.e., the stop). If the closure, burst, frication, and aspiration are combined and regarded as one interval this would be a "phonemic" segment. This is not a problem with segments such as vowels, where "subsegments" are not likely to be identified. However, when dealing with spectrograms produced by speakers with speech disorders this can be a problem, and it is wise to keep in mind that segmentation may result in two or more pieces that actually relate to the same phoneme. The opposite case is also true, that two or more consecutive phonemes may not be segmentable as two separate "pieces," as described above for vowel-vowel, vowel-semivowel, and other sequences for which clear boundaries cannot be identified.[4]

Spectrographic segmentation of the utterance, "The blue spot is a normal dot," spoken by a 53-year-old male, is shown in Figure 9–9. A broad phonetic transcription is provided below the spectrogram, with the phonetic symbols located along the time axis roughly in the middle of the acoustically identified segments. The vertical lines immediately below the baseline mark the segmentation boundaries, determined according to the rules outlined above. The

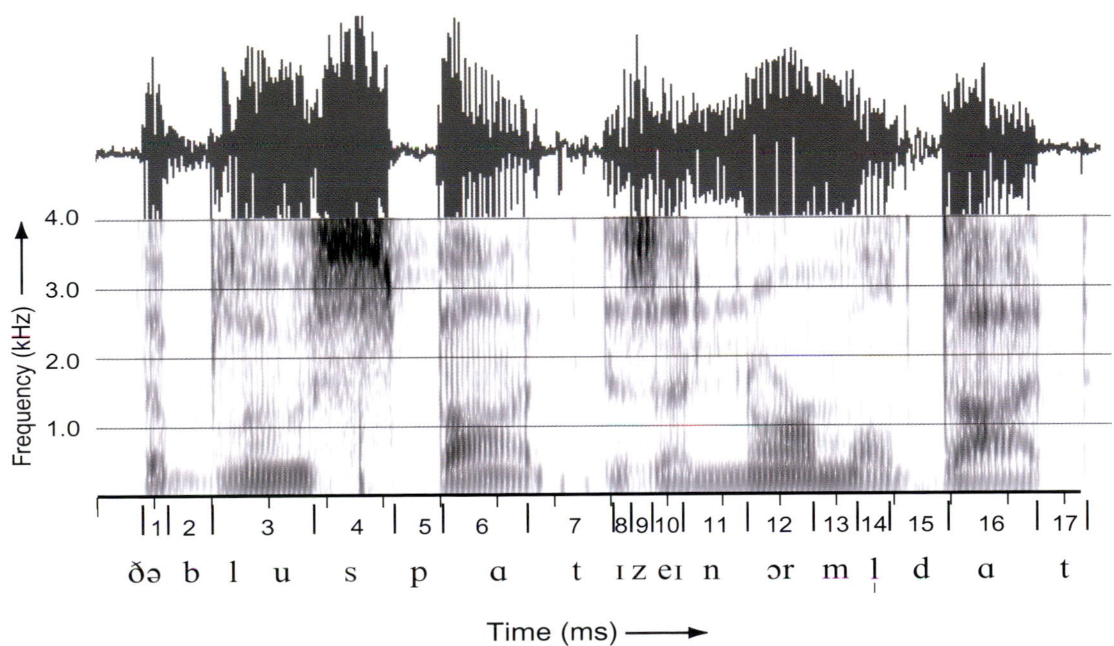

Figure 9–9. Spectrogram segmented according to the rules described in the text. The vertical lines immediately below the baseline of the spectrogram show the onsets and offsets of the segments, and the sound class corresponding to a segment is shown between the segment boundaries.

[4]Segmentation of a spectrogram does not have to be guided by sound classes (the approach described here), although that is certainly the most typical strategy. Segmentation could be guided by the underlying vocal tract gestures, an example of which is the vocalic articulatory gesture for the /uɪ/ sequence in the utterance, "The stew is good" (/ðəstuɪzgʊd/). Here the interest is in the relatively rapid and smoothly executed transition from a high-back (/u/) to a high-front (/ɪ/) configuration. These sorts of articulatory sequences, for which the "units" (segments) are defined on the basis of gestures rather than sound classes, have not been explored much in the clinical literature but are potentially of great diagnostic and theoretical value in understanding speech disorders.

1980s required a recording of speech on some permanent medium and, of course, the instrument itself. Typically, a speech sample would be recorded on a tape recorder (the tape being the permanent medium) and at some later time "fed into" the spectrograph for production of a spectrogram. All processing of the signal—the frequency analysis, the type of display, and so forth—was done by the fixed electronic circuitry of the instrument. That circuitry processed and displayed the *continuous* fluctuations of the magnetic field's strength recorded on the tape and then stored temporarily on the tape loop of the spectrograph. These continuous fluctuations in the strength of the magnetic field were converted to continuous fluctuations in the voltage applied to the marking stylus, which then burned patterns of relative darkness onto the paper in proportion to the strength of the voltage. The word *continuous* is important to this discussion: everything in this process was based on original recordings and transformations of the signal (i.e., from voltage to magnetic field, and then back to voltage, and ultimately to the darkness of the burned pattern) that did not change the continuous nature of the speech signal. A process such as this, in which the transforms and representations (magnetic, voltage, darkness of the trace, and so forth) are in the same form as the input signal—in this case the speech signal—is called an *analog process*. Computer analysis of speech requires a conversion of this analog representation to digital form.

Speech Analysis by Computer: From Recording to Analysis to Output

Figure 9–11 presents a simple block diagram of the important steps in speech analysis by computer. A microphone must be used to transduce the continuously varying pressure waveform of speech into a continuously varying electrical signal. High-quality microphones achieve this transduction in a number of different ways, producing an electrical replica of the pressure wave in all respects, including frequency, amplitude, and time. The microphone signal can be used as input to a tape recorder, or to the hard disk of the computer. The left side of Figure 9–11 shows these two different input paths for the microphone signal. When a tape recorder (assumed to be an analog device for this discussion) is the destination for the microphone signal, at some point the tape-recorded signal has to be input to the computer.

Computers (or digital tape recorders, essentially simple computing devices dedicated to sampling and storing analog signals) perform *digital* transformations of input signals, in which the analog signals are converted to a series of discrete numbers, each of which has the form of sequences of zeros (0s) and ones (1s). How that transformation is done is all important in computer-based speech analysis. The important factors in this transformation are (a) sampling rate, (b) filtering, and (c) quantization.

Digital Speech Samples and the Aural Flip Book

When speech is synthesized by computer, or when a natural speech signal is digitized, the computerized form of the signal is a series of discrete time points—samples—each of which contains a spectrum. When these time points are output from a computer—when they undergo digital-to-analog conversion—the human ear will connect the discrete samples and hear them as a smoothly-flowing speech signal. It is just like the flip books you enjoyed, and perhaps created, as a child (and maybe even as an adult). Each individual picture in the flip book is like a digital sample. When the stack of individual pictures is flipped, the human visual system connects the sequence of images and voilà! We have animation! Think of the process of digital-to-analog conversion as aural animation.

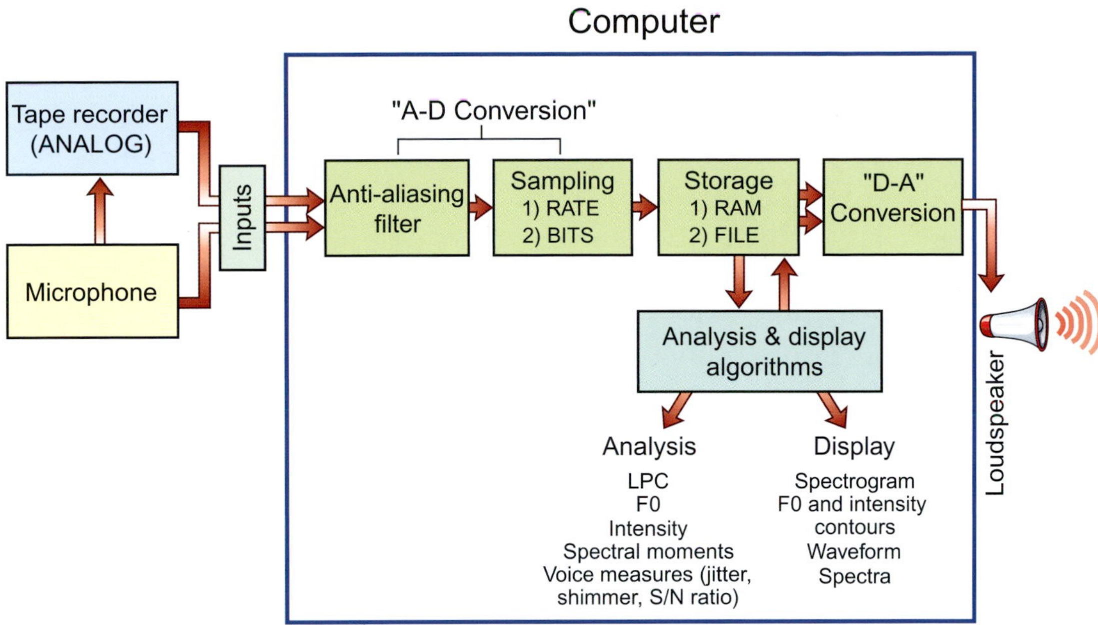

Figure 9–11. Block diagram of speech analysis by computer. See text for details

Sampling Rate

Because the computer stores an acoustic waveform as a series of discrete numbers, a decision must be made concerning how frequently the computer will "pick" and store a value from the continuously varying waveform. The conversion of analog to digital representation—A-to-D conversion, as indicated in Figure 9–11—is done by a piece of hardware called a sound card. The *sampling rate* determines how frequently numbers are picked off the analog event. Most computer programs and sound cards allow the sampling rate to be adjusted according the user's needs. These needs can be summed up pretty easily: What is the highest frequency in the analog waveform that is of interest for analysis, or perhaps playback to a listener?

Figure 9–12 illustrates the concept of sampling rate and how it is tied to the highest frequency of interest in a speech signal. For simplicity, a sinusoidal signal is used for this illustration, but the concept applies to complex waveforms. Panels A, B, and C of Figure 9–12 show one complete cycle of the same 1000-Hz sinusoidal signal, in its analog form, sampled by a computer at three different rates. Locations along the waveforms where samples would be taken by the computer are shown by the red circles for sampling rates of 500 Hz (500 samples per second; panel A), 2000 Hz (panel B), and 5000 Hz (panel C). In panel A, the 500 Hz sampling rate extracts only a single sample from the cycle. The location of this sample, indicated by the red circle slightly before the completion of the first half-cycle, is arbitrary. However, for this 1000-Hz sinusoid, a 500-Hz sampling rate will result in only one sample extracted per cycle, regardless of where the sample is located. This is because a 500-Hz sampling rate picks samples from the analog waveform every 2 ms (that is, the period of 500 Hz), which is *twice the duration of a 1000-Hz cycle*. In other words, the 500-Hz sampling is simply much too slow (i.e., selects samples too infrequently) to produce a correct digital estimate of the frequency of this 1000-Hz signal. This sampling rate could never produce two samples *within* a single cycle of this 1000-Hz waveform, regardless of where during the cycle a first sample is taken. The next (or previous) sample would always be taken in the next (or previous) cycle.

The example in panel A reveals an important axiom of computer sampling of analog waveforms.

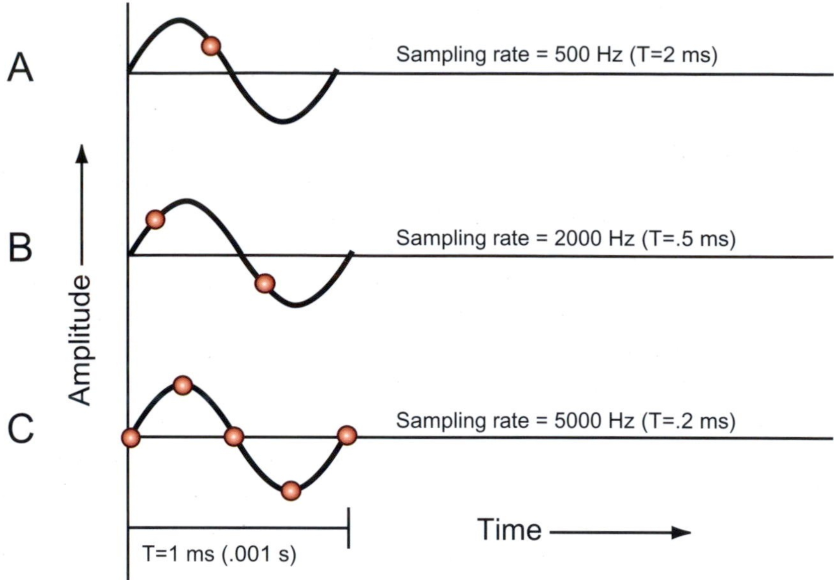

Figure 9–12. The concept of sampling rate, and its relation to the frequencies being sampled. Panels A, B, and C show how progressively higher sampling rates (computer samples of analog signal indicated by red circles on the waveforms) extract samples from a 1000-Hz sinusoid. "T" refers to the period of successive computer samples (the inverse of sampling rate). The "T" of 1 ms, shown under the sinusoidal waveforms, is the period of the signal being sampled. See text for explanation.

The axiom is directly related to the discussion in Chapter 6 of the relationship between frequency and period. A period (T) is a time interval along a repeating waveform whose inverse is frequency. The measurement of such a time *interval* requires at least two points—one to identify the start of the interval, the second to identify the end of the interval. With this in mind, the sampling axiom is as follows: *An accurate determination of a given frequency (not necessarily of the waveform details; see below) requires a sampling rate that extracts at least* ***two*** *samples from each individual cycle of the waveform*. The two samples then allow estimation of the period of the cycle, and thus its frequency. The way to ensure that two samples are obtained per cycle is to use a sampling rate that is twice the frequency one wishes to measure. Panel B shows how a sampling rate of 2000 Hz, with samples extracted from the analog waveform every 0.5 ms (half the time it takes to complete a single 1000-Hz cycle), results in the two samples-per-cycle required for an accurate estimate of the period. As in panel A, the placement of the first sample is arbitrary, but with a 2000-Hz sampling rate the next sample must fall within this particular cycle.

A general lesson from this discussion is that the sampling rate should always be at least twice the highest frequency that needs to be measured. According to information on vowels and consonants presented in Chapters 7 and 8, across *all* speech sounds there is phonetically relevant frequency information at least in the 0- to 8.0-kHz range, and for a limited number of sounds definitely up to 10.0 kHz. If one takes 10.0 kHz as the highest frequency of interest for most speech analysis applications, a sampling rate of no less than 20.0 kHz is required. Many speech analysis programs use 22.05 or 44.10 kHz as the default sampling rate (44.10 kHz is the standard sampling rate for digital audio equipment such as DAT tape recorders and compact disk players). Obviously, the more times per second a waveform is sampled, the more accurate the match between the analog waveform and its digital representation. In the absence of any other considerations, a high sampling rate is always desirable to increase the match between the analog and digital versions of the signal.

Sampling Rate Sidebar: Anti-Aliasing Filters

Figure 9–11 shows the input to the computer, whether from tape recorder or microphone, going through an *anti-aliasing filter* before the sampling phase of A-to-D conversion. The anti-aliasing filter is necessary to eliminate mistakes arising from the digital sampling process when no filter is used. These mistakes take the form of frequencies derived from the sampled signal, estimated from an *apparent* period between two sample points, that are not really in the signal but are natural results of a very specific (undesired) condition of sampling. That condition is in effect *when the sampling rate is not at least twice the highest frequency in the signal being sampled*. This may seem like a restatement of the sampling rate rule given above, but there is an important difference. To restate that rule: The sampling rate must be at least twice the highest frequency of *interest* to estimate it correctly. The aliasing rule says that if there are frequencies in the signal greater than *half* the sampling rate, the sampling process will estimate these frequencies erroneously—that is, the process will produce alias frequencies, which are not truly in the signal.

Why does this occur? A reconsideration of panel A of Figure 9–12 helps to answer the question. In this example, the frequency being sampled (1000 Hz) is, in fact, greater than half the sampling rate of 500 Hz. As stated above, with this sampling rate only one sample will be picked from the 1000-Hz waveform and the signal frequency will not be estimated correctly. However, because there are samples occurring every 2 ms, *something* will be estimated because the process will produce successions of points and, therefore, time intervals that will masquerade as real periods in the signal, even though the true signal does not contain those periods.

In a spectral analysis of the 1000-Hz sinusoid shown in Figure 9–12, the aliased frequency would be easily recognized, but in a complex signal, such as speech, aliasing can present a major problem if not addressed correctly. And even though 10.0 kHz was identified as the highest frequency of interest for *phonetic relevance*, the speech signal contains frequencies well above 10.0 kHz, especially for certain consonants. These very high frequencies are prevalent for some fricatives (Tabain, 1998), as well as when speakers have very short vocal tracts (e.g., when analyzing infant speech; see Bauer & Kent, 1987). This is where the anti-aliasing filter comes into play. To prevent frequencies greater than half the sampling rate from creating an aliasing problem, the signal is *filtered* before it is submitted to the A-to-D process. The anti-aliasing filter should have a low-pass configuration (i.e., passing frequencies from 0 Hz to some high frequency cutoff), with the cutoff frequency at half, or slightly less than half, the sampling rate. The object is to remove all frequencies more than half the sampling rate and so prevent aliasing—hence the name *anti-aliasing filter*.

Speech analysis systems with sampling rates of 22.05 kHz usually set the cutoff frequency of the anti-aliasing filter somewhere between 8.0 and 10.0 kHz. The actual filters may be resident on the sound card, as a hardware solution, or may be implemented with software. The exact details of cutoff frequencies are beyond the scope of this discussion; ask your instructor if you have a sudden, burning interest in the intricacies of anti-aliasing filters.

There is a familiar example of aliasing, familiar not from speech analysis but rather from the movies. Everyone has seen a movie scene in which a vehicle accelerates and the wheels initially appear to spin in the right direction (forward). As the vehicle continues to pick up speed, however, the wheels appear to freeze, as if they have stopped spinning, or may seem to spin in *reverse* even as the vehicle continues to move forward. The perception of frozen or reverse wheel motion is a case of aliasing. The illusion of no motion, or reverse motion, is produced by a sampling process like the one described above. Think of the motion of a rotating wheel on a car or stagecoach as an analog event, and the process of filming the motion as a sampling problem. Motion pictures are constructed from a series of individual frames, photographed at a fairly high rate—typically 24 frames per second (fps). Each frame is a sample picked from the analog motion, just like a sample taken by a sound card from an acoustic waveform. When the discrete motion picture frames are played back for viewing, the visual system connects the discrete frames and interprets them as continuous motion (because of a phenomenon called "persistence of vision"). As long as the sampling rate—24 fps—is twice as great as the frequency of wheel rotation, there will be two sampling points per rotation to allow a correct visual estimation of the relative speed and direction of the wheel's motion. When the wheel rotation frequency (~12 rotations per second) reaches half the sampling frequency (24 fps), however, the wheel rotation is illuminated over and over at exactly the same point in the rotation cycle and the wheel motion appears to stop. As the frequency of the wheel rotation increases past the one-half sampling frequency point, the sampling points occur across several cycles of the wheel motion and the direction of that motion seems to reverse. These alias motions (clearly the wheel is not frozen in time, nor spinning in reverse as the car speeds toward some spectacular encounter with a wall, the Hulk, or garden-variety James Bond villain) are a byproduct of the sampling process. In film, it is no big deal, but in the analysis of speech it could lead to the "finding" of signal frequencies not truly there.

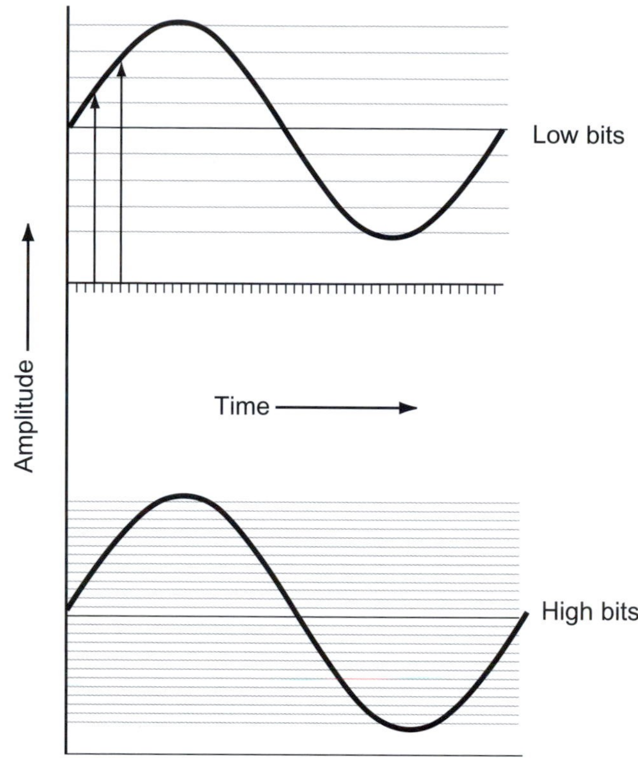

Figure 9–13. Quantization of analog waveform during the A-to-D process. Quantization levels are shown by the series of horizontal lines extending from the top to bottom of the amplitude scale. Time samples for conversion of the analog signal to digital form are shown on the *x*-axis of the upper graph. *Upper panel* = few quantization levels, low bit rate. *Lower panel* = many quantization levels, high bit rate. On the upper, low-bit chart, arrows pointing upward from the third and sixth samples show samples for which an exact quantization level is not available.

Quantization (Bits)

The preceding discussion describes how a computer implements A-to-D conversion along the time scale, but not the amplitude scale. Information concerning waveform amplitude must also be coded in digital form, a process called quantization. The number of *bits* used in A-to-D conversion determines how accurately the amplitude of an analog waveform is represented in digital form. Quantization is illustrated by the schematic diagrams in Figure 9–13. A 1000-Hz sinusoid having an arbitrary peak-to-peak amplitude is shown in both the upper and lower panels. In both panels, the sinusoid is shown with a series of equidistant, horizontal lines spanning the entire amplitude scale. In the upper panel these horizontal lines are less closely spaced than in the lower panel. Think of these horizontal lines as amplitude levels that can be digitized by the sound card. These are called quantization levels. At points along the sinusoid where a horizontal line—a quantization level—crosses the waveform, the amplitude stored by the computer will be faithful to the amplitude in the analog waveform. But what happens for points sampled along the time domain for which the analog waveform amplitude is between two quantization levels? For example, if the 1000-Hz sinusoid is sampled at a high rate (e.g., 22.05 kHz; individual sample times in Figure 9–13 marked by the short vertical lines along the *x*-axis) with the quantization levels shown in the upper panel in Figure 9–13, there will be a number of time samples along the waveform for which a quantization level is not available. These are shown in Figure 9–13, upper panel, by the time samples falling in between two of the adjacent amplitude levels available for digital storage (arrows extending upward from the third and sixth time samples). The value stored by the computer for an amplitude of an analog waveform that is "between" quantization levels will be the one corresponding to the closest quantization level. This means that, during the digitization process, some real (analog) amplitudes will "jump up," and some will "jump down," to the nearest quantization level. The absence of a quantization level at a given point along the amplitude variation of a waveform, therefore, does not prevent storage of that sample, which seems like a good thing. The amplitude represented for such a sample, however, is not the correct one and, in fact, produces a digital representation that distorts the shape of the analog waveform. This is not desirable, although in some cases it may be unavoidable. The ideal solution to the problem is to have the quantization levels spaced as closely as possible along the amplitude scale, as simulated in the lower panel of Figure 9–13. In this case, the quantization offered produces a digital representation of the sinusoid amplitudes much more like the analog waveform, because more analog amplitude variations can be stored directly, at the available quantization levels, and the "jumps" for in-between time samples will be smaller than the ones required in the upper panel of Figure 9–13.

The number of quantization levels available in A-to-D conversion is generally described by the number of bits (bits = binary digits) used to store amplitudes in digital form. The greater the number of bits, the more quantization levels available for storing waveform amplitudes. It follows that a greater number of bits will produce a better match between the amplitudes of the analog and digital versions of the waveform. The A-to-D conversion illustrated in the lower panel of Figure 9–13 has a greater number of bits compared to the upper panel because it allows more amplitudes to be represented during the conversion process. Speech waveforms have been digitized (that is, undergone the process of A-to-D conversion) at 8, 12, 16, and 32 bits. Sixteen bits provides very good representation of the amplitude fluctuations in a speech waveform. Speech digitized with 8 bits of amplitude resolution is fairly intelligible, but the overall quality of the signal is noticeably improved when a 16-bit conversion is used.

Analysis and Display

Most speech analysis programs have algorithms for display, editing, and analysis of speech waveforms. The basic display of a speech analysis program is the speech waveform, shown above the spectrograms in Figures 9–8 and 9–9. A waveform of the utterance *To feed the cat one must shoo the dog* is shown in Figure 9–14. This utterance was produced by one of the authors as a direct-to-disk recording (microphone input directly into the computer; see Figure 9–11), with a sampling rate of 22.05 kHz and 16 bits of amplitude resolution. The utterance waveform was displayed in near-real time as it was spoken, and immediately stored as a file. The waveform display at the top of Figure 9–14 is essentially identical to the one that appeared on the screen as it was being recorded.

Speech analysis programs allow the user to manipulate and process waveforms in many different ways, and to display the results of those processes. As listed in Figure 9–11, the typical speech analysis program allows linear predictive code analysis of formant frequencies (see below), different types of F0 and intensity measurement, computation of spectral moments (see Chapters 8 and 10), as well as other analyses beyond the scope of this book. Programs can generate a digital spectrogram, F0 contours, intensity contours, spectra for different "chunks" of a waveform, measures of voice production (jitter, shimmer, signal-to-noise ratio), and so forth. As a case study of computer analysis of speech and as a teaser for information on vowels presented in Chapter 10, consider Figure 9–14 from top to bottom as a demonstration of computer analysis of vowel formant frequencies.

The utterance whose speech waveform is shown in Figure 9–14 contains an example of each of the corner vowels of English (the phonetic symbol for the vowel in *dog* is given as /ɔ/, but the low-back corner vowel is usually thought to be /ɔ/'s near neighbor /ɑ/. In the dialect of the individual who produced the display shown in Figure 9–14, a weird farrago of Philadelphia origin and Cheesehead spirit, the vowel in *dog* sounds to most listeners as something between /ɔ/ and /ɑ/). Formant frequencies are often measured for the corner vowels as a way to map out, in acoustic terms, the limits of vowel articulation for a given speaker. The conventional way to make formant frequency measures is to locate and segment the vowel of interest, select for analysis a relatively brief piece ("window") from the overall vowel waveform, and calculate for this piece the values of F1, F2, and F3.

Modern, digital techniques for processing and analyzing speech waveforms were presented.

An important caution is that digital techniques can sometimes produce incorrect analyses, and that the likelihood of such errors is greater in speakers with noisy voice sources and hypernasality, two speech characteristics encountered often in speech disorders.

REFERENCES

Atal, B., & Hanauer, S. (1971). Speech analysis and synthesis by linear prediction. *Journal of the Acoustical Society of America*, *50*, 637–655.

Bauer, H., & Kent, R. (1987). Acoustic analyses of infant fricative and trill vocalizations. *Journal of the Acoustical Society of America*, *81*, 505–511.

Byrd, D. (1993). 54,000 American stops. *UCLA Working Papers in Phonetics*, *83*, 97–116.

Crystal, T., & House, A. (1988). The duration of American-English stop consonants: An overview. *Journal of Phonetics*, *16*, 285–294.

Klatt, D. (1976). Linguistic uses of segmental duration in English: Acoustic and perceptual evidence. *Journal of the Acoustical Society of America*, *59*, 1208–1221.

Solzhenitsyn, A. (1969). *The first circle*. New York: Bantam Books.

Tabain, M. (1998). Non-sibilant fricatives in English. Spectral information above 10 kHz. *Phonetica*, *55*, 107–130.

Umeda, N. (1977). Consonant duration in American English. *Journal of the Acoustical Society of America*, *61*, 846–858.

Zue, V., & Cole, R. (1979). Experiments on spectrogram reading. *Acoustics, Speech, and Signal Processing, IEEE International Conference on ICASSP '79*, *4*, 116–119.

10

Acoustic Phonetics Data

INTRODUCTION

This chapter provides a selective summary of acoustic phonetics data. The presentation must be selective because the research literature is voluminous. The large quantity of data available reflects the many uses of acoustic phonetics research—the discipline of acoustic phonetics serves many masters. For example, acoustic phonetics data are used by linguists who wish to enhance their phonetic description of a language; by speech communication specialists who are interested in developing high-quality speech synthesis and recognition systems; by scientists who wish to test theories of speech production, and prefer to use the speech acoustic approach to the interpretation of articulatory patterns obtained using one of the more invasive and time-consuming physiological approaches (such as x-ray tracking of articulatory motions); by speech perception scientists who want to understand the acoustic cues used in the identification of vowels and consonants by normal hearers and persons with hearing loss and prosthetic hearing devices; and by speech-language pathologists who want information concerning a client's speech production behaviors —information that can be documented quantitatively and, in some cases may be too subtle or transient to be captured by auditory analysis.

The majority of this chapter is concerned with the acoustic characteristics of *speech sound segments* —the vowel and consonant segments of a language. A brief discussion of the acoustic characteristics of prosody concludes the chapter.

VOWELS

The upper part of Figure 10–1 shows a spectrogram of two vowels, /æ/ and /i/, spoken by a 57-year-old healthy male in the disyllable frames /əˈhæd/ and /əˈhid/. The /əˈhVd/ frame (where V = vowel) is a famous one in speech science, originally used by Peterson and Barney (1952) in their landmark study of vowel formant frequencies produced by men, women, and children. Peterson and Barney (1952) wanted to measure formant frequencies in vowels under minimal influence from the surrounding phonetic context—that is, with little or no coarticulatory effects. The obvious way to get this kind of "pure" information on vowel articulation, and the resulting formant frequencies, is to have speakers produce isolated, sustained vowels. However, when participants are asked to do this, they have a tendency to sing, rather than speak, the vowels. Peterson and Barney, therefore, designed a more natural speech task in which the unstressed schwa preceded a stressed syllable initiated by the glottal fricative /h/. The reasoning was that a segment whose articulation required primarily laryngeal gestures would minimally influence the vocal tract gestures required for a following vowel. The /d/ at the end of the syllable was necessary to provide a "natural" ending to the syllable, and also accommodated the production of lax vowels such as /ɪ/, /ɛ/, and /ʊ/, which in English do not occur in open syllables.

Clearly, the /d/ at the end of the syllable might have some influence on the vowel articulation. But Peterson and Barney (1952) made their formant

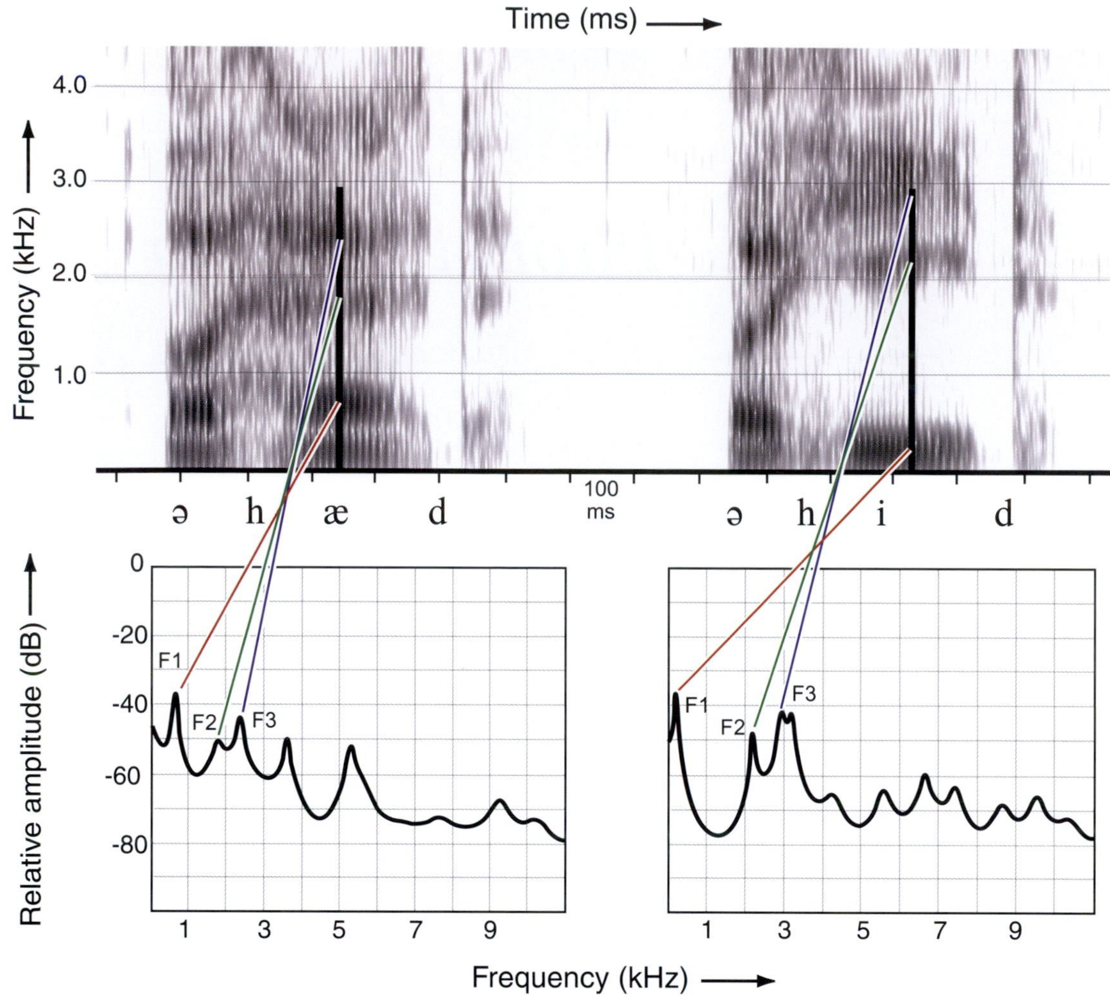

Figure 10–1. Spectrograms of two vowels (*top part of figure*), /æ/ and /i/, spoken by a 57-year-old healthy male in the disyllable frames /əˈhæd/and /əˈhid/. Bottom part of the figure shows LPC spectra for the two vowels, measured at the temporal middle of the vowels. The colored lines connect the middle of the formant bands on the spectrograms to the peaks in the LPC spectra.

frequency measurements at a location where the formants were "steady" (not changing in frequency), which they believed minimized any influence from the final /d/. Conveniently, this measurement point also seemed likely to capture the "target" location of the vowel. In other words, the point at which formant frequencies were stable was likely to coincide with the articulatory configuration aimed at by the speaker when trying to produce the best possible version of the vowel. Also, the inclusion of the schwa as the first syllable provided some control over the prosodic pattern of the disyllable, placing stress on the /hVd/ syllable.

Forty-three years following the publication of Peterson and Barney's (1952) classic work, Hillenbrand, Getty, Clark, and Wheeler (1995) published a replication of the study using updated analysis methods. Like Peterson and Barney, Hillenbrand et al. studied men ($N = 45$), women ($N = 48$), and children aged 10 to 12 years ($N = 46$, both girls and boys) producing the twelve monophthong vowels of English (/i,ɪ,e,ɛ,æ,ɑ,ɔ,o,ʊ,u,ʌ,ɝ/ in an /hVd/ frame.[1] Hillen-

[1]The vowel inventory of English is not always described as having twelve monophthongs. In particular, /e/ and /o/ are diphthongized in many dialects, but less often in the upper Midwest dialects included in the Hillenbrand et al. (1995) study.

brand et al. measured the first four formants (F1-F4) at their most stable point, in much the same way as shown in Figure 10–1 (in the figure, measurement of the fourth formant is omitted). The heavy vertical line through the spectrogram shows the point in time at which the formant frequencies were measured (in these cases, roughly in the middle of the vowel duration). Formant frequencies were estimated using linear predictive code (LPC) analysis, discussed in Chapter 9. The LPC spectra for the measurement point shown on the spectrograms are provided in the lower half of Figure 10–1. Lines point from the middle of the formant bands to the corresponding peaks in the LPC spectra. For these vowels, values of the first three formant frequencies for /æ/ are approximately 700, 1750, and 2450 Hz, and for /i/ are roughly 290, 2200, and 2950 Hz.

Figure 10–2 shows some of Hillenbrand et al.'s (1995, p. 3104) data in the form of an F1-F2 plot. Each phonetic symbol represents an F1-F2 coordinate for a given speaker's production of that vowel. Two of the vowels (/e/ and /o/) are not plotted to reduce crowding of the data points. The ellipses drawn around each vowel category enclose roughly 95% of all the observable points for that vowel. These data show clearly how a single vowel can be

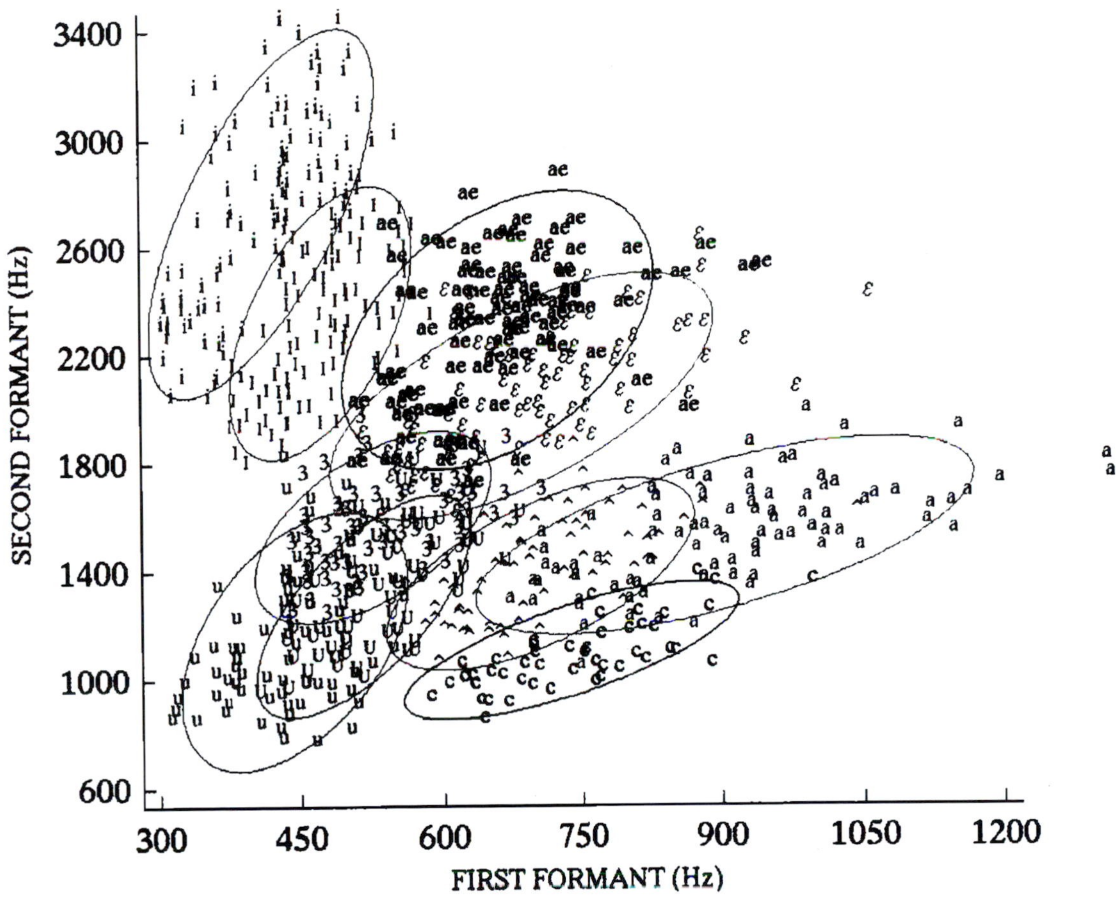

Figure 10–2. F1-F2 plot of American English vowels from Hillenbrand et al. (1995, p. 3104). Each phonetic symbol represents an F1-F2 coordinate for a given speaker's production of that vowel. Two vowels (/e/ and /o/) are not plotted to reduce crowding of the data points. The ellipses drawn around each vowel category enclose roughly 95% of all the observable points for that vowel. Reproduced with permission.

/ɝ/ is sometimes also not included as an English monophthong, but may be considered a rhotacized (/ɹ/-colored) vowel. Also note that Hillenbrand et al. did not use the schwa preceding the /hVd/syllable, as in Peterson and Barney (1952).

represented by a wide range of F1-F2 values. For example, the vowel /i/ shows points ranging between (approximately) 300 to 500 Hz on the F1 axis and 2100 to 3400 Hz on the F2 axis. The ellipse enclosing the /i/ points is oriented upward and leaning slightly to the right. Points in the lower part of the ellipse are almost certainly from men, points in the middle from women, and points at the upper part and to the right from children. This follows from the material presented in Chapters 6 and 7 on resonance patterns of tubes of different lengths, and age and sex-related differences in vocal tract length. The same general summary can be given for almost any vowel in this plot, even though the degree of variation and orientation of the ellipses varies from vowel to vowel. Despite the wide variation across speakers in formant frequencies for a given vowel, Hillenbrand et al. (1995) replicated Peterson and Barney's (1952) finding that the vowel intended by a speaker was almost always perceived correctly—consistent with the speaker's intention—by listeners. Somehow listeners heard the same vowel category even when confronted with a wide variety of formant patterns.

Figure 10–2 also shows that the formant frequency patterns of one vowel often overlap with those of another vowel. There is a small region of overlap between the ellipses of /i/ and /ɪ/, and a larger region of overlap between /æ/ and /ɛ/. In the lower left-hand part of the plot, roughly around F1 = 525 Hz and F2 = 1400 Hz, there is a three-way overlap of the vowels /u/, /ʊ/, and /ɝ/. In many cases, these areas of overlap are for vowels produced by speakers with vocal tracts of different lengths. For example, a good portion of the overlap between /æ/ and /ɛ/ seems to come from adult male /æ/ values with adult female, or child /ɛ/ values. But there are many cases where the overlap is not so clearly explained by differing vocal tract lengths. Still, the question remains, how do we hear the *same* formant frequencies produced by different speakers as *different* vowels? For the time being, Hillenbrand et al.'s (1995) data, like those of Peterson and Barney (1952), demonstrate that knowing a pattern of formant frequencies does not necessarily provide sufficient information to identify the intended (spoken) vowel category. At the least, the identity of the speaker, including age, sex, and almost certainly dialect, must be known to link a specific formant pattern to a vowel category.

Figure 10–3 plots a summary of a subset of the data reported by Hillenbrand et al. (1995). The subset includes averaged F1-F2 data from men, women, and children, for corner vowels that were "well-identified" by a panel of listeners. Corner vowels define the limits of vowel articulation, with /i/ the highest and most front vowel, /æ/ the lowest and most front, /ɑ/ the lowest and most back, and /u/ the highest and most back. If these are the most extreme articulatory configurations for vowels in English, the formant frequencies should also be at the most extreme coordinates in F1-F2 space. By including only data from "well-identified" vowels, the plotted data can be regarded as excellent exemplars of these vowel categories. When the average F1-F2 coordinates for each of the four corner vowels are connected by a line for each of the three speaker groups, three vowel quadrilaterals are formed. In an F1-F2 plot, the area enclosed by such a quadrilateral is called the acoustic vowel space.

Three general characteristics of these F1-F2 plots are noteworthy. First, the vowel quadrilaterals for men, women, and children move from the lower left to upper right part of the graph, respectively. This is because the vocal tract becomes progressively shorter across these three speaker groups, and shorter vocal tracts produce higher resonant frequencies. Second, the area of the vowel quadrilaterals—the acoustic vowel space—appears to be larger for children, as compared to women, and larger for women as compared to men. This probably has little to do with articulatory differences between the groups, but rather is another consequence of the different-sized vocal tracts. Exactly the same articulatory configurations for the corner vowels in a shorter, as compared to longer vocal tract, not only generate higher formant frequencies in the shorter vocal tract but also greater distances between F1-F2 points for the different vowels. The larger vowel space for the children, as compared to the men, therefore, does not mean the children use more extreme articulatory configurations for vowels. Third, the acoustic vowel quadrilateral for one group of speakers cannot be perfectly fit to the quadrilateral for a different group by moving it to the new location and uniformly expanding or shrinking it until an exact

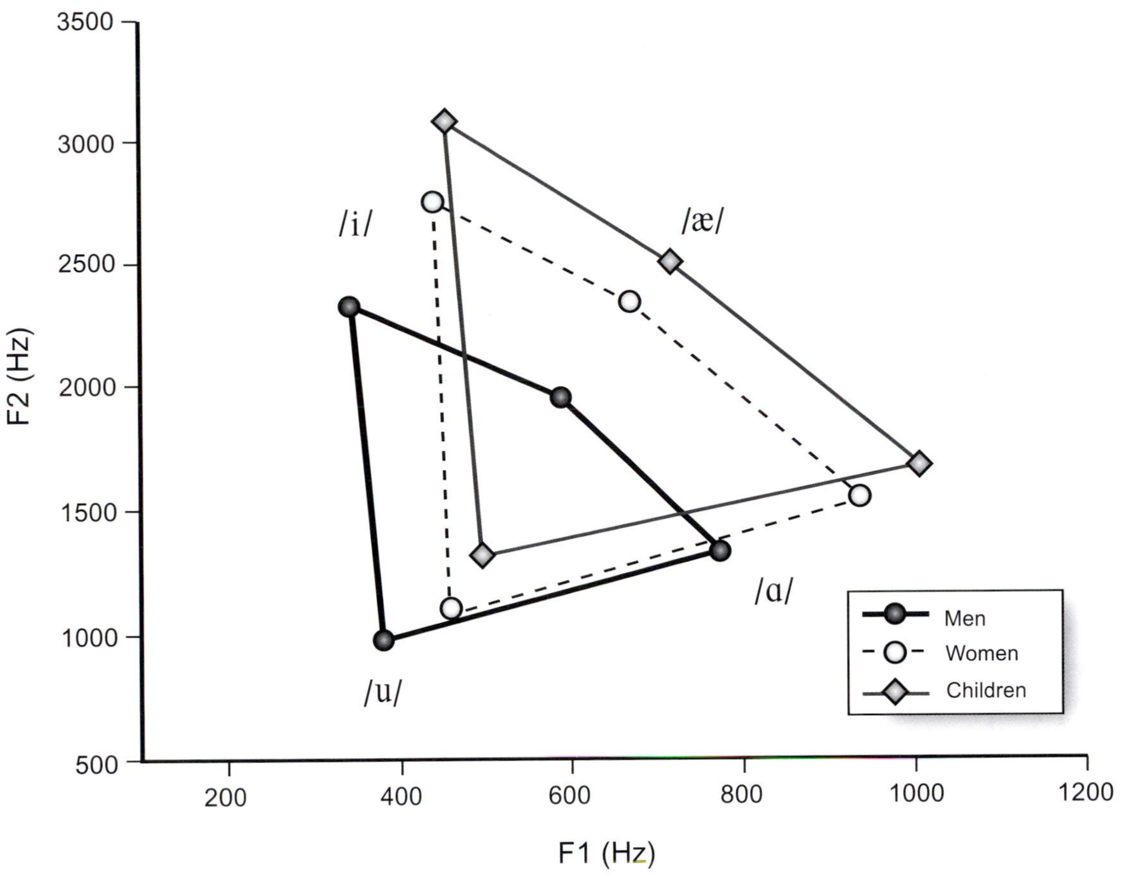

Figure 10–3. Vowel spaces constructed from corner vowels (/i/, /æ/, /ɑ/, /u/) of American English for men (*filled circles connected by solid lines*), women (*unfilled circles connected by dashed lines*), and children aged 10 to 12 years (*lightly shaded diamonds connected by solid lines*). These data are replotted from Hillenbrand et al. (1995, Table V., p. 3103) and are averages of vowels that were well identified by a crew of listeners.

match is achieved. Imagine the quadrilateral for men in Figure 10–3 moved into the position of the quadrilateral for women, followed by a uniform expansion of the male space to "fit" the female space. This attempt to scale the male quadrilateral to the female quadrilateral fails because the magnitudes of the sex-related vowel differences are not the same for each vowel. For example, note the relative closeness in F1-F2 space of the male and female /u/, as compared to the other three vowels. A similar inability to scale the vowels of one group to another is seen in Figure 10–4, which is an F1-F2 plot for the lax vowels (/ɪ/, /ʊ/, /ɛ/) reported by Hillenbrand et al. (1995). The group differences in these vowel triangles are very much like the ones shown for the corner vowel quadrilaterals (Figure 10–3), including vowel-specific differences across groups. Note especially the small difference between males and females for /ʊ/, as compared to the much larger male-female differences for /ɪ/ and /ɛ/. The lax-vowel triangle for men clearly cannot be scaled in a simple way to obtain the triangle for women.

The acoustic vowel space for corner vowels has a potential clinical application as an index of speech motor integrity. Evidence from several studies of speakers with dysarthria (speech disorders resulting from neurological disease (see Turner, Tjaden, & Weismer, 1995; Weismer, Jeng, Laures, Kent, & Kent, 2001; Liu, Tsao, & Kuhl, 2005), glossectomy (removal of tongue tissue, usually because of a cancerous tumor (see Sammam, 2006; Whitehill, Ciocca, Chan, & Samman, 2006), and even neurologically normal

vowel. In contrast, the F1-F2 points for the [ɪ]-[e] and [u]-[ʊ] English vowel pairs produced by Taiwanese speakers are very close together, differing only by small amounts along the F1 dimension. These vowel pairs in Mandarin-accented English are, therefore, closer together than any other vowel pair in the graph. It is as if the Mandarin speakers are treating the two English vowels of both pairs as members of a single vowel class.

There are complicated and competing theories of why the patterns in Figure 10–6 occur. Without pursuing in too much depth these very complex explanations of L2 phonetic performance, in both cases described above the Mandarin speakers produced a "new" vowel ([ɪ] in one case, [ʊ] in the other) almost as if it were a member of one of the "shared" vowels ([e] and [u]). Because the formant frequencies for the "shared" vowels are not identical across the two languages (see above), perhaps it may be more accurate to say the Mandarin speakers took the "shared"-"new" vowel pairs, and treated them as one category by producing F1-F2 values for both the "shared" and "new" vowels at an intermediate location between the American's well-separated F1-F2 points for the two vowels. Think of it as a phonetic compromise when the skill of producing two nearby, but separate, vowels is not yet available to a speaker.

Within-Speaker Variability in Formant Frequencies

The formant frequencies plotted in Figures 10–3 to 10–6 are averages across speakers. Figure 10–2, from Hillenbrand et al. (1995), presents a more realistic picture of variability in formant frequencies for a given vowel, but even this presentation shows only *across*-speaker variability. Within a speaker, vowel formant frequencies vary with a number of factors. These factors include—but may not be limited to—speaking rate, syllable stress, speaking style, and phonetic context.

Traditionally, the effects of these different factors on vowel formant frequencies have been referenced to a speaking condition in which the vowel is produced in a more or less pure form. Presumably, the best way to obtain a "pure" vowel production would be to have a speaker produce it in isolation, perhaps much like the sustained vowel often used in a clinical evaluation of the speech production apparatus. A problem with this is the tendency of speakers to sing, rather than speak the vowel. As mentioned above, in their original study of vowel formant frequencies, Peterson and Barney (1952) designed the /əˈhVd/ frame as a speech production event similar to real speech but largely free of many of the influencing factors noted above. Stevens and House (1963), in their classic paper on phonetic context effects on vowel formant frequencies, demonstrated in three sophisticated speakers the lack of any difference in F1 and F2 for isolated vowels and vowels spoken in the /hVd/ frame. This result, as well as some other data reviewed by Stevens and House, suggest that formant frequencies measured at the midpoint of a vowel in the /hVd/ frame are representative of vowels articulated under minimal influence from factors such as context, rate, and so forth. Because of this, vowels measured in the /hVd/ frame are often referred to as *null context vowels.*

When null context vowels are plotted in F1-F2 space together with the same vowels produced in varied phonetic contexts, at different rates, and in different speaking styles, an interesting pattern emerges. Figure 10–7 shows such a plot for the corner vowels (/i/, /æ/, /ɑ/, /u/) whose formant frequencies were derived for male speakers from several different sources in the literature. Two sets of "null context" data are plotted, one from Peterson and Barney (1952; filled circles connected by solid lines), the other from Hillenbrand et al. (1995; open circles connected by dashed lines). The decision to include F1-F2 data for null context vowels from two different data sets underscores the potential variability in these kinds of measurements. The two sets of null context data are most different for the low vowels /æ/ and especially /ɑ/. The speakers in the two studies were from the same geographical region (Michigan, with a few speakers from other areas), but their recordings are separated in time by close to 50 years. A likely explanation for the difference in the low vowel formant frequencies is changing patterns of vowel pronunciation over the period from about 1950 to 1990.

How do formant frequencies deviate from null context values when they are produced under different speaking conditions? The data shown in Figure 10–7 include F1-F2 data for the corner vowels

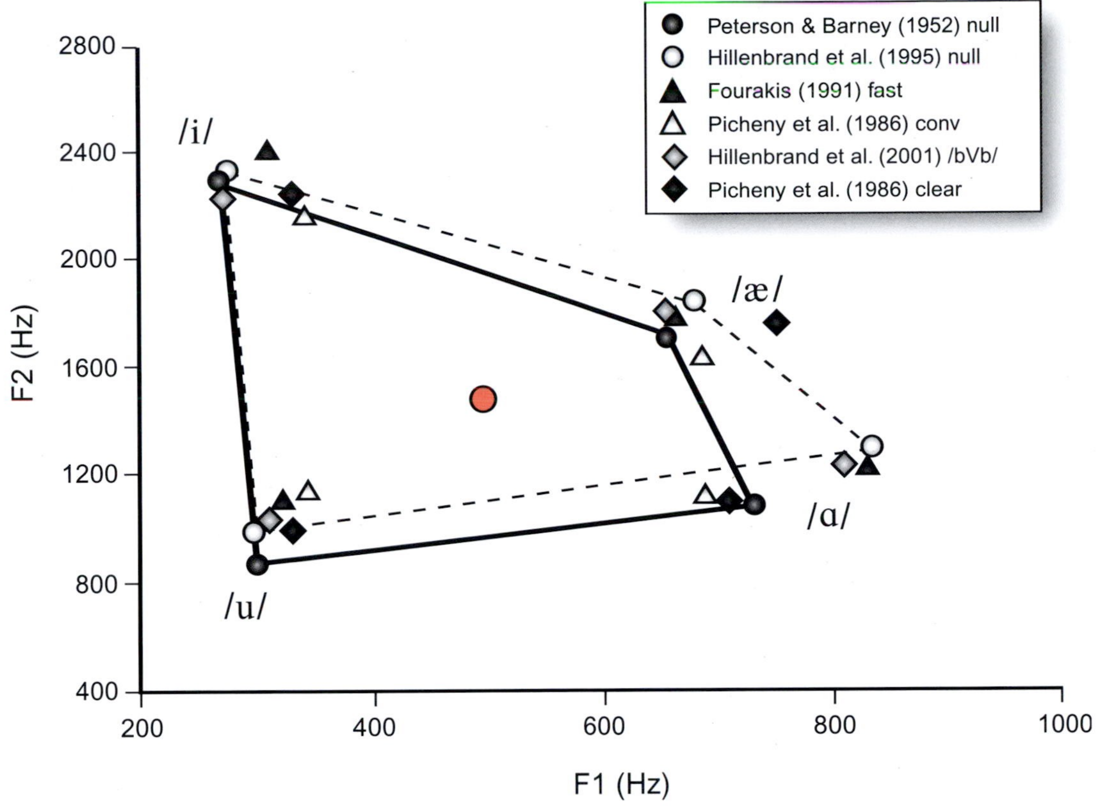

Figure 10–7. F1-F2 plot showing two vowel spaces for the "null context" corner vowels, plus corner-vowel data from studies in which the vowels were produced in other speaking conditions. Null context data are from tabled means published by Peterson and Barney (1952) and from careful pencil-and-ruler estimates of figures shown in Hillenbrand et al. (1995). Data from Fourakis (1991) are from tabled formant frequencies for fast-speech, stressed vowels pooled across various phonetic contexts. Values plotted from Picheny, Durlach, and Braida (1986) are for vowels extracted from sentence productions in conversational and clear-style speech and were estimated by the pencil-and-ruler technique from their published figures. The same estimation technique was used to obtain the /bVb/ data from Hillenbrand et al. (2001). The red circle in the middle of the plot is the F1-F2 pattern expected from a male vocal tract with uniform cross-sectional area from glottis to lips (the expected vocal tract shape for schwa). All plotted data points are from male speakers.

for vowels spoken at a fast rate, but with syllable stress (Fourakis, 1991; filled triangles), in conversational-style production of sentences (Picheny et al., 1986; unfilled triangles), in a "clear-speech" production style of sentences (Picheny et al., 1986; filled diamonds), and in a /bVb/ context (Hillenbrand, Clark, & Nearey, 2001; lightly shaded diamonds).

With certain exceptions,[2] and especially when the Hillenbrand et al. (1995) null context vowel space is used as a reference, vowels spoken in any of the other conditions tend to have F1-F2 points that move "inside" of the vowel space created by the null context quadrilateral. Somewhat more specifically, the F1-F2 points for the different conditions seem to move away from the null context points for any of the corner vowels in the direction of a point roughly in the center of the quadrilaterals, indicated by the red circle. This point plots F1 = 500 Hz, F2 = 1500 Hz, the first two formant frequencies associated with the "neutral vowel" configuration, or a vocal

[2]The most notable exceptions are the points from Fourakis (1991) for /ɑ/ and /i/.

tract with uniform cross-sectional area from the glottis to the lips. As discussed in Chapter 7, this is the vocal tract configuration most closely associated with schwa (/ə/). The F1 = 500 Hz, F2 = 1500 Hz pattern is appropriate for an adult male.

One way to interpret the overall pattern seen in Figure 10–7 is to regard the null context formant frequencies (and underlying vocal tract configuration) for a given vowel as an idealized target. In this view, described most explicitly by Bjorn Lindblom (1963, 1990), the speaker always aims for the idealized target, but misses it in connected speech by varying degrees because the articulators do not have sufficient time to reach the target before transitioning to the target for the next sound. For example, the target vocal tract shape (the area function) for the vowel /i/ would have a relatively tight constriction in the front of the vocal tract, and a very wide opening in the pharyngeal region. This vocal tract shape is a significant deviation from the straight-tube configuration of schwa, and, of course, fits the description of /i/ as a high-front vowel. In Lindblom's view, when a vowel such as /i/ is produced in a condition other than the null context, the idealized target will be missed in a specific way, namely, by producing a vocal tract configuration (and resulting formant frequencies) that reflects a slightly lesser deviation from the schwa configuration. It is as if all vowels are viewed as deviated vocal tract shapes (and formant frequencies) from the straight-tube configuration of schwa. Under optimal conditions, these deviations are maximal. In connected speech, however, the deviations from the schwa configuration are not as dramatic. By not producing the most extreme configuration associated with the sound, the speech production apparatus has more time to produce a sequence of sounds in an acceptable manner. An /i/ in connected speech is still a high-front vowel, but not quite as high and front as in the null context.

Lindblom (1963) called this phenomenon "articulatory undershoot." Undershoot, in his opinion, occurred as a result of phonetic context, increased speaking rate, reduced stress, and casual speaking style, but all these different causes could be explained by a single mechanism. Simply put, the shorter the vowel duration, the greater the undershoot. In the language of phonetics, vowels experience greater reduction as vowel duration decreases, regardless of the condition in which the shorter vowel duration is elicited. Although this is not a universally accepted interpretation of undershoot, it often explains a good deal of variation in formant frequencies for a given vowel produced by a specific speaker. Most likely, factors other than vowel duration may, in some cases, have an independent effect on formant frequencies. For example, in Figure 10–7, the vowels /ɑ/ and /i/ from Fourakis (1991) do not fit the duration explanation of undershoot because they fall outside the null context quadrilaterals, even though the "fast condition" vowel durations were relatively short (as reported by Fourakis, 1991, Table III, p. 1821). Because these vowels were stressed, an independent effect of stress on vowel formant frequencies must be considered a possibility.

Summary of Vowel Formant Frequencies

The take-home messages from this discussion of vowel formant frequencies and their variability across and within speakers are as follows. First, sex and age have a dramatic effect on the formant frequencies for a given vowel because these variables are closely associated with differences in vocal tract size and length. In general, the longer and larger the human vocal tract, the lower the formant frequencies for all vowels. This explains why, for a given vowel, there is such a large range of formant frequencies across the population (see Figure 10–2). The issue of how humans recognize a wide range of F-patterns as the same vowel is taken up in Chapter 11. Second, even when vocal tract length/size factors are held roughly constant, the formant frequencies for a given vowel may vary for several reasons. One of these reasons may reflect the inherent constraints on a phonetic symbol system. Even though a vowel may be transcribed as /u/ in several different languages, the F-pattern associated with these vowels may be substantially different (see Figure 10–5). The same conclusion can almost certainly be made about the same vowel produced by speakers of different dialects of the same language (Clopper, Pisoni, & de Jong, 2005). Additional reasons for variation with constant vocal tract length include the effects of phonetic context, syllable stress, speaking rate, and speaking style.

All this means that if one is asked the question, "What are the formant frequencies for the vowel ____?" An answer cannot be supplied without additional information on the speaker, the nature of the speech material, the language being spoken, and so forth. Even with all these questions answered, a definitive, precise answer is probably not feasible. It is more likely that a definitive, precise answer is not necessary because vowels may be perceived by focusing on relations among the formant frequencies, rather then absolute values of individual formants. These and other issues concerning vowel perception are discussed in Chapter 11.

A Brief Note on Vowel Formant Frequencies Versus Formant Trajectories

The discussion above presented what can be called a "slice-in-time" view of vowel formant frequencies. In this view, the formant frequencies measured *at a given point in time* during the vowel nucleus provide a good representation of the vowel articulation—and presumably, the contribution of the vowel to speech intelligibility—if the time point for measurement is chosen wisely. Typically, speech scientists have tried to select the time point for formant frequency measurement by estimating the location of the vowel "target." These target locations have sometimes been estimated at the temporal middle of the vowel, where the formants seem to remain steady (the steady state of the vowel) after the initial transition from the consonant preceding the vowel, or perhaps one-third of the distance from the beginning to the end of the vowel. Each of these measurement points, when used alone, is likely to separate vowels with a high degree of success. This has been demonstrated in experiments in which single-slice measurements have been used to obtain either human classifications of vowels or classifications by statistical routines (Hillenbrand & Nearey, 1999). However, when single-slice formant frequencies are supplemented with information on formant movement throughout the vowel nucleus, identification/classification accuracy increases, sometimes substantially (Assman, Nearey, & Hogan, 1982; Hillenbrand & Nearey, 1999). Simply put, both single-slice formant frequencies *and* formant movement throughout a vowel nucleus make important contributions to vowel identity.

This comes as no surprise to anyone who has studied tongue, lips, and jaw motions during speech for even the simplest CVC syllable. Figure 10–8 shows these motions for the vowel [ɪ] in the word [sɪp] produced by a young adult female. These data were collected with the x-ray microbeam instrument

Articulatory and Acoustic Phonetics

When speech scientists use the term "articulatory phonetics," they have in mind the positions and movements of the articulators, and the resulting configuration of the vocal tract, as they relate to speech sound production. The term "acoustic phonetics," of course, describes the relations between the acoustic signal (resulting from those positions, movements, and configurations) and speech sounds. Many scientists have studied the relations between articulatory and acoustic phonetics, and found them to be fantastically complex. Why is this so? There are many reasons, but here are two prominent ones: First, exactly the same acoustic phonetic effect can be produced by very different articulatory maneuvers. For example, the low F2 of /u/ can be produced by rounding the lips, backing the tongue, or lowering the larynx. And second, certain parts of the vocal tract—the pharynx, for instance—are exceedingly difficult to monitor during speech production, yet play a very important role in the speech acoustic signal. Scientists who study the relations between articulatory and acoustic data often use very advanced mathematical and experimental techniques to determine just how an articulatory phonetic event "maps on" to an acoustic phonetic event.

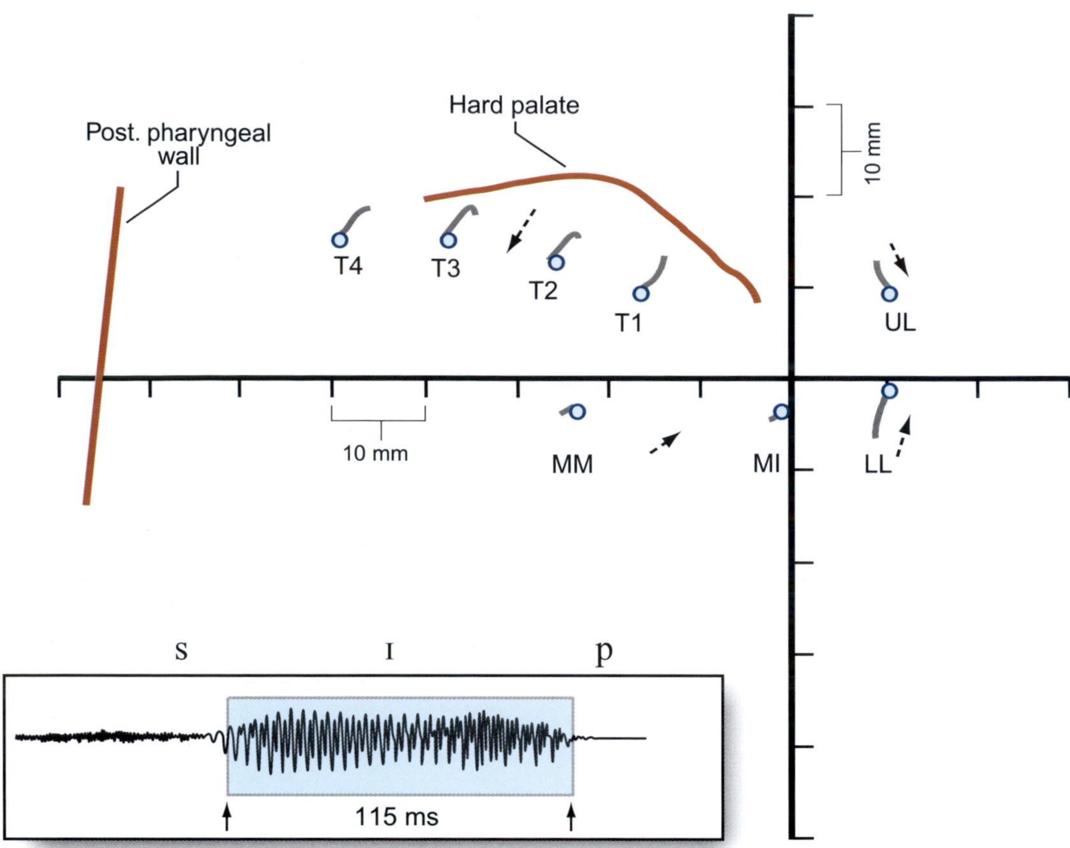

Figure 10–8. Tongue, jaw, and lip pellet motions for the vowel [ɪ] in the word [sɪp], produced by a young adult female. The directions of the pellet motions throughout the vowel are shown by dashed arrows, and the final pellet positions are marked by circles at the end of the motion tracks. Data are shown in the x-ray-microbeam coordinate system (Westbury, 1994), with the *x*-axis defined by a plate held between the teeth and the *y*-axis by a line perpendicular to the *x*-axis and running through the maxillary incisors. The portion of the speech waveform for which the motions are shown is highlighted by the shaded box on the waveform in the lower part of the figure.

which allows an investigator to track the motions of very small gold pellets attached to the tongue, jaw, and lips. In Figure 10–8 the lips are to the right and the outline of the hard palate is seen in the upper part of the *x-y* coordinate system. The motions of two lip pellets (UL = upper lip; LL = lower lip), two mandible (jaw) pellets (MM = mandible at molars; MI = mandible at incisors), and four tongue pellets (T1-T4 arranged front to back roughly from tip [T1] to dorsum [T4]) are shown for the vowel [ɪ]. The shaded portion on the waveform in the lower part of the figure corresponds to the time period of the motions shown in the upper part of the figure (arrows pointing up to the waveform indicate the onset and offset of the vowel, hence the beginning and end of the displayed motions of the various pellets). This interval lasts approximately 115 ms. The direction of the pellet motions throughout the vowel is shown by the arrows with dashed lines. The final position of each pellet, at the last glottal pulse of the vowel before the lip closure for [p], is marked by a small circle at the end of the motion track. All tongue pellets move down throughout the vowel, with the exception of the small upward motions in T2 and T3 at the beginning of the vowel. Throughout the syllable, the mandible moves up very slightly and the lips come together, as would be expected when a vowel is followed by a labial consonant. Although this display does not show the motions as a function of time, they are more or less continuous throughout the vowel nucleus and do not have obvious steady-state portions where the motion "freezes." This is especially so for the tongue pellets, for which the downward motion is smooth and continuous from the beginning to end of the vowel.

The continuous motions of the articulators for the simple, relatively short-duration vowel [ɪ] are consistent with changing formant frequencies throughout the vowel nucleus. Based on these motions and the resulting formant transitions, it is not surprising that portions of the vowel in addition to the "slice-in-time" target measurement contribute to vowel identification. One future area of research is to generate better descriptions of these simple vowel motions, and to understand the role of such motions in vowel identity. This is an important area of research because of the significant contribution of vowel articulation to speech intelligibility deficits in the speech of individuals who are hearing impaired (Metz, Samar, Schiavetti, Sitler, & Whitehead, 1985) and who have dysarthria (Weismer & Martin, 1992), among other disorders.

Vowel Durations

Vowel durations have been studied extensively because of the potential for application of the data to speech synthesis, machine recognition of speech, and description and possibly diagnosis of speech rate disorders. What follows is a brief discussion of the major variables known to affect vowel durations.

Intrinsic Vowel Durations

An "intrinsic" vowel duration is one deriving from the articulation of the vowel segment itself, as opposed to an external influence on its duration (as described more fully below). The easiest way to understand this is to imagine a fixed syllable such as a consonant-vowel-consonant (CVC) frame, with vowel durations measured for all vowels inserted into the "V" slot of the frame. Figure 10–9 shows three sets of vowel duration values from a /CVC/ frame, as reported by Hillenbrand et al. (2001). In this experiment the Cs included /p,t,k,b,d,g,h,w,r,l/, in all combinations (consonants such as /h/ and /w/ were restricted to initial position). In Figure 10–9 vowel duration in ms (*y*-axis) is presented for each vowel (*x*-axis), averaged across all consonant contexts (filled circles, solid lines), across vowels surrounded only by voiceless Cs (unfilled circles, dotted lines), and only by voiced Cs (lightly filled diamonds, solid lines). The pattern of durations across vowels is essentially the same for these three contexts. Because the contexts stay constant for any one of the three curves, any differences in vowel duration must be a property of the vowels themselves—precisely what is meant by an "intrinsic" property. Clearly, for each of the curves, low vowels such as /æ/ and /ɑ/ have greater durations than high vowels such as /i/, /ɪ/, /ʊ/, and /u/. The differences between low and high vowel durations typically are on the order of 50 to 60 ms, a very large effect in the world of speech timing. The explanation for the intrinsic difference in the duration of low versus high vowels has typically pointed to the greater articulatory distance required for the consonant-to-vowel-to-consonant path when the vowel is low, as compared to high. Greater articulatory distance to be traveled requires more time. This may explain part of the high-low intrinsic duration difference, but doesn't seem to account for all of the 50- to 60-ms difference.

The data in Figure 10–9 also show one other well-known intrinsic vowel duration difference, between tense and lax vowels. In any one of the three consonant contexts, tense vowels are longer than their lax vowel "partners" (compare the durations of the /i/-/ɪ/ and /u/-/ʊ/ pairs for any of the three curves). The difference in the duration of tense and lax vowels has a wide range (from about 22 to 65 ms in the data shown in Figure 10–9, depending on the consonant context), but always favors tense vowels when the consonant environment is held constant. This very consistent difference between tense and lax vowel durations is not easy to explain, and may be related to the spectral similarity of tense-lax pairs.[3]

Listeners are sensitive to the high-low and tense-lax intrinsic differences in vowel duration. When

[3]The thinking is that /i/ and /ɪ/, and /u/ and /ʊ/ have formant frequencies that are only subtly different, so vowel duration may have evolved in phonological systems to create an additional cue to the tense-lax vowel distinction.

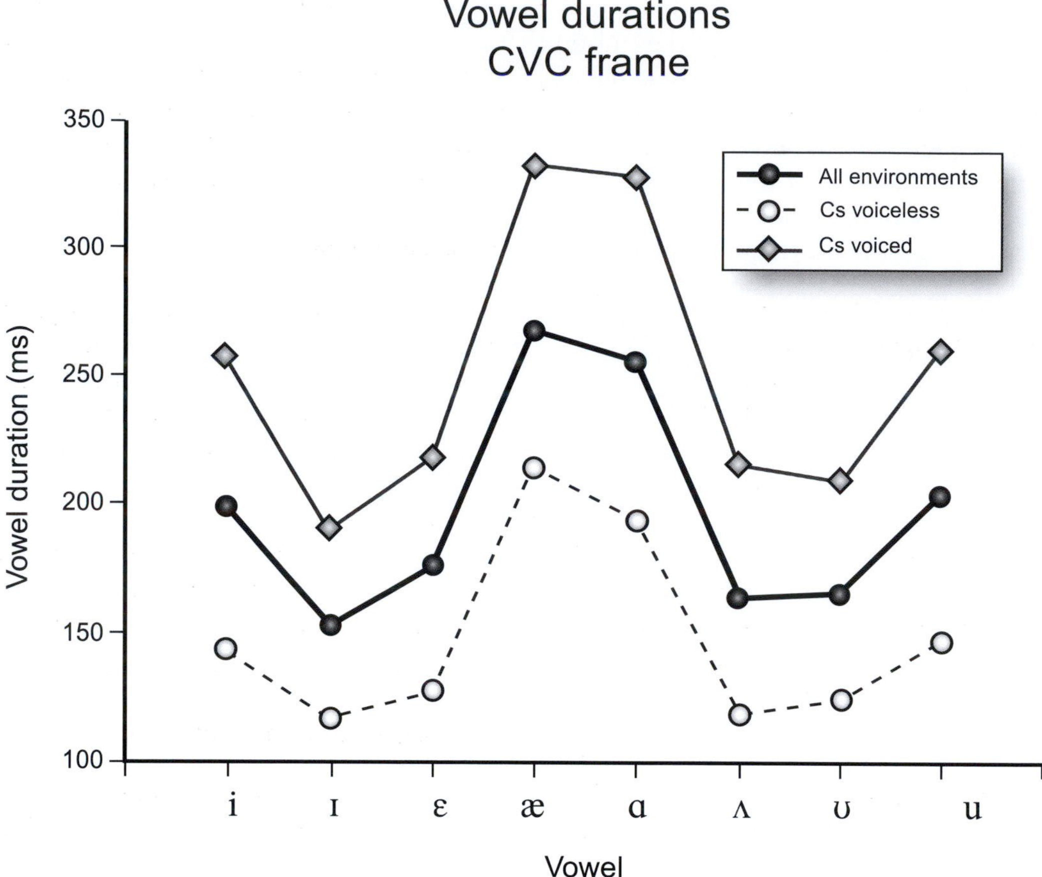

Figure 10–9. Vowel durations in fixed CVC frames for eight vowels in American English. Data are shown for environments in which all C environments are combined (*filled circles*, C = voiceless (*unfilled circles*), C = voiced (*lightly shaded diamonds*). Data replotted from Hillenbrand et al. (2001).

high-quality speech synthesizers are programmed, for example, the differences just described are built into the algorithms to generate natural-sounding speech.

Extrinsic Factors Affecting Vowel Durations

Many factors influence vowel duration, certainly many more than can be covered in this chapter. What follows is a brief discussion of a few of the often-studied influences on vowel duration. Readers interested in comprehensive surveys of how and why vowel duration varies in speech production can consult House (1961), Klatt (1976), Umeda (1975), the series of papers by Crystal and House (1982, 1988a, 1988b, 1988c) and Van Santen (1992).

Consonant Voicing

Vowels are typically longer when surrounded by voiced, as compared to voiceless consonants. This effect is seen clearly in Figure 10–9 by comparing the "Cs voiceless" curve (unfilled circles, dashed lines) to the "Cs voiced" curve (lightly shaded diamonds, solid lines). The effect varies from vowel to vowel, but a reasonable generalization from the Hillenbrand et al. (2001) data is that vowels surrounded by voiced consonants are about 100 ms longer than vowels surrounded by voiceless consonants. The voicing of both the initial and final C in the CVC frame contributes to changes in vowel duration, but the largest influence is the voicing status of the final consonant of the syllable. If the syllable frame is marked as C_1VC_2, a voiced C_1 will lengthen a vowel by somewhere between 25 to 50 ms as compared to a voiceless C_1, whereas a voiced C_2 will lengthen a vowel by 50 to 90 ms relative to a voiceless C_2. The magnitude of these effects is lessened in more natural speaking conditions (Crystal & House, 1988a, 1988b).

Stress

Lexical stress is a characteristic of multisyllabic words in many languages, the best known examples in English being noun-verb contrasts such as "rebel-rebel" (/ˈrɛbl/-/rəˈbɛl̩/), and "contract-contract" (/ˈkɑntrækt/-/kənˈtræːkt/). Of course, many other multisyllabic words have alternating patterns of stressed and unstressed syllables as in "California" /kæləˈfɔrnjə/), where the first and third syllables have greater stress than the second and fourth syllables. When single syllables are stressed for emphasis or contrast ("Bob stopped by earlier"; "Did you say *Barb* stopped by?" "No, *Bob* stopped by"), the vowel in the emphasized syllable has greater duration than the original, lexically stressed production. All other things being equal, vowels in lexically or emphatically stressed syllables have greater duration than vowels in unstressed or normally stressed syllables (Fourakis, 1991). The magnitude of the duration difference between stressed and unstressed syllables, or between contrastively stressed and "normally stressed" syllables, is quite variable across speakers (Howell, 1993; Weismer & Ingrisano, 1979).

Speaking Rate

Vowel duration varies over a large range when speakers change their speaking rate. Slow rates result in longer vowel durations, fast rates in shorter vowel durations. Speaking rate also varies widely *across* speakers. Some speakers have naturally slow rates, some fast. Speakers who have habitually slow speaking rates have longer vowel durations than speakers with habitually fast rates (Tsao & Weismer, 1997). Perhaps these speaker-specific vowel durations should be considered intrinsic, rather than extrinsic influences on vowel duration.

Utterance Position Effects

The same vowel has variable duration depending on its location within an utterance. If the duration of

Are We Wired for Rate?

Imagine you had a large sample of talkers—say, 100 people—each of whom reads a passage from which speaking rates (in syllables per second) are measured acoustically. If the talkers were chosen randomly, you would find a huge range of "typical" speaking rates, from very slow talkers, to talkers of average rate, to very fast talkers. These experimental measurements would confirm the everyday observation that some people speak very slowly, some very rapidly. Now imagine that you chose the slowest and fastest talkers in this sample, and asked them to produce the passage as fast as possible. If all talkers were able to produce the passage at the same, maximally fast speaking rate, regardless of their "typical" rate, that would indicate that the very slow or fast "typical" rates were a kind of conscious choice on the part of individual talkers. However, if the slow talkers couldn't speak as fast as the fast talkers, that would suggest that speaking rates reflect some basic neurological "wiring" that determines the "typical" rate. This experiment was performed by Tsao and Weismer (1997), who found that the maximal speaking rates of slow talkers were, in fact, less than the maximal rates of fast talkers. It seems we are not all wired the same for typical speaking rate, and probably a bunch of other stuff, as well.

in duration. The left-most window is the murmur piece, the middle window the piece straddling the boundary between murmur offset and vowel onset (murmur + transition piece), and the right-most window the transition piece, or the piece of the vowel containing transitions from the consonant to the vowel.

These waveform pieces can be used to address the question, "Which piece(s) of the waveform, or which acoustic characteristics within each piece, allow a classification of place of articulation (bilabial vs. lingua-alveolar) for the nasal consonant?" The classification can be performed by a statistical procedure (see below) or by human listeners. Stated in a different way: "Do the three pieces allow equivalent accuracy in classifying place of articulation for nasals, or is one piece 'better' than another?" For example, if the nasal murmur piece (the left-most box) is presented to listeners, can they use just this acoustic information to assign place of articulation accurately? Alternatively, if certain acoustic characteristics are extracted from the murmur window for /m/ and /n/, can these measures be used by an automatic classification algorithm to separate the two places of articulation? These types of experiments appear several times in the speech acoustics literature (e.g., Harrington, 1994; Kurowski & Blumstein, 1984, 1987; Repp, 1986). The results of the various experiments, although not always precisely consistent, suggest that *any* of these three pieces, when presented alone to human listeners or classified statistically, allow fairly accurate identification of place of articulation for syllable-initial nasals. Moreover, when two or more of the pieces are presented (or classified) together, the accuracy of place identification improves.

First consider the results for isolated murmurs. If nasal place of articulation can be identified (classified) accurately from just the murmur, something about its acoustic characteristics must be systematically different for labials versus lingua-alveolars. The duration of the murmur can be ruled out as a measure that separates /m/ from /n/, but there are almost certainly spectral differences. The spectral differences are a result of different resonances and antiresonances of the coupled pharyneal and oral tracts. In Chapter 8, the frequency locations of the antiresonances for /m/ versus /n/ were discussed, the former having a lower region (according to Fujimura [1962], roughly 750–1250 Hz), the latter a higher region (1450–2200 Hz). The unique resonances for /m/ in Fujimura's study included a two-formant cluster in the vicinity of 1000 Hz, and for /n/ a similar cluster above 2000 Hz. Qi and Fox (1992), in an analysis of the first two resonances of nasal murmurs for /m/ and /n/ produced by six speakers, reported average second resonances for /m/ and /n/ of 1742 and 2062 Hz, respectively. A careful examination of the /m/ and /n/ murmurs in Figure 10–15 shows formant patterns, and inferred antiresonance locations, generally consistent with the observations of Fujimura and Qi and Fox. Both /m/ and /n/ have the expected first formant around 300 Hz, but in the frequency range above this formant, the spectra are different. Between the F1 and the next evidence of a higher resonance, both murmurs have an obvious "white space." For /m/, the white space extends roughly from 500 to 1150 Hz, and for /n/ it is located between 500 and 1600 Hz. Under the assumption that the exact antiresonance frequencies are approximately in the middle of these white space ranges, their center frequencies are 850 Hz for /m/ and 1050 Hz for /n/. Immediately above the antiresonance, the /m/ murmur has a second and perhaps third resonance around 1500 Hz, and above that a resonance around 2300 Hz. In comparison, the /n/ murmur has a second resonance around 1800 Hz, and what appears to be a cluster of two resonances around 2500 Hz. Clearly, the two murmurs have different spectral characteristics. It is reasonable to expect that listeners can use these differences to identify place of articulation.[6] In Repp (1986), listeners made accurate place judgments for /m/ and /n/ when given only the mumur piece of CV syllables, and Harrington (1994) obtained excellent

[6]The antiresonance and upper resonance locations for the murmurs in Figure 10–15 are different from those reported by Fujimura (1962) based on his theoretical calculations and data from two subjects, but the spectral relations (e.g., higher antiresonance for /n/ as compared to /m/, different patterns of resonances above the constant F1 at 300 Hz) are consistent with Fujimura's general description. Fujimura, and many other authors, have pointed to the wide range of variability expected across speakers for nasal murmur spectra as a result of variations in nasal tract and sinus cavity morphology (Dang & Honda, 1995).

statistical classification for these two nasals when using acoustic information from single spectrum "slices" taken from the murmur.

The spectrograms in Figure 10–15 also show different patterns of formant transitions as the murmur is released into the following /ɛ/. There is a long history of considering formant transitions at CV boundaries as strong cues to consonant place of articulation. This history originated in the late 1940s and early 1950s, at the Haskins Laboratories, where experiments showed that synthesized formant transitions cued place of articulation in the absence of consonant spectra (Liberman, Delattre, Cooper, & Gerstman, 1954). Figure 10–16 shows a spectrogram of the utterance /əŋɛ/ to contrast its transitions with those of /əmɛ/ and /ənɛ/ in Figure 10–15. The

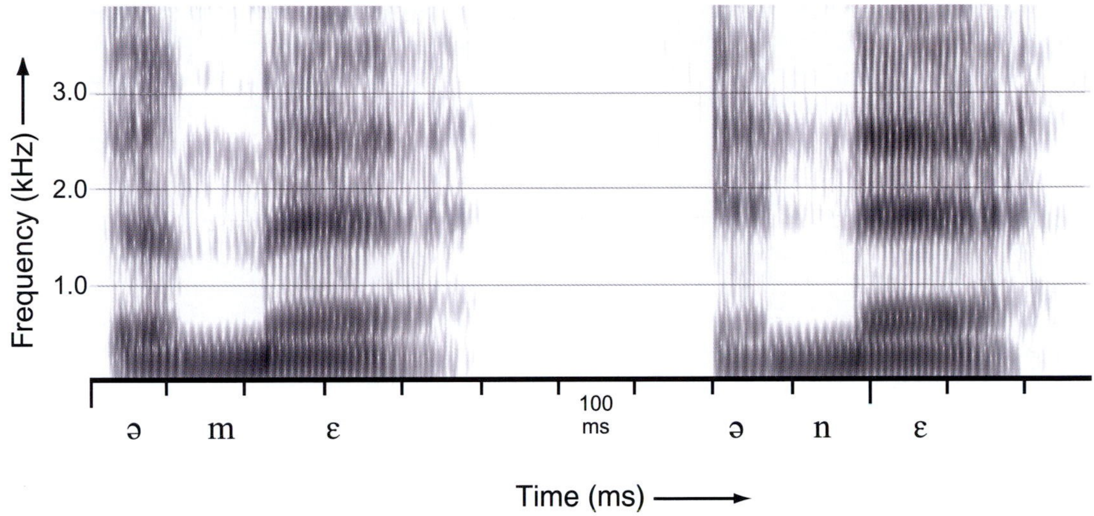

Figure 10–15. Spectrograms of the utterances /ə'mɛ/ and /ə'nɛ/, produced by a 57-year-old, healthy male. Note between-place differences in the murmur spectrum and the pattern of formant transitions as the nasal is released into the vowel.

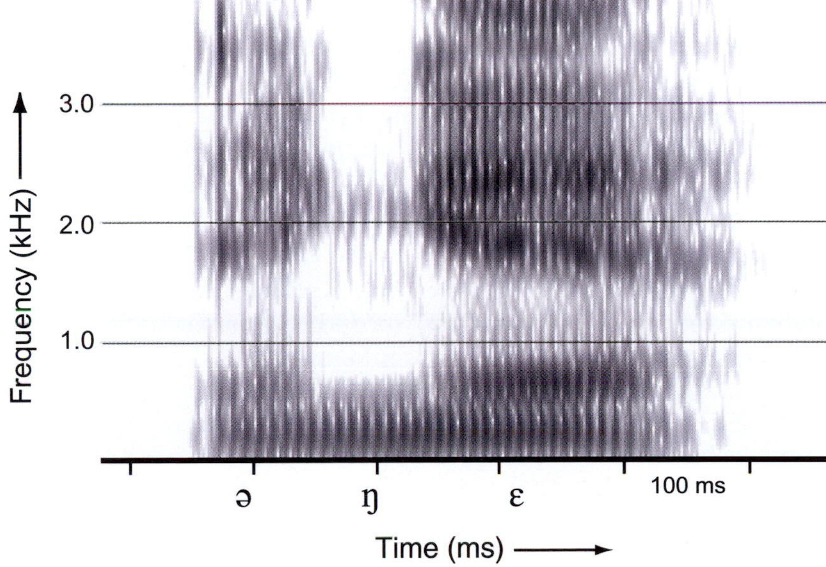

Figure 10–16. Spectrogram of the VCV utterance /ə'ŋɛ/, produced by a 57-year-old, healthy male. Note the F2-F3 transition pattern immediately following release of the nasal murmur.

pattern of F2 and F3 transitions over the first 40 or 50 ms following release of the murmur are unique to the different places of nasal articulation. For the transitions coming out of the /m/ murmur both F2 and F3 are rising, from /n/ they are more or less flat, and from /ŋ/ F2 is falling and F3 rising. This latter pattern (see Figure 10–16) seems to show F2 and F3 starting at nearly the same frequency and separating throughout the transition. The details of these F2-F3 transition patterns change depending on the identity of the vowel following the murmur, but in most cases the patterns are uniquely different for the three places of articulation. Of course, in English the velar nasal /ŋ/ does not appear in the prestressed position shown in Figure 10–16, but this is not a physiological limitation—there are languages in which the sound can appear in this position—so the point concerning place-specific transition patterns is a valid one.

Place of articulation information is present in these unique transition patterns, as demonstrated for listeners (Repp, 1986) and statistical classification (Harrington, 1994). The accuracy of place identification from the transitions (i.e., from the "transition piece" of the spectrogram shown in Figure 10–14) is essentially similar to the accuracy from the "murmur piece," as described above. Place information for nasals, therefore, seems to have acoustic correlates in at least two different locations in a CV syllable, and these correlates are both sufficiently stable to be reliable for listener and statistical classification of nasals.

Finally, in Figure 10–14 the middle "piece" straddles the boundary where the murmur ends and the transition begins. This interval would be expected to have a very rapid change from the low-energy, unique resonance patterns associated with murmurs to the high-energy formant patterns for vowels. Several scientists (Kurowski & Blumstein, 1984, 1987; Seitz, McCormick, Watson, & Bladon, 1990) have argued that each place of articulation is associated with a unique frequency pattern for this rapid change. Whether or not this particular "piece" is more important in the classification of nasal place of articulation, as compared to the murmur or transitions alone, is a matter of considerable debate.

Nasalization

Nasalization, as reviewed in Chapter 8, is a concept with broad application in general and in clinical phonetics. Nasalization of vowels, which is of concern here, involves complex acoustics as a result of the mix of oral and nasal tract formants with antiresonances originating in the sinus cavities.[7] Because measurement and interpretation of the spectrum of nasalized vowels is challenging, only a few studies have reported data on nasalization acoustics. Interesting theoretical treatments of vowel nasalization can be found in Stevens, Fant, and Hawkins (1987) and Feng and Castelli (1996).

Chen (1995, 1997) developed two acoustic measures of nasalization, one of which is described here. Recall that a Fourier spectrum of a vowel shows the amplitude of the consecutive harmonics (where the first harmonic = F0) produced by the vibrating vocal folds. Further, the amplitude variation of these harmonics reflects, in part, the resonance characteristics of the vocal tract. When a vowel is produced with an open velopharyngeal port and is, therefore, nasalized, some glottal harmonics in the region of the nasal resonances have increased amplitude (relative to the amplitudes when the vowel is not nasalized), and some harmonics in the region of oral formants have reduced amplitudes, as a result of nearby antiresonances and the extra damping due to increased absorption of sound energy in the nasal cavities (see Chapter 8). Chen (1995) took advantage of these facts and constructed a spectral measure of nasalization in which the amplitude of the harmonic closest to the first formant is compared to the amplitude of a harmonic close to the location of the second nasal resonance. The technique is illustrated in Figure 10–17.

[7]Recall that nasalization occurs when the velopharyngeal port is open at the same time the oral tract opens for vowel production. This combination of events is characteristic of "normal" speech production in at least two ways. First, vowels are typically not produced with perfect velopharyngeal port closure, but have a variable amount of small opening that depends on tongue height (higher the vowel, tighter the closure). Second, the coarticulatory patterns of nasal-vowel and vowel-nasal sequences almost always involve some velopharyngeal port opening during the vowel that reflects the open port requirement of the nasal consonant.

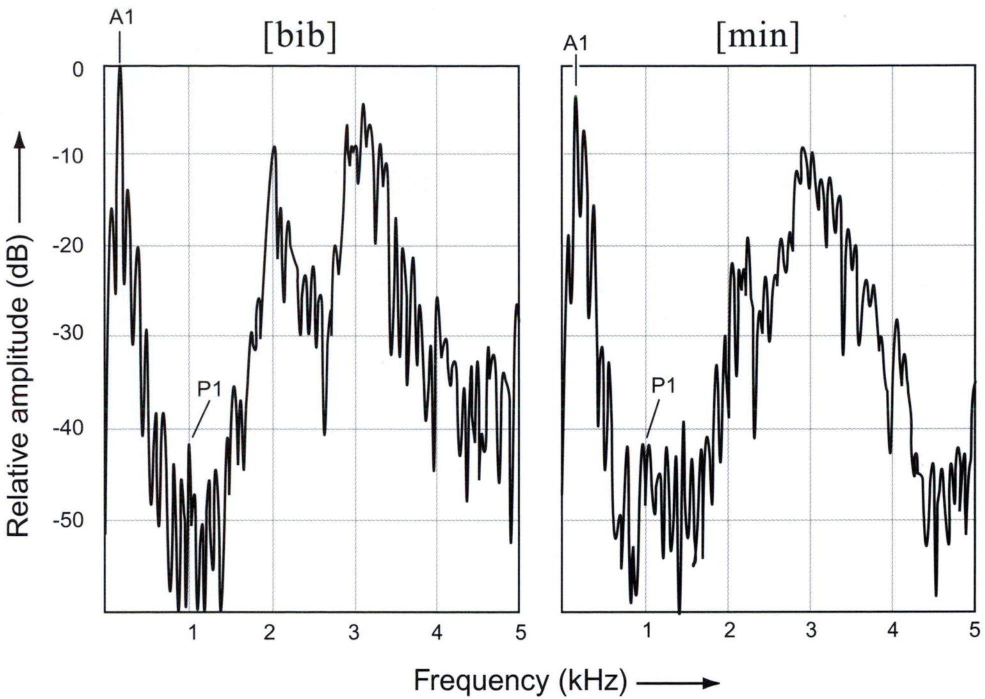

Figure 10–17. Two /i/ spectra showing the application of Chen's (1995) acoustic technique for quantifying the degree of vowel nasalization. The left spectrum is for /i/ in a non-nasal context, the right spectrum for /i/ in a nasal context. "A1" is the highest-amplitude harmonic in the vicinity of the F1 for /i/, "P1" a harmonic around 950 Hz, associated with a nasal resonance. The acoustic measure is the amplitude difference, in dB, between A1 and P1.

Figure 10–17 shows two FFT spectra, both for the middle 30 ms of the vowel /i/ in the CVC [bib] (left spectrum) and [min] (right spectrum). In both spectra, two harmonics are of interest. One, labeled "A1," is the harmonic in the immediate vicinity of the low-frequency F1 of the vowel /i/. As expected, the A1 harmonic in the two spectra has relatively high amplitude as compared to the other harmonics. This makes sense because the amplitude of this harmonic is "boosted" by the typical first resonant frequency (that is, F1) of /i/. The other harmonic of interest is the one labeled "P1." Chen (1995) identified this harmonic as one "boosted" when the oral and nasal cavities are coupled via opening of the velopharyngeal port. The P1 harmonic is in the vicinity of the second resonance associated with the nasal cavity. In theory, the amplitude of the P1 harmonic should be quite small when the velopharyngeal port is closed and relatively greater when the port is open. Based on theoretical and experimental work, Chen recommended identifying the P1 harmonic by locating the FFT peak closest to 950 Hz.

Chen's (1995) index of nasalization requires measurement of the A1-P1 amplitude difference within a vowel spectrum. In Figure 10–17, the A1 and P1 *relative* amplitudes for [i] surrounded by [b] are roughly 0 and –42 dB, respectively, yielding an A1-P1 index of 42 dB. When [i] is surrounded by nasal consonants (right spectrum), and therefore likely to be partially nasalized due to coarticulatory influences, A1 = –4 dB, P1 = –42 dB, giving an A1-P1 index of 38 dB. As expected, the A1-P1 index for the vowel in a nasal environment is smaller than the index when the vowel is between non-nasal consonants.

The 4-dB difference between the A1-P1 amplitudes in oral and nasal consonant environments is small, and probably at the low end of the distribution for normal speakers. This oral versus nasal difference can be referred to as the $(A1\text{-}P1_{oral}) - (A1\text{-}P1_{nasal})$ index. For the vowel /i/, Chen (1997) reported the

(A1-P1_{oral}) – (A1-P1_{nasal}) index to range between 4.2 and 22.3 dB across 10 normal speakers producing CVCs like the ones used for the example in Figure 10–17. The magnitude of this index also depends on which vowel is measured. Chen reported the greatest average index for /i/ (15 dB), with average indices for /u/, /ɛ/, and /ʌ/ of 11, 10, and 12 dB, respectively.

Why would the measure vary across vowels? The amplitudes of A1 and P1 depend on the proximity of a formant to the FFT peaks of interest. For example, if P1 is always located as the harmonic peak closest to 950 Hz, it follows that its amplitude is affected by its distance from an oral formant. In a vowel such as /i/, the relatively low F1 (around 300 Hz) and high F2 (above 2000 Hz) are distant from the target region of 950 Hz, and so have only a small influence, if any, on the P1 amplitude. But a vowel such as /u/, for which F2 is likely to be somewhere in the 1000- to 1200-Hz range, may have a greater effect on P1 amplitude. Low-back vowels such as /ɑ/, which have a relatively high F1 and low F2 and therefore virtually surround the 950-Hz target region for the P1 amplitude measure, are even more problematic (Chen [1997]) found the average [A1-P1_{oral}] – [A1-P1_{nasal}] index to be only 5.2 dB for /ɑ/).[8] A clinician interested in establishing a normative data base of the (A1-P1_{oral}) – (A1-P1_{nasal}) index for comparison to clients with suspected or known velopharyngeal incompetence would do well to use speech materials in which low vowels are avoided.

Although a large-scale, normative database does not exist for A1-P1 amplitude differences in non-nasal environments, there is preliminary evidence for the clinical potential of this measure. Chen (1995) measured A1-P1 amplitude differences for vowels produced in non-nasal environments by children with impaired and normal hearing. She chose children with impaired hearing for this comparison because an important component of their reduced speech intelligibility is thought to be excessive nasalization of vowels. The children with normal hearing had A1-P1 differences for these vowels ranging from about 10 to 30 dB, with an average around 20 dB. In contrast, the children with impaired hearing had A1-P1 amplitude differences ranging from about 1 to 15 dB, with the mean of these values clearly below 10 dB (values estimated from Chen, 1995, Figure 3, p. 2448). Of particular interest is Chen's finding of a relatively strong, neg-

Spectrographic Challenges

Experienced acoustic phoneticians know that some spectrograms are easy to analyze, others are much more difficult. The "goodness" of a spectrographic display is usually easy to predict, based on characteristics of the person whose speech is being analyzed. Talkers with very high F0s and/or breathy voices are notoriously difficult to analyze, as are persons with a lot of nasal resonance. The low-amplitude, broad bandwidth formants in hypernasal speech complicate the precise identification of formant frequencies. Moreover, the most popular computer technique for formant frequency identification—linear predictive code (LPC) analysis—is based on a mathematical model that neglects the antiresonance "dips" described in Chapter 8. LPC formant estimates for a nasalized vowel are, therefore, often incorrect, and must be checked carefully on a spectrogram-by-spectrogram basis. This obviously complicates the use of LPC analysis in many speech disorders associated with velopharyngeal incompetence.

[8]Chen (1997) described an approach to correcting for these vowel influences. Interested readers are encouraged to consult her paper for details.

ative correlation between A1-P1 differences and perceptual ratings of nasality for the children with hearing impairment. As the A1-P1 amplitude difference decreased, children were perceived as increasingly nasal.

Because nasalization is a pervasive problem in a wide range of speech disorders, measures such as the Chen index (1995) should be pursued as supplements to other forms of nasality assessment. As presented in Figure 10–17, the measure is fairly simple, but the identification of the A1 and P1 peaks is not always easy, especially when voice quality is poor and the glottal harmonics are not well defined. The technique may, therefore, have limited utility in clients with co-occurring velopharyngeal and laryngeal (voice) dysfunction.

SEMIVOWELS

In this chapter, /w/, /ɹ/, /l/, and /j/ are considered semivowels. /w/ and /j/ are also referred to as glides, /ɹ/ and /l/ as liquids, and the latter two sounds are also called rhotic and lateral, respectively. The term "semivowel" is a convenient way to group all four sounds because it captures a shared aspect of their production. All four sounds require movement to and away from a vocal tract constriction tighter than that for vowels, but not nearly so tight as required for obstruents (fricatives, stops, and affricates).

Figure 10–18 shows spectrograms of the four semivowels in VCV frames where V = /ɛ/. A quick

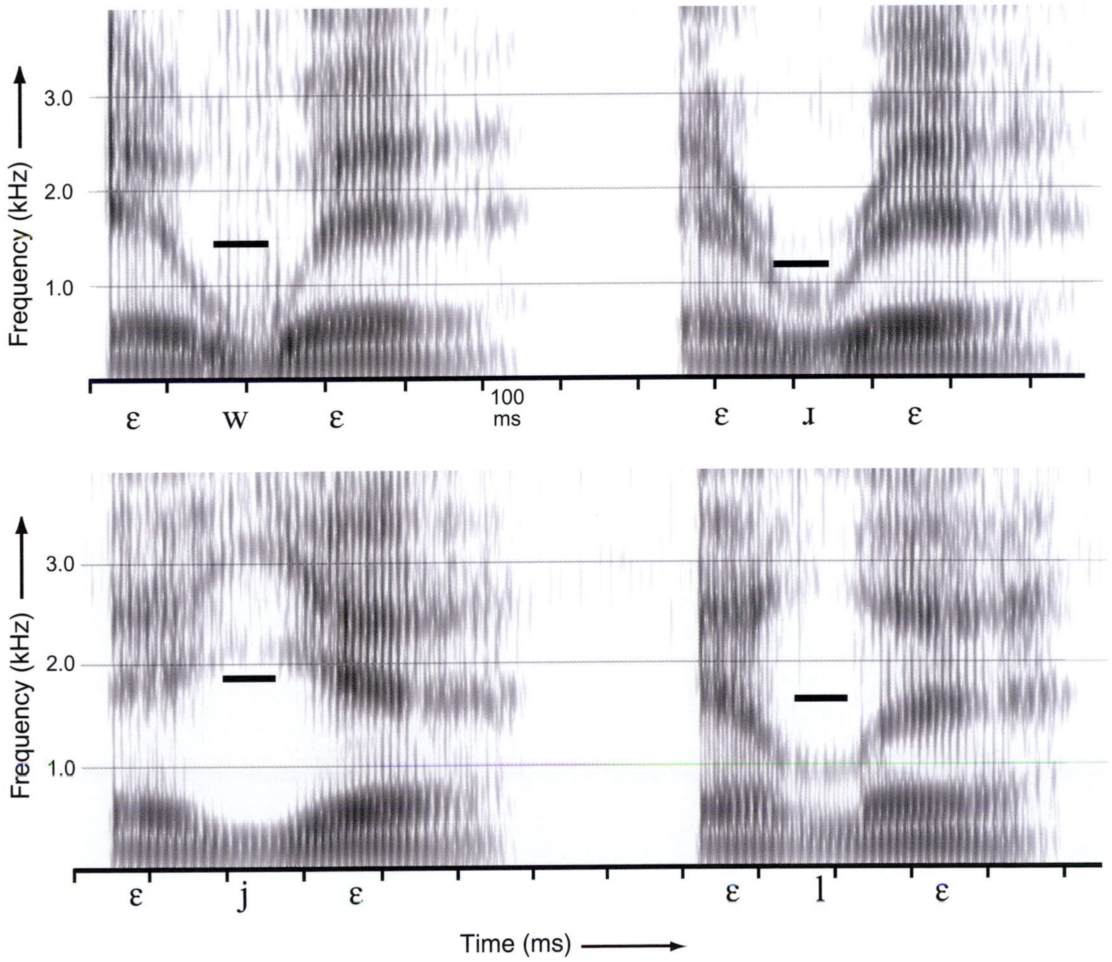

Figure 10–18. Spectrograms of English semivowels in VCV frames where V = /ɛ/. The horizontal bar located between 1.0 and 2.0 kHz in each spectrogram shows the approximate time interval corresponding to the constriction interval of each semivowel. See text for further explanation.

glance at these spectrograms suggests a few prominent acoustic features of all semivowels. An interval during which F1, F2, and F3 are more or less constant (i.e., at steady frequencies) is surrounded by relatively large transitions in at least one of the first three formants. The interval of relatively "flat" formants is called the *constriction interval,* and it is assumed to correspond to the articulatory phase of semivowel articulation when the vocal tract is *most* constricted. The length of the constriction interval for each semivowel is marked in Figure 10–18 by a horizontal bar between the 1.0- and 2.0-kHz calibration lines (the precise location of the horizontal bar along the frequency scale is not important; the position is different from semivowel to semivowel to avoid obscuring formants within the constriction interval). The duration of the constriction intervals in Figure 10–18 is always under 100 ms and in less carefully articulated speech is probably about 40 to 50 ms, on average (Dalston, 1975).

The constriction interval has a formant pattern in much the same sense as a vowel. The relative stability of these formant frequencies allows target values to be measured for the different semivowels. Do these formant frequencies distinguish the semivowels from each other? F1 is quite similar across the semivowels, but unique F2-F3 patterns seem to characterize each of the sounds. Figure 10–19 shows how the semivowels in Figure 10–18 are separated in F2-F3 space. These formant frequencies, estimated by eye at the temporal midpoint of the horizontal bars in Figure 10–18, are plotted in Figure 10–19 (filled circles) together with values reported for young adult speakers by Dalston (1975; unfilled triangles = males, filled triangles = females) and Espy-Wilson (1992; *unfilled squares*). The values for a given semivowel

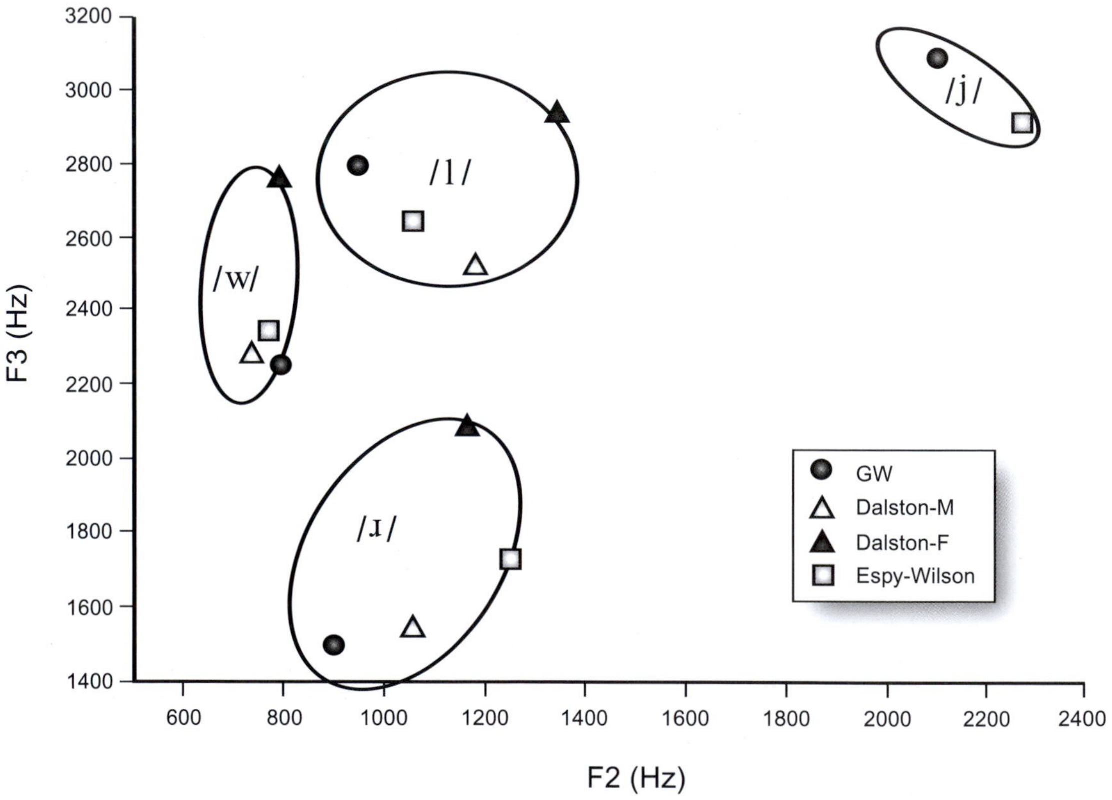

Figure 10–19. F2-F3 plot of constriction interval formant frequencies from three data sources. GW points (*filled circles*) are estimated formant frequencies (by eye) from the semivowels shown in Figure 10–18. Dalston-M and Dalston-F points (*unfilled and filled triangles, respectively*) are averages from Dalston (1975) for semivowels spoken as word-initial consonants in isolated words by three adult males and two adult females. Espy-Wilson (1992) points (*unfilled boxes*) are averages for intervocalic semivowels produced by two adult males and two adult females.

are fairly consistent across the three different data sources, even though there are differences in speaker sex, age, and phonetic context of the constriction intervals (see Figure 10–19 caption). The ellipses are included to show the separation of the points for the four semivowels. Most obvious in this plot is the low F3 associated with /ɹ/, clearly different from the F3s of the other semivowels. A distinguishing acoustic characteristic of rhotic articulation is an F3 very close to F2, with F3 lower than (about) 2000 Hz. Figure 10–19 shows just such a pattern. In Figure 10–19, a horizontal line at roughly 2100 Hz could be drawn across the graph to separate /ɹ/ data from the other three semivowels. /w/ and /l/ both have a wide frequency separation between F2 and F3, as indicated by their general location in the upper left quadrant of the plot. /w/ and /l/ are distinguished from each other, however, by the generally lower F2 and F3 of /w/ as compared to /l/. Overall, this typically results in a greater F2-F3 separation between /l/ as compared to /w/. Finally, /j/ has a much higher F2 than the other semivowels. F3 of /j/ is also higher than the F3 of /w/, /ɹ/, and /l/. /j/ appears to occupy its own corner of the F2-F3 plot, clearly separated from the other semivowels.

The pattern of formant transitions into and out of the constriction intervals also distinguishes among the semivowels. In very general terms, the important characteristics of these patterns are (a) which formants show large transitions into and out of the constriction interval, and (b) the direction (rising versus falling) of the transitions. For the purposes of this discussion, the direction of transitions is always referenced to the constriction interval. For example, in Figure 10–18, the VC (V = /ɛ/, C = semivowel) F1 transitions for all semivowels are falling into the constriction interval, and are rising for the CV part. With a special-case exception described below, the F1 transitions do not seem to distinguish among the four semivowels.

The direction of the F2 transitions into and out of the constriction interval easily separates /j/ from the other three semivowels. For /j/ the transition is rising into the constriction, and falling out of it. For /w/, /ɹ/, and /l/, there are fairly large, falling transitions into the constriction interval, and rising transitions out of it. The magnitude of these transitions—the frequency range covered from the onset of the transition to its end—and the transition rate (transition magnitude/transition duration) are affected by the vowel context in which the semivowel is articulated. These context effects are very detailed and numerous. Interested readers should consult Espy-Wilson (1992, 1994) for relevant information.

The F3 transitions allow further distinction of /w/, /ɹ/, and /l/. /ɹ/ has a large falling (VC) and rising (CV) transition. This F3 transition is often immediately above (of greater frequency than) the F2 transition. The F3 transition seems to follow the F2 transition closely, especially just prior to and after the constriction interval. An F3 transition is often absent for /w/, or possibly has only very slight movement. The large F3 transition for /ɹ/ effectively separates its acoustic characteristics from those of /w/. The F3 transition for /l/, as shown in Figure 10–18, is rising slightly into the constriction interval and falling slightly out of it.

CV transition characteristics when C = semivowel are summarized in Table 10–2. When semivowels are in a symmetric VCV frame as in Figure 10–18, the VC and CV transitions are mirror images of each other. Table 10–2 uses a simple classification approach to transition type, much like that published by Espy-Wilson (1994). In this classification scheme, no two semivowels have exactly the same pattern of transitions to or from the following or preceding vowel. To be sure, the F1 and F2 transitions in this classification system are identical for /w/, /ɹ/, and /l/, but the F3 transition distinguishes among them. Note, however, the qualifications in Table 10–2 concerning the F3 transition of /w/ and the F1 and F3 transitions of /l/. These transitions

Table 10–2. Classification of CV Transition Type for the CV Sequence of a VCV Frame Where V = /ɛ/ and C = Semivowel.

SEMIVOWEL	F1	F2	F3
/w/	rising	rising	flat[a]
/ɹ/	rising	rising	rising
/l/	rising[b]	rising	falling[c]
/j/	rising	falling	falling

[a]Some may rise, some may fall depending on context.
[b]Rise may look like a 'jump'; see text.
[c]Very context-sensitive; some may be flat, some may rise.

may be especially sensitive to the identity of the following or preceding vowels. The F1 transition for /l/ + vowel sequences often appears to "jump" from the constriction interval to the following vowel. Figure 10–18 shows this in the CV part of /ɛlɛ/.

When the constriction interval and transition acoustics of semivowels are taken together, there is ample reason to believe the acoustic information is rich enough to distinguish among these sounds. Much like the case of nasals, discussed above, if the acoustic information is sufficient to distinguish among the semivowels, an automatic classification based on these acoustic characteristics should be successful in getting the sounds "right." As reported by Espy-Wilson (1994), however, there are frequent classification confusions between /w/ and /l/. These confusions occur because /w/ and /l/ are so similar acoustically (note the proximity of /w/ and /l/ data in Figure 10–19), and different phonetic contexts blur the subtle acoustic distinctions between them.[9]

The speech-language pathologist should know about semivowel acoustics because semivowel errors are frequent during phonological development. In both typical and delayed phonological development, /w/ for /ɹ/, /w/ for /l/, and /j/ for /l/ errors are not unusual. Perhaps the unique gesture characteristics of semivowels, of fairly rapid articulatory movement to and away from a constriction greater than required for vowels, but not so great as fricatives, make the sounds highly confusable. A somewhat different perspective is that the difficulty of mastering these sounds is not due to the similarity of their articulatory gestures, but rather to the similarity of the acoustic models of semivowels heard by the child as she is trying to connect perceptual representations of speech sounds with their production requirements. In this latter view, the child could produce the semivowels correctly if she were able to distinguish between them on a consistent basis.

This issue has been given some attention in the literature, by asking a simple question. When, for example, a child produces what appears to be a [w] for /ɹ/ error (as when a child is heard to say [waɪt] for the word "right"), is the error [w] acoustically similar or identical to a correctly produced [w] (when a child says [waɪt] for the word "white")? The question has been asked in two ways, when both the error and correct versions of the sound are obtained from the same child, or when the error sound is obtained from a single child and is compared to acoustic characteristics of the correctly produced sound collected from a group of children with normal articulation. Either approach seems to yield the same result: The acoustics of a [w] in a [w] for /ɹ/ error (or any other substitution error) are often *not* like the acoustics of normally articulated [w] (Chaney, 1988; Dalston, 1972; Hoffman, Stager, & Daniloff, 1983). In these analyses, the error [w] is different from correct [w] by having acoustic characteristics more or less between the error sound and the correct sound. A distinction is made by the child, but is perhaps too subtle for human listeners who may not be able to hear it or may have a tendency to place it in a "comfortable" phoneme category even if they do notice the subtle difference.

This finding seems to be consistent with the child's ability to hear the differences between the semivowels, but to have a limited ability to reproduce those distinctions. Acoustic characteristics that distinguish error [w] from correct [w] provide evidence for the child's knowledge of the required distinction between [w] and other semivowels. This knowledge is presumably obtained from the distinctions heard by the child, as produced by normally articulating adults and children. The kinds of acoustic analyses described above provide a level of understanding of a child's articulation behavior that appears to be unavailable when perceptual analyses alone are used to understand speech sound errors.[10]

[9]Speech-language pathologists are familiar with the distinction between light and dark /l/ ([l] vs.[ɫ]). Dark /l/ usually involves an articulatory configuration with a tighter constriction in the velar region or more posterior tongue position, as compared to light /l/. The dark /l/ constriction interval, therefore, has a higher F1 and lower F2 as compared to light /l/ (Narayanan, Alwan, & Haker, 1997). The higher F1 and lower F2 of dark /l/ may make it more confusable than the light /l/ with /w/, especially because of the lowered F2 in dark /l/ (see Figure 10–19, and notice how a lowering of F2 for /l/ would move it toward the /w/ region).

[10]The [w] for /ɹ/ examples presented here were chosen because of their clarity and frequency as errors in normal and delayed phonology. Many other examples could have been described; interested readers should consult Weismer, Dinnsen, and Elbert (1981), Weismer (1984), and Forrest, Weismer, Hodge, Dinnsen, and Elbert (1990) for additional examples.

Semivowel Durations

It is difficult to provide specific data on semivowel durations because it is challenging to segment semivowels from adjacent vowels (see Chapter 9). When constriction intervals can be segmented from the surrounding transitions—essentially a *phonetic* segmentation, as described in Chapter 9—these will have durations of 30 to 70 ms, with the majority of the values toward the lower end of this range (Dalston, 1975). The duration of transitions into and out of the constriction interval are also in the 30- to 70-ms range. The combined time for the transitions and constriction intervals of semivowels may, therefore, be very brief (as short as 100 ms). This gives the impression of very rapid, complex articulatory gestures occurring in a short amount of time, perhaps explaining, in part, why children master these sounds relatively late in the overall scheme of phonological development.

FRICATIVES

Fricatives are characterized by an interval of aperiodic energy whose spectrum and overall amplitude depend on place of articulation and, in some cases, voicing status. In English, fricatives are categorized as sibilants (/s,z,ʃ,ʒ/) and nonsibilants (/f,v,θ,ð/) (the glottal fricative /h/ is discussed toward the end of this section). The sibilant-nonsibilant distinction is acoustically and perceptually meaningful because sibilants are more intense and have better-defined spectra than nonsibilants. "Better defined spectra" implies the presence of more easily identified spectral peaks and concentrations of spectral energy.

A general illustration of the acoustic bases of the sibilant-nonsibilant distinction is shown in Figure 10–20. Spectrograms are shown of the fricatives /s/ and /f/ in a VCV frame where V = /ɛ/. Superimposed LPC spectra for /s/ and /f/, computed over a 50-ms time interval centered at the midpoint of the frication noise, are shown immediately below the spectrogram. Along the baseline of the spectrogram, upward-pointing arrows show the frication onsets and offsets, based on the last glottal pulse preceding, and the first glottal pulse following the frication noise, respectively. The /s/ and /f/ durations are 174 ms and 154 ms, respectively.

The intensity difference between the sibilant /s/ and nonsibilant /f/ is seen easily in the spectrogram by the much darker frication noise for /s/. Note in the superimposed spectra the overall higher level of /s/ as compared to /f/. This kind of intensity difference is consistent for any sibilant-nonsibilant comparison, such as the /ʃ/ versus /θ/ comparison. Behrens and Blumstein (1988) reported a typical intensity difference of 14 dB between voiceless sibilant and nonsibilant frication noises. Data reported by Jongman, Wayland, and Wong (2000) suggest a slightly smaller difference of about 9 to 10 dB. The sibilant-nonsibilant intensity difference applies to voiced fricatives (e.g., /z/ vs. /v/, or /ʒ/ vs. /ð/) as well, but the difference is probably not as great as in the case of voiceless fricatives (see Jongman et al., 2000, Table V, p. 1259). The higher intensity for sibilants is largely due to the presence of an obstacle, the teeth, in the path of the airstream emerging from the fricative constriction for /s,ʃ,z,ʒ/. As discussed in Chapter 8, the airstream striking the teeth creates a second turbulent flow source and boosts the overall energy of the source spectrum for these fricatives. The nonsibilants /f,θ,v,ð/ typically are produced with little or no obstacle in front of the constriction, and, therefore, have a weaker source spectrum than sibilants.

The difference in sibilant versus nonsibilant spectra is further appreciated by studying the superimposed spectra of the two sounds. The /f/ and /s/ spectra in Figure 10–20 differ by the prominence (that is, the definition) of their peaks. The /s/ spectrum has two distinct, intense peaks, one around 4.3 and the other just above 5.0 kHz. Both peaks are roughly 35 dB more intense than the lowest amplitude in the spectrum. In contrast, the /f/ spectrum has its greatest peaks just above 9.0 kHz and just below 10.0 kHz, roughly 30 dB more intense than the lowest energy in its spectrum (close to 0 kHz). Basically, the /f/ spectrum can be described as flatter than the /s/ spectrum (or the /s/ spectrum can be described as "peakier" than the /f/ spectrum). Sibilants typically have peakier spectra than nonsibilants, as shown in Figure 10–21 for the /ʃ/-/θ/ (left) and /z/-/v/ (right) contrasts.

As discussed in Chapter 8, quantification of the frequency characteristics of fricative spectra is not straightforward. Fricative spectra have sometimes been characterized with a single number, the peak frequency, defined as the frequency in the spectrum

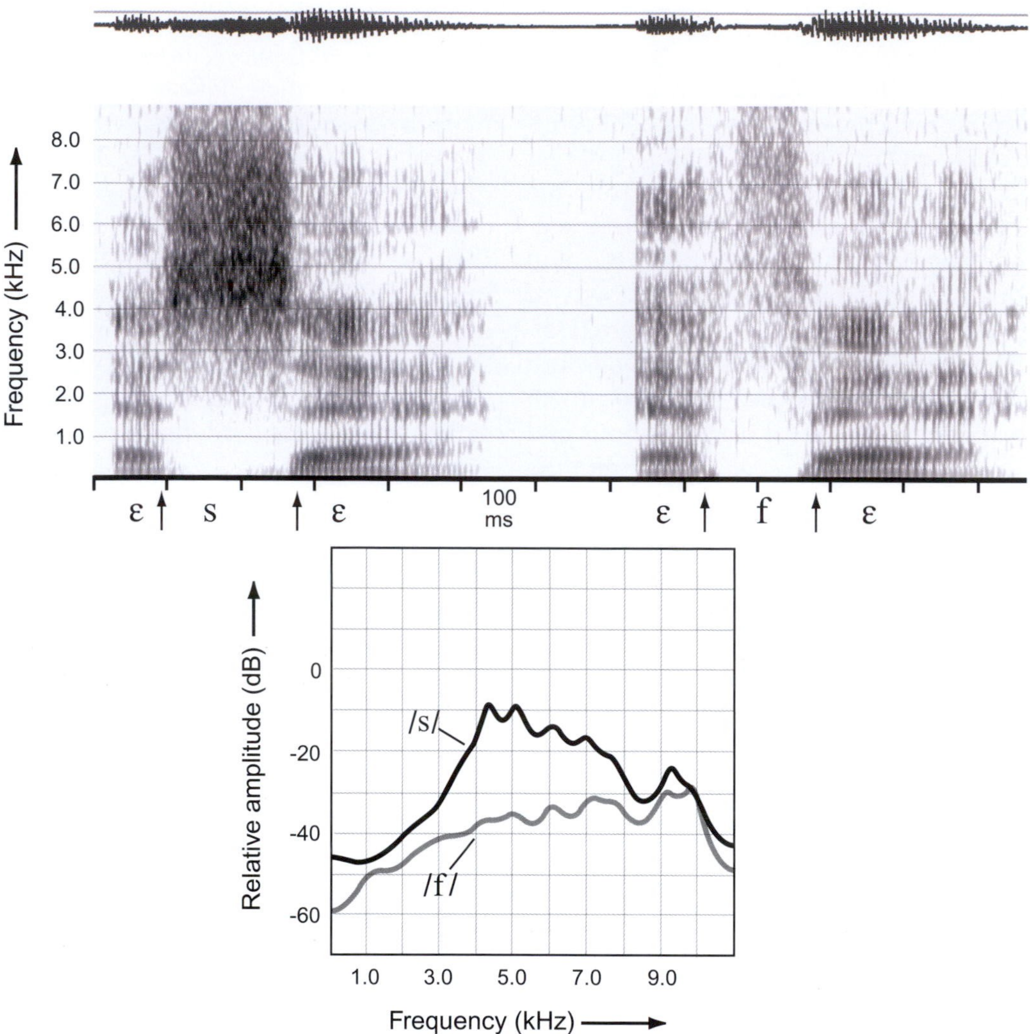

Figure 10–20. Spectrograms of the fricatives /s/ and /f/ in VCV frames where V = /ɛ/. Note the 0 to 8.4-kHz frequency range in these displays, to demonstrate the characteristic higher-frequency energy of frication noise. The upward-pointing arrows indicate the onsets and offsets of the fricatives, indicated by the last glottal pulse preceding the frication noise (*onset*) and the first glottal pulse following the frication noise (*offset*), respectively. Below the spectrograms LPC spectra are shown for the middle 50 ms of the frication noise; lighter line = /f/ spectrum, darker line = /s/ spectrum.

with maximum amplitude. For example, in Figure 10–21 the peak frequency for /ʃ/ is roughly 5.8 kHz, for /θ/ 9.2 kHz, for /z/ 4.5-5.0 kHz (there is a broad peak spanning this frequency range), and for /v/ 10.0 kHz. Jongman et al. (2000) reported that the simple measurement of peak frequency *statistically* distinguished fricative place of articulation when data were averaged across 20 speakers. The average, peak frequencies obtained by Jongman et al. for the four places of English fricative articulation are shown in Table 10–3. These peaks decrease in frequency as place of articulation moves backward in the vocal tract. As discussed in Chapter 8, this makes theoretical sense because the primary resonance of the vocal tract in fricative production derives from the cavity in front of the constriction, whose size increases as the place of articulation becomes more posterior. Larger resonators mean lower resonant frequencies.

The match between Jongman et al.'s (2000) peak frequency data and speech acoustic theory, however, should be approached with a certain degree of

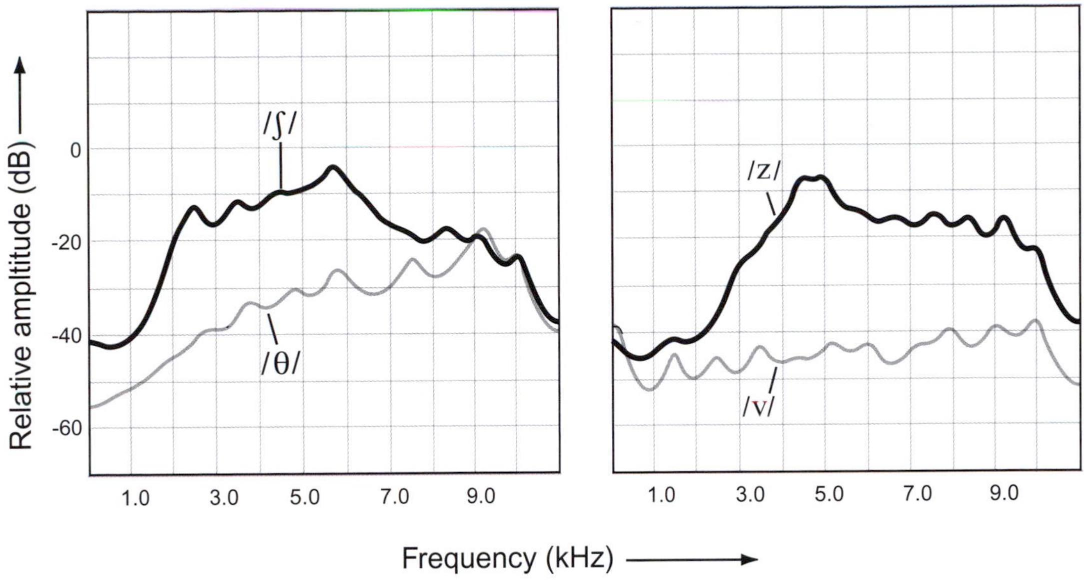

Figure 10–21. Left panel: LPC spectra for /θ/ (*light trace*) and /ʃ/ (*dark trace*). Right panel: LPC spectra for /v/ (*light trace*) and /z/ (*dark trace*). All fricatives were produced in a VCV frame where V = /ɛ/. Spectra were computed from the middle 50 ms of the frication noise.

Table 10–3. Average Peak Frequencies for Four Fricative Places of Articulation Reported by Jongman et al. (2000) for 20 Speakers Producing CVC Words in a Carrier Phrase

PLACE		PEAK FREQUENCY (Hz)
Labiodental	/f,v/	7733
Dental	/θ,ð/	7470
Alveolar	/s,z/	6839
Palatoalveolar	/ʃ,ʒ/	3820

Note: Data are for the first C in the CVC word. Peak frequencies were derived from spectra computed from the center 40 ms of the frication noise. Measurements were made from inspection of both FFT and LPC spectra.

caution. The data, averaged across speakers (including sex) and vowel contexts, hide the substantial variation in spectral details occurring from repetition to repetition for a given speaker, and across different speakers. One of these spectral details is the location of the peak frequency. In Figure 10–21, for example, the peak frequency of one of the author's /ʃ/ spectrum (left panel) is approximately 1000 Hz higher than that of his /z/ spectrum (right panel). Not only are these numbers inconsistent with the *direction* of the effect reported by Jongman et al., in which alveolar fricatives have higher peak frequencies as compared to palato-alveolar fricatives,[11] but the actual values of the peak frequencies shown in Figure 10–21 are quite different from those listed in Table 10–3. For example, the peak frequency in Figure 10–21 for /ʃ/ is 5800 Hz, as compared to an average for /ʃ/ and /ʒ/ of 3820 Hz reported by Jongman et al. (2000). Substantial intra- and inter-speaker variation in fricative spectrum details has been described by Narayanan (1995). Peak frequency as a descriptor of fricative spectra may separate fricative place of articulation with statistical reliability, but there is a great deal of error variation (unexplained data noise) in the statistical findings, and as Figure 10–21 shows it is easy to find exceptions to the trends reported in Table 10–3.

[11]The reversal of the direction expected from Jongman et al.'s (2000) data, and from speech acoustic theory, still holds even when the Figure 10–21 comparison is adjusted for mixing of place and voicing. Jongman et al. reported that voiced fricatives had somewhat lower peak frequencies than voiceless fricatives—about 300 Hz on average—but even when this is applied to the Figure 10–21 spectra the peak frequency difference is still around 700 Hz, and in the wrong direction.

characteristics of these sounds. Many classification errors, however, involved /s/ and /ʃ/ productions classified as /f/ or /θ/. Forrest et al. noted that the use of the four moments to classify fricatives neglects an important difference between sibilants and nonsibilants, namely, intensity of the frication noise. Many of the classification errors in Forrest et al., where sibilants were classified as nonsibilants, could have been avoided if frication intensity was included as a fifth classification variable.

Jongman et al. (2000), in a more extensive study of fricative acoustics, obtained spectral moments for all English fricatives produced by men and women in a variety of vowel contexts. Their moments data, averaged across speakers and vowels, are reproduced in Table 10–4. The data for the first moment (M1), which are given in units of Hz, are consistent with the theoretical discussion of fricative acoustics presented in Chapter 8.[12] M1 is nearly 2000 Hz higher for /s,z/ as compared to /ʃ,ʒ/, reflecting the difference in size of the resonator in front of the fricative constriction. The nearly identical M1 values for /f,v/ and /θ,ð/ are consistent with the absence of a resonating cavity in front of the constrictions for these nonsibilants. The M1s for /f,v,θ,ð/ are located roughly in the center of the analyzed frequency band (approximately 1–11,000 Hz). In the absence of a resonating cavity to shape the source spectrum, nonsibilant output (source × filter) spectra tend to resemble the source spectra (see Chapter 8), which are relatively flat. This is why the M1s are so close to 5000 Hz, close to the center frequency of the analysis band.[13]

The M2 values listed in Table 10–4 also contrast the nonsibilants with the sibilants. Sibilant spectra have much smaller variances than nonsibilant spectra, which follows from the tendency of sibilant spectra to be peaky (that is, to have energy concentrated in peaks) and nonsibilant spectra to be flat (to have energy spread out across the entire spectrum).

Table 10–4. Spectral Moments Data for Fricatives.

	M1	M2	M3	M4
/f,v/	5108	6.37	0.007	2.11
/θ,ð/	5137	6.19	–0.083	1.27
/s,z/	6133	2.92	–0.229	2.36
/ʃ,ʒ/	4229	3.38	0.693	0.42

Source: Data from Jongman et al. (2000, Table I, p. 1257).
Note: M1 = mean, M2 = variance, M3 = skewness, M4 = kurtosis. M1 values are in Hz, M2 values in MHz, and M3 and M4 values have no units (they are dimensionless, having been normalized). See Forrest et al. (1988) for computational details.

The M3 data show a dramatic contrast between /s,z/ and /ʃ,ʒ/, the former having negative skewness, the latter positive skewness. This skewness contrast can be seen by comparing the /z/-/ʃ/ spectra displayed in Figure 10–21. The peaks for the palato-alveolar /ʃ/ are pushed to the lower-frequency, left-hand side of the spectrum, as compared to the higher-frequency peaks of the alveolar /z/. If the two spectra are thought of as distributions, the /z/ spectrum is tilted much more to the right than the /ʃ/, hence the negative skew value for /z/ and positive skew value for /ʃ/. The M3 values for /f,v,θ,ð/ are very close to zero, consistent with the essential flatness of their spectra.

In contrast to the values of the first three moments, values for M4 (kurtosis) reported by Jongman et al. (2000) are less easy to connect with known or expected characteristics of fricative spectra. The M4 values in Table 10–4 suggest that /f,v/ spectra are peakier than /ʃ,ʒ/ spectra, but this seems at odds with the large resonance peaks observed around 2000 to 4000 Hz for /ʃ,ʒ/ as compared to the typically flattened spectrum of /f,v/.

Some time has been spent explaining spectral moments and reviewing the relationship of values

[12]Although the mean of a normal distribution is zero, computation of the first spectral moment is based on frequency (Hz) and is not normalized like the zero mean of the normal distribution. M1 is computed by taking each frequency in the analysis band and weighting it by its amplitude. Thus, frequencies with greater amplitude are given more weight than frequencies with lesser amplitude in determining the M1 value of the spectrum. M1 can be interpreted as the primary energy concentration within the spectrum.

[13]Spectral moments are calculated within fixed frequency bands; the end frequencies of the moments reported in Table 10–4 are 1 Hz on the low end, and 11,000 Hz on the high end. The width of the band can be varied in whatever way an investigator desires, but it is typically dictated by the sampling rate and the low-pass filter cutoff frequency used when digitizing speech waveforms. For example, the moments reported in Table 10–4 (Jongman et al., 2000) were derived from waveforms sampled at 22,000 Hz and filtered with a cutoff frequency of 11,000 Hz.

reported by Jongman et al. (2000) to spectral characteristics of exemplar fricatives presented in Figures 10–20 and 10–21, or to characteristics expected from theoretical considerations. Spectral moments have become quite popular as a way to characterize fricative and stop-burst spectra. Most speech analysis programs, such as the one used to generate the spectrograms and spectra shown in this chapter, include algorithms to compute moments. One keystroke and four moments are reported. There are, however, three main problems with spectral moments that should be kept in mind when these measures are used as acoustic indices of fricative (or stop) production. First, the actual value of the moments is quite variable across different studies, and highly variable across speakers within a study. The reader is encouraged to compare fricative moments data published by Jongman et al., Fox and Nissan (2005), Tjaden and Turner (1997), Newman, Clouse, and Burnham (2001), and Tabain (2001) to gain a sense of the cross-study variation in these measures. Second, although moments quantify a lot of information in fricative spectra, they have not been successful in classifying fricative place of articulation. Forrest et al. (1988), Jongman et al., and Fox and Nissan all obtained the same results when classifying fricatives with moments (and some other variables). Typically, correct classification rates are about 90% for sibilants but only 60 to 70% for nonsibilants.[14] If spectral moments were the most inclusive and best way to represent the fricative spectrum, higher classification rates would be obtained.

The third problem with spectral moments consists of two interrelated subproblems. One of these subproblems is the tendency for high correlations between the moments, suggesting a lack of independence of the different measures. For example, because spectral moments are computed from a fixed analysis band, an M1 (spectral mean) of higher frequency is likely to have a more negative M3 (skewness). Stated otherwise, as the concentration of energy is "pushed" to the right of the analysis band (higher M1, as in /s/) the spectrum is tilted more to the right (more negative M3). Similarly, a more positive M4 (kurtosis), reflecting a spectrum in which there are very prominent peaks, likely has a smaller M2 (variance) because the energy is concentrated in a small frequency range (see bottom graph of Figure 10–22). The extent to which the moments are intercorrelated has not been reported in the literature in a formal, large-scale analysis, but speech scientists who have used the analysis are aware of the potential for lack of independence among the four measures.

The other subproblem is a lack of uniqueness between the numbers obtained in a moments analysis, and the actual shape of the observed spectrum. To understand this issue, consider the following thought experiment. A speech scientist is shown a list of formant frequencies in which each row consists of F1, F2, and F3 values. Based on these three formant frequencies, the speech scientist is asked to identify a vowel category. For example, the values F1 = 310, F2 = 2000, and F3 = 2800 would most likely be assigned the vowel category /i/. This would be a fairly easy task for a person with experience in acoustic phonetics. Even when the wrong vowel category was chosen it would almost certainly be adjacent in the vowel diagram to the correct category. Now, assume a similar experiment with the four spectral moments, the speech scientist's task being to select the most likely fricative category, or to draw the approximate spectral shape based on the numbers. This would be a daunting task for even the most seasoned expert. The difficulty of the task derives from the lack of independence of the moment values, as described above, and because a particular moment value can be associated with very different spectral shapes. This latter issue is especially relevant to the M2, M3, and M4 values.

These cautionary comments are not meant to negate the use of moments in describing fricative spectra. Spectral moments capture more information

[14]The frequent confusions in classification experiments between /f/ and /θ/ and /v/ and /ð/ are almost certainly due to the similarity of their spectra and their weak intensity. Sounds that are not easily distinguished, or in the language of phoneticians, that do not meet a reasonable criterion of acoustic contrast, are often merged over time and lose their contrastive value. In English, for example, there are many dialects where the /ɪ/-/ɛ/ distinction is not made (in southern Indiana, for example, one both writes with a [pɪn] "pen" and wears a [pɪn] "pin"). A similar merger seems to be occurring between the labiodental and dental fricatives in African-American English, where forms such as [bof] "both" and [bɚfdeɪ] "birthday" are commonly heard (Craig, Thompson, Washington, & Potter, 2003). It is reasonable to assume the merger is being "provoked," in part, by the lack of discriminability between these sounds.

The Ultimate Social Consequence

The literature on speech sound development makes frequent reference to the negative social consequences faced by children who have speech sound errors. These are, of course, important, but none results in such extreme punishment as was metered out for an /s/-/ʃ/ confusion to the Ephramites of Biblical fame. As told in the Book of Judges in the Old Testament, a battle between the Gileadites and Ephramites resulted in the passages of Jordan being held by the Gileadites. Ephramites who desired safe passage were required to pass a verbal screening test that revealed whether or not they were friend or foe. Chapter 12, Verse 6 says "Then said they unto him, Say now Shibboleth: and he said Sibboleth: for he could not frame to pronounce it right. Then they took him, and slew him at the passages of Jordan." Verse 6 goes on to say that 42,000 fell at the time. There is no record of how many went because their speech revealed them to be foe. The concept of a specific utterance that marks a person's geographical home was borrowed from this biblical story for the TIMIT (Texas Instruments/MIT) speech database, a huge collection of utterances from many different speakers, carefully transcribed and recorded for research use by speech scientists. The dialect group of the speakers in this database is revealed by two "shibboleth sentences," designed to be phonetically sensitive to dialect variation around the United States.

about a fricative spectrum than a peak frequency measure, and for certain distinctions, such as /s/-/ʃ/, seem to function quite well and are useful in revealing aspects of articulatory dysfunction in motor speech disorders and their response to clinical manipulations (Tjaden & Wilding, 2004). Care should be taken, however, in the use and interpretation of these measures.

Formant Transitions and Fricative Distinctions

In the earlier section on nasal acoustics, the role of formant transitions at the release (CV) or onset (VC) of the nasal murmur was discussed as an acoustic correlate of place of articulation. Interest in formant transitions as a reliable marker of place of articulation for fricatives has often been driven by concerns with the lack of a consistent distinction in fricative *spectra* between /f,v/ and /θ,ð/. The fricative spectra of /s,z/ and /ʃ,ʒ/ are sufficiently distinctive from each other, and from /f,v/ and /θ,ð/, to cue place of articulation for listeners, but some other part (or parts) of the acoustic signal must contain the information to distinguish labiodentals from dental nonsibilants.[15] In an early experiment on fricative perception, Harris (1958) showed that the primary cue for the labiodental-dental distinction was the pattern of formant transitions at the release of the fricative. This idea has been accepted in the speech science community for many years, even in the absence of supporting data from acoustic measurements of actual speaker productions. As reviewed

[15]Most spectral analyses of frication noises have been confined to a highest frequency of 10.0 to 11.0 kHz, so there is always the possibility that /f,v/ could be distinguished from /θ,ð/ noise on the basis of spectral features above 10 kHz. Tabain (1998) examined just this hypothesis for speakers of Australian English and found no evidence for consistent spectral distinctions between the labiodental and dental fricatives in the frequency region above 10 kHz.

by Jongman et al. (2000), the evidence for the importance of formant transitions in distinguishing place of articulation for nonsibilant fricatives is mixed. Indeed, Jongman et al. failed to identify formant transition patterns that consistently separated the four places of fricative articulation, including the critical labiodental-dental distinction. Perhaps these sounds are inherently confusable and will disappear, over time, as a useful contrast in English (see footnote 14).

Fricative Duration

The literature on fricative duration has produced a fair amount of agreement on some basic facts. First, voiceless fricatives are longer than voiced fricatives, all other things being equal. The "all other things being equal" qualifier is important, because such factors as position-in-word (e.g., /ʃæk/ "shack" versus /kæʃ/ "cash"), stress level of the syllable in which the fricative occurs, speaking rate, immediate phonetic context (e.g., /sæk/ "sack" versus /stæk/ "stack"), among other variables, modify the duration of a particular segment. Second, among the voiceless fricatives and possibly also voiced fricatives, sibilants have slightly greater duration than nonsibilants.

Figure 10–23 is a spectrogram of the syntactically well-formed but semantically curious utterance, "Two scenes at the zoo failed to verify the shame." This utterance was constructed solely to illustrate fricative duration measures. Precise measures of fricative duration were made using a speech analysis program (TF32: Milenkovic, 2001) and the segmentation rules presented in Chapter 9. The actual durations for the eight fricatives marked in Figure 10–23 are provided in the legend. Fricative onsets and offsets are marked by arrows at the spectrogram baseline, and a horizontal bar connecting

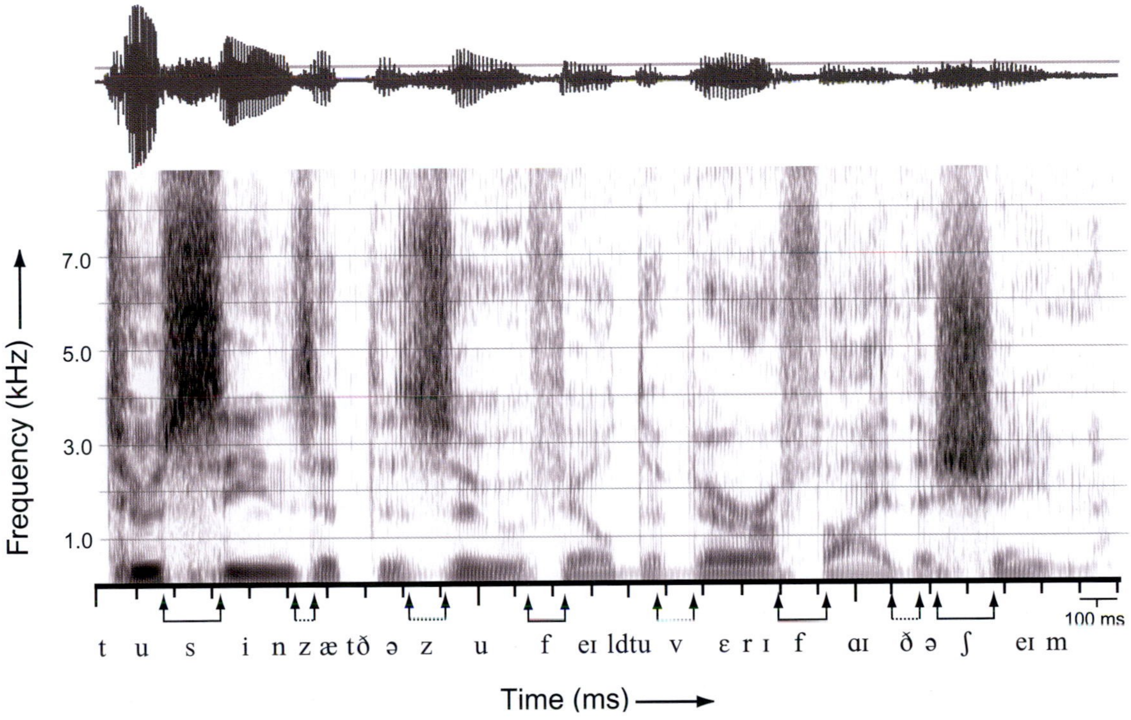

Figure 10–23. Spectrogram of the utterance "Two scenes at the zoo failed to verify the shame," constructed to show aspects of fricative duration. Eight fricatives in the utterance have been marked for duration; from left to right the fricative durations (all in milliseconds) are /s/ = 165; /z/ = 59; /z/ = 127; /f/ = 114; /v/ = 88; /f/ = 130; /ð/ = 71; /ʃ/ = 162 (the /ð/ in /ætðə/ was not measured because the preceding stop makes it impossible to locate the /ð/ onset). Solid horizontal bars connecting the onset and offset arrows are for voiceless fricatives, dotted bars for voiced fricatives.

the base of the arrows shows the duration (solid lines = voiceless fricatives; dotted lines = voiced fricatives). The two voiceless sibilant durations (/s/ = 165 ms, /ʃ/ = 162 ms) are clearly a good deal longer than the voiceless nonsibilants (/f/ = 114 ms; /f/ = 130 ms). And, although one /z/ (in "zoo") has a duration of 127 ms, the other three voiced fricatives all have durations less than 100 ms. Even these single examples of fricatives, in a connected-speech utterance (as compared to citation forms: see below) with variation in phonetic context and stress level, show patterns of duration largely consistent with the generalizations noted above. Voiceless fricatives are longer than voiced fricatives, sibilants are longer than nonsibilants.

A summary of published fricative duration data is provided in Table 10–5. Consideration of these data does not contradict the general outline of the two generalizations about fricative duration, but it does show that the magnitude of the voiceless/voiced and sibilant/nonsibilant difference varies a good deal across studies. For example, among the three studies in which both /s/ and /ʃ/ were compared to /f/ and /θ/ durations (Behrens & Blumstein, 1988; Jongman et al., 2000; Umeda, 1977), only one (Behrens & Blumstein, 1988) reported findings supporting a decisive difference between sibilant and nonsibilant durations. The difference is slightly more convincing for the voiced sibilant-nonsibilant difference. Similarly, the difference in fricative duration for voiceless versus voiced stops is quite large in some studies (Jongman et al., 2000) and more subtle in others (Baum & Blumstein, 1987).

Two reasonable questions arise from this review of fricative duration. First, are there good explanations for the two general effects identified above? Is there a straightforward reason why sibilants would be longer than nonsibilants, and voiceless fricatives longer than voiced fricatives? Second, why do fricative duration values and the magnitude of the sibilant-nonsibilant and voicing effects vary so much across studies?

Explanations for the effects are tentative, but may reveal something about the relationship of fricative duration measures to underlying speech physiology. More specifically, the process of making the measurements from acoustic records may explain part or all of the effects. For example, the longer duration of sibilants, as compared to nonsibilants, could reflect the generation of longer-duration, turbulent noise sources for sibilants. As presented in Chapter 8 and reiterated above, sibilants have more intense frication noise than nonsibilants largely because of the obstacle (teeth) effect. Perhaps the

Table 10–5. Selected Fricative Durations from Sources in the Literature.

	/f/	/v/	/θ/	/ð/	/s/	/z/	/ʃ/	/ʒ/
Umeda[a]	122	78	119		129	85	118	85*
Baum & Blumstein[b]	149	116	134	107	174	152		
Behrens & Blumstein[c]	149		134		174		175	
Crystal & House[d]			72	41				
Jongman et al.[e]	166	80	163	88	178	118	178	123

Note: All data are for prestressed (fricatives preceding stressed vowels) fricatives, and are reported in milliseconds.
[a]Umeda (1977); *N* = 1 speaker, connected speech (reading).
[b]Baum & Blumstein (1987); *N* = 3 speakers, citation form syllables.
[c]Behrens & Blumstein (1988); *N* = 3 speakers, citation form syllables.
[d]Crystal & House (1988d); *N* = 6 speakers, connected speech (reading).
[e]Jongman et al. (2000); *N* = 20 speakers, citation form syllables.

turbulent source is not only stronger, but also active over a longer period of time for /s,z,ʃ,ʒ/ as compared to /f,v,θ,ð/. This may be a reasonable explanation when scientists use the onset and offset of *frication noise* as the criterion for marking the boundaries of a fricative duration. Many scientists use this approach to measure fricative durations (e.g., Baum & Blumstein, 1987; Behrens & Blumstein, 1988; Jongman et al., 2000). The possible impact of this approach is illustrated by the subtle case shown in Figure 10–24, which shows two VCVs spoken by one of the authors with V = /ɑ/ and C = /θ/ (left) and /ʃ/ (right). Every attempt was made to pro-duce these VCVs at the same rate and with stress on the second syllable. The vertical lines mark off the frication interval, defined by the onset (left line) and offset (right line) of the visible frication noise. When the measurements were made with maximal time expansion of the spectrographic display (to provide the best temporal resolution), the frication intervals of /θ/ and /ʃ/ were 114 and 124 ms, respectively. This difference is fairly consistent with the sibilant-nonsibilant duration difference reported by Umeda (1977) and Jongman et al. If the duration of the frication noise is taken to reflect directly the duration of the fricative articulatory configuration, data shown in Table 10–5 and Figure 10–24 suggest that sibilants are indeed longer than nonsibilants.

As suggested above, however, fricative durations measured from a spectrographic or waveform display may not capture the entire duration over which a fricative configuration is maintained. Turbulent airflow, the source of aperiodic energy seen in acoustic displays of fricatives, occurs when an airflow of sufficient magnitude is driven through a sufficiently narrow constriction or strikes an edge of a sharp object. It is easy to imagine a situation in which a fricative configuration is maintained but aperiodic energy is either not generated or is of such weak intensity as to be undetected in a spectrographic or waveform display. For example, the lingual nonsibilants /θ/ and /ð/ have a very broad, loose constriction (Tabain, 2001) which may not always be tight enough to generate turbulence, even though the fricative configuration is produced. Moreover, the conditions under which these loose constrictions occur may be more likely at the onset and offset of the fricative, when the constriction is being formed and released, respectively.

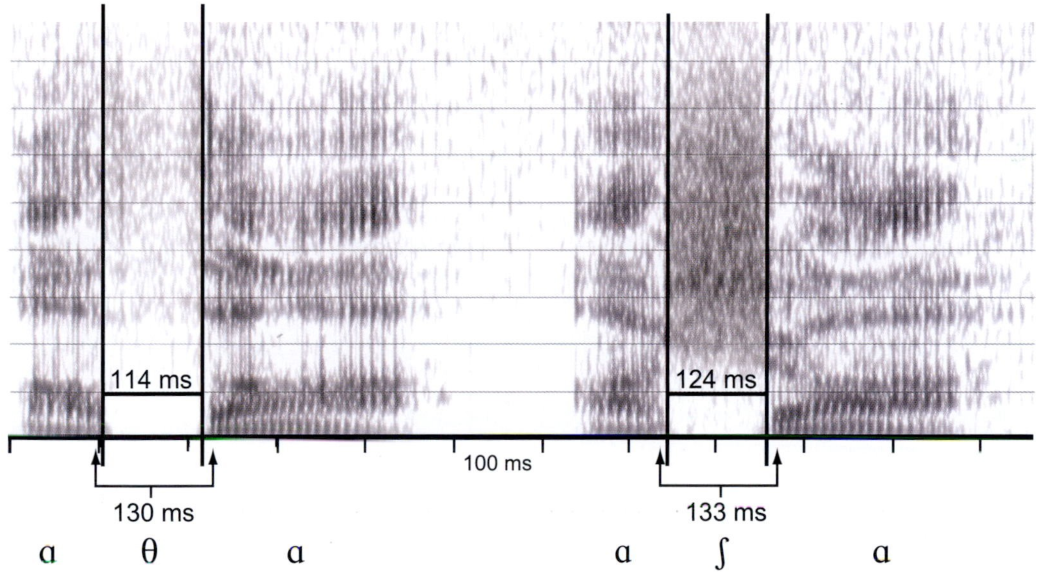

Figure 10–24. Spectrograms of the utterances /ɑθɑ/ (*left*) and /ɑʃɑ/ (*right*), illustrating the measurement of fricative duration under two criteria, one where the onsets and offsets of frication noise define the segment boundaries (*vertical lines running the length of the spectrogram*), the other where the preceding and following glottal pulses define the segment boundaries (*upward-pointing arrows*).

One way to address the possible mismatch of onset and offset of frication noise versus onset and offset of fricative *configuration* is to measure fricative durations from the last glottal pulse preceding the frication noise to the first glottal pulse following the noise. From an articulatory point of view, this makes sense because the last glottal pulse preceding frication is often timed to coincide with the onset of the supraglottal constriction (see review in Weismer, 2006, and below). In Figure 10–24, /θ/ and /ʃ/ durations measured with the glottal pulse criterion (boundaries marked by upward-pointing arrows) are 130 and 133 ms, respectively. Weismer (1980), using the glottal pulse criterion to measure fricative durations for nine speakers, reported mean, citation-form durations for /f/, /s/, and /ʃ/ of 180, 189, and 182 ms, respectively. These means were statistically indistinguishable from each other.

These considerations are offered to the reader in the spirit of an interesting scientific problem, rather than an endorsement of one measurement approach relative to another. The scientific problem shows how a measurement decision may affect conclusions about underlying articulatory processes. In particular, this issue shows how interpretation of acoustic data may require a good working knowledge of speech physiology. In the current case, the relevant physiology concerns the aeromechanics associated with fricative production.[16]

The second general effect for fricative durations, of consistently longer voiceless as compared to voiced fricatives, also requires a working knowledge of speech physiology. Data in Table 10–5 from Umeda (1977) and Jongman et al. (2000) suggest that voiceless fricatives in the prestressed position (in a CV or VCV frame where the vowel following the fricative is stressed) are nearly twice the duration of voiced fricatives. Why should there be such a large difference between the durations of cognate fricatives? The answer is most likely found in the different laryngeal behavior for voiceless versus voiced fricatives. Voiceless fricatives require the laryngeal devoicing gesture (LDG), an opening-closing movement of the vocal folds observed in many languages for virtually all voiceless obstruents (e.g., Hirose, 1977; Löfqvist, 1980). The LDG differs from the opening-closing motions of the vocal folds during phonation in two important ways. First, the opening and closing movements of the LDG are produced under muscular control—the ***posterior cricoarytenoid*** muscle producing the opening, the ***interarytenoid*** (perhaps assisted by the ***lateral cricoarytenoid***) the closing, with perhaps some assistance from the ***cricothyroid*** muscle to stiffen the folds and contribute to the cessation of phonation (Hirose, 1976; Löfqvist, Baer, McGarr, & Story, 1989). In contrast, the opening and closing movements during phonation are the result of aerodynamic and mechanical forces acting against the background forces exerted by laryngeal muscles (see Chapter 3). Second, the opening and closing motion of the LDG produces a very long event compared to the short-duration, opening and closing motion of a single cycle of vocal fold vibration. The LDG typically takes roughly 120 to 150 ms, whereas a "long" period for one phonatory cycle would be roughly 10 ms in duration (for an F0 = 100 Hz, a rather low, average speaking fundamental frequency). The relatively long duration of the LDG is critical to understanding the relatively long duration of voiceless, as compared to voiced, fricatives.

The laryngeal and supralaryngeal events shown schematically in Figure 10–25 for a VCV where C = /f/, /θ/, /s/, or /ʃ/, explain the relatively long duration of voiceless fricatives. Laryngeal events are shown as a function of time on the line labeled A_g, or "area of the glottis." These data are collected through an endoscope positioned directly above the vocal folds and connected to a recording device. The opening and closing motions of the vocal folds produce closely related variations in the area of the glottis (i.e., the area of the opening between the vocal folds). Upward deflections of the trace reflect opening of the vocal folds, downward deflections reflect closing of the vocal folds. The baseline represents full vocal fold approximation, such as occurs at the end of every phonatory cycle. The short dura-

[16]There is, at least in theory, a simple answer to the problem posed here. When fricative configurations are evaluated *directly* (by electropalatography techniques, or perhaps x-ray or electromagnetic techniques), are sibilant configurations longer than nonsibilant configurations, all other things being equal? This seems to be a straightforward question that might have been answered over the last 50 years of speech research, but, in fact, an answer requires very precise technical tools and measurement decisions. This is a fancy way to say that the relevant experiment has not been done.

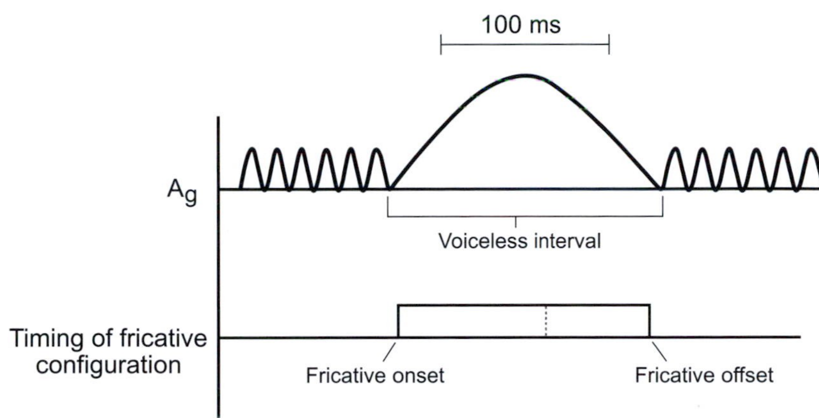

Figure 10–25. Schematic representation of laryngeal and supralaryngeal events for a VCV utterance in which C = a voiceless fricative. A_g = area of the glottis; upward movement on this trace indicates opening motions of the vocal folds, downward movement closing motions of the folds. The short-duration cycles are phonatory motions of the folds, the long-duration motion is the LDG. Voiceless interval = the duration of the laryngeal devoicing gesture. "Timing of fricative configuration" indicates the onset, duration, and offset of the supralaryngeal configuration required for fricative production. See text for additional details.

tion cycles of opening-closing movements are the phonatory cycles associated with the vowels and the long-duration, larger opening-closing movement is the LDG. The time course of the LDG can be compared to events on the line labeled "Timing of fricative configuration." This is a schematic representation of the onset, duration, and offset of the grooved fricative configuration made by the tongue in contact with parts of the palate, or between the lower lip and upper teeth. This contact is shown as a raised box meant to represent the timing of the fricative configuration relative to the laryngeal events depicted on the top line. When the joint timing of laryngeal and supralaryngeal events is considered, the following conclusions can be drawn. First, the onset of the fricative configuration is synchronous with the onset of the LDG. Second, the offset of the fricative configuration, presumably when the fricative is released into the following vowel, occurs approximately at the same time as the return of the vocal folds to the phonation-ready position (the closed position that permits aerodynamic and mechanical forces to create repeated oscillations of the vocal folds for phonation). Third, the LDG is in excess of 100 ms, as indicated by comparison of the LDG duration to the time-scale indicated above the trace. In Figure 10–25 the duration of the LDG is labeled as the voiceless interval because it is the time during which the vocal folds are prevented from vibrating for phonatory purposes.

The LDG seems to "run off" as a preprogrammed gesture for production of a voiceless obstruent. The gesture does not seem to be subject to precise voluntary control (Löfqvist, Baer, & Yoshioka, 1981), suggesting that its amplitude and duration is relatively fixed, at least for a given stress condition and speaking rate. If the LDG is implemented for production of a voiceless fricative (as it should be for correct production of the sound class), and if its "programmed" duration is a fair amount in excess of 100 ms as shown in Figure 10–25, the duration over which the fricative configuration is maintained would also have to be in excess of 100 ms and, in fact, would have to nearly match the duration of the LDG. This is because an earlier release of the fricative, such as the point in time shown in Figure 10–25 by the dotted, vertical line, slightly past the most open phase of the LDG, would result in a substantial period of aspiration noise. The aspiration noise would extend from the time of fricative release until the LDG brought the vocal folds back to midline in preparation for phonation. This would clearly not be desirable because aspiration noise following release of an English obstruent is a hallmark of voiceless stops and the single voiceless affricate. An extended interval of fricative aspiration could result in misidentifications of fricatives as stops or affricates and ultimately affect speech intelligibility.

The explanation for the relatively long duration of voiceless fricatives is, therefore, the need to "match" the duration of the supralaryngeal fricative configuration to the duration of the LDG—that is, to the voiceless interval duration. This duration is almost always in excess of 100 ms, and is likely to be somewhere within the 120- to 150-ms range, on average. Because voiced fricatives are not produced with an LDG, their duration is not required to be so long. The duration of most voiced fricatives is around 100 ms or even a little less.

/h/ Acoustics

/h/ is often described as a glottal fricative because an aperiodic, continuant-type source is generated in and around the glottis. The glottis is partially or largely open during the production of /h/, and the aperiodic source is produced when the air jet emerging from the constriction between the vocal folds strikes the edges of the ventricular folds and epiglottis, generating turbulent airflow (Stevens, 1998, pp. 428–436). This is like the teeth-obstacle model presented above for fricatives /s/, /z/, /ʃ/, and /ʒ/, except in the case of /h/ the obstacles are structures immediately above the vocal folds.

The source-filter acoustics for /h/ are quite complex (Stevens, 1998). Here, /h/ acoustics are summarized in a few major points with reference to spectrograms of the utterances "Ohio" (/ohaɪjo/) and /ə'he/ (Figure 10–26). In both utterances, /h/ is in the intervocalic position, and the approximate onsets and offsets of the /h/-intervals are indicated by upward-pointing arrows at the spectrographic baseline. The /h/-interval clearly contains aperiodic energy, as expected when the sound source is the result of turbulent airflow. Careful examination of the /h/-intervals indicates evidence of relatively weak glottal pulses—compared to the pulses in the surrounding vowels—mixed in with the noise. Intervocalic /h/ often has a combination of aperiodic and weakly periodic energy, suggesting that the abducted vocal folds are still vibrating weakly, with minimal or absent closed phases (Ladefoged, 2005).

Formants can be detected during the /h/-intervals. These regions of dark, aperiodic-plus-voicing energy seem to line up with the formants of

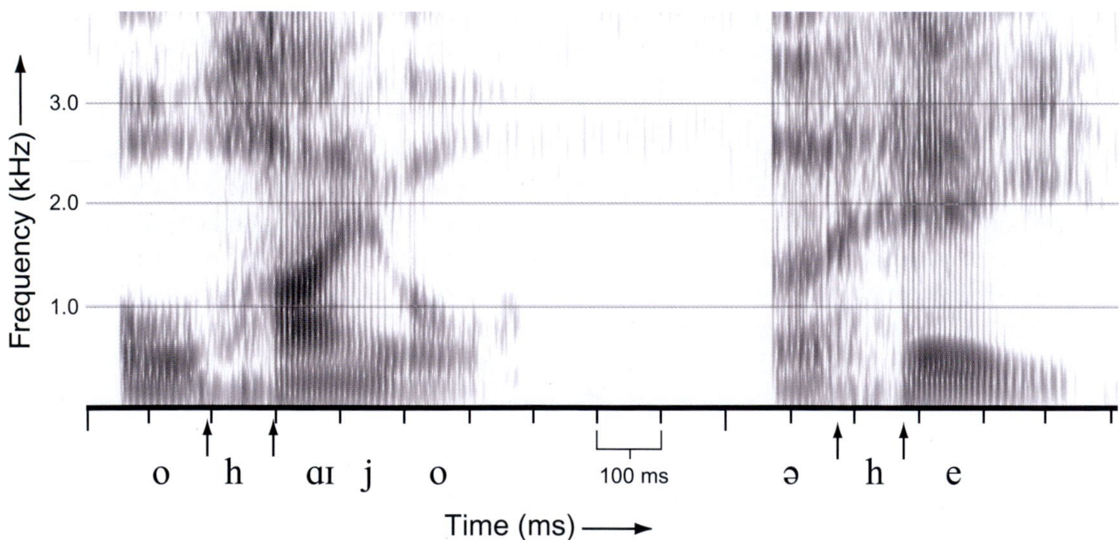

Figure 10–26. Spectrograms of the utterances /ohaɪjo/ (*left*) and /ə'he/ (*right*), illustrating the acoustics of /h/. The onsets and offsets of the /h/ interval are indicated by upward-pointing arrows.

Survival of the Phonetic Fittest

Speech and language are constantly changing, always evolving. This is certainly the case in phonetics, where "strong" phonetic segments maintain their contrastive identity, weak phonetic segments do not. In Chapter 8 the ongoing merger of the /f/-/θ/ contrast in African-American English was cited as one such case. /h/ qualifies as phonetically "weak" for the same reason as /f/ and/θ/—it has very low amplitude. The sound is, therefore, subject to possible disappearance from sound inventories or deletion in connected speech. The weak energy of /h/ gives it poor survival potential in, say, noisy or difficult communication settings. Mielke (2003) reported an experiment in which Turkish speakers deleted /h/ at fast speaking rates, but only in phonetic environments where the /h/ energy was most likely to be extremely weak and, therefore, hard to perceive. It is almost as if speakers recognized the phonetic conditions in which /h/ was likely not to be heard, and took advantage of this knowledge by deleting the sound production from their utterances. /h/ deletion is common in other languages as well, the best known example being Cockney English (Norman, 1973).

the following (and to some extent, preceding) vowel. This makes sense under the assumption that /h/ is produced with the vocal tract shape of the surrounding vowel(s), except with a largely aperiodic source. Perhaps this is why Ladefoged (2005, p. 58) described /h/ as a "noisy vowel." The most complete treatment of the formant structure of /h/-intervals is found in Lehiste (1964, pp. 141–180).

A dramatic feature of this noisy, formant-bearing interval is the relative weakness of energy around F1 as compared to the much more intense energy of the upper formants. This intensity difference is shown clearly in both /h/s in Figure 10–26. The weak energy in the F1 region of the /h/ noise is the result of sound absorption in the trachea. Interestingly, this fact explains why a person with a breathy voice may also suffer intelligibility problems as a result of indistinct vowels. The loss of F1 energy due to vocal fold vibration characterized by poor closure, a physiological correlate of breathy voice, may result in a loss of vowel distinctiveness. The effect of a breathy voice on communication may, therefore, be more than just a voice problem. The effect may extend to segmental (acoustic) integrity and, therefore, speech intelligibility.

STOPS

Stop consonants enjoy a special status in speech acoustics. Their acoustic characteristics have been the subject of much study and debate, and their role in the perception of speech has a very long and contentious history. Stops are also attractive for acoustic-phonetic study because they are the only consonant type to occur in *all* languages of the world (Ladefoged & Maddieson, 1996). Within languages, stops are among the most frequently occurring consonant segments (Maddieson, 1997). Study of the acoustic phonetic characteristics of stops can, therefore, be considered as a "high-yield" effort in understanding both speech production and perception.

Spectrograms illustrating the basic properties of stop consonants are shown in Figure 10–27. The stops /t/ and /d/ are shown in VCV frames, where V = /ɑ/. The upper spectrograms show the stops produced with stress on the second syllable (/ɑ'tɑ/, /ɑ'dɑ/), whereas the lower spectrograms show stops with stress on the first syllable (/'ɑtɑ/, /'ɑdɑ/). The frequency range for these spectrograms is roughly 0 to 8.5 kHz.

Table 10–6. Selected Stop Closure Durations from Sources in the Literature. All data are reported in milliseconds.

	p	b	t	d	k	g	Voiceless	Voiced
Umeda[a]	89	90	77	83	69	69	78	81
Umeda[b]	67	57	25	26	61	53	51	45
Stathopoulous & Weismer[c]	96	92	82	76	72	68	83	79
Stathopoulous & Weismer[d]	87	66	44	41	71	56	67	54
Luce & Charles-Luce[e]	93	61	68	51	84	52	82	55
Luce & Charles-Luce[f]	89	77	89	62	75	60	84	66
Crystal & House[g]	66	55	—	—	61	60	54	52
Byrd[h]	69	64	53	52	60	54	59	56

[a]Umeda (1977); *N* = 1 speaker, connected speech (long reading passage), V'CV environment.

[b]Umeda (1977); *N* = 1 speaker, connected speech (long reading passage), 'VCV environment.

[c]Stathopoulos & Weismer (1983); *N* = 6 speakers, CVCVC citation forms in carrier phrase, V'CV environment.

[d]Stathopoulos & Weismer (1983); *N* = 6 speakers, CVCVC citation forms in carrier phrase, 'VCV environment.

[e]Luce & Charles-Luce (1985); *N* = 4 speakers, CVC citation forms in long carrier phrases, closure for second C measured preceding vowel /ɪ/, stops, therefore, in 'VCV environment, with C = word final.

[f]Luce & Charles-Luce (1985); *N* = 4 speakers, CVC citation forms in long carrier phrases, closure for second C measured preceding fricative /s/, stops, therefore, in 'VC/s/ environment, with C = word final.

[g]Crystal & House (1988b); *N* = 6 speakers, connected speech (two reading passages), data for /p,b,k,g/ are for stops in prevocalic, word-initial stops; voiced/voiceless data are for stops in all positions.

[h]Byrd (1993); *N* = 630 speakers, connected speech (sentences), all phonetic contexts pooled.

case of voiced stops, however, voicing of the closure interval is often incomplete. The typical pattern, illustrated nicely by /ɑ'dɑ/ in Figure 10–27, is for voicing to be present at the start of the closure interval but to terminate some milliseconds prior to the burst (voicing terminates roughly 30 ms prior to the burst in this example). As discussed in Chapter 8, this may occur when the oral air pressure developed in the vocal tract approximates the magnitude of the tracheal pressure. If there is an insufficient pressure difference across the vocal folds, they will not vibrate, and it makes sense for the pressure difference to become insufficient later, rather than earlier in the closure interval.

Flap Closures

The case of /t/ and /d/ in the intervocalic, post-stressed position of words is particularly interesting, and serves to illustrate how the style of speech—formal versus less formal—can influence speech segment durations. The single speaker studied by

Umeda (1977) produced /t/ and /d/ closure durations in the 'VCV context of 25 and 26 ms, respectively (Table 10–6, note b). For the same kind of context, Luce and Charles-Luce (1985) reported /t/ and /d/ closure durations of 68 and 51 ms (Table 10–6, note e). At first glance, Umeda's (1977) values seem very short compared to other closure durations in Table 10–6, but, in fact they are almost identical to intervocalic, poststressed flap durations (/t/ = 26 ms; /d/ = 27 ms) reported by Zue and LaFerriere (1979) for six speakers producing words such as "rater" (/reɪɾɚ/) and "matter" (/mæɾɚ/). Luce and Charles-Luce's much longer intervocalic, poststressed closure durations for /t/ and /d/ almost certainly reflect, in part, the more formal speech style associated with citation form. Luce and Charles-Luce's lingua-alveolar closure durations also reflect the word-final position from which their stop closure durations were measured (see Table 10–6, notes e and f). As Byrd (1993) has reported, flaps occur in this word-final position when they are intervocalic and poststressed, but are less likely to occur than when the lingua-alveolar stop is located *within* a word (e.g., flaps would be expected in the words "rooter" and "ruder," but perhaps not so frequently in "root a lot," where the lingua-alveolar stop occurs in word-final position).

Closure Duration and Place of Articulation

Data in Table 10–6 can be used to evaluate the effect of place of articulation on stop closure duration. When closure duration values in the two columns for labial stops are compared to the lingua-alveolars and dorsals, there is clearly a tendency for labials to have the longest durations. Differences between lingua-alveolar and dorsal closure durations are less convincing.

Stop Voicing: Some Further Considerations

The acoustics of stop consonant voicing are complex. A famous article by Lisker (1986) listed *16* potential acoustic measures that could differentiate the /p/ and /b/ in minimal pairs such as "rapid" versus "rabid." It seems, therefore, as if there are multiple "candidate" acoustic cues to the voicing distinction for stop consonants. According to Lisker, the notion of "candidate" cues for stop voicing means that they *may* signal the difference between voiced and voiceless stops, but are not *all* necessary to make the distinction a good one. In fact, the particular cues that may signal the voicing status of a stop are context dependent. This context dependency includes not only where the stop is located relative to other sounds and the prevailing prosodic conditions (e.g., word medially versus word-initially?) pre- or post-stressed?), but also the relational status of the candidate cues to the voicing distinction. Lisker provides an excellent example of the latter dependency, noting that even though the duration of the closure interval can signal the difference between "rabid" and "rapid," it will not do so if the [b] closure interval is fully voiced. In this case, the word will be heard as "rabid" no matter how long or short the closure interval.

In fact, the simplest acoustic cue to the voicing of stop consonants would seem to be this most straightforward one, namely, whether or not the closure interval contains glottal pulses. It seems logical to expect voiced stops to be produced with closure intervals containing glottal pulses, and voiceless stops to have no voicing during the closure. Whereas the absence of glottal pulses during a voiceless closure interval is almost always the case, the presence of glottal pulses during the closure interval of a voiced stop is a more complicated phenomenon. First, as discussed earlier in the chapter, glottal pulses do not always fill the entire closure interval of a voiced stop closure. The pulses may begin at the onset of the closure interval but terminate well before the stop is released. Depending on how much of the closure interval is actually voiced (i.e., contains periodic energy generated by the vibrating vocal folds) as well as the intensity of the pulses that are present, the closure may have a voiced or voiceless quality when judged by a listener. In the absence of consideration of other potential cues to the stop voicing distinction, the voiced stops could, therefore, be considered more vulnerable to perceptual errors (i.e., voiceless-for-voiced stop errors) than voiceless stops (voiced-for-voiceless errors). Interestingly, literature on stop voicing errors in dysarthria and apraxia of speech is consistent with this asymmetry, that speakers are more often heard to produce voiceless-for-voiced than voiced-for-voiceless errors (Marquardt, Reinhart, & Peterson, 1979; Platt, Andrews, & Howie, 1980). The extent to which this asymmetry reflects true substitution errors, as compared to phonetic errors in which voiced closure intervals are only partially voiced and, therefore, perceptually ambiguous and judged by listeners as voiceless stops, is unknown.

The potential ambiguity of a partially voiced closure interval may be reduced or eliminated as a result of the value(s) of one or more of the other cues to stop voicing. The best-studied cue to stop voicing is voice-onset time (VOT), defined as the time interval between the burst and the first glottal pulse of a following vowel. Because the value of VOT is grossly correlated with the presence or absence of glottal pulses within the closure interval, VOT may remove any ambiguity concerning the voicing status of a stop. This is true in English (at least) and for stops preceding stressed vowels (at least). Why should the value of VOT be associated with the presence versus absence of glottal pulses within the closure interval?

The answer has to do with the laryngeal devoicing gesture, discussed above with reference to the voicing distinction for fricatives (see Figure 10–25). Figure 10–28 repeats the schematic presentation of Figure 10–25, but with the vocal tract timing (labeled as "Timing of stop closure") now appropriate for a voiceless stop closure (rather than a voiceless fricative constriction). The LDG is identical to the one shown in Figure 10–25 for a voiceless fricative. In particular, note how the onsets of the LDG and supralaryngeal closure for the stop are synchronized, as well as the LDG duration of well over 100 ms. All this is the same as in Figure 10–25. The striking difference in Figure 10–28, as compared to Figure 10–25, is the release of the stop consonant closure interval roughly 60 to 70 ms after its onset (as compared to the maintenance of the fricative constriction for the entire duration of the LDG in Figure 10–25). This earlier release, shortly after the widest separation of the vocal folds during the LDG, means that a significant interval of time will elapse after the stop release and before the vocal folds are brought together to resume vibratory activity. This interval is the VOT, and its relatively long duration results because the stop is released well before the LDG has completed its opening-closing movement. Voiced stops do not have an LDG. During the closure interval, the vocal folds remain more or less in the midline, in the phonation-ready position. The vocal folds will vibrate and cause glottal pulses to appear within the closure interval as long as there is a sufficient pressure differential (tracheal pressure minus

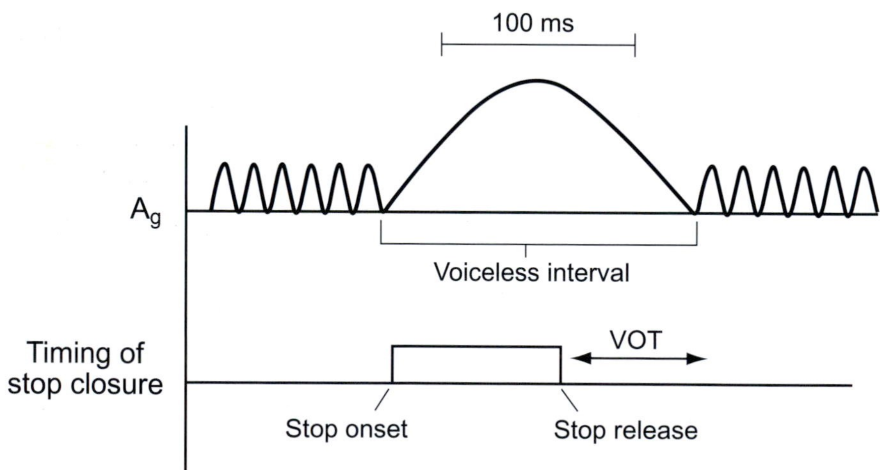

Figure 10–28. Schematic representation of laryngeal and supralaryngeal events for a VCV utterance in which C = a voiceless stop. A_g = area of the glottis. See Figure 10–25 legend for other details. "Timing of stop closure" indicates the onset, duration, and offset of the supralaryngeal configuration required for stop consonant production.

oral pressure) across the vocal folds. But even if vocal fold vibration ceases halfway through the closure interval, when the supralaryngeal stop closure is released, the vocal folds will be in the midline position and ready to resume vibrating almost immediately. This is the reason why the value of VOT is grossly correlated with the presence versus absence of glottal pulses within a stop closure interval. The absence of glottal pulses throughout the closure interval implies the presence of the LDG, which in turn results in a relatively long VOT. Glottal pulses within the closure interval, even if ceasing well before the stop release, imply the absence of the LDG and, therefore, the readiness of the vocal folds to resume vibrating very soon after the stop release.

VOT values have been reported many times since the classic study of Lisker and Abramson (1964) defined the measure and showed how it varied in different languages and speaking conditions. Extensive reviews of VOT data are available in Cho and Ladefoged (1999), Auzou et al. (2000), and Weismer (2006). Figure 10–29 summarizes VOT data for English by showing typical values along with selected factors known to modify the measured values. The VOT continuum shown in Figure 10–29 ranges between –30 and 50 ms and is marked off in 10-ms steps. Immediately above the horizontal time line phonetic symbols indicate typical VOT values for stops in sentences, as reported by Lisker and Abramson for four speakers. For example, Lisker and Abramson (their Table 17) reported average VOT's for /p/, /t/, and /k/ of 28, 39, and 43 ms, respectively. Each of the voiced stops has two entries along the VOT time line. One set is in the positive part of the continuum (7, 9, and 17 ms for /b/, /d/, and /g/, respectively), the other shows the three sounds grouped together with an arrow pointing to values more negative than -30 ms. Lisker and Abramson (1964) noted that some voiced stops are produced with voicing beginning *before* their release, and designated these as prevoiced with negative VOT values. Just as positive VOT values represent the delay between the burst and first glottal pulse of the following vowel, negative VOT values represent the time by which glottal pulses within the closure interval *precede* the burst. Both positive and negative VOT values are common in voiced stop production. The prevoiced, voiced stops reported by Lisker and Abramson all had VOTs more negative than -30 ms, the last negative value on the continuum shown in Figure 10–29.

Figure 10–29 shows a vertical dotted line at 25 ms along the VOT continuum. This line designates a boundary between typical positive VOTs for voiced

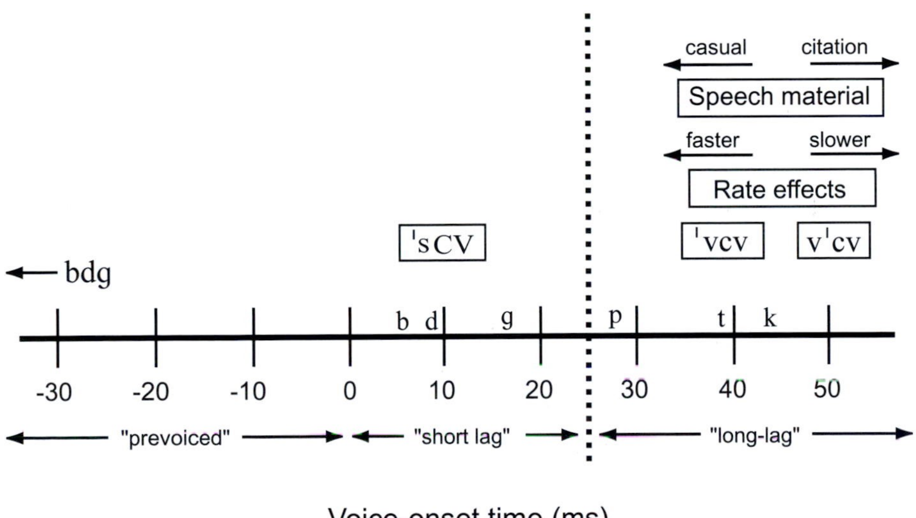

Figure 10–29. Graphic summary of VOT data from English speakers. A VOT continuum ranging from –30 ms to +50 ms is shown, and effects are indicated by the phonetic symbols and boxes above the continuum line. See text for additional detail.

and voiceless stops. Voiceless stops can be expected to have VOTs exceeding 25 ms (*long-lag* VOTs), whereas voiced stops have VOT's less than 25 ms (*short-lag* VOTs) (Weismer, 2006).

The boxes above the VOT continuum and to the right of the 25-ms boundary identify factors that cause VOT to vary in systematic ways. These boxes are in the long-lag range of the VOT continuum because the effects are typically most prominent for voiceless stops, with much smaller effects on the short-lag VOTs of voiced stops. VOT is affected by the position of a voiceless stop relative to a stressed vowel. Longer VOTs are measured when the stop precedes, as compared to follows, a stressed vowel. The box containing the V'CV frame has been placed to the right (longer VOTs) of the 'VCV box to indicate this effect. In fact, VOTs for voiceless stops in 'VCV frames may be so short as to place them in the short-lag range (Umeda, 1977). The effect of speaking rate on VOT, indicated in Figure 10–29 by the box and arrows immediately above the stress effects, are predictable from the direction of rate change. Slower rates produce longer VOTs for voiceless stops (shown by the arrow pointing to the right), and faster rates produce shorter VOTs (left-pointing arrow) (Kessinger & Blumstein, 1997). The reduction (shortening) of long-lag VOTs at very fast speaking rates, however, is rarely so dramatic as to encroach on the short-lag range (Kessinger & Blumstein, 1997; Summerfield, 1975). Finally, the topmost box indicates that speaking style affects the value of long-lag VOTs. Longer VOTs for voiceless stops are produced in more formal speaking styles, sometimes referred to as citation form or "clear" speech (Krause & Braida, 2004; Smiljanic & Bradlow, 2005). Casual speech styles yield shorter VOTs. The difference between formal and casual speaking styles is likely to involve a difference in speaking rate. Formal speaking styles typically have slower rates than casual styles (Picheny et al., 1986).

A special case of VOT modification for voiceless stops is indicated by the "'sCV" box above the short-lag range. "'sCV" stands for prestressed s+stop clusters, in words such as "<u>st</u>op," "<u>sk</u>ate," "<u>sp</u>eech," "a<u>st</u>ounding," and so forth. Voiceless stops in s+stop clusters have short-lag VOTs (Umeda, 1977), as illustrated by the spectrograms in Figure 10–30. The first two words in this spectrogram are "peach" and "speech," with the VOT measurement for the two /p/s shown along the baseline. These

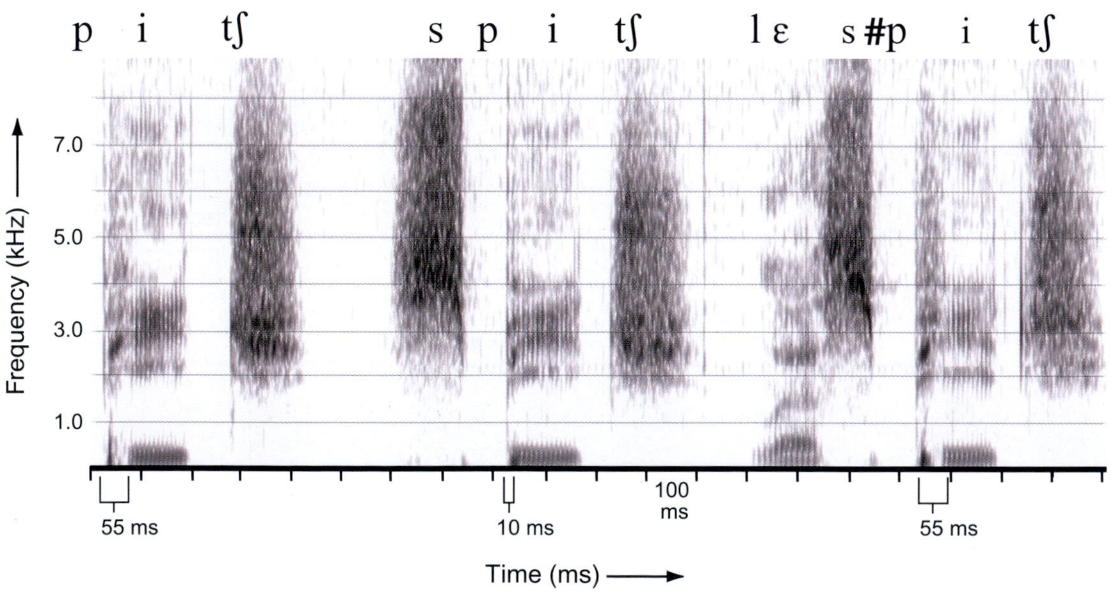

Figure 10–30. Spectrograms of the utterances /pitʃ/, /spitʃ/, and /lɛs#pitʃ/, showing how VOT varies when preceded by an /s/ in the same syllable (/spitʃ/) and across a word boundary (/lɛs#pitʃ/). VOT intervals are shown on the baseline.

intervals have a left-hand boundary at the /p/ burst and a right-hand boundary at the first glottal pulse of the following vowel. The 55-ms VOT for the /p/ in /pitʃ/ clearly fits the long-lag expectation for voiceless stops, whereas the 10–ms VOT for /p/ in /spitʃ/ illustrates the short-lag outcome of producing a voiceless stop in an s+stop cluster. This shortening effect seems to require that the s+stop cluster be part of one syllable, however (Davidsen-Nielsen, 1974). In Figure 10–30, the right-most spectrographic pattern is for the sequence /lɛs#pitʃ/, where the s + stop cluster crosses a word boundary (symbolized by "#"). In this case, the VOT for /p/ is in the long-lag range, essentially the same as the /p/ VOT in "peach."

In summary, the value of VOT can be used in many cases as a correlate of the voicing status of a stop consonant. Long-lag stops are typically voiceless, and short-lag stops are typically voiced. The "mismatches" between VOT values and the voicing status for stops usually occur only for voiceless stops whose VOT values are measured in the short-lag range. This can occur when voiceless stops are in the poststressed position of a word, and should occur with near certainty when a voiceless stop is part of an s + stop cluster within a single syllable.

Finally, something must be said about VOT values in other languages. Many languages have stop voicing distinctions, but "cut up" the VOT range in different ways as compared to English. For example, Korean has a three-way voicing distinction for each place of articulation, with the VOT range of roughly +20 to 120 ms "cut up" in three ways for the contrast (Cho, Jun, & Ladefoged, 2002). In contrast, French has a two-way voicing contrast in which the VOT continuum is "cut up" differently than in English. The voiced stops of French all have negative VOTs (i.e., they are prevoiced), and *short-lag*, positive VOTs for voiceless stops (Kessinger & Blumstein, 1997). This is why the voiceless stops of French are said to be unaspirated. Cho and Ladefoged (1999) provide an excellent analysis and interpretation of how very many different languages exploit the VOT continuum to "implement" their unique voicing contrasts.[17]

Bursts

Material presented in Chapter 8 describes the burst as the acoustic result of the sudden and rapid loss of oral air pressure at the release of a stop constriction. In practice, the isolation of a burst from the following frication interval (see Chapter 8) is exceedingly difficult. Theoretical analyses (Stevens, 1998; and see Johnson, 2003) suggest a duration of less than 5 ms for the actual burst of a stop. In the acoustic phonetics literature, the term "burst" is often used in a somewhat broader sense to include the burst plus the following 10 to 20 ms into the frication interval. This broader use of the term "burst" is justified by the following summary of material from Chapter 8. Although the aeromechanical bases of the burst source and frication source are different, their spectra are quite similar. Because both source spectra are shaped by the resonator in front of the source, the output spectra for the actual burst and the following frication interval tend to be very similar. The use of the term "burst" to include the burst plus a brief part of the frication interval is, therefore, not a case of mixing apples and oranges. For the discussion that follows, the term "burst" is used in this broader sense.

Bursts are considered one of the hallmarks of the stop manner of production. In laboratory experiments involving citation-form speech, stops are almost always produced with a clear burst. Interestingly, in more connected forms of speech such as reading, a significant number of stop consonants have no identifiable burst even when perception suggests a "good" stop has been produced (Byrd, 1993; Crystal & House, 1988c). This is yet another example of how speech style can modify acoustic phonetic phenomena.

Stop bursts have been the focus of a great deal of research. In particular, the spectrum of stop bursts has been studied in an attempt to demonstrate that each of the three places of stop articulation in English is associated with a unique spectral shape. This problem was framed early in the history of speech acoustics research by Halle, Hughes, and Radley (1957) who measured spectra for stop bursts in

[17]Voicing contrasts may be implemented in several different ways, including manipulation of the VOT continuum. This is not to say that VOT is not the only way to effect a voicing contrast, just one of the more popular, at least among speech scientists who enjoy measuring it and perhaps among speakers of different languages, too (Kingston & Diehl, 1994).

simple CV syllables, where C = each of the English stops and V = /i/, /ɪ/, /ʌ/, /ɑ/, and /u/. Their analyses were similar to ones shown in Figure 10–31, where speech waveforms are shown for /pʌ/, /tʌ/, and /kʌ/ and a 20-ms increment beginning at the burst is marked off for spectral analysis. This interval is shown below each waveform in Figure 10–31 by the horizontal line whose endpoints are indicated by upward pointing arrows. Halle et al. isolated these 20-ms intervals and for each one computed a Fourier spectrum for the frequency range 250 to 10,000 Hz (the Fourier spectra shown in Figure 10–31 have a slightly wider analysis band, namely 0 to 11,000 Hz).

Halle et al.'s (1957) observations concerning the spectra of these burst intervals have been replicated (with some minor differences) in several studies. Halle et al.'s observations were stated in terms of spectral shapes, that is, the relative distribution of energy across frequency. They described labial bursts as having primary concentration of energy in the lower frequencies, lingua-alveolar bursts with flat spectra or an emphasis of energy in the high frequencies (by which they meant, above 4.0 kHz), and dorsal stops as having prominent energy peaks in the midfrequency regions, meaning roughly between 1.5 and 4.0 kHz. In Figure 10–31, the /p/ burst has a relatively flat spectrum between 0 and 5.0 kHz

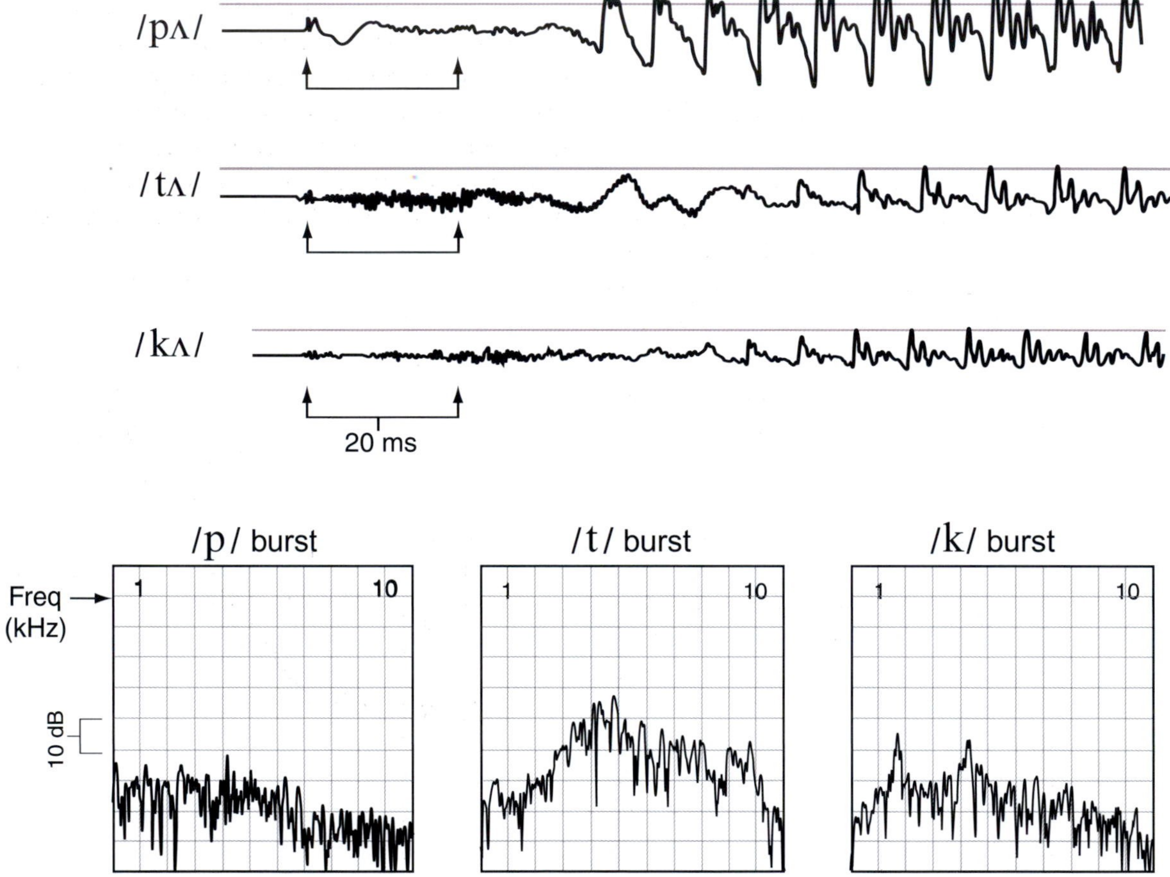

Figure 10–31. Waveforms (*three upper traces*) and spectra (*lower three panels*) for the stop consonants and initial part of vowels in /pʌ/, /tʌ/, and /kʌ/. A 20-ms interval, beginning at the stop burst, is indicated in the upper three traces by the horizontal line whose endpoints are marked by upward pointing arrows. This is the interval over which Halle et al. (1957) computed spectra for the stop burst. The Fourier spectra shown at the bottom of the figure are computed for the 0- to 11-kHz range. Each division along the frequency axis is a 1.0-kHz increment, each division along the intensity axis a 10-dB increment.

and decreasing energy between 5.0 and 11.0 kHz; the /t/ burst has clearly increasing energy from 0 to 5.0 kHz and decreasing energy at the higher frequencies; and the /k/ burst has two large, midfrequency peaks of energy, one around 1.8 kHz and the other at 4.2 kHz. Despite the difference in speakers and (probably more importantly) the different frequency analysis bands, the spectral shapes in Figure 10–31 are very consistent with the major summaries offered by Halle et al. in their study of stop burst spectra. Based on these observations, it would seem reasonable to claim that place of articulation is differentiated by the spectrum of the stop burst. If this is true, listeners presumably can use this information to identify place of articulation for stop consonants.

Perhaps it seems obvious that the burst would have unique spectral characteristics for the three different places of articulation. After all, the acoustic theory of speech production predicts different resonant frequencies depending on the location of a constriction in the vocal tract. Clearly, the different constriction locations for the three places of articulation are accompanied by differences in vocal tract shape over the first few milliseconds following the release of a stop. Reliable differences in stop burst spectra as a function of place of articulation should, therefore, be expected. Speech scientists use the term *acoustic invariance* to refer to the stable, place-specific acoustic characteristics discussed here. An acoustically invariant characteristic of a particular speech sound is one that is always found in the waveform, regardless of who is producing the utterance or under what conditions the utterance is spoken.

This view, although attractive and apparently logical, neglects the well-known phenomenon of coarticulation. There are different ways to define coarticulation, but a more or less conventional definition will make the point: Coarticulation is the influence of one segment on another. Stated otherwise, the articulatory (and hence acoustic) characteristics of a particular segment depend on the articulatory (acoustic) characteristics of adjacent, and in some cases nonadjacent, segments. In the case of stop burst spectra, the important question is: How stable is the spectrum for a particular stop place of articulation when the following vowel (or any preceding or following segment) varies? If stop burst spectra vary in a significant way depending on the following vowel, the claim of unique spectral characteristics for the three different places of stop articulation may be difficult to defend. Vowel induced variation could result in highly variable stop burst spectra for a given place of articulation, with too little acoustic stability to serve as a reliable cue to place identification.

Figure 10–32 shows an example of a vowel effect on a burst spectrum. Two spectra are shown, both calculated for a 26-ms interval starting at the burst of the /t/ in /ɑti/ (light trace) and /ɑtu/ (dark trace). The analysis band is limited to 0 to 5 kHz and the spectra have been smoothed. The smoothing of the spectra, which eliminates the detail of individual Fourier-spectrum components as if a continuous line were drawn to connect the many energy peaks while ignoring the dips and other details, was performed by calculating the LPC spectrum for the 26-ms interval (see Chapter 9). These two spectra have obvious differences, but are also very similar in an important way. The main difference between the spectra is the emphasis of lower frequencies for /tu/ as compared to /ti/. The /tu/ spectrum has rather large peaks at 2.8 and 3.7 kHz, whereas the /ti/ spectrum lacks dramatic peaks below

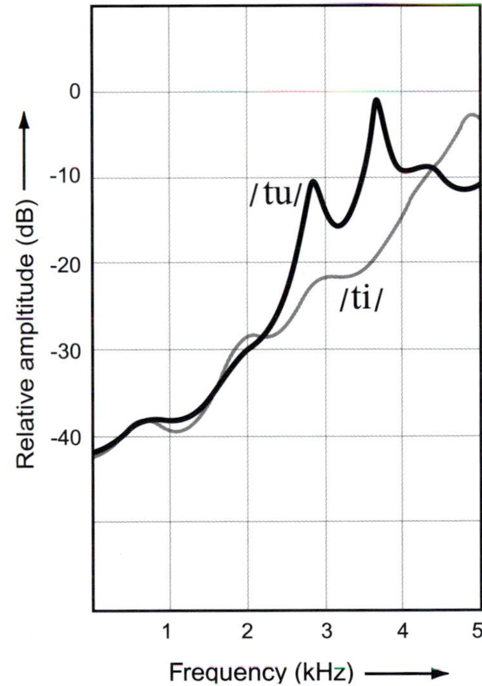

Figure 10–32. Two LPC spectra (0–5.0 kHz) for /t/ bursts produced before an /u/ (*dark line*) and an /i/ (*light line*). A comparison between these spectra shows the effects of vowel coarticulation on /t/ burst acoustics.

4.0 kHz but has steadily increasing energy up to roughly 5.0 kHz, where a peak seems to be present. Stated more generally, the /t/ burst followed by /u/ has more low-frequency energy when compared to the /t/ burst followed by /i/, at least for this 0- to 5.0-kHz analysis band. From the perspective of coarticulation this makes sense because the formants of /u/ concentrate more energy in the low frequencies, whereas the formants of /i/ have more high-frequency concentration. These different concentrations of vowel energy influence the concentration of energy in the burst spectra.

The commonality in these two spectra is the steadily increasing energy from 0 to nearly 4.0 kHz, despite the difference in the location of prominent peaks. In this analysis band, both spectra are tilted to the higher frequencies. Perhaps the gross, upward tilt for /t/ bursts is the critical acoustic correlate to this place of articulation, and is always present even when the following vowel influences details of peak location and magnitude. The auditory system may be able to strip away all spectral detail and use the gross spectral shape to identify stop place of articulation.

In a classic acoustic phonetics study, Blumstein and Stevens (1979) attempted to demonstrate the uniqueness of such spectral shapes for the three different places of stop articulation. After examining LPC burst spectra for a 26-ms interval starting at the burst and for the 0- to 5.0-kHz analysis band, as produced by a small number of speakers, Blumstein and Stevens designed "spectral templates" for each of the three places of articulation. These templates were meant to allow spectral variation in the burst spectrum due to speaker differences and coarticulation (that is, as a result of a particular stop being articulated with a variety of vowels) while preserving the more global spectral shape that was presumably the constant, or invariant acoustic characteristic of the stop burst. The templates were named *diffuse-falling* for bilabials, *diffuse-rising* for lingua-alveolars, and *compact* for dorsals. Examples of LPC spectra consistent with these templates are shown in Figure 10–33.

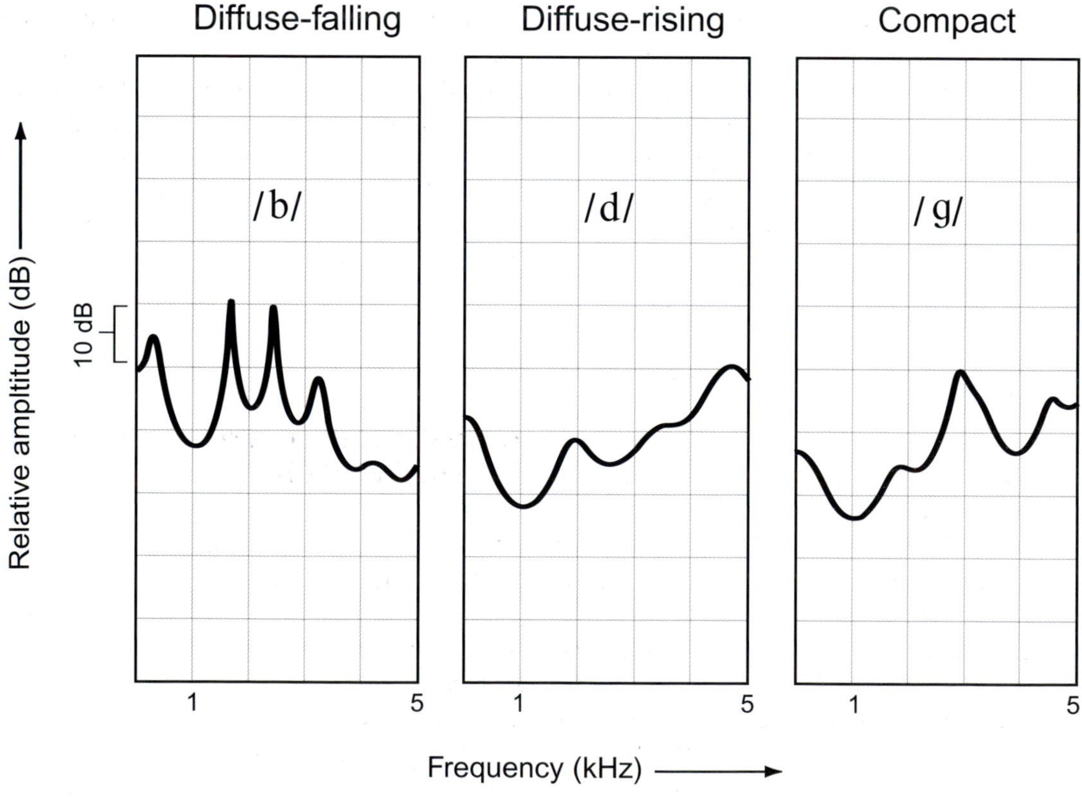

Figure 10-33. Examples of spectral templates for stop place of articulation, based on 26-ms burst spectra (LPC). The three templates—diffuse-falling, diffuse-rising, compact—were developed by Blumstein and Stevens (1979).

According to Blumstein and Stevens (1979), the diffuse-falling template fit most of the bilabial bursts, the diffuse-rising template the lingua-alveolar bursts, and the compact template the dorsal bursts. The diffuse-falling template had peaks between 0 and 5.0 kHz of roughly equivalent magnitude or with somewhat decreasing energy as frequency increased. In contrast, the diffuse-rising template showed peaks increasing in amplitude with increasing frequency. Both the diffuse-falling and diffuse-rising templates were likely to have multiple peaks of energy (energy diffusely spread across the spectrum), but with essentially opposite tilts: the falling template was tilted down and the rising template was tilted up. The compact template, however, had energy focused in a single, mid-frequency peak somewhere between 1200 and 3500 Hz. Burst spectra shown in Figure 10–33 for the voiced stops /b/, /d/, and /g/, followed by the vowel /ɛ/, are more or less consistent with these descriptions. It is not too difficult to see the /b/ burst spectrum as flat or falling at higher frequencies, the /d/ burst as rising, and the /g/ burst as having a central peak of energy around 3.0 kHz. The stops from which these bursts were extracted were produced by one of the authors in V'CV frames, and the spectral analysis was derived from a 26-ms interval starting at the burst, just as in the Blumstein and Stevens study.

Blumstein and Stevens' (1979) description of these place-specific spectral templates for stop consonant bursts is very much consistent with the more qualitative observations of Halle et al. (1957), reviewed above. Blumstein and Stevens, however, were the first scientists to quantify the *consistency* of these spectral templates in the classification of stop place of articulation. After the templates were finalized, six speakers produced 900 CV stops where C = /b,d,g,p,t,k/ and V = /i,e,ɑ,o,u/, in all combinations and with each combination repeated five times (6 stops × 5 vowels × 5 repetitions × 6 speakers = 900 stops). Every stop, therefore, was produced with a wide variety of vowels to create a large amount of burst spectrum variation due to coarticulation. Stevens and Blumstein asked the following, two questions: Even with vowel-induced variation (see example in Figure 10–32) do the templates still capture a consistent spectral characteristic related to place? And are these consistencies found for different speakers? LPC spectra were prepared for each of the 900 stops and then *visually* classified by fitting each spectrum to each template and judging it as a match, or not a match. The results of this rather complicated procedure can be stated in simple terms, even if the interpretation is not so simple. Roughly 85% of the burst spectra were both correctly matched to the "correct" place template and correctly rejected by the "incorrect" templates. The last point needs some clarification. Each burst spectrum was compared to *each* template and a decision of "match" or "no match" was made. Blumstein and Stevens were looking for "match" when a burst spectrum from a particular place fit that place's template, and "no match" when the same burst was compared to the two other place templates. This implies that one burst spectrum might fit more than one of the three templates, and indeed this occurred in a small number of cases.

Is an 85% "correct match" and "correct rejection" performance good? Blumstein and Stevens (1979) thought so, concluding that their visual spectrum-matching experiment demonstrated the existence of acoustic invariants for stop place of articulation, at least in CV syllables. Later experiments measuring different types of smoothed burst spectra also demonstrated successful classification of place of articulation (85–95% correct rates), either by visual matching or using automatic (statistical) classification procedures (Forrest et al., 1988; Kewley-Port, 1983; Kobatake & Ohtani, 1987; Nossair & Zahorian, 1991). The question, therefore, is not whether classification of stop place from burst spectra can be done with reasonable success, but *is the success good enough*? More generally, *why does the answer to this question matter*?

Acoustic Invariance and Theories of Speech Perception

The answer to the question of acoustic invariance for stop place of articulation is so important because of the profound role it has played in the development of theories of speech perception. Here, a brief summary of the issues is provided. More detail is provided in Chapter 11.

Early in the history of speech research, many speech scientists did not believe there were consistent acoustic characteristics for a given stop place of articulation. These scientists were convinced that the influence of different vowels on stop consonant acoustics was too great to allow something constant to remain in the acoustic signal that indicated reliably which place of articulation had been produced. Interestingly, this conclusion of "no acoustic invariance" (note the curious, double negative; despite the literary inelegance, this is a famous phrase in the speech science literature) was mostly derived from a series of well-known *perceptual* experiments conducted at the Haskins Laboratories (located originally in New York City, now for many years in New Haven, Connecticut). These experiments used something called a *pattern-playback machine* to convert painted replicas of spectrographic patterns into sound. This device, described in more detail in Chapter 11, allowed an experimenter to create spectrographic patterns of any type to determine how these patterns, or variants of them, affected a listener's perception of sound identity.

When the Haskins scientists painted a pattern based on a real spectrogram, they typically did not reproduce every spectrographic detail. In a sense, the painted patterns were somewhat like stick-figure or schematic representations of real spectrographic patterns. In the course of preparing these patterns, the scientists discovered something interesting. They could elicit perception of a stop-vowel syllable with a pattern having only F1-F2 transitions and following steady states. Stated otherwise, a painted representation of a burst was not necessary to create the auditory impression of a stop consonant (see Liberman, Cooper, Shankweiler, & Studdert-Kennedy, 1967, for a review of this work and relevant citations).

Examples of two burstless, painted patterns are shown in Figure 10–34. The schematic F1 and F2 in both patterns contain transitions followed by a steady state, the latter defined as the interval during which the formant frequencies remain constant. When the pattern on the left was converted to sound and played to listeners, they heard /di/. The pattern on the right was heard as /du/. If the transition portions were eliminated and only the steady states played to listeners, they clearly heard the vowels /i/ (left) and /u/ (right).

Note in Figure 10–34 how different the F2 transition is for the perception of the /d/ in /di/ versus /du/. The reader, after an examination of these two patterns, may have already asked the following question, relevant to the discussion of acoustic

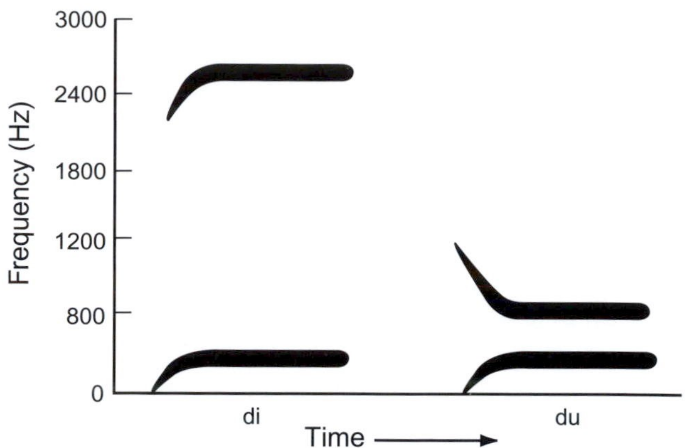

Figure 10–34. Burstless, painted patterns of formant transitions and steady states used in early Haskins Laboratories experiments to elicit perception of the consonant /d/ in two vowel environments. Adapted from Liberman et al. (1967).

invariance: Why did two such different patterns of formant transitions result in the perception of the *same* stop consonant? The Haskins scientists determined, in fact, that for any place of articulation a wide variety of F2 transition patterns was associated with the perception of the same stop. The different F2 transitions depended on which vowel was paired with a particular stop consonant. If the vowel context had such a profound influence on the acoustic characteristics related to place of articulation of a stop, the Haskins scientists argued that there was no acoustic invariance for the place feature of stop consonants. This conclusion led to the development of a theory of speech perception, discussed more fully in Chapter 11, that downplays (if not eliminates) a primary role for auditory acoustic analysis in the perception of speech.

Blumstein and Stevens (1979), as well as other investigators who have had success in classifying stop place of articulation using the burst spectrum, argued against the position taken by the Haskins scientists. The demonstrated ability to assign 85 to 95% of burst spectra to the "correct" place of articulation seemed to point to a sufficient amount of acoustic invariance for the listener to rely on for important phonetic decisions, at least in the case of stop place of articulation. Researchers interested in the issue of acoustic invariance, or the lack of it, could reasonably argue that the Haskins studies were bound to find what appeared to be unmanageable variability in the acoustic manifestation of a given stop consonant. This is because they focused almost all their attention on the transition patterns, not the spectrum of the burst interval, a classic case of looking for the right thing in the wrong place. In defense of the Haskins scientists, though, they did recognize the importance of the burst spectrum for *some* vowel contexts (Liberman et al., 1967), but never investigated the actual stability of those burst spectra in spoken utterances. The Haskins conclusions concerning the lack of acoustic invariance for stop acoustics were, in fact, based almost exclusively on perceptual, not production experiments.

Acoustic Invariance at the Interface of Speech Production and Perception

The issue of acoustic invariance has focused on stop consonants, but a more general question is the stability of the acoustic characteristics for *any* speech sound. A given sound may have very different acoustic characteristics, in both the temporal and spectral domains, depending on who produces the speech sample and the conditions under which it is produced. A speech sound has acoustic variability depending on the age, dialect, sex, size, and possibly race of the speaker. In addition, phonetic context, speaking rate, and speaking style can also have major effects on a speech sound's acoustic characteristics. If the acoustic characteristics of a speech sound are so variable, exactly what is meant by the term "acoustic invariance"?

The Haskins scientists apparently defined acoustic invariance in a very strict way. For them, almost any degree of acoustic variability for a particular aspect of a speech sound (such as the cues for place of articulation of stops) was an undesirable aspect of a communication signal. Scientists such as Blumstein and Stevens (1979), and several others who followed them, had a slightly looser approach to this problem. These scientists allowed that a sufficient degree of acoustic invariance was demonstrated when a relatively small percentage (5–15%) was misclassified according to their analysis criteria. This work has sometimes been criticized for two reasons, one having to do with the arbitrary nature of the analysis criteria, the second with the failure to explain the classification errors and how they are treated in the perception of speech.

The arbitrary analysis criteria can be illustrated with the following, simple questions: Does the 26-ms burst interval used by Blumstein and Stevens (1979) bear any relationship to the way the auditory system processes speech spectra? Is there good evidence for spectral shape analysis by the auditory system? Does the auditory system use a straightforward frequency analysis such as suggested by the work of Blumstein and Stevens, and others, or does it change the way frequency is represented as the signal travels the auditory pathways from the ear canal to the auditory cortex? These questions cannot be pursued in detail in this chapter, but it can be said that the answers to the questions are not simple. The point is, speech acoustic analysis strategies may not always be well-matched to known aspects of auditory, and presumably speech perception, analysis. The second issue, of classification errors and how they are handled, has not been addressed in the series of articles on classification of stop burst spectra. Five to 15% does not seem like a lot of errors, but how often do listeners experience such perceptual errors when listening to speech? The answer is, not very often at all, unless speech is being produced and perceived in a very noisy environment or is heard by a listener with a hearing loss. So, how are classification errors explained within a perspective on "normal" speech perception?

An alternative view to this problem has been formulated by Lindblom (1990). For Lindblom, the issue is not the strict acoustic invariance of a particular speech sound, but rather how much its acoustic characteristics can vary and still remain distinctive relative to neighboring sounds. Lindblom (1990; see also Moon & Lindblom, 1994) pointed to the known variability in acoustic characteristics of speech sounds as an asset, not a liability, in a theory of speech production and perception. Speakers often vary the precision with which they produce sound segments. Under more formal circumstances, they produce speech very carefully, but in casual situations they are likely to be rather imprecise. Formal speech styles, referred to in contemporary literature as "clear speech" (Ferguson & Kewley-Port, 2007), are characterized by acoustic characteristics of speech sounds that are maximally distinct from each other. However, casual speech styles decrease the distance between these acoustic characteristics, but leave them far enough apart to retain their

The speaker who produced the utterance in Figure 10–35 was not instructed to speak in a particular way. The F0 contour was produced by natural reading, and is a "real" reflection of how F0 was organized by this speaker within and across declarative phrases. The same pattern may not be seen, however, for every speaker and even for this particular speaker under different communication conditions. Phrase-level F0 contours can be highly variable, and may be affected by several linguistic and paralinguistic factors. The most obvious of these are the different F0 contours associated with declarative and interrogative utterances. An interrogative F0 contour typically has a *rising* F0 at the end of an utterance, not the falling F0 shown within and across the phrases in Figure 10–35. The utterance-final rise of F0 is a cue to the listener, along with other cues (lexical, syntactic, situational), that a question is being asked. F0 contours may also rise at the end of a declarative utterance when the speaker is intending to continue speaking. These F0 rises tend to be less dramatic than the rise for questions, but they are effective in signaling the listener that the talker is not finished (Lea, 1973). When a talker is finished and wants to signal the listener to respond, he or she is likely to produce a phrase-final F0 contour with a very steep and rapid fall.

F0 contours may also be modified by the level of stress produced on a specific syllable or syllables throughout a phrase or series of phrases. In English, multisyllabic words have lexical stress patterns (such as "frequency" /ˈfrikwənsi/ and "approach" /əˈproʊtʃ/) in which one or more syllables has greater stress than the other syllables. In words such as "frequency" and "approach," the stressed syllable typically has a greater F0 than the unstressed syllable or syllables. The magnitude of the F0 difference between stressed and unstressed syllables is highly variable across speakers (Howell, 1993; Sereno & Jongman, 1995). Syllables can also be stressed to focus attention on a specific word within an utterance. For example, in the utterance "Put these two back" (Wang, Kent, Duffy, & Thomas, 2005), speakers can add stress to any of the words (e.g., "Put THESE two back" versus "Put these TWO back") to signal their importance in conveying a message. This is called sentence stress (sometimes emphatic stress, or contrastive stress), and the syllable receiving extra emphasis typically has a higher F0 as compared to the syllable spoken without any extra stress. As in the case of lexical stress, the magnitude of the F0 difference between the emphatic and normally-stressed syllable is quite variable across speakers (McRoberts, Studdert-Kennedy, & Shankweiler, 1995; Wang et al., 2005). More is said in the section titled "Stress" about the role of F0 in both lexical and sentence stress.

A phase-level F0 contour will also be affected, albeit at a subtle (but systematic) level, by the identity of the specific segments in a phrase. For example, all other things being equal, the F0 of high vowels is 7 to 15 Hz higher than the F0 of low vowels (Lea, 1973; and see Whalen & Levitt, 1995). Also, all other things being equal, the F0 following a voiceless consonant is up to 20 Hz higher than the F0 following a voiced consonant (Ohde, 1984; Silverman, 1987). These influences of segmental identity on F0 contours may appear to be small, but they change the form of the contour enough to allow listeners to detect them (Silverman, 1987).

Finally, F0 contours are subject to a variety of paralinguistic influences. The term *paralinguistics* is used to describe nonverbal aspects of speech, usually related to prosodic variation, that convey emotion and physiological status. Paralinguistic aspects of vocal communication can be thought of as a backdrop against which a message is transmitted. This vocal backdrop conveys a meaning in parallel to the meaning conveyed by the spoken words (that is, the same words can be spoken in a happy and sad voice). Studies of variation in F0 contours with natural emotional variation are not easy because they require an experimenter to "be there" when there is an emotional change, and to identify reliably which emotional state is the correct description for a speaker. Scientists have tried to develop paralinguistic models of F0 contours by using actors to simulate different emotions and measuring the resulting variation in phrase-level F0. This work has revealed subtle changes between the F0 contours of simulated emotions such as anger, joy, and sadness (Bänziger & Scherer, 2005). "Sad" F0 contours tend to be flatter than angry or joyful F0 contours, but there is no clear evidence of sharp (categorical) distinctions between them (see review in Pell, 2001).

In summary, phrase-level F0 contours are subject to a number of influences, but the basic form of declarative and interrogative contours is clear, as are segmental influences on local F0 changes throughout an utterance. A general understanding of F0 contours and the influences on them is important because prosody plays a role in clinical issues. For example, F0 variation across words or phrases has been identified as a potentially important aspect of diagnosing developmental verbal apraxia (Shriberg et al., 2003) and characterizing neurogenic speech disorders in adults (Kent & Rosenbek, 1982). Treatment of persons with various speech disorders may have to account for paralinguistic influences on F0 contours, as in Parkinson disease where depression is known to be common.

Phrase-Level Intensity Contours

Phrase level intensity contours have not been studied as extensively as F0 contours, but clinical considerations suggest the need for more data on this aspect of prosody. In a connected speech sample, an intensity contour varies over time primarily because consonants are less intense than vowels. A reasonable estimate of typical intensity differences between consonants and vowels is 7 to 14 dB. The degree to which consonants are less intense than vowels depends on many factors, including type of consonant and vowel, position of the consonant in a word, syllable stress level, overall vocal effort level, and sex of the speaker (Fairbanks & Miron, 1957). In more recent data from conversational speech, the standard deviation of intensity across utterances (pauses, and therefore zero intensity intervals, were excluded in this analysis) was found to be about 6.5 dB (Rosen, Kent, Delaney, & Duffy, 2006). This figure seems to be generally consistent with the 7- to 14-dB range reported by Fairbanks and Miron because the standard deviation reflects intensity variation across an utterance between relatively high-intensity vowels and lower intensity consonants (± 1 standard deviation, a conventional way to estimate the "primary" variability of a measure, is 13 dB in this case). Figure 10–36 shows a relative intensity trace, scaled in decibels, for the same utterance shown in Figure 10–35. Selected relative intensities have been marked to show the typical differences between consonants (red arrows) and vowels (black arrows). For example, in the phrase "the short rays of the sun," the relative intensity of /ʃ/ is roughly 6 dB less than the following vowel, and the relative

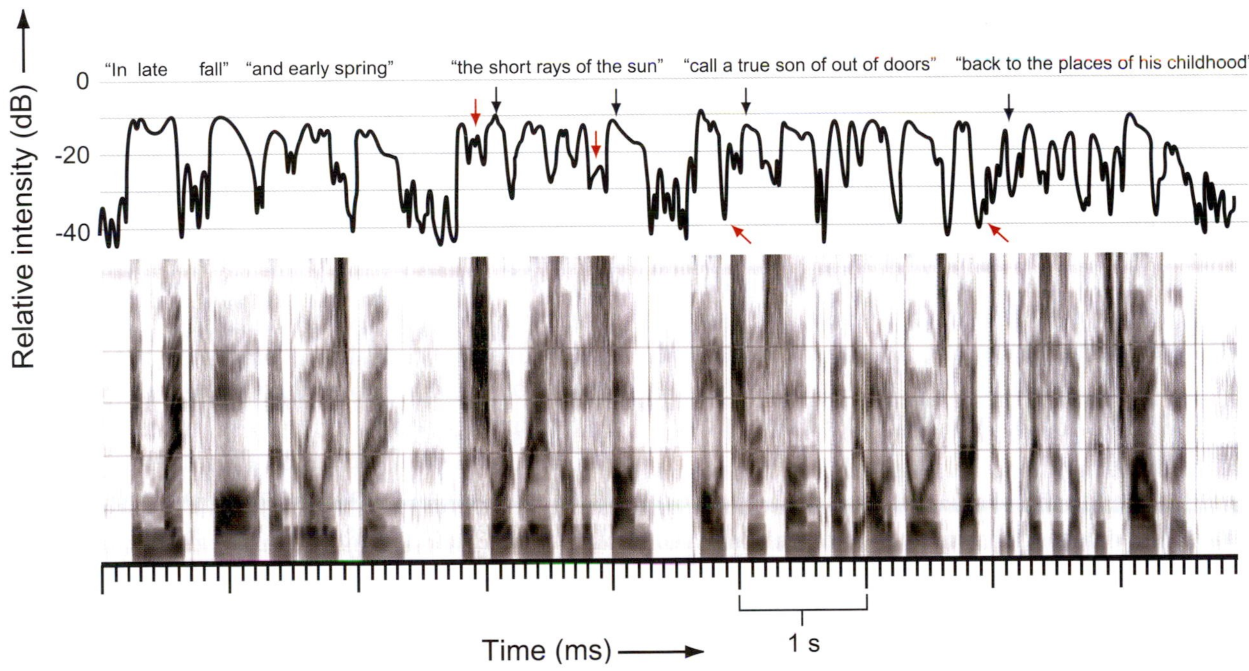

Figure 10–36. Spectrogram (*lower part of figure*) and time-synchronized intensity contour (*upper part of figure*) showing intensity variation across five phrases from a connected reading by an adult female. Selected vowel intensities are shown by downward-pointing, dark arrows; selected consonant intensities are shown by downward-pointing, red arrows. The two slanted, upward-pointing red arrows indicate intensities during stop closure intervals.

Chen, M. (1997). Acoustic correlates of English and French nasalized vowels. *Journal of the Acoustical Society of America, 102*, 2360–2370.

Chen, Y., Robb, M., Gilbert, H., & Lerman, J. (2001). Vowel production by Mandarin speakers of English. *Clinical Linguistics & Phonetics, 15*, 427–440.

Cho, T., Jun, S-A., & Ladefoged, P. (2002). Acoustic and aerodynamic correlates of Korean stops and fricatives. *Journal of Phonetics, 30*, 193–228.

Cho, T., & Ladefoged, P. (1999). Variation and universals in VOT: Evidence from 18 languages. *Journal of Phonetics, 27*, 207–229.

Clopper, C., Pisoni, D., & de Jong, K. (2005). Acoustic characteristics of the vowel systems of six regional varieties of American English. *Journal of the Acoustical Society of America, 118*, 1661–1676.

Craig, H., Thompson, C., Washington, J., & Potter, S. (2003). Phonological features of child African American English. *Journal of Speech, Language, and Hearing Research, 46*, 623–635.

Crystal, T., & House, A. (1982). Segmental durations in connected-speech signals: Preliminary results. *Journal of the Acoustical Society of America, 72*, 705–716.

Crystal, T., & House, A. (1988a). The duration of American-English vowels: An overview. *Journal of Phonetics, 16*, 263–284.

Crystal, T., & House, A. (1988b). The duration of American-English stop consonants: An overview. *Journal of Phonetics, 16*, 285–294.

Crystal, T., & House, A. (1988c). Segmental durations in connected-speech signals: Current results. *Journal of the Acoustical Society of America, 83*, 1553–1573.

Crystal, T., & House, A. (1988d). A note on the durations of fricatives in American English. *Journal of the Acoustical Society of America, 84*, 1932–1935.

Dalston, R. (1972). *A spectrographic analysis of the spectral and temporal acoustic characteristics of English semivowels spoken by three year old children and adults.* Doctoral Dissertation, Northwestern University, Evanston, IL.

Dalston, R. (1975). Acoustic characteristics of English /w,r,l/ spoken correctly by young children and adults. *Journal of the Acoustical Society of America, 57*, 462–469.

Dang, J., & Honda, K. (1995). Acoustic characteristics of the paranasal sinuses derived from transmission characteristic measurement and morphological observation. *Journal of the Acoustical Society of America, 100*, 3374–3383.

Darley, F., Aronson, A., & Brown, J. (1975). *Motor speech disorders.* Philadelphia: W. B. Saunders.

Davidsen-Nielsen, N. (1974). Syllabification in English words with medial sp, st, sk. *Journal of Phonetics, 2*, 15–45.

Espy-Wilson, C. (1992). Acoustic measures for linguistic features distinguishing the semivowels /wjrl/ in American English. *Journal of the Acoustical Society of America, 92*, 736–757.

Espy-Wilson, C. (1994). A feature-based semivowel recognition system. *Journal of the Acoustical Society of America, 96*, 65–72.

Fairbanks, G., & Miron, M. (1957). Effects of vocal effort upon the consonant-vowel ratio within the syllable. *Journal of the Acoustical Society of America, 29*, 621–626.

Feng, G., & Castelli, E. (1996). Some acoustic features of nasal and nasalized vowels: A target for vowel nasalization. *Journal of the Acoustical Society of America, 99*, 3694–3706.

Ferguson, S., & Kewley-Port, D. (2007). Talker differences in clear and conversational speech: Acoustic characteristics of vowels. *Journal of Speech, Language, and Hearing Research, 50*, 1241–1255.

Fletcher, S. (1989). Palatometric specification of stop, affricate, and sibilant sounds. *Journal of Speech and Hearing Research, 32*, 736–748.

Forrest, K., Weismer, G., Hodge, M., Dinnsen, D., & Elbert, M. (1990). Statistical analysis of word-initial /k/ and /t/ produced by normal and phonologically disordered children. *Clinical Linguistics & Phonetics, 4*, 327–340.

Forrest, K., Weismer, G., Milenkovic, P., & Dougall, R. (1988). Statistical analysis of word-initial voiceless obstruents: Preliminary data. *Journal of the Acoustical Society of America, 84*, 115–124.

Fourakis, M. (1991). Tempo, stress, and vowel reduction in American English. *Journal of the Acoustical Society of America, 90*, 1816–1827.

Fox, R., & Nissan S. (2005). Sex-related acoustic changes in voiceless English fricatives. *Journal of Speech, Language, and Hearing Research, 48*, 753–765.

Fry, D. (1955). Duration and intensity as physical correlates of linguistic stress. *Journal of the Acoustical Society of America, 27*, 765–768.

Fujimura, O. (1962). Analysis of nasal consonants. *Journal of the Acoustical Society of America, 34*, 1865–1875.

Gay, T. (1968). Effect of speaking rate on diphthong formant movements. *Journal of the Acoustical Society of America, 44*, 1570–1573.

Gottfried, T., Miller, J., & Meyer, D. (1993). Three approaches to classification of American English diphthongs. *Journal of Phonetics, 21*, 205–229.

Halle, M., Hughes, G., & Radley, J.-P. (1957). Acoustic properties of stop consonants. *Journal of the Acoustical Society of America, 29*, 107–116.

Harrington, J. (1994). The contribution of the murmur and vowel to the place of articulation distinction in nasal consonants. *Journal of the Acoustical Society of America, 96*, 19–32.

Harris, K. (1958). Cues for the discrimination of American English fricatives in spoken syllables. *Language and Speech, 1*, 1–7.

Henrich, J., Lowit, A., Schalling, E., & Mennen, I. (2006). Rhythmic disturbance in ataxic dysarthria: A comparison of different measures and speech tasks. *Journal of Medical Speech-Language Pathology, 14*, 291–296.

Hillenbrand, J., Clark, M., & Nearey, T. (2001). Effects of consonant environment on vowel formant patterns. *Journal of the Acoustical Society of America, 109*, 748–763.

Hillenbrand, J., Getty, L., Clark, M., & Wheeler, K. (1995). Acoustic characteristics of American English vowels. *Journal of the Acoustical Society of America, 97*, 3099–3111.

Hillenbrand, J., & Nearey, T. (1999). Identification of resynthesized /hVd/ utterances: Effects of formant contour. *Journal of the Acoustical Society of America, 105*, 3509–3523.

Hirose, H. (1976). Posterior cricoarytenoid as a speech muscle. *Annals of Otology, Rhinology, and Laryngology, 85*, 334–343.

Hirose, H. (1977). Laryngeal adjustments in consonant production. *Phonetica, 34*, 289–294.

Hoffman, P., Stager, S., & Daniloff, R. (1983). Perception and production of misarticulated /r/. *Journal of Speech and Hearing Disorders, 48*, 210–215.

Holbrook, A., & Fairbanks, G. (1962). Diphthong formants and their movements. *Journal of Speech and Hearing Research, 5*, 38–58.

House, A. (1961). On vowel duration in English. *Journal of the Acoustical Society of America, 33*, 1174–1178.

Howell, P. (1993). Cue trading in the production and perception of vowel stress. *Journal of the Acoustical Society of America, 94*, 2063–2073.

Hughes, G., & Halle, M. (1956). Spectral properties of fricative consonants. *Journal of the Acoustical Society of America, 28*, 303–310.

Johnson, K. (2003). *Acoustic and auditory phonetics*. Oxford, UK: Blackwell.

Jongman, A., Fourakis, M., & Sereno, J. (1989). The acoustic vowel space of Modern Greek and German. *Language and Speech, 32*, 221–248.

Jongman, A., Wayland, R., & Wong, S. (2000). Acoustic characteristics of English fricatives. *Journal of the Acoustical Society of America, 108*, 1252–1263.

Kent, R., & Rosenbek, J. (1982). Prosodic disturbance and neurologic lesion. *Brain and Language, 15*, 259–291.

Kessinger, R., & Blumstein, S. (1997). Effects of speaking rate on voice-onset time in Thai, French, and English. *Journal of Phonetics, 25*, 143–168.

Kewley-Port, D. (1983). Time-varying features as correlates of place of articulation in stop consonants. *Journal of the Acoustical Society of America, 73*, 322–335.

Kimble, C., & Seidel, S. (1991). Vocal signs of confidence. *Journal of Nonverbal Behavior, 15*, 99–105.

Kingston, J., & Diehl, R. (1994). Phonetic knowledge. *Language, 70*, 419–454.

Klatt, D. (1975). Vowel lengthening is syntactically determined in a connected discourse. *Journal of Phonetics, 3*, 129–140.

Klatt, D. (1976). Linguistic uses of segmental duration in English: Acoustic and perceptual evidence. *Journal of the Acoustical Society of America, 59*, 1208–1221.

Kobatake, H., & Ohtani, S. (1987). Spectral transition dynamics of voiceless stop consonants. *Journal of the Acoustical Society of America, 81*, 1146–1151.

Kochanski, G., Grabe, E., Coleman, J., & Rosner, B. (2005). Loudness predicts prominence: Fundamental frequency lends little. *Journal of the Acoustical Society of America, 118*, 1038–1054.

Krause, J., & Braida, L. (2004). Acoustic properties of naturally produced clear speech at normal speaking rates. *Journal of the Acoustical Society of America, 115*, 362–378.

Kurowski, K., & Blumstein, S. (1984). Perceptual integration of the murmur and formant transitions for place of articulation in nasal consonants. *Journal of the Acoustical Society of America, 76*, 383–390.

Kurowski, K., & Blumstein, S. (1987). Acoustic properties for place of articulation in nasal consonants. *Journal of the Acoustical Society of America, 81*, 1917–1927.

Labov, W. (1991). The three dialects of English. In P. Eckert (Ed.), *New ways of analyzing sound change* (pp. 1–44). New York: Academic Press.

Ladefoged, P. (2005). *Vowels and consonants* (2nd ed.). Oxford, UK: Blackwell.

Ladefoged, P., & Maddieson, I. (1996). *The sounds of the world's languages*. Oxford, UK: Blackwell.

Lea, W. (1973). Segmental and suprasegmental influences on fundamental frequency contours. In L. Hyman (Ed.), *Consonant types and tone* (pp. 15–70). Los Angeles: University of Southern California.

Lehiste, I. (1964). Acoustical characteristics of selected English consonants. *International Journal of American Linguistics, 30*, 1–197.

Lehiste, I. (1970). *Suprasegmentals*. Cambridge, MA: MIT Press.

Lehiste, I. (1973). Rhythmic units and syntactic units in production and perception. *Journal of the Acoustical Society of America*, 54, 1228–1234.

Lehiste, I. (1975). The phonetic structure of paragraphs. In A. Cohen & S. Nooteboom (Eds.), *Structure and process in speech perception* (pp. 195–206). New York: Springer-Verlag.

Lehiste, I. (1977). Isochrony reconsidered. *Journal of Phonetics, 5*, 153–163.

Lehiste, I., & Peterson, G. (1961). Transitions, glides, and diphthongs. *Journal of the Acoustical Society of America, 33*, 268–277.

Lenden, J., & Flipsen, P., Jr. (2007). Prosody and voice characteristics of children with cochlear implants. *Journal of Communication Disorders, 40*, 66–81.

Liberman, A., Cooper, F., Shankweiler, D., & Studdert-Kennedy, M. (1967). Perception of the speech code. *Psychological Review, 74*, 431–761.

Liberman, A., Delattre, P., Cooper, F., & Gerstman, L. (1954). The role of consonant-vowel transitions in the perception of stop and nasal consonants. *Psychological Monographs, 68*, 1–13.

Lindblom, B. (1963). Spectrographic study of vowel reduction. *Journal of the Acoustical Society of America, 35*, 1773–1781.

Lindblom, B. (1990). Explaining phonetic variation: A sketch of the H&H theory. In W. Hardcastle & A. Marchal (Eds.), *Speech production and speech modeling* (pp. 403–440). Dordrecht, Netherlands: Kluwer Academic Publishers.

Lisker, L. (1957). Closure duration and the intervocalic voiced-voiceless distinction in English. *Language, 33*, 42–49.

Lisker, L. (1986). "Voicing" in English: A catalogue of acoustic features signaling /b/ versus /p/ in trochees. *Language and Speech, 29*, 3–11.

Lisker, L., & Abramson, A. (1964). A cross-language study of voicing in initial stops. *Word, 20*, 384–442.

Liu, H-M., Tsao, F.-M., & Kuhl, P. (2005). The intelligibility of reduced vowel working space on speech intelligibility in Mandarin-speaking young adults with cerebral palsy. *Journal of the Acoustical Society of America, 117*, 3879–3889.

Löfqvist, A. (1980). Interarticulator programming in stop production. *Journal of Phonetics, 8*, 475–490.

Löfqvist, A., Baer, T., McGarr, N., & Story, R. (1989). The cricothyroid muscle in voicing control. *Journal of the Acoustical Society of America, 85*, 1314–1321.

Löfqvist, A., Baer, T., & Yoshioka, Y. (1981). Scaling of glottal opening. *Phonetica, 38*, 236–251.

Low, L., Grabe, E., & Nolan, F. (2000). Quantitative characterizations of speech rhythm: Syllable-timing in Singapore English. *Language and Speech, 43*, 377–401.

Luce, P., & Charles-Luce, J. (1985). Contextual effects on vowel duration, closure duration, and the consonant/vowel ratio in speech production. *Journal of the Acoustical Society of America, 78*, 1949–1957.

Maddieson, I. (1997). Phonetic universals. In W. Hardcastle & J. Laver (Eds.), *The handbook of phonetic sciences* (pp. 619–639). Oxford, UK: Blackwell.

Marquardt, T., Reinhart, J., & Peterson, H. (1979). Markedness analysis of phonemic substitution errors in apraxia of speech. *Journal of Communication Disorders, 12*, 481–494.

McRoberts, G., Studdert-Kennedy, M., & Shankweiler, D. (1995). The role of fundamental frequency in signaling linguistic stress and affect: Evidence for a dissociation. *Perception & Psychophysics, 52*, 159–174.

Metz, D., Samar, V., Schiavetti, N., Sitler, R., & Whitehead, R. (1985). Acoustic dimensions of hearing-impaired speakers' intelligibility. *Journal of Speech and Hearing Research, 28*, 345–355.

Mielke, J. (2003). The interplay of speech perception and phonology: Experimental evidence from Turkish. *Phonetica, 60*, 208–229.

Milenkovic, P. (2001). *TF32*. Computer program. http://userpages.chorus.net/cspeech/

Moon, S-J., & Lindblom, B. (1994). Interaction between duration, context, and speaking style in English stressed vowels. *Journal of the Acoustical Society of America, 96*, 40–55.

Most, T., Amir, O., & Tobin, Y. (2000) The Hebrew vowels: Raw and normalized acoustic data. *Language and Speech, 43*, 295–308.

Narayanan, S. (1995). *Fricative consonants: An articulatory, acoustic, and systems study*. Doctoral Dissertation, University of California, Los Angeles.

Narayanan, S., Alwan, A., & Haker, K. (1997). Toward articulatory-acoustic models for liquid approximants based on MRI and EPG data. Part I. The laterals. *Journal of the Acoustical Society of America, 101*, 1064–1077.

Newman, R., Clouse, S., & Burnham, J. (2001). The perceptual consequences of within-talker variability in fricative production. *Journal of the Acoustical Society of America, 109*, 1181–1196.

Norman, L. (1973). Rule addition and intrinsic order. *Minnesota Working Papers in Linguistics and Philosophy of Language, 1*, 135–159.

Nossair, Z., & Zahorian, S. (1991). Dynamic spectral shape features as acoustic correlates for initial stop consonants. *Journal of the Acoustical Society of America, 89*, 2978–2991.

Ohala, J. (1980). *The acoustic origin of the smile*. Paper presented at the 100th meeting of the Acoustical Society of America, Los Angeles.

Ohde, R. (1984). Fundamental frequency as an acoustic correlate of stop consonant voicing. *Journal of the Acoustical Society of America, 75*, 224–230.

Pell, M. (2001). Influence of emotion and focus location on prosody in matched statements and questions. *Journal of the Acoustical Society of America, 109*, 1668–1680.

Penner, H., Miller, N., Hertrich, I., Ackermann, H., & Schumm, F. (2001). Dysprosody in Parkinson's disease: An investigation of intonation patterns. *Clinical Linguistics & Phonetics, 15*, 551–566.

Peterson, G., & Barney, H. (1952). Control methods used in a study of the vowels. *Journal of the Acoustical Society of America, 24,* 175–184.

Picheny, M., Durlach, N., & Braida, L. (1986). Speaking clearly for the hard of hearing II: Acoustic characteristics of clear and conversational speech. *Journal of Speech and Hearing Research, 29,* 434–446.

Platt, L., Andrews, G., & Howie, P. (1980). Dysarthria of adult cerebral palsy. II. Phonemic analysis of articulation errors. *Journal of Speech and Hearing Research, 23,* 41–55.

Port, R. (2003). Meter and speech. *Journal of Phonetics, 31,* 599–611.

Pruthi, T., & Espy-Wilson, C. (2004). Acoustic parameters for automatic extraction of nasal manner. *Speech Communication, 43,* 225–239.

Qi, Y., & Fox, R. (1992). Analysis of nasal consonants using perceptual linear prediction. *Journal of the Acoustical Society of America, 91,* 1718–1726.

Repp, B. (1986). Perception of the [m]-[n] distinction in CV syllables. *Journal of the Acoustical Society of America, 79,* 1987–1999.

Rosen, K., Kent, R., Delaney, A., & Duffy, J. (2006). Parametric quantitative acoustic analysis of conversation produced by speakers with dysarthria and healthy speakers. *Journal of Speech, Language, and Hearing Research, 49,* 395–411.

Seitz, P., McCormick, M., Watson, I., & Bladon, A. (1990). Relational spectral features for place of articulation in nasal consonants. *Journal of the Acoustical Society of America, 87,* 351–358.

Sereno, J., & Jongman, A. (1995). Acoustic correlates of grammatical class. *Language and Speech, 38,* 57–76.

Shriberg, L., Campbell, T., Karlsson, H., Brown, R., McSweeny, J., & Nadler, C. (2003). A diagnostic marker for childhood apraxia of speech: The lexical stress ratio. *Clinical Linguistics & Phonetics, 17,* 549–574.

Silverman, K. (1987). *The structure and processing of fundamental frequency contours.* Doctoral Dissertation. Cambridge: Cambridge University.

Smiljanic, R., & Bradlow, A. (2005). Does clear speech enhance the voice onset time contrast in Croatian and English? *Journal of the Acoustical Society of America, 118,* 1900.

Stathopoulos, E., & Weismer, G. (1983). Closure duration of stop consonants. *Journal of Phonetics, 11,* 395–400.

Stevens, K. (1993). Modelling affricate consonants. *Speech Communication, 13,* 33–43.

Stevens, K. (1998). *Acoustic phonetics.* Cambridge, MA: MIT Press.

Stevens, K. (2002). Toward a model for lexical access based on acoustic landmarks and distinctive features. *Journal of the Acoustical Society of America, 111,* 1872–1891.

Stevens, K., Fant, G., & Hawkins, S. (1987). Some acoustical and perceptual correlates of nasal vowels. In R. Channon & L. Shockey (Eds.), *In honor of Ilse Lehiste* (pp. 241–254). Dordrecht, Netherlands: Foris.

Stevens, K., & House, A. (1963). Perturbation of vowel articulations by consonantal context: An acoustical study. *Journal of Speech and Hearing Research, 6,* 111–128.

Summerfield, Q. (1975). How a full account of segmental perception depends on prosody and vice versa. In A. Cohen & S. Nooteboom (Eds.), *Structure and process in speech perception* (pp. 51–66). New York: Springer-Verlag.

Tabain, M. (1998). Non-sibilant fricatives in English: Spectral information above 10 kHz. *Phonetica, 55,* 107–130.

Tabain, M. (2001). Variability in fricative production and spectra: Implications for the hyper- and hypo- and quantal theories of speech production. *Language and Speech, 44,* 57–94.

Tjaden, K., & Turner, G. (1997). Spectral properties of fricatives in amyotrophic lateral sclerosis. *Journal of Speech, Language, and Hearing Research, 40,* 1358–1372.

Tjaden, K., & Wilding, G. (2004). Rate and loudness manipulations in dysarthria: Acoustic and perceptual findings. *Journal of Speech, Language, and Hearing Research, 47,* 766–783.

Tsao, Y.-C., & Weismer, G. (1997). Interspeaker variation of habitual speaking rate: Evidence for a neuromuscular component. *Journal of Speech, Language and Hearing Research, 40,* 858–866.

Turner, G., Tjaden, K., & Weismer, G. (1995). The influence of speaking rate on vowel space and speech intelligibility for individuals with amyotrophic lateral sclerosis. *Journal of Speech, Language, and Hearing Research, 38,* 1001–1013.

Umeda, N. (1975). Vowel duration in American English. *Journal of the Acoustical Society of America, 58,* 434–445.

Umeda, N. (1977). Consonant duration in American English. *Journal of the Acoustical Society of America, 61,* 846–858.

Van Santen J. (1992). Contextual effects on vowel duration. *Speech Communication, 11,* 513–546.

Wang, Y., Kent, R., Duffy, J., & Thomas, J. (2005). Dysarthria associated with traumatic brain injury: Speaking rate and emphatic stress. *Journal of Communication Disorders, 38,* 231–260.

Watson, C., & Harrington, J. (1999). Acoustic evidence for dynamic formant trajectories in Australian English vowels. *Journal of the Acoustical Society of America, 106,* 458–468.

Weismer, G. (1980). Control of the voicing distinction for intervocalic stops and fricatives: Some data and theoretical considerations. *Journal of Phonetics, 8,* 427–438.

Weismer, G. (1984). Acoustic analysis strategies for the refinement of phonological analyses. In M. Elbert, D.

for their next experimental move. Whalen and Liberman had obtained duplex perception for /dɑ/ and /gɑ/ syllables in which the "base" and "chirp" (isolated third formant transition, as in Figure 11–6) were played into the *same* ear, but the "chirp" was raised in intensity relative to the "base." When the "chirp" intensity was relatively low in comparison with the "base," listeners heard a good /dɑ/ or /gɑ/ depending on which F3 transition was used, but as the F3 "chirp" was increased in intensity a threshold was reached at which listeners heard both a good /dɑ/ or /gɑ/ *plus* a "chirp." In other words, they perceived the signal as duplex, just as in the earlier experiments described above in which the "base" and "chirp" were in opposite ears. Fowler and Rosenblum repeated this experiment except with the 0- to 3.0-kHz signal as the "base" and the 3.0- to 11.0-kHz signal as the "chirp." Relatively low "chirp" intensities produced a percept of a slamming metal door, a percept consistent with listening to the original, intact signal (top spectrum in Figure 11–8). As the "chirp" intensity was raised, a threshold was reached at which listeners heard the slamming metal door *plus* the shaking can of rice/tambourine/jangling keys. Fowler and Rosenblum (1991) had evoked a duplex percept exactly parallel to the one described above for /dɑ/ and /gɑ/, except in this case for nonspeech sounds.

If the original duplex perception findings (Liberman & Mattingly, 1985; Mann & Liberman, 1983; Whalen & Liberman, 1987) seemed like compelling evidence for a special speech perception module in humans, the demonstration of duplex perception for a slamming metal door is devastating evidence *against* the idea of the speech module. As Fowler and Rosenblum (1991) pointed out, if the phonetic member of duplex perception was taken as the output of a special speech module, the slamming metal door percept in response to presentation of the two lower signals in Figure 11–8 had to be taken as evidence of a special human module for the perception of such doors being slammed shut. It is not ridiculous to imagine a human biological endowment for perceiving speech signals as an evolutionary adaptation, but it is impossible to imagine an adaptive advantage for modular (automatic) processing of the sound of a slamming metal door. Perhaps there is a special biological endowment for perceiving speech, but duplex perception is not the critical test for its existence.

Acoustic Invariance

The lack of acoustic invariance for speech sounds was an important catalyst for the development of the motor theory of speech perception. As discussed in Chapter 10, Blumstein and Stevens (1979) performed an acoustic analysis of stop burst acoustics that led them to reject this central claim of the motor theorists. Blumstein and Stevens used the stop burst spectrum to classify correctly 85% of word-initial stop consonants in a variety of vowel contexts. They regarded this finding as a falsification of the motor theorists' claim that there was too much context-conditioned acoustic variability to allow listeners to establish a consistent and reliable link between speech acoustic characteristics and phonetic categories. For the motor theorist, consistency associated with speech sound categories was found in the underlying articulatory gestures for specific sounds, even when the context of a sound was changed. For the motor theorist, the "underlying articulatory gesture" meant the neural code for generating the gesture. This code was assumed to be the same for a particular gesture, regardless of its phonetic context. Whatever changes occurred to the *actual* articulatory gesture—the collective movements of the lips, tongue, mandible, and so forth—for a given sound in different phonetic contexts were not relevant to the motor theory. In the motor theory, perception of speech depended on these more abstract neural commands, higher up in the process, so to speak, that were not coded for phonetic context. These invariant commands were assumed to be part of the special speech module.

The falsification of the lack of acoustic invariance for sound categories is a bit more involved than a simple demonstration of consistency between a selected acoustic measure (such as the shape of a burst spectrum) and a particular sound. Liberman and Mattingly (1985), in a very fine review of why they believed the acoustic signal was not consistent enough to establish and maintain speech sound categories in perception (where "categories" = "phonemes"), identified a whole set of complications with so-called "auditory theories" of speech perception. Auditory theories claim that information in the speech acoustic signal is sufficient, and sufficiently consistent, to support speech perception. These theories regard the auditory mechanisms for speech perception to be the same as mechanisms for the perception of environmental sounds, music, or any acoustic signal. One specific auditory perspective on speech perception (Diehl, Lotto, & Holt, 2004; Kingston & Diehl, 1994) claims that speakers control their speech acoustic output to produce speech signals well-matched to auditory processing capabilities.

Why were Liberman and Mattingly (1985) so adamant in rejecting auditory theories of speech perception? First, Liberman and Mattingly pointed to what they termed "extra-phonetic" factors that cause variation in the acoustic characteristics of speech sounds. These factors include (among others) speaking rate and speaker sex and age. The speaker sex/age issue is particularly interesting because the same vowel has widely varying formant frequencies depending on the size of a speaker's vocal tract. An auditory theory of speech perception either requires listeners to learn all these different formant patterns, or employs some sort of cognitive process to place all formant patterns on a single, "master" scale. This issue, of how one hears the same vowel (or consonant) when so many different-sized vocal tracts produce it with different formant frequencies, is called the "speaker normalization" issue (interesting papers on speaker normalization are found in Johnson and Mullenix [1997]). The motor theory, however, finesses this problem by arguing that the perception of different formant patterns is mediated by a special mechanism that perceives intended articulatory gestures. For example, the motor theory assumes that the intended gestures (the neural code for the gestures) for the vowel in the word "bad" are roughly equivalent for men, women, and children, even if the outputs of their different-sized vocal tracts are not. The special speech perception module registers the same intended gesture for all three speakers, and hence the same vowel perception. The motor theory makes the speaker normalization problem go away.

A second reason to reject auditory theories, according to Liberman and Mattingly (1985), is the interesting case of trading relations in the acoustic cues for a given sound category. For any given sound, there are at least several different acoustic cues whose values (such as the value of a formant frequency, or of a stop closure duration) can contribute to the proper identification of the sound. As Liberman and Mattingly pointed out, none of these individual values are necessarily critical to the proper identification of a sound segment, but the *collection* of the several values may be. More interesting for the present discussion, among these several cues, the acoustic value of one can be "offset" by the acoustic value of another to yield the same phonetic percept. For example, Figure 11–9 shows spectrograms of a single speaker's production of the words

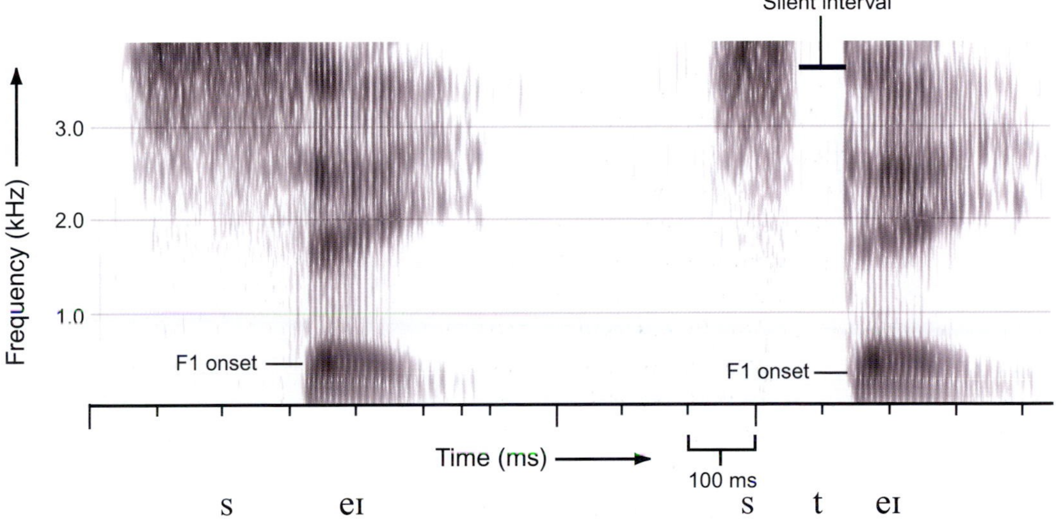

Figure 11–9. Spectrograms of the utterances "say" and "stay" showing two acoustic differences that distinguish the syllables with and without the /t/. One difference is the presence of the silent (closure interval) for /t/ (*right*), the other is the slightly lower F1 starting frequency in "stay," as compared to "say." See text for details.

"say" and "stay." These two words can be described as a minimal-pair opposition defined by the presence or absence of the stop consonant /t/. In "stay" (but not "say") there is the obvious silent closure interval of approximately 60 to 90 ms, but the "say"-"stay" opposition also involves a subtle difference in the starting frequency of the F1 transition for /eɪ/. Figure 11–9 shows the F1 starting frequency in "stay" to be somewhat lower than the starting frequency in "say" (compare frequencies labeled "F1 onset"). The lower starting frequency in "stay" is consistent with theoretical and laboratory findings of F1 transitions pointing toward the spectrographic baseline—that is, 0 Hz—at the boundary of a stop consonant and vowel (Fant, 1960).

In an often cited experiment, Best, Morrongiello, and Robson (1981), took advantage of these two cues to the difference between "say" and "stay"—the closure interval, and the lower F1 starting frequency following the stop closure—to demonstrate the "trading relations" phenomenon. Figure 11–10 shows the kinds of stimuli used by Best et al. to make their point. The gray, stippled interval represents the voiceless fricative /s/, the narrow rectangles the closure intervals for /t/, and the two solid lines the F1-F2 trajectories for /eɪ/. Best et al. synthesized these sequences in two ways, one with an F1 starting frequency of 230 Hz (Figure 11–10, left side), the other with an F1 starting frequency of 430 Hz (Figure 11–10, right side). Best et al. changed the duration of the stop closure interval between 0 (no closure interval) and 136 ms, sometimes with the lower F1 starting frequency, and sometimes with the higher frequency, and discovered something interesting. When the pattern was synthesized with one of the longer closure intervals, close to 136 ms, listeners clearly heard the sequence as "stay." When the pattern was synthesized with a very short or nonexistent closure interval, "say" was heard. None of this is surprising and is consistent with the real spectrographic patterns shown in Figure 11–9.

The interesting findings occurred when the length of the closure interval between the /s/ and /eɪ/ was rather short (~30–50 ms) and, therefore, produced roughly equal "say" and "stay" responses (that is, the presence or absence of a /t/ was

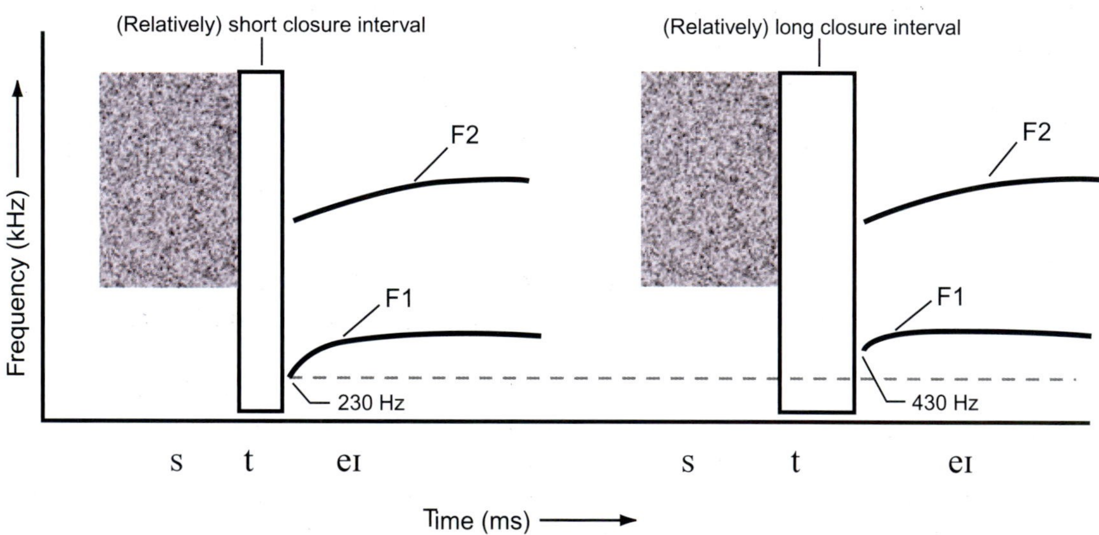

Figure 11–10. Two schematic spectrograms, showing how two different cues can "trade off" against each other to maintain a single phonetic percept. The phonetic percept is the presence of the stop consonant /t/ between an /s/ and /eɪ/. The two cues manipulated in these schematic spectrograms are (a) the duration of the closure interval (the width of the narrow rectangles), and (b) the starting frequency of the F1 transition. Longer closure intervals and lower F1 starting frequencies tend to produce more /t/ responses. The tendency for more /t/ responses with longer closure intervals can be offset by a higher starting frequency for F1. In the left spectrogram, a shorter closure requires a lower F1 starting frequency for the /t/ percept. In the right spectrogram, which shows a longer closure interval, the F1 starting frequency can be higher.

Speech Synthesis and Speech Perception

The pattern-playback machine allowed speech scientists to synthesize speech signals, but the quality of these signals was—let's be gracious—not particularly good. Developments in computer technology, knowledge of acoustic phonetics, and programming skills have greatly improved speech synthesis. Current synthetic speech signals are so good they sometimes cannot be distinguished from natural speech. These developments have allowed speech perception researchers to make very fine adjustments in signals to learn about speech perception while avoiding the problem of the fuzzy speech signals produced by the pattern-playback machine. In 1987, Dennis Klatt from the Massachusetts Institute of Technology published a wonderful history of speech synthesis, and provided audio examples of synthetic speech signals from 1939 to 1987 (Klatt, 1987). You can hear these examples at http://www.cs.indiana.edu/rhythmsp/ASA/Contents.html

ambiguous). Best et al. determined that when the F1 starting frequency was the higher one (430 Hz in Figure 11–10), a longer closure interval was required for listeners to hear "stay." When the F1 starting frequency was the lower one (230 Hz in Figure 11–10), a shorter closure interval allowed the listeners to hear "stay." In other words, the two cues to the presence of a /t/ between the /s/ and /eɪ/—closure interval duration and the F1 starting frequency—seemed to "trade off" against each other to produce the same percept—a /t/ between the fricative and the following vowel. Both patterns shown in Figure 11–10 produced the same percept of a "good" /t/. There was a "trading relation" between the two cues to the presence or absence of /t/ between the /s/ and /eɪ/.

For Liberman and Mattingly (1985), the trading relations phenomenon proved the point about the inability to connect a particular acoustic characteristic with a particular sound category. The potential multiple acoustic cues to a given phonetic category were simply too numerous to be used by a listener to develop and maintain the category identification. In the particular case of "say"-"stay," the lower versus higher F1 starting frequency, or the precise value of the closure interval, was not by itself sufficient to serve as an acoustic constant of a phonetic category. The *collection* of these several cues, however, was a reflection of the underlying gesture for the sound category. Small variations in one cue could be compensated for by a different cue, but in the end the sum of these various cues yielded a single percept which was the phonetic category (e.g., a /t/ associated with a constant and consistent articulatory gesture). In support of Liberman and Mattingly's theoretical cause, trading relations have been demonstrated for many different phonetic distinctions. It is not just a "say"-"stay" phenomenon (see Repp [1982] and Repp and Liberman [1987] for excellent reviews of trading relations in phonetic perception).

The Competition: General Auditory Explanations of Speech Perception

An obvious approach to understanding speech perception is to regard the speech acoustic signal as a sufficiently rich source of information for a listener's needs. In this view, the speech acoustic signal contains reliable, learnable information for a listener to identify the sounds, words, and phrases intended by a speaker. A *general auditory explanation* of speech perception seems simple, and perhaps the logical starting point—like a default perspective—for scientists who study speech perception. On the contrary, general auditory explanations have fought an uphill scientific battle since the motor theory was formulated in the 1950s.

The information presented above described the reasons for the development of the original and revised motor theories of speech perception. Those reasons led to one overarching assumption concerning speech perception. A special perceptual processor is required because general auditory mechanisms were not up to the task of perceiving speech (Remez, Rubin, Berns, Pardo, and Lang [1994] offer yet another perspective on the essential difference between perceiving speech and nonspeech sounds). In contrast, a central theme of general auditory explanations of speech perception is that special perceptual mechanisms are not required. Indeed, the speech acoustic signal is assumed to be processed in precisely the same way as other acoustic signals.

As in the published work on the motor theory, a set of reasons in support of a general auditory account of speech perception has been carefully articulated in the scientific literature. These are summarized below.

Sufficient Acoustic Invariance

As noted earlier, Blumstein and Stevens (1979) demonstrated a fair degree of acoustic consistency for stop consonant place of articulation, and many of the successful, automatic classification experiments described in Chapter 10 imply something consistent in the acoustic signal for vowels, diphthongs, nasals, fricatives, and semivowels. Recall from Chapter 10 that Lindblom (1990) argued for a more flexible view of speech acoustic variability. In this view, listeners do not need absolute acoustic invariance for a speech sound, but rather only enough to maintain discriminability from neighboring sound classes.

General auditory accounts of speech perception rely on this more flexible view of acoustic distinctiveness for the perception of speech sounds. Presumably, an initial front-end acoustic analysis of the speech signal by general auditory mechanisms is supplemented by higher level processing which can resolve any ambiguities in sound identity. The front-end analysis is like a hypothesis concerning the sequence of incoming sounds, and the higher-level processes include knowledge of the context in which each sound is produced, plus syntactic, semantic, and pragmatic constraints on the message. Clearly, listeners bring more to the speech perception process than just a capability for acoustic analysis. These additional sources of knowledge considerably loosen the demand for strict acoustic invariance for each sound segment.

Scientists often refer to the front-end part of this process as "bottom-up" processing, and the higher level knowledge part of this process as "top-down" processing. Stevens (2005) has proposed a speech perception model in which bottom-up, auditory mechanisms analyze the incoming speech signal for segment identity and top-down processes resolve ambiguities emerging from this front-end analysis. When an account of speech perception is framed within the general cognitive abilities of humans and includes these top-down processes, a role for general auditory analysis in the perception of speech becomes much more plausible (Lotto & Holt, 2006). Clearly, the lack of strict acoustic invariance for a particular speech sound cannot be used as an argument against a role for general auditory mechanisms in speech perception.

Replication of Speech Perception Effects Using Nonspeech Signals

Many categorical perception effects have been demonstrated using synthetic speech stimuli. Several of these experiments were reviewed above. There have also been many demonstrations of similar effects using nonspeech signals. Categorical perception of speech signals has been a centerpiece of the original and revised motor theory. The demonstration of the same effects with nonspeech signals, however, seems to damage the proposed link between speech production and speech perception implied by findings of categorical perception for speech signals.

The approach employed by scientists interested in a general auditory theory of speech perception is to take a categorical perception experiment using speech signals and "mirror" it using nonspeech signals. If the nonspeech "mirror" experiment turns out the same way as the speech experiment, the categorical perception effect is attributed to auditory, not speech-special perceptual mechanisms. A famous example of such an experiment was published by Pisoni (1977) who showed that categorical perception functions for the voiced-voiceless contrast were probably due to auditory, not speech-special mechanisms.

Pisoni (1977) reviewed speech perception experiments in which labeling and discrimination data (as reviewed above) suggested categorical perception of voiced and voiceless stops. A typical set of data for this experiment is shown in Figure 11–11, where VOT is plotted on the x-axis and labeling (red points, left axis) and discrimination (blue points, right axis) are plotted as two y-axes. In this experiment, the stimulus is synthesized to sound like a stop-vowel syllable, and all features are held constant except for the VOT. Assume the transitions are synthesized to evoke a bilabial stop, and that VOT is varied from lead values (negative VOT values) to long-lag values in 5-ms steps. For each VOT value, listeners are asked to label the stimulus as either /b/ or /p/. In the discrimination experiments, two stimuli from the VOT continuum are presented, always separated by 20 ms along the continuum (e.g., one stimulus with a VOT of 0 ms, the other with a VOT of 20 ms), and listeners are asked if they are the same or different. The results in Figure 11–11 show only /b/ labels for stimuli with VOT's from −10 ms to +15 ms, half /b/ and half /p/ for the stimulus with VOT of 20 ms, and all /p/ labels for stimuli with VOT = 30 ms or more. The change from /b/ to /p/ labels occurs quickly in the 20- to 30-ms range of VOTs, as required for an interpretation of categorical perception. The discrimination data (blue points) show perfect discrimination when the two VOT stimuli cross the labeling "boundary," but much poorer discrimination when the two stimuli are within a category, In short, these VOT data meet the requirements for categorical perception as reviewed above for stop place of articulation. The interpretation of categorical perception of VOT was consistent with the motor theory of speech perception. Speakers cannot produce continuous changes in VOT, so they cannot perceive them.

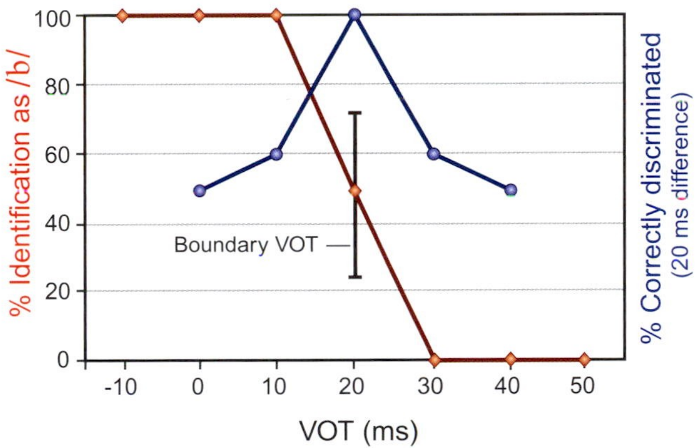

Figure 11-11. Labeling (identification) and discrimination functions for a VOT continuum, showing expected pattern for an interpretation of categorical perception of the voicing distinction for stops. The x-axis is VOT. Two y-axes are shown, one for identification (*left y-axis, red points*), one for discrimination (*right y-axis, blue points*). The categorical boundary, where the labeling function shifts rapidly between /b/ and /p/, is shown as 20 ms. Discrimination across this 20 ms-boundary is 100%. Within the categories it is close to 50%. See Figure 11–12 and discussion in text.

Pisoni (1977) knew that the synthesis of VOT differences for the same place of stop articulation involved variable asynchronies between two acoustic events. Re-examination of Figure 11–2 shows that the two-formant patterns for the three cognate pairs /bɑ-pɑ/, /dɑ-tɑ/, and /gɑ-kɑ/ differ only in the onset time of the first formant relative to the second formant. Listeners were made to hear the voiceless member of each pair by delaying the onset of the first formant by approximately 50 ms relative to the onset of the second formant. A synthetic VOT continuum, such as the one just described, was generated in early studies by varying the starting time of the first format relative to the starting time of the second formant. Pisoni "mirrored" this situation with stimuli like those shown in Figure 11–12. Each stimulus consisted of a pair of sinusoids, one at a lower frequency (500 Hz), the other at a higher frequency (1500 Hz). Stimulus 1 shows the two tones with simultaneous onsets, which in a synthetic speech signal corresponds to simultaneous onset of the first two formant frequencies or a VOT = 0 ms. Stimuli 2 through 6 have increasing asynchronies between the two tones, with the onset of the lower-frequency tone lagging that of the higher-frequency tone by increasing amounts. The stimulus progression from 2 through 6 represents increasing, positive VOTs.[3]

[3]Readers will note that the manipulation of VOT in the synthetic speech signals of Figure 11–2, and the "mirror signals" illustrated in Figure 11–12, depend on modification of an acoustic variable that is somewhat different from the typical definition of VOT. VOT for natural speech signals is defined as the time difference between a stop burst and the onset of vocal fold vibration for the following vowel. The synthetic signals used to construct VOT continua, however, typically did not have a burst. Rather, the percept of the voiced-voiceless contrast could be elicited with the "F1 cutback" technique described in the text and illustrated in Figure 11–2.

and "representation" (as examples), was not much more than a convenient set of descriptive terms. The terms, for Gibson, did not have ecological validity—that is, they did not represent "real" things, "real" mechanisms that were the stuff of perception.

Motor theory requires operations of a special module to "convert" an unstable acoustic signal to a stable articulatory representation. A general auditory approach to speech perception requires some processing stages to match the incoming acoustics to stored templates or features (Klatt, 1989; Stevens, 2005). In both cases, cognitive operations of varying degrees of automaticity are required for perception of incoming sounds. Fowler (1986, 1996), the leading proponent of direct realism in speech perception, rejects cognitive "constructions" in the perception of speech sounds. She argues for direct perception of articulatory gestures. In this case, the speech acoustic signal is linked directly with the articulatory gesture that produced it. Listeners learn these links and do not need to construct the percepts of sounds. They literally hear articulatory gestures (or, on another interpretation, the sounds they hear *are* the articulatory gestures). The parallel with Gibson's (1969, 1970) view of visual perception is easy to see.

How is direct realism different from the motor theory? Both theories focus on perception of articulatory gestures, but motor theory requires a special, completely automatic mechanism (a module) to transform acoustic signals into articulatory mechanisms. Direct realism proposes no special mechanisms, and, in fact, claims that the same principles apply to visual, auditory, and haptic (sense of touch) perception. In all cases, the source of the stimulation is what is perceived, without mediation by cognitive processing of the signals produced by that source.

How is direct realism different from an auditory approach to speech perception? This is a more interesting question, and one with a more complicated (and hotly debated) answer (see the exchange between Lotto and Holt [2006] and Fowler [2006]). The simplest answer is, in direct realism listeners hear the articulatory gestures, whereas in a general auditory approach listeners hear the acoustic signal. Is there really a difference between these two? One difference, noted above, is that a general auditory approach presumably requires a listener to perform some kind of operation on the incoming speech acoustic signal such as matching it to a stored acoustic prototype, or transforming it to a more phonetically useful format (such as a binary or trinary feature), before it can be perceived as a particular sound. Direct realism, however, claims direct perception of the gestures that (in the language of direct realists) "structured" the acoustic signal. Perceptions are not "constructed" in direct realism—they are direct. In the comparison between these two approaches, is there an advantage of the direct realist perspective over the general auditory approach?[4]

As reviewed in Chapter 10, the speech acoustic signal for a given sound varies depending on its phonetic context (and other factors as well). For example, the /s/ spectra in the utterances [su] and [si] are quite different, because speakers typically produce some lip rounding during the /s/ in [su], but not [si]. The acoustic effect of lip rounding during the /s/ in [su] is to emphasize much lower frequencies in the aperiodic fricative spectrum, as compared to the /s/ spectrum in [si]. Direct realists argue that a general auditory approach to speech perception is cumbersome and overly complicated because a listener must learn and store all these different variants of spectra for a given sound. In direct realism, listeners are not burdened with this learning and storage problem because they "hear" the lingual fricative gesture combined, or coproduced, with the lip rounding gesture. Moreover, in direct realism the degree to which two articulatory gestures, such as lingual and labial gestures, are "coproduced" is perceived directly. In a general auditory approach, the large number of slight variations (for example, of how much of the /s/ in [su] is lip-rounded) presumably introduce acoustic variability for a given sound that may complicate the learning of speech sound categories and the mature form of speech perception. In short, direct realists see their theory of speech perception as much simpler than general auditory approaches.

---

[4]Many direct realists, including Fowler (Fowler et al., 2003), believe that their theory has the advantage of being preferable on *philosophical* grounds, in addition to any scientific advantages that may be demonstrated. This is to say that direct realism unifies perceptual behavior across the senses, discards the (in their view) awkward theoretical constructs of much of cognitive psychology (such as the notion of mental representations, or specialized modules), and may be easier to integrate with general evolutionary theory than the "constructed perceptions" of so many psychological theories.

Growing Up in the 1950s and Speech Perception

Many of us who grew up in the 1950s went to the picture show every Saturday and sat through double features of perfectly awful science fiction movies. The music that was meant to convey the weirdness of on-screen aliens was equally awful, usually a kind of singing, multitonal whistling you might associate with attempts to tune in a distant radio station. Professor Robert Remez of Barnard University (and his colleagues) used such sounds to prove a point about speech perception. They looked at the first three formants of a natural utterance and mimicked their time-dependent frequency changes using sinusoids (you can hear these signals, plus the sentences they were based on, at http://www.haskins.yale.edu/featured/sws/swssentences/sentences.html). When listeners heard these sounds, some described them just as suggested above—as weird outer space signals. But when people were told to listen to the signals as if they were speech, many heard the sentence as originally spoken, even though the signal was composed only of three time-varying sinusoids. Remez and his associates concluded that this finding disproved the idea of a speech-specific module that was *automatically* engaged by speech signals. It was as if listeners could hear the signals as speech, *if instructed to do so*. A dedicated speech perception module would not allow that kind of choice (see Pardo & Remez, 2006, pp. 207–208).

Speech Perception and Word Recognition

The three major theories (or approaches) discussed above are all concerned with phonetic perception. They attempt to account for the way in which speech sounds are identified. Clearly, an important part of speech perception involves speech sound identification, but just as clearly the goal of speech perception is to recognize words, their combinations, and ultimately the message they convey.

Speech sound identification, however it is accomplished, is seen by many scientists as the "trigger" that initiates the process of word identification. A simple way to think about the link between sound and word identification is to imagine the lexicon as consisting of word "units" represented by strings of abstract phonological symbols (phonemes). In a very general sense, when the incoming sounds are identified and well-matched to one of these abstract, stored word units, spoken word recognition occurs.

This simple view glosses over some important details. First, it is known that spoken word recognition does not require a complete analysis of all the sounds in the word. Listeners can make decisions concerning word identity before all the sounds are known, or even before any analysis of some remaining component sounds has been undertaken. This is especially the case for longer, multisyllabic words (Dahan & Magnuson, 2006; Nooteboom & van der Vlugt, 1988). In broad terms, spoken word recognition unfolds over time, by a *continuous* process as sound analysis and top-down information becomes increasingly available (Dahan & Gareth Gaskell, 2007; Grosjean, 1980). The ability of listeners to make correct word identifications in the absence of all the relevant "data" highlights the substantial role of top-down processing in spoken word recognition. Top-down processes may include, but are not limited to, a listener's knowledge of possible word candidates with a similar phonetic structure (see below) or similar frequencies of occurrence, the meaning of previously recognized words in an extended utterance, the topic under discussion, and even the identity of the person who is speaking. Second, there is a fair amount of disagreement concerning the specific processes involved in transforming an initial sound analysis to the form of the abstract word representation. For example, when a man and acoustic signal. More specifically, signal integrity was important at the sound segment level. If the acoustic characteristics of individual speech sounds were in good shape, the speech intelligibility score would be high. Disruption of speech sound acoustics, by a low presentation level, filtering (restriction of frequencies transmitted by the communication system), or competing noise, lowered the speech intelligibility score in proportion to the extent of the disruption (Weismer, 2008).

It is easy to see how this kind of information could be extended past the evaluation of a communication system, to the case of a person with a *hearing* disorder. Speech intelligibility tests, in various forms, have been used for years in the determination of speech reception thresholds, speech discrimination scores, the fitting of hearing aids, and programming of implantable devices (Katz, 2002). Whereas the early speech intelligibility tests were designed to evaluate communication systems, the application of such tests in clinical audiology demonstrated how the tests could be used in the case of the receiver (hearer) as well.

An extension of speech intelligibility tests to evaluate the *speaker* (sender) also makes sense. When speech is impaired and the communication system and receiver are in good shape, it seems logical that a speech intelligibility score serves as an index of the speaker's communication impairment. Speech intelligibility tests developed specifically for the evaluation of speech impairment were initially aimed primarily at clients with hearing impairment and dysarthria (Monsen, 1983; Weismer & Martin, 1992). Kent, Weismer, Kent, and Rosenbek (1989) reviewed these tests and concluded that most were merely indices of severity. Moreover, as demonstrated earlier by Monsen for speech intelligibility among persons with severe to profound hearing impairment, an intelligibility score depended on many factors extrinsic to the speaker. These factors included the identity of the listener (the degree of experience with specific speech characteristics of persons with hearing impairment) and the phonological and (in the case of sentence tests) syntactic complexity of the test utterances. Additional extrinsic factors also contribute variation to the speech intelligibility score for a particular individual with a speech impairment. In short, the statement, "Mr. Jones has a speech intelligibility score of 75%" is nearly impossible to interpret unless additional information is available about the test, the listening conditions (including the specific speech materials), and the listeners. This potential ambiguity in the meaning of a percentage value derived from a speech intelligibility test seemed to limit the utility of the measure even for simple estimates of speaker severity.[5]

"Explanatory" Speech Intelligibility Tests

Kent et al. (1989) had the idea to extend the interpretation of speech intelligibility testing by isolating the particular phonetic deficits that contributed to an intelligibility deficit. This idea emerged from a common clinical observation that two clients with the same overall speech intelligibility score (e.g., 60%) may have very different reasons for their speech intelligibility deficits. For example, one client's intelligibility deficit may be primarily a result of velopharyngeal incompetency, whereas another may derive from problems with consonant place of articulation. The Kent et al. test was designed as a single-word, multiple choice instrument in which the response alternatives were related to the target by carefully manipulated phonetic contrasts. By analyzing not only the total number of incorrect words, but also the phonetic contrast errors underlying the incorrect choices, a profile of "vulnerable" contrasts—those frequently involved in word choice errors—was available. These "vulnerable" contrasts would be targeted in therapy because they presumably made a large contribution to the intelligibility deficit. In a sense, identification of "vulnerable" contrasts was like a prescription for primary attention in speech-language management. The concept of "vulnerable" contrasts also provided an explanation for the two clients who sounded so different but received the same overall speech intelligibility score. The clients differed in their "vulnerable" contrasts, and, therefore, should have different therapy priorities.

[5]Such limitations could be eliminated by national or international standards for speech intelligibility testing, but these do not exist.

Earlier in this section, the original speech intelligibility tests were described as a way to test the contribution of speech signal integrity to the goodness of a communication system. There is a direct link between this idea and the phonetic contrast approach to speech intelligibility testing, in which the *speaker* is the variable. In the original approach, speech intelligibility scores reflected the sum of the acoustic characteristics of the speech sounds in the test words. Any degradation of the acoustic characteristics of a particular sound contributed to a decrease in an overall speech intelligibility score. The greater the number of sounds affected (degraded) by the communication system, the lower the intelligibility score. Similarly, the phonetic contrast approach of Kent et al. (1989) considered speech intelligibility as a sum of "good" phonetic contrasts produced by the speaker. The smaller the number of these "good" contrasts (the greater the number of "vulnerable" contrasts), the lower the speech intelligibility score. In addition, the ability to identify specific "vulnerable" contrasts provides an explanation of the intelligibility deficit.

Different clients, in fact, may have different "vulnerable" contrasts revealed by the Kent et al. (1989) test (Weismer & Martin, 1992). Different "vulnerable" contrasts may be seen in different dysarthria types and may depend on the sex of the speaker (Kent et al., 1992). Although the concept of the Kent et al. (1989) test seems sound, there are problems in the interpretation of "vulnerable" contrasts. Specifically, the idea that the "good" phonetic contrasts sum up to produce the intelligibility score (much as the good acoustic characteristics sum up to show the integrity of a communication system) is overly simple. This is because the different phonetic contrasts, such as the high-low and front-back contrasts for vowels, the voiced-voiceless and palatal-alveolar contrasts for consonants, and glottal-null (e.g., "hate" vs. "ate") contrast for syllable shape, are apparently *not* independent. A simple way to say this is, if one of these contrasts is revealed to be vulnerable by the Kent et al. (1989) test, the others will be as well (Weismer & Martin, 1992). Even though the contrasts may appear to have different "vulnerabilities" in different speakers or clinical populations, they are all highly correlated with each other and may not furnish the kind of prescription for management imagined when the test was developed.

The kinds of speech intelligibility tests described above are probably of greatest use when a single speaker's progress (or decline) is being tracked across therapy or progression of a disease. In this case, all measures involve the same individual, who in a sense serves as his or her own control in evaluating the effects of management or disease progression. What is needed are measures of speech intelligibility motivated by more sophisticated knowledge of speech perception, and especially by factors that truly tap into language comprehension. For example, the ability of listeners to identify word onsets in connected speech produced by persons with speech disorders, and to access the lexicon to extract the meaning of a client's message, seems to be the next step in enhancing the clinical relevance of these measures of perception.

REVIEW

The modern era of speech perception research was initiated by experiments using the pattern-playback machine, a device that synthesized speech signals and was used to create small changes in the signals to evaluate the effect on listeners' phonetic decisions.

The motor theory of speech perception was based on the finding of categorical perception for stop consonant place of articulation.

Additional findings, including duplex perception and trading relations, were used to support the motor theory.

Motor theory was based on the idea that speech production and perception in humans were part of a special "code," and required a special mechanism in the brain for the perception of speech.

Categorical perception can be demonstrated in infants and animals, findings that may be interpreted as support for, or against, the motor theory.

The general auditory approach competes with motor theory as an explanation of speech perception and takes the perspective that the speech acoustic signal is sufficiently consistent to support speech sound perception, and that general auditory mechanisms (not special mechanisms) are used in the perception of speech signals.

Direct realism, a competing theory inspired by J. J. Gibson's ecological approach to perception, says that articulatory gestures are perceived directly (not by special mechanisms), and that listeners actually hear gestures, not acoustic representations of speech sounds that must be processed by cognitive mechanisms for proper recognition.

Speech perception involves not only the perception of speech sounds, but the use of those sounds to access words from the lexicon through a combination of bottom-up and top-down processes that probably account for the interplay between sound analysis and word choices in the understanding of a spoken message.

Speech intelligibility testing, a subtype of the general category of speech perception phenomena, has a clear role in speech-language pathology, even though specific tests have rarely been constructed according to principles derived from the speech perception literature.

REFERENCES

Andoni, S., Li, N., & Pollak, G. (2007). Spectrotemporal fields in the inferior colliculus revealing specificity for spectral motion in conspecific vocalizations. *Journal of Neuroscience*, *27*, 4882–4893.

Best, C., Morrongiello, B., & Robson, R. (1981). Perceptual equivalence of acoustic cues in speech and nonspeech perception. *Perception and Psychophysics*, *29*, 191–211.

Blumstein, S., & Stevens, K. (1979). Acoustic invariance in speech production: Evidence from measurements of the spectral characteristics of stop consonants. *Journal of the Acoustical Society of America*, *66*, 1001–1017.

Cleary, M., & Pisoni, D. (2001). Speech perception and spoken word recognition: Research and theory. In E. Goldstein (Ed.), *Blackwell handbook of perception* (pp. 499–534). Oxford, UK: Blackwell.

Cole, R., & Rudnicky, A. (1983). What's new in speech perception? The research and idea of William Chandler Bagley, 1874–1946. *Psychological Review*, *90*, 94–101.

Cooper, F., Liberman, A., & Borst, J. (1951). The interconversion of audible and visible patterns as a basis for research in the perception of speech. *Proceedings of the National Academy of Sciences*, *37*, 318–325.

Cutler, A., Dahan, D., & van Donselaar, W. (1997). Prosody in the comprehension of spoken language: A literature review. *Language and Speech*, *40*, 141–201.

Dahan, D., & Gareth Gaskell, M. (2007). The temporal dynamics of ambiguity resolution: Evidence from spoken word recognition. *Journal of Memory and Language*, *57*, 483–501.

Dahan, D., & Magnuson, J. (2006). Spoken word recognition. In M. Traxler & M. Gernsbacher (Eds.), *Handbook of psycholinguistics* (2nd ed., pp. 249–283). New York: Academic Press.

Davies, N., Madden, J., & Butchart, S. (2004). Learning fine-tunes a specific response of nestlings to the parental alarm calls of their own species. *Proceedings of the Royal Society of London B*, *271*, 2297–2304.

Diehl, R., Lotto, A., & Holt, L. (2004). Speech perception. *Annual Review of Psychology*, *55*, 149–179.

Duffy, J. (1995). *Motor speech disorders: Substrates, differential diagnosis, and management*. St. Louis, MO: Mosby.

Eimas, P., Miller, J., & Jusczyk, P. (1990). On infant speech perception and the acquisition of language. In S. Harnad (Ed.), *Categorical perception: The groundwork of cognition* (pp. 161–195). Cambridge, UK: Cambridge University Press.

Fant, G. (1960). *Acoustic theory of speech production*. Hague, Netherlands: Mouton.

Fowler, C. (1986). An event approach to the study of speech perception from a direct-realist perspective. *Journal of Phonetics*, *14*, 3–28.

Fowler, C. (1996). Listeners do hear sounds, not tongues. *Journal of the Acoustical Society of America*, *99*, 1730–1741.

Fowler, C. (2006). Compensation for coarticulation reflects gesture perception, not spectral contrast. *Perception and Psychophysics*, *68*, 161–177.

Fowler, C., Galantucci, B., & Saltzman, E. (2003). Motor theories of perception. In M. Arbib (Ed.), *The handbook of brain theory and neural networks* (pp. 705–707). Cambridge, MA: MIT Press.

Fowler, C., & Rosenblum, L. (1991). The perception of phonetic gestures. In I. Mattingly & M. Studdert-Kennedy (Eds.), *Modularity and the motor theory of speech perception* (pp. 33–59). Hillsdale, NJ: Lawrence Erlbaum.

Gibson, J. (1968). *The senses considered as perceptual systems*. Boston: Houghton Mifflin.

Gibson, J. (1979). *The ecological approach to visual perception*. Boston: Houghton Mifflin.

Goldinger, S. (1998). Echoes of echoes? An episodic theory of lexical access. *Psychological Review*, *105*, 251–279.

Grosjean F. (1980). Spoken word recognition processes and the gating paradigm. *Perception and Psychophysics*, *28*, 267–283.

Hirsh, I. (1959). Auditory perception of temporal order. *Journal of the Acoustical Society of America*, *31*, 759–767.

Johnson, K., & Mullenix, J. (1997). *Talker variability in speech processing*. New York: Academic Press.

Katz, J. (Ed.). (2002). *Handbook of clinical audiology* (5th ed.). Baltimore: Lippincott Williams & Wilkins.

Kent, R. (Ed.) (1992). *Intelligibility in speech disorders: Theory, measurement, and management*. Amsterdam, Netherlands: John Benjamin.

Kent J., Kent R., Rosenbek J., Weismer G., Martin R., Sufit R., & Brooks B. (1992). Quantitative description of the dysarthria in women with amyotrophic lateral sclerosis. *Journal of Speech and Hearing Research, 35*, 723–733.

Kent, R., Weismer, G., Kent, J., & Rosenbek, J. (1989). Toward phonetic intelligibility testing in dysarthria. *Journal of Speech and Hearing Disorders, 54*, 482–499.

Kingston, J., & Diehl, R. (1994). Phonetic knowledge. *Language, 70*, 419–454.

Klatt, D. (1987). Review of text-to-speech conversion for English. *Journal of the Acoustical Society of America, 82*, 737–793.

Klatt, D. (1989). Review of selected models of speech perception. In W. Marslen-Wilson (Ed.), *Lexical representation and process* (pp. 169–226). Cambridge, MA: MIT Press.

Kluender, K. (1994). Speech perception as a tractable problem in cognitive science. In M. Gernsbacher (Ed.), *Handbook of psycholinguistics* (pp. 173–217). San Diego, CA: Academic Press.

Kluender, K., & Kiefte, M. (2006). Speech perception within a biologically realistic information-theoretic framework. In M. Traxler & M. Gernsbacher (Eds.), *Handbook of psycholinguistics* (2nd ed., pp. 153–199). London: Elsevier.

Kuhl, P. (1986). Theoretical contribution of tests on animals to the special mechanisms debate in speech. *Experimental Biology, 45*, 233–265.

Kuhl, P., & Miller, J. (1975). Speech perception by the chinchilla: Voiced-voiceless distinction in alveolar plosive consonants. *Science, 190*, 69–72.

Kuhl, P., & Padden, D. (1983). Enhanced discriminability at the phoneme boundaries for place of articulation in macaques. *Journal of the Acoustical Society of America, 73*, 1003–1010.

Liberman, A., Cooper, F., Shankweiler, D., & Studdert-Kennedy, M. (1967). Perception of the speech code. *Psychological Review, 74*, 431–461.

Liberman, A., Harris, K., Hoffman, H., & Griffith, B. (1957). The discrimination of speech sounds within and across phoneme boundaries. *Journal of Experimental Psychology, 54*, 358–368.

Liberman, A., & Mattingly, I. (1985). The motor theory of speech perception revised. *Cognition, 21*, 1–36.

Lieberman, P. (1996). Some biological constraints on the analysis of prosody. In J. Morgan & K. Demuth (Eds.), *Signal to syntax: Bootstrapping from speech to grammar in early acquisition* (pp. 55–66). Hillsdale, NJ: Lawrence Erlbaum.

Lindblom, B. (1990). Explaining phonetic variation: A sketch of the H&H theory. In W. Hardcastle & A. Marchal (Eds.), *Speech production and speech modeling* (pp. 403–440). Dordrecht, Netherlands: Kluwer Academic.

Liss, J. (2007). The role of speech perception in motor speech disorders. In G. Weismer (Ed.), *Motor speech disorders* (pp. 187–219). San Diego, CA: Plural.

Liss, J., Spitzer, S., Caviness, J., Adler, C., & Edwards, B. (2000). Lexical boundary error analysis in hypokinetic and ataxic dysarthria. *Journal of the Acoustical Society of America, 107*, 3415–3424.

Lotto, A., & Holt, L. (2006). Putting phonetic context effects into context: A commentary on Fowler (2006). *Perception and Psychophysics, 68*, 178–183.

Luce, P., & McLennan, C. (2005). Spoken word recognition: The challenge of variation. In D. Pisoni & R. Remez (Eds.), *The handbook of speech perception* (pp. 591–609). Malden, MA: Blackwell.

Mann, V., & Liberman, A. (1983). Some differences between phonetic and auditory modes of perception. *Cognition, 14*, 211–235.

Miller, J., & Jusczyk, P. (1989). Seeking the neurobiological basis of speech perception. *Cognition, 33*, 111–137.

Monsen, R. (1983). The oral speech intelligibility of hearing-impaired talkers. *Journal of Speech and Hearing Disorders, 48*, 286–296.

Mullenix, J., Pisoni, D., & Martin, C. (1989). Some effects of talker variability on spoken word recognition. *Journal of the Acoustical Society of America, 85*, 365–378.

Nooteboom, S., & van der Vlugt, M. (1988). A search for a word-beginning superiority effect. *Journal of the Acoustical Society of America, 84*, 2018–2032.

Pardo, J., & Remez, R. (2006). The perception of speech. In M. Traxler and M. Gernsbacher (Eds.), *Handbook of psycholinguistics* (2nd ed., pp. 201–248). London: Elsevier.

Patterson, D., & Pepperberg, I. (1998). Acoustic and articulatory correlates of stop consonants in a parrot and a human subject. *Journal of the Acoustical Society of America, 103*, 2197–2215.

Pisoni, D. (1977). Identification and discrimination of the relative onset time of two complex tones: Implications for voicing perception in stops. *Journal of the Acoustical Society of America, 61*, 1352–1361.

Popper, K. (2002a). *Conjectures and refutations: The growth of scientific knowledge*. London: Routledge Classics.

Popper, K. (2002b). *The logic of scientific discovery*. London: Routledge Classics.

Repp, B. (1982). Phonetic trading relations and context effects: New experimental evidence for a speech mode of perception. *Psychological Bulletin, 92*, 81–110.

Repp, B., & Liberman, A. (1987). Phonetic category boundaries are flexible. In S. Harnad (Ed.), *Categorical perception: The groundwork of cognition* (pp. 89–112). Cambridge, UK: Cambridge University Press.

Remez, R., Rubin, P., Berns, S., Pardo, J., & Lang, J. (1994). On the perceptual organization of speech. *Psychological Review, 101*, 129–156.

Saffran, J. (2003). Statistical language learning: Mechanisms and constraints. *Current Directions in Psychological Science, 12*, 110–114.

Saffran, J., & Thiessen, E. (2007). Domain-general learning capacities. In E. Hoff & M. Shatz (Eds.), *Handbook of language development* (pp. 68–86) Cambridge, UK: Blackwell.

Sommers, M., & Barcroft, J. (2006). Stimulus variability and the phonetic relevance hypothesis: Effects of variability in speaking style, fundamental frequency, and speaking rate on spoken word identification. *Journal of the Acoustical Society of America, 119*, 2406–2416.

Stevens, K. (2005). Features in speech perception and lexical access. In D. Pisoni & R. Remez (Eds.), *The handbook of speech perception* (pp. 125–155). Malden, MA: Blackwell.

Studdert-Kennedy, M., & Shankweiler, D. (1970). Hemispheric specialization for speech perception. *Journal of the Acoustical Society of America, 48*, 579–594.

Watkins, K., & Paus, T. (2004). Modulation of motor excitability during speech perception: The role of Broca's area. *Journal of Cognitive Neuroscience, 16*, 978–987.

Weismer, G. (2008). Speech intelligibility. In M. Ball, M. Perkins, N. Müller, & S. Howard (Eds.), *Handbook of clinical linguistics*. Oxford, UK: Blackwell.

Weismer, G., & Martin, R. (1992). Acoustic and perceptual approaches to the study of intelligibility. In R. Kent (Ed.), *Intelligibility in speech disorders: Theory, measurement, and management* (pp. 67–118). Amsterdam, Netherlands: John Benjamin.

Whalen, D., & Liberman, A. (1987). Speech perception takes precedence over nonspeech perception. *Science, 237*, 169–171.

Yorkston, K., Beukelman, D., Strand, E., & Bell, K. (1999). *Management of motor speech disorders in children and adults* (2nd ed.). Austin, TX: Pro-Ed.

12

Swallowing

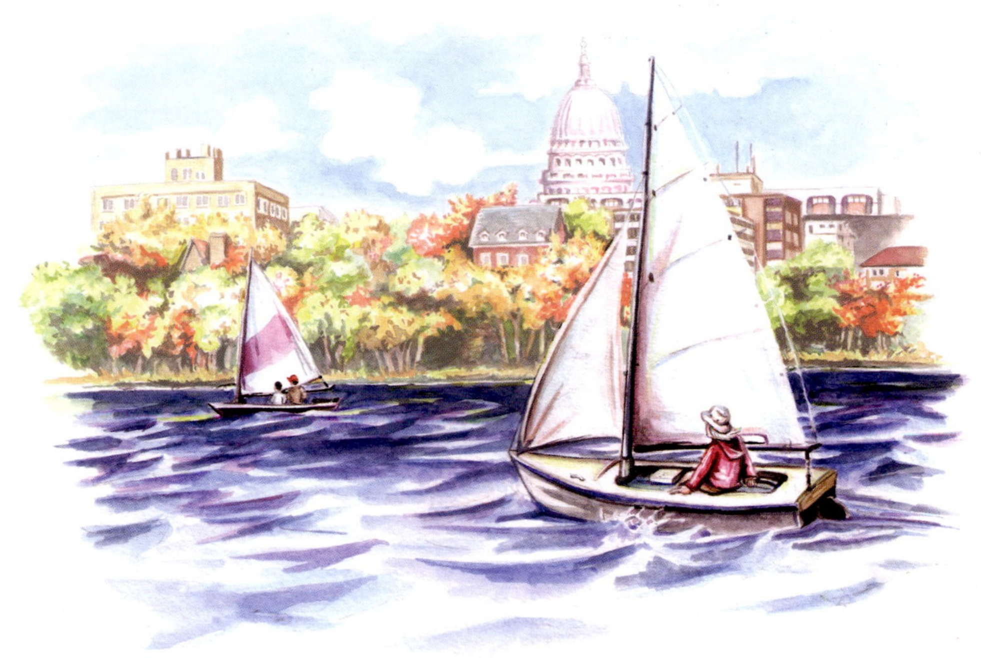

Scenario

She stepped on her skiff and things somehow felt a little different. There was no wind and the lake was as smooth as glass, yet she seemed to be gently rolling and pitching. The feeling was very brief and she thought nothing of it. By the time her skiff was rigged, the wind picked up, as if at her command. Lake Mendota and the signs of fall were especially calming to her. Her life was good. She had a new granddaughter to dote on, and her retirement from the university was coming into sight.

A week later she stumbled but caught herself as she walked in her living room. The incident was registered but then ignored. Within the next month she noticed occasional cramps in her legs and some twitching now and then in her right hand, just near the junction where her thumb and index finger came together. Probably nothing. But was it? She began to wonder only after she found herself struggling to get up out of an overstuffed chair in front of the television set. There was something wrong. It had crossed a threshold. She mentioned the events to her husband and they agreed that she should talk with her physician.

From this time on until her condition was diagnosed, other things about her movements began to concern her. She occasionally choked when eating, something she rarely did before. She seemed to tire more easily than usual. And she seemed to be losing some of the power in her voice. Within 3 months, a neurologist had fixed the diagnosis and the words were numbing. She had Lou Gehrig's disease or amyotrophic lateral sclerosis, and no matter which she chose to call it, her future was set. Only the time course and the manner of devastation were uncertainties.

Two years passed and her condition worsened. By then, she had moderate breathing discomfort, a wet and gurgly sounding voice, and her speech was difficult to understand in conversation. She had trouble swallowing and had lost much of her enjoyment of eating. She could no longer walk and was confined to a wheelchair during the day. All of her movements were slow and weak and she gave the impression of running on a dying battery. Her plight had rendered her almost completely dependent and only occasionally was her clear mind able to lift her above her quiet despair. Her best moments were when her new granddaughter was in sight.

She began to lose weight because of her swallowing problem, her speech was nearly unintelligible, and her breathing was becoming more of a struggle. Her neurologist referred her to a local medical center with the request that a speech-language pathologist evaluate her swallowing and speech and that a pulmonologist evaluate her breathing, both with an eye toward palliative management.

INTRODUCTION

Some of the most enjoyable activities of daily living involve eating and drinking. These include meals (where eating and drinking are the purpose of the activity), special events such as receptions (where eating and drinking enhance the celebration), and relaxation activities such as going to the movies (where eating popcorn and drinking soda are an integral part of the experience for some people). Figure 12–1 is a cartoon that depicts the anticipation of a good meal and the social context in which it is enjoyed.

The ease of eating and drinking is deceptive. They are complicated activities that require intricately coordinated actions of the lips, mandible, tongue, velum, pharynx, larynx, esophagus, and other structures. Because eating and drinking engage many of the same structures and much of the same airway as are used for speaking and breathing, it is not uncommon for competition to exist or for tradeoffs to occur when attempting to execute them simultaneously. For example, there are certain times when chewing must stop for speaking to occur and when speaking and breathing must stop for swallowing to occur.

The entire act of placing food or liquid in the oral cavity, moving it backward to the pharynx, propelling it into the esophagus, and allowing it to make its way to the stomach is called deglutition. Although the word swallowing is sometimes used as a synonym for deglutition, swallowing actually includes only certain phases of deglutition. Nevertheless, to simplify the explanations that follow, the term swallowing is used in place of deglutition and is meant to include all phases of deglutition.

ANATOMY

Figure 12–2 shows the structures that participate in swallowing. These structures extend from the lips to the stomach. Many of these same structures also participate in speech production, except for the esophagus and stomach.

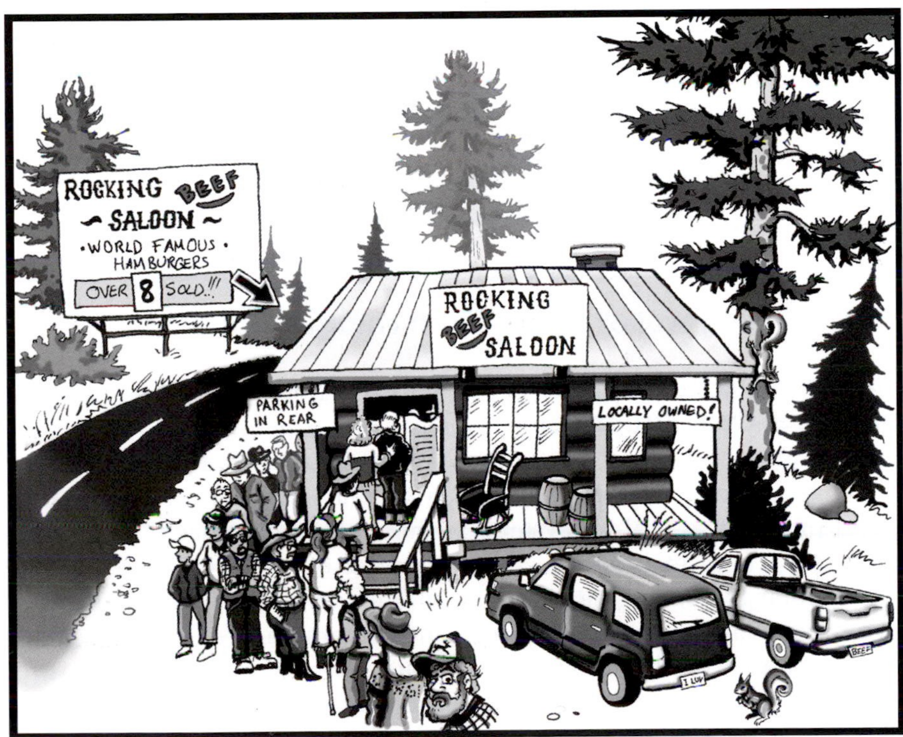

Figure 12–1. Cartoon depicting the anticipation of a good meal and the social context in which it is enjoyed.

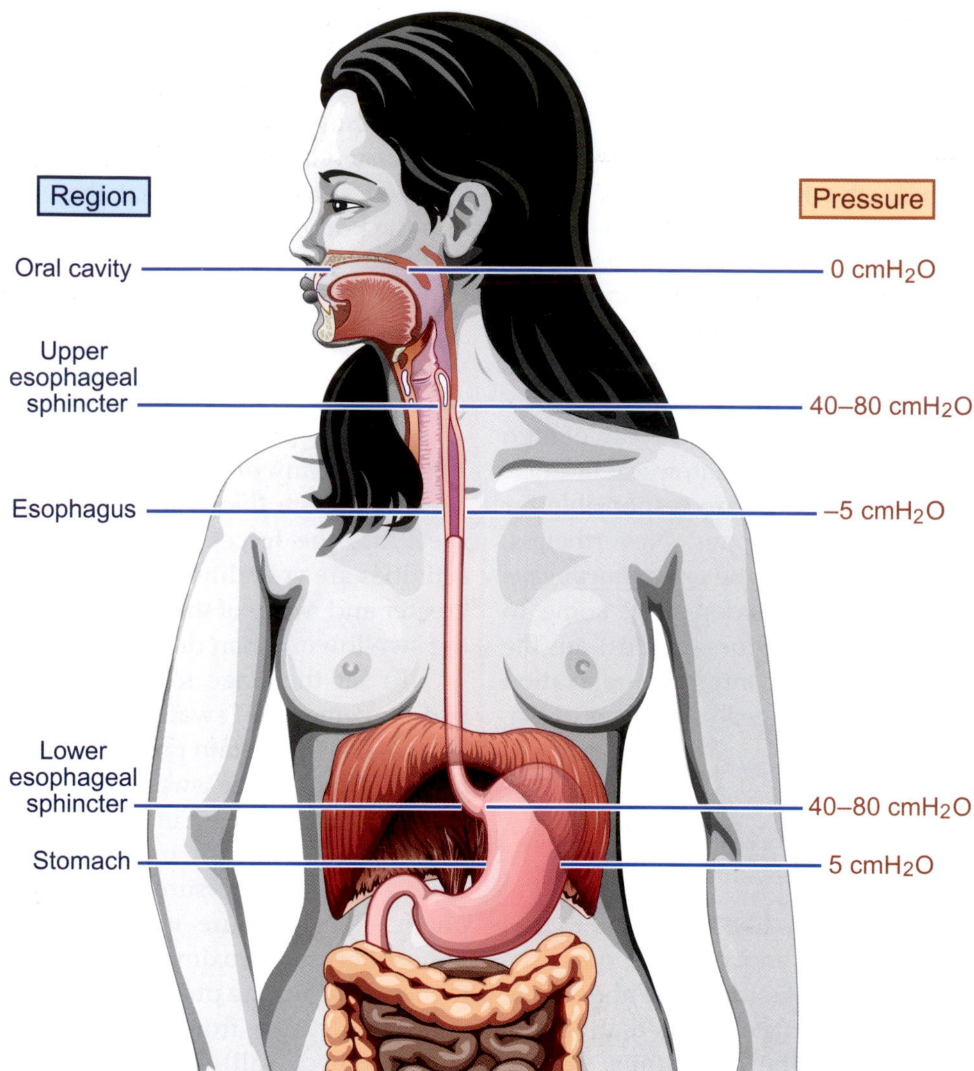

Figure 12-3. Relevant mechanical pressures associated with the resting state of the swallowing apparatus.

above atmospheric (approximately 5 cmH_2O) and results from the "muscle tone" of the wall of the stomach and the hydrostatic properties of the stomach contents. In contrast to these relatively low pressures, the pressures within the upper and lower esophageal sphincters are high (a typical range is 40 to 80 cmH_2O in the resting state). Their absolute magnitudes depend on the measurement approach used as well as a variety of physiological factors (Goyle & Cobb, 1981; Linden, Hogosta, & Norlander, 2007). The relatively high pressures in the upper and lower esophageal sphincters allow these regions to function like forcefully closed valves while at rest. It is important that the pressure in the lower esophageal sphincter remains substantially higher than the pressure in the stomach. Otherwise, substances from the stomach may reflux (flow back) into the esophagus.

Both passive and active forces contribute to swallowing. Passive force comes from many sources including (a) the natural recoil of connective tissues (ligaments and membranes), cartilages, and bones, (b) the surface tension between structures in apposition, (c) the pull of gravity, and (d) aeromechanical factors. Active force results from the activation of breathing, laryngeal, velopharyngeal-nasal, and pharyngeal-oral muscles in various combinations. These contributions to active force are described in

Chapters 2, 3, 4, and 5, and are discussed here as they relate to swallowing.

Forces and movements of swallowing can be considered in association with four phases of swallowing, as shown schematically in Figure 12–4. These are the oral preparatory phase, oral transport phase, pharyngeal transport phase, and esophageal transport phase and are used to describe the movement of a bolus through the oral, pharyngeal, and esophageal regions of the apparatus. Bolus is the word used to refer to the mass of food or the volume of liquid to be swallowed.

Oral Preparatory Phase

The oral preparatory phase is depicted in Figure 12–5. This phase begins as liquid or food makes contact with the structures of the anterior oral vestibule. The mandible lowers and the lips abduct to allow liquid or food to enter. What happens next is largely dependent on the nature of the substance to be swallowed.

If the substance is liquid, the mandible elevates and the lips adduct, forming an anterior seal to contain the bolus. The bolus is contained in the anterior region of the oral cavity by actions of the tongue and other structures, and held there momentarily (usually on the order of 1 s). The anterior tongue depresses and the sides of the tongue elevate to form a "cup" for the bolus. The bolus may be cupped in one of two ways, depending on the person. Some people hold the bolus with the tongue tip elevated and contacting the back surface of the maxillary incisors, and other people hold the bolus on the floor of the oral cavity in front of the tongue. These two holding positions have been dubbed "dipper" and "tipper" type swallows (Dodds et al., 1989). The back of the tongue elevates to make contact with the velum to form a back wall that separates the oral from the pharyngeal cavities and helps to ensure that no substance can slip by and into the pulmonary airways. The velopharynx is open so that breathing can continue. Nevertheless, many people stop breathing momentarily (called the apneic interval) at this point in the swallow, or even before the cup of liquid reaches the lips (Martin, Logemann,

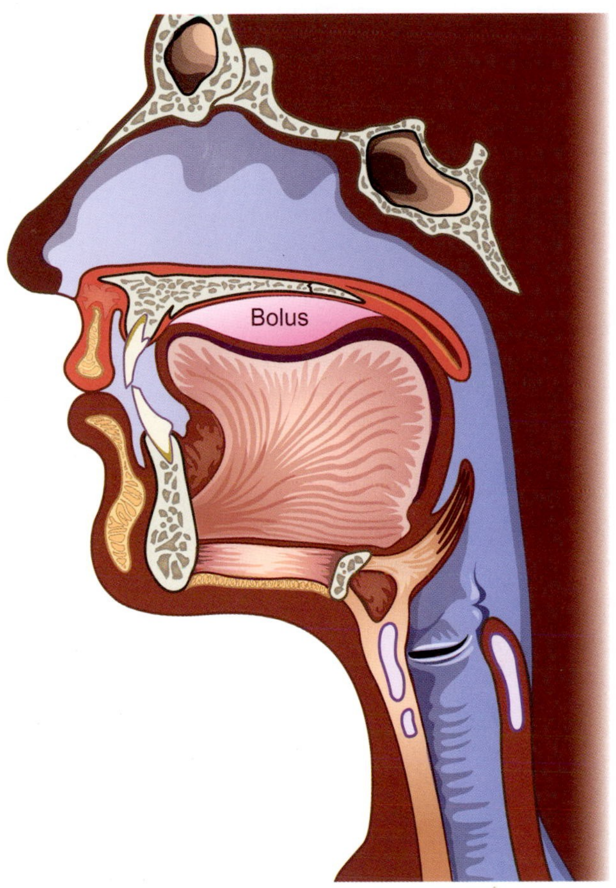

Figure 12–5. Oral preparatory phase of swallowing.

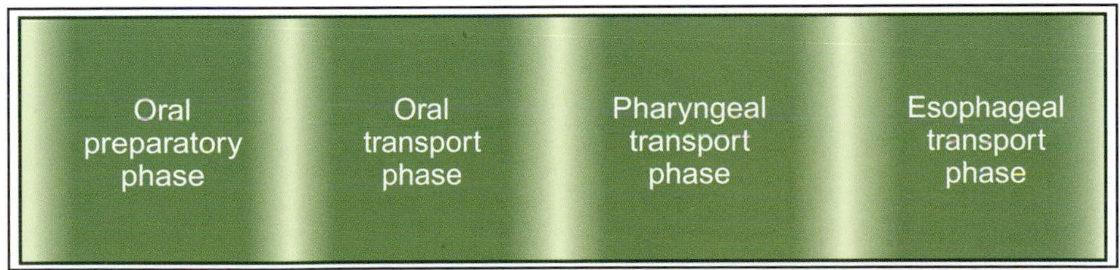

Figure 12–4. Schematic depiction of the four phases of swallowing.

Shaker, & Dodds, 1994; Martin-Harris, Brodsky, Price, Michel, & Walters, 2003; Martin-Harris, Michel, & Castell, 2005b). This apneic interval serves to reduce the risk of aspiration (defined as invasion of substances below the vocal folds).

These initial events are quite different when the substance to be swallowed is food, rather than liquid, because solid substances need to be masticated (chewed) into smaller pieces and mixed with saliva before being transported toward the esophagus. Actions of the mandible (and teeth), lips, tongue, and cheeks grind and manipulate the food into a cohesive bolus (lump) and position it on the surface of the anterior tongue. The lips may remain fully adducted (though this is not necessary) while the mandible moves to grind the food. During chewing, the mandible moves up and down, forward and backward, and side to side. This is in contrast to speech production, during which the mandible moves primarily up and down. The velum makes contact with the back part of the tongue to seal off the oral from the pharyngeal cavity to prevent the bolus from moving into the pharynx and larynx. The velopharynx is open during preparation of the bolus, and breathing may either continue or be interrupted by apnea (McFarland & Lund, 1995; Palmer & Hiiemae, 2003). The duration of the oral preparatory phase may last from as short as 3 s, when chewing a soft cookie, to as long as 20 s, when chewing a tough piece of steak.

At the end of the oral preparatory phase, the substance in the oral cavity is ready for consumption. Usually it is transported back toward the pharynx (oral transport phase) immediately. There are choices at this point, however, including that the substance can be (a) savored for awhile by continued manipulation, (b) squirreled in the cheeks, or (c) expelled. In fact, the expulsion option is used when performing a "sham" feeding test to study the actions of the stomach in anticipation of receiving food.

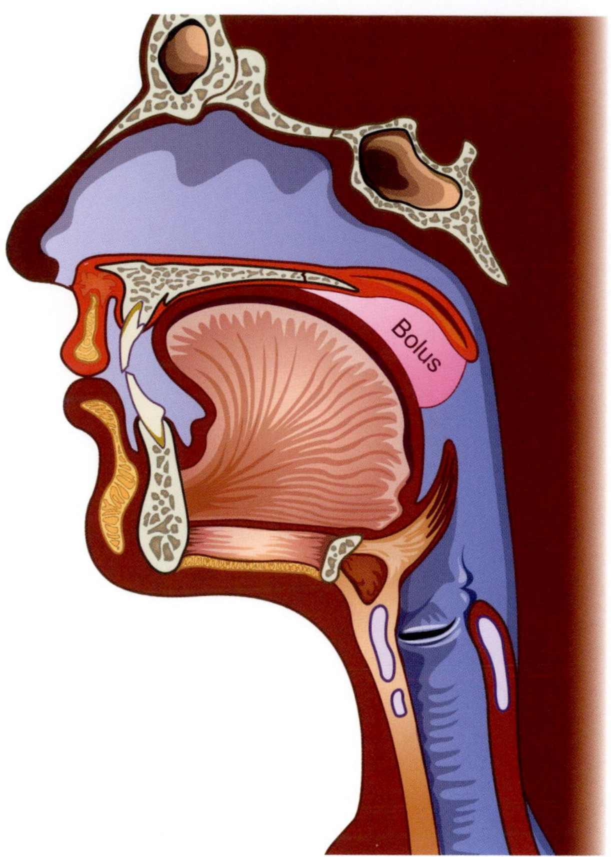

Figure 12–6. Oral transport phase of swallowing.

Oral Transport Phase

Once the bolus is in the ready position (either the "dipper" or "tipper" position for liquids), it is usually transported back toward the pharynx, as illustrated in Figure 12–6. This is accomplished by elevating the tongue tip and squeezing the bolus against the hard palate. The fact that the tongue behaves like a muscular hydrostat (in that it can move and change shape in an almost infinite number of ways—see Chapter 5) makes it especially effective in moving and clearing the bolus. The force used to propel the bolus varies with bolus viscosity. The lips usually press together firmly (although this is not necessary) and the cheeks are pulled inward slightly to keep the bolus positioned over the tongue. At the same time, the velum begins to elevate and the pharyngeal walls begin to constrict. The oral transport phase is generally short, lasting less than 0.5 second (Cook et al., 1994; Tracy et al., 1989).

Pharyngeal Transport Phase

The pharyngeal transport phase of the swallow is usually "triggered" when the bolus passes the anterior faucial pillars, although sometimes the location of the trigger point is closer to the esophagus, depending on the bolus type and the age of the individual. During this phase, depicted in Figure 12–7,

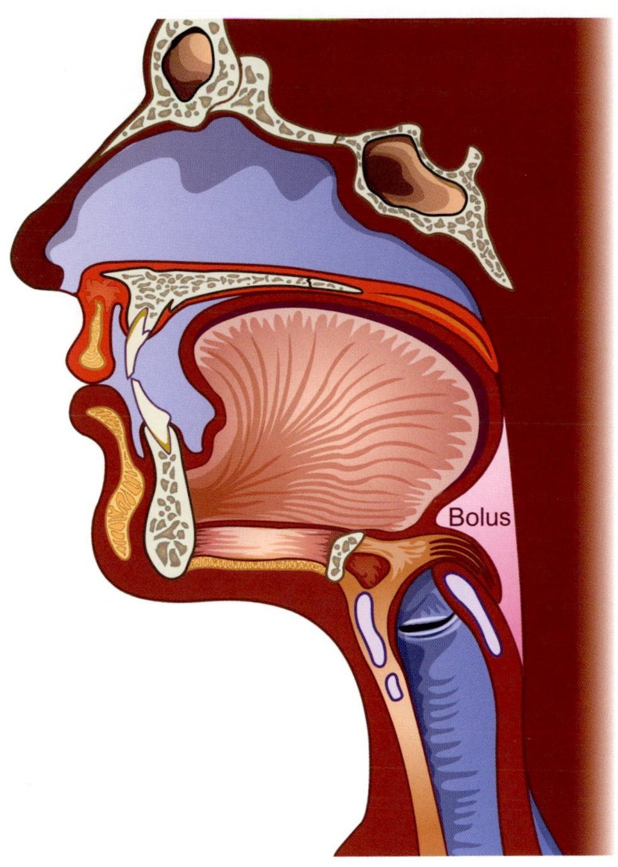

Figure 12–7. Pharyngeal transport phase of swallowing.

several events occur rapidly and nearly simultaneously to move the bolus quickly through the pharynx while protecting the airway. This phase is under "automatic" control, so that once triggered, it proceeds as a relatively fixed set of events that cannot be altered voluntarily (except in the magnitude and duration of the pressures generated). These events occur within about 0.5 s or less (Cook et al., 1994; Tracy et al., 1989) and include adjustments related to velopharyngeal closure, elevation of the hyoid bone and larynx, laryngeal closure, pharyngeal constriction, and opening of the upper esophageal sphincter, as described below.

The velopharynx closes like a flap-sphincter valve by elevation of the velum and constriction of the pharyngeal walls. This closure is forceful (more forceful than for speech production) so as to prohibit passage of substances into the nasopharynx.

The hyoid bone and larynx move upward and forward as a result of contraction of extrinsic tongue muscles (recall that several extrinsic muscles of the tongue attach to the hyoid bone). As the hyoid bone is pulled upward and forward, the larynx is pulled along with it via its muscular connections to the hyoid bone. In fact, because of these anatomical connections and the tendency to move as a unit, this group of structures is often called the hyolaryngeal complex. Elevation of the larynx also causes the pharynx to shorten.

Closure of the larynx for swallowing has been described as a folding of the laryngeal apparatus (Fink & Demarest, 1978) that forms a seal to the entrance of the trachea to protect the pulmonary airways. Closure occurs at multiple levels, which include the vocal folds, the ventricular folds, and the aryepiglottic folds and epiglottis. Both the vocal folds and ventricular folds adduct firmly, whereas the epiglottis is forced down over the laryngeal aditus like a trap door and serves as a first line of defense against substances entering the larynx and pulmonary airways. The epiglottis moves from a relatively upward pointing position, through a horizontal position, to a relatively downward pointing position. Both passive and active forces appear to be responsible for downward movement of the epiglottis during swallowing (Ekberg & Sigurjonsson, 1982; Fink & Demarest, 1978; VanDaele, Perlman, & Casell, 1995). The passive force derives from backward movement of the tongue and upward and forward movement of the hyoid bone and larynx, which mechanically deflect the epiglottis backward and downward. Upward and forward movement of the larynx simultaneously contributes to airway protection by tucking the larynx against the root of the tongue and deflecting the trachea away from the digestive pathway. The active force is somewhat less certain (Fink, Martin, & Rohrmann, 1979; Ramsey, Watson, Gramiak, & Weinberg, 1955; VanDaele et al., 1995), but is argued to derive from contraction of the ***aryepiglottic*** muscles (and possibly from vertically ascending lateral fibers of the ***thyroarytenoid*** muscles), which purportedly pull the epiglottis downward to complete the seal with the laryngeal aditus (Ekberg & Sigurjonsson, 1982). Whatever the relative contribution of passive and actives forces to downward displacement of the epiglottis, it can be stated with considerable certainty that the structure plays a key role in protection of the pulmonary airways during swallowing.

As the tongue propels the bolus into the pharynx, the pharynx undergoes segmental contraction (from top to bottom). The tongue root moves backward and the pharyngeal walls constrict to "squeeze" the bolus toward the esophagus. The bolus often divides at the epiglottis as it passes through the left and right epiglottic valleculae (lateral channels between the root of the tongue and the epiglottis) and into the left and right pyriform sinuses (recesses bounded by the pharynx and larynx), or it flows down one side or through the midline of the covered laryngeal aditus (Dua, Ren, Bardan, Xie, & Shaker, 1997; Logemann, Kahrilas, Kobara, & Vakil, 1989).

The final step of the pharyngeal swallow is the opening of the upper esophageal sphincter to allow the passage of the bolus into the esophagus. This is accomplished by relaxation of the ***cricopharyngeus*** muscles and simultaneous stretching of the esophageal opening by movement of the hyolaryngeal complex.

The bolus is propelled through the pharynx to the esophagus during the pharyngeal transport phase by a combination of mechanical (structural) forces and aeromechanical forces. The mechanical forces consist of the tongue pushing the bolus back into the pharynx and the pharynx contracting segmentally against the tongue root, as just described. The aeromechanical forces are in the form of regional air pressure changes that help to move the bolus along. Specifically, backward movement of the tongue and constriction of the pharyngeal walls serve to narrow the airway in that region and reduce the airway volume, thereby causing the air pressure to rise in that region. At the same time, dilation of the upper esophageal sphincter lowers the air pressure below the bolus. The pressure differential (higher pressure behind the bolus than in front of it) helps to drive the bolus toward its destination.

The pharyngeal transport phase of the swallow is invariably short (generally 0.5 s or less) and is characterized by a series of actions that move the bolus quickly through the pharynx and, at the same time, protect the pulmonary airways from invasion by substances. The final phase of swallowing is initiated as the bolus moves into the esophagus.

Esophageal Transport Phase

The esophageal transport phase, illustrated in Figure 12–8, begins when the bolus enters the upper esophageal sphincter and ends when it passes into the stomach through the lower esophageal sphincter. This phase may last anywhere from 8 to 20 s (Dodds, Hogan, Reid, Stewart, & Arndorfer, 1973). As described above, the bolus is pushed into the esophagus by muscles of the tongue and pharynx and by pressure differentials, and the upper esophageal sphincter opens so that the bolus can pass into the esophagus (the lower esophageal sphincter relaxes at the same time). The bolus is then propelled by peristaltic actions (alternating waves of contraction and relaxation) of the esophageal walls. Peristaltic contraction raises pressure behind the bolus and relaxation lowers pressure in front of the bolus creating the pressure differential needed to propel it toward the stomach. The nature of the peristaltic action varies somewhat depending on the nature of the bolus (solid or liquid), body position (relation of esophagus and bolus to gravity), and other factors. When a substance is left behind following the primary peristalsis, it is cleared by subsequent peristaltic action (called secondary peri-

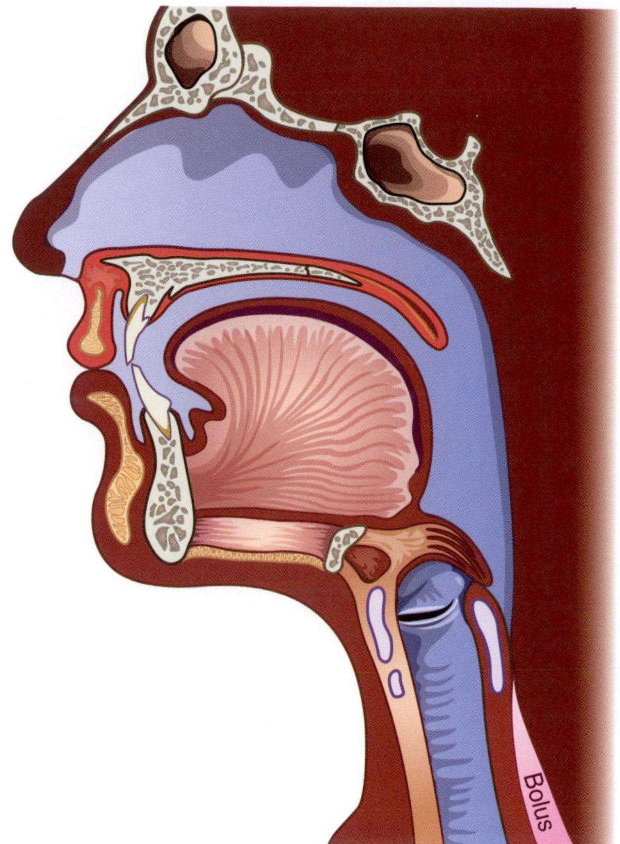

Figure 12–8. Esophageal transport phase of swallowing.

GERD

Your stomach is rich with chemicals that have about the same acidity as the battery acid in your car. That's right, that's the same battery acid that will burn a hole in your clothes if you splash some of it on you. GERD, an acronym for gastroesophageal reflux disease, is a chronic condition in which acid from the stomach backs up into the esophagus when the lower esophageal sphincter (the valve that separates the esophagus and stomach) fails to do its job properly. Two of the symptoms of GERD are heartburn and regurgitation of acid that has a foul taste. When stomach acid in the esophagus spills onto the larynx, it can irritate and erode laryngeal tissue. If symptoms are chronic, get medical attention. If symptoms occur only occasionally, you may just need to modify some of your habits. Don't stuff yourself before you go to bed, lay off foods that make it worse, and sleep with your body inclined so that your head is higher than your feet.

stalsis). Although the esophagus usually transports substances toward the stomach, it can also transport substances or gas away from the stomach (as in the case of vomiting or burping).

Overlap of Phases

Although the phases of swallowing are described above as though they are discrete and occur one after the other, they can overlap. When eating solid foods, for example, preparation of part of the bolus in the oral cavity may continue while another part of the bolus moves into the pharyngeal area, as illustrated in Figure 12–9. This partial bolus may remain in the epiglottic valleculae as long as 10 s before it merges with the remainder of the bolus and the pharyngeal transport phase of the swallow is triggered (Hiiemae & Palmer, 1999).

Overlap of phases is also apparent if swallowing is viewed in relation to the actions of individual structures, rather than in relation to the status of the bolus. Whereas the traditional description of swallowing (used in this chapter) focuses on the preparation and transport of the bolus to define the phases of swallowing, there are schema that attempt to segment physiological events along somewhat different conceptual lines and to categorize them across different levels of observation (Martin-Harris

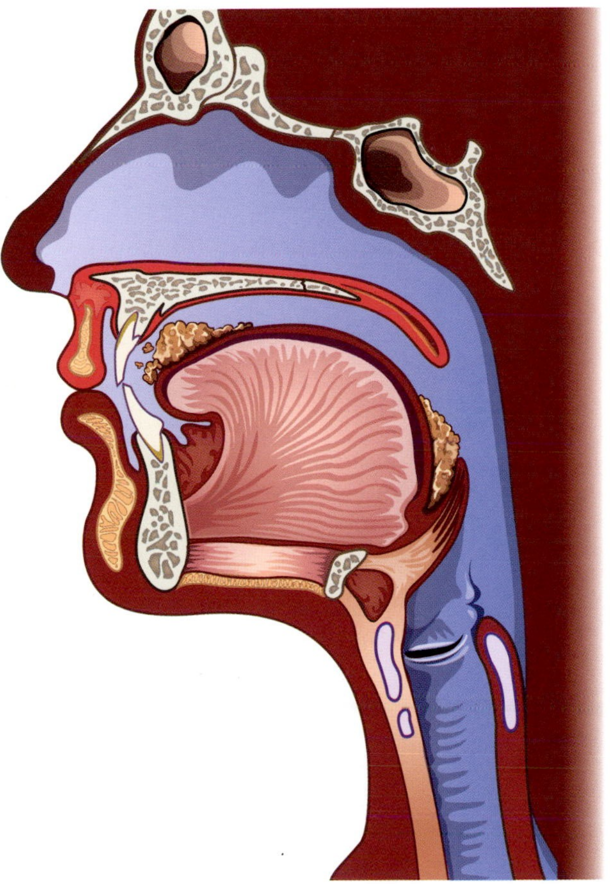

Figure 12–9. An illustration of eating, in which part of the bolus continues to be chewed while another part moves to the pharynx.

et al., 2005b). Such notions have emerged relatively recently and rely on the coordination of temporal events across structures that traditionally have been thought of in sequential terms. Schema that are based on cross-structure analyses speak to common and overlapping elements of swallowing behavior and hold promise for better understanding the function of the swallowing apparatus as a whole and interactions among its components.

BREATHING AND SWALLOWING

Protection of the pulmonary airways during swallowing is dependent, in large part, on the coordination of breathing and swallowing. Without such coordination, inspiration might occur just as a substance is being transported through the pharynx and that substance might be "sucked" through the larynx into the pulmonary airways (aspiration). This is avoided by closing the larynx for a brief period during the swallow. The risk of aspiration appears to be further reduced by timing the swallow in relation to the inspiratory-expiratory flow of the breathing cycle.

Swallowing usually occurs during the expiratory phase of the breathing cycle, with the most common pattern being expiration-swallow-expiration. That is, expiration begins, the swallow occurs (accompanied by apnea), and then expiration continues (Martin et al., 1994; Martin-Harris, 2006; Nishino, Yonezawa, & Honda, 1985; Perlman, Ettema, & Barkmeier, 2000; Selley, Flack, Ellis, & Brooks, 1989; Smith, Wolkove, Colacone, & Kreisman, 1989). This pattern, shown in Figure 12–10, is the predominant one for swallowing over a broad range of bolus volumes and consistencies and under a variety of serving condi-

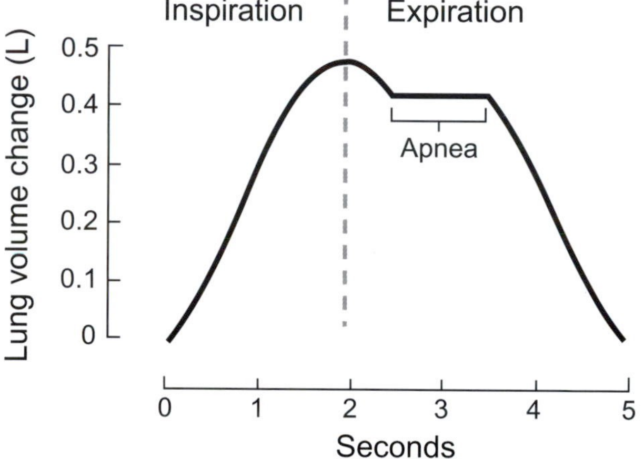

Figure 12–10. Swallow-related apnea (cessation of breathing) during expiration.

One Tug and Two Consequences

Breathing and swallowing cooperate in healthy individuals to prevent unwanted substances from entering the pulmonary airways. This cooperation can be more difficult with certain diseases. Chronic obstructive pulmonary disease (COPD) is one of these. A characteristic of this disease in advanced states is that the pulmonary apparatus expands and the diaphragm rides low and flat because air is trapped in the alveoli and airways. The abnormal positioning of the diaphragm has two potential consequences for swallowing. One is that a downward tug is placed on the larynx that tends to abduct the vocal folds and diminish their ability to protect the pulmonary airways. A second possible consequence is that the same downward tug lowers the laryngeal housing and tethers it from below. This means that the larynx may have difficulty moving up during a swallow because it has farther to go and because it must work against the downward pull of the diaphragm.

tions, such as presenting a liquid bolus with a syringe, drinking from a cup or straw, or eating solid food (Preiksaitis & Mills, 1996). This appears to be a protective mechanism for potentially "blowing" any foreign substance away from the pulmonary airways. Nevertheless, it is interesting to note that not every swallow is followed by expiration, and that some healthy individuals inspire occasionally immediately after a swallow. This is particularly prevalent in people over age 65 years (Martin-Harris et al., 2005a). Thus, it is not absolutely necessary to expire after swallowing.

Although the apneic interval during swallowing typically lasts about 1 s, it can range from less than a second to several seconds (Klaun & Perlman, 1999; Martin et al., 1994; Martin-Harris et al., 2003, 2005a; Palmer & Hiiemae, 2003; Perlman et al., 2000; Preiksaitis & Mills, 1996). In some people, the duration of the apneic period is influenced by variables such as bolus volume (Preiksaitis, Mayrand, Robins, & Diamant, 1992). Nevertheless, most of the variability in apnea duration can be attributed to variability in the onset of apnea relative to the eating or drinking event. For example, one person may stop breathing as the food or liquid is approaching the mouth, whereas another person may continue to breathe until immediately before the larynx begins to elevate for the pharyngeal transport phase of the swallow (Martin et al., 1994).

NEURAL CONTROL OF SWALLOWING

The neural control of swallowing is complex and not completely understood. Nevertheless, studies of humans and animals have offered important insights into how swallowing is controlled by the nervous system. Some of the salient features of that control are discussed below as they relate to peripheral nervous system and central nervous system participation.

Role of the Peripheral Nervous System in Swallowing

Nearly all the structures involved in swallowing are the same as those involved in speech production (the most notable exceptions being the esophagus and stomach). Those structures that participate in both swallowing and speech production are innervated by the spinal nerves and cranial nerves described in Chapters 2, 3, 4, and 5 and summarized in Table 12–1. As can be seen in the table, half of the cranial nerves (6 of 12) and most of the spinal nerves (22 of 31) are potential participants in swallowing (and speech production). The cranial nerves are involved in swallowing through their innervation of the lips, mandible, tongue, velum, pharynx, and

A Sidetrack to a Sidetrack

The previous sidetrack focused on chronic obstructive pulmonary disease (COPD) and how certain mechanical consequences of advanced stages of the disease affect swallowing. These mechanical consequences are important contributors to swallowing problems, but there is another (perhaps less obvious) problem associated with COPD that may be equally important to swallowing. People with COPD are plagued by dyspnea (breathing discomfort), a condition that causes them to avoid activities that compete with their already strong drive to breathe. Most healthy people have no idea that they hold their breath when they swallow. But, for people with severe COPD, it's quite a different story. Eating may be an unpleasant chore because the swallowing associated with it may lead to "air hunger." Do everything you can to avoid COPD and your life will be happier. Have you quit smoking yet?

Table 12–1. Summary of Motor and Sensory Nerve Supply to the Breathing Apparatus, Laryngeal Apparatus, Velopharyngeal-Nasal Apparatus, and Pharyngeal-Oral Apparatus. Spinal nerves are designated by their segmental origins (C = cervical, T = thoracic, L = lumbar). Cranial nerves are V (trigeminal), VII (facial), IX (glossopharyngeal), X (vagus), XI (accessory), and XII (hypoglossal).

	INNERVATION	
APPARATUS	MOTOR	SENSORY
Breathing	C1-C8, T1-T12, L1-L2	C1-C8, T1-T12, L1-L2
Laryngeal	V, VII, X, XI, XII, C1-C3	X*
Velopharyngeal-Nasal	V, VII, Pharyngeal Plexus**	V, VII, IX, X
Pharyngeal-Oral	V, VII, XI, XII, Pharyngeal Plexus	V, VII, IX, X

*Sensory innervation of extrinsic and supplementary laryngeal muscles includes other cranial nerves, such as V and VII.

**The pharyngeal plexus is a network that includes cranial nerves IX, X, and possibly XI.

larynx, whereas the spinal nerves are primarily involved in breathing and its cessation as they relate to swallowing.

Peripheral innervation of the esophagus differs along its length. The upper (cervical) region is made up of striated muscle, the type of muscle found in other structures of the swallowing apparatus (lips, mandible, tongue, velum, pharynx, and larynx). The cervical region, which includes the upper esophageal sphincter, is innervated by the recurrent branch of the vagus nerve (cranial nerve X), the same branch that innervates most of the intrinsic muscles of the larynx. Thus, the same peripheral nerve is responsible for the simultaneous actions of closing the larynx and opening the upper esophageal sphincter. This means that there is a strong neural link between actions that serve to protect the airway and actions that allow substances to pass into the esophagus. This strong link has obvious advantages for the coordination of the normal swallow, but also has the disadvantage that damage to the recurrent branch of the vagus nerve can have serious consequences for both voice production and swallowing (Corbin-Lewis, Liss, & Sciortino, 2005).

In lower regions of the esophagus, where smooth muscle intermingles with striated muscle (thoracic esophagus) and where smooth muscle is the only type of muscle present (abdominal esophagus), a different form of neural control operates. This control comes from the autonomic nervous system, which is generally considered to be under automatic (as opposed to voluntary) control. The autonomic nervous system has two parts, the parasympathetic and sympathetic subdivisions. The parasympathetic subdivision is important for maintaining gastrointestinal motility so that a swallowed substance moves through the esophagus easily and quickly. In contrast, the sympathetic subdivision, best known for its importance in fight-or-flight responses to stressful situations, tends to inhibit gastrointestinal motility. This is one reason why gastrointestinal problems are associated with physical and emotional stress. Many of the nerve fibers of the autonomic nervous system travel with the vagus nerve.

Role of the Central Nervous System in Swallowing

Although swallowing and speech production are executed using many of the same peripheral nerves, the central nervous system control of these two activities is quite different. This means that a given structure, such as the tongue, is under one form of neural control during swallowing and under another form of neural control during speech production. Because of this, it is entirely possible to have central nervous system damage that impairs the function of a structure for speech production but not swallowing, and vice versa.

There are two major regions within the central nervous system that are responsible for the control of swallowing. One is in the brainstem and the other is in cortical and subcortical areas. The brainstem center is located primarily in the medulla, the structure that is contiguous with the uppermost part of the spinal cord. There are two main groups of brainstem neurons that participate in swallowing, one that appears to be primarily responsible for triggering the swallow and shaping its temporal pattern and another group that appears to allocate neural drive to the various motor nerves that participate in swallowing (Jean, 2001). The brainstem center has primary control over the more automatic phases of swallowing (pharyngeal and esophageal phases).

There are also cortical and subcortical regions that may contribute to the generation and shaping of swallowing behaviors. Cortical areas include the primary motor cortex, premotor cortex, and primary sensory cortex, among others, and subcortical areas include the insular cortex and the anterior cingulate cortex, with probable contributions from basal nuclei, thalamus, and cerebellum, among others (Humbert & Robbins, 2007). Activity from these areas has a strong influence over the control and modulation of the more voluntary phases of swallowing (oral preparatory phase, including mastication, and oral transport phase). However, studies of people with cortical damage from strokes indicate that the cortex may also exert influence over what have traditionally been thought of as the automatic phases (pharyngeal and esophageal phases) of swallowing (Martin & Sessle, 1993).

Afferent input is critical to the generation of a normal swallow. The sources of afferent input are numerous and include, but are not limited to, information related to (a) muscle length and rate of length change, (b) muscle tension, (c) joint position and movement, (d) surface and deep pressures, (e) surface deformation, (f) temperature, (g) taste, and (h) noxious stimuli. Afferent activity is generated by receptors in the swallowing apparatus and sent to the brainstem, where such activity may trigger the motor output required to elicit the pharyngeal phase of the swallow or it may modulate the motor output to accommodate a larger-than-expected bolus. Afferent activity may also be sent on to subcortical regions (such as the thalamus) or cortical regions (such as the sensorimotor cortex) where it may be consciously perceived. Often the perception is a pleasant experience, such as savoring the flavor and texture of ice cream, or it may be unpleasant (see Figure 12–11 and sidetrack on sphenopalatineganglioneuralgia).

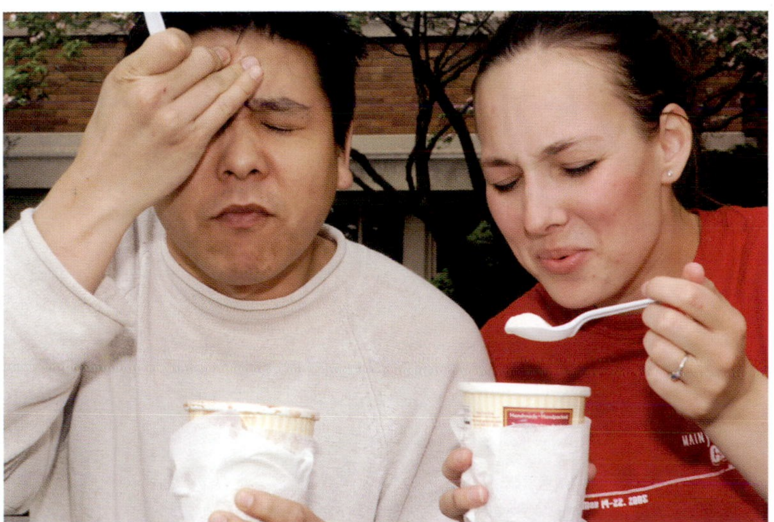

Figure 12–11. Sphenopalatineganglioneuralgia (or so-called "brain freeze") caused by placing something cold against the roof of the mouth. Image provided courtesy of the University of Cincinnati. Reproduced with permission.

Sphenopalatineganglioneuralgia

Boy, that sounds like something you wouldn't want to meet in the dark. But it comes from something really good. As a child (or even as an adult) you may have said the phrase, "I scream, you scream, we all scream for ice cream." Scream has a meaning of anticipation in this context, but it can also have a meaning of hurting. You know the feeling. You take a bite of ice cream and momentarily hold it against the roof of your mouth before you swallow it. Then suddenly you get an intense, stabbing pain in your forehead. What's up? The pain is caused as your hard palate warms up after you made it cold. Cold causes vasoconstriction (reduction in blood vessel diameter) in the region, which is followed by rapid vasodilation (increase in blood vessel diameter). It's the rapid vasodilation that hurts and gets your attention. Fortunately, the pain lasts only a few seconds. Be thankful. There's all that ice cream still waiting to be eaten.

VARIABLES THAT INFLUENCE SWALLOWING

A number of variables influence swallowing. Some relate to the characteristics of the bolus, the swallowing mode, and the prevailing body position. There are also developmental and aging effects on swallowing, but essentially no influence of sex.

Bolus Characteristics and Swallowing

Although the act of swallowing occurs generally as described near the beginning of this chapter, the precise nature of the swallow is determined, in part, by what exactly is being swallowed. Bolus consistency, volume, and taste are three variables that have been found to influence the act of swallowing.

Consistency

One of the most important consistency contrasts that determines swallowing behavior is the difference between liquids and solids. Whereas a liquid bolus is usually held briefly in the front of the oral cavity before being propelled to the pharynx, chewed food may be moved to the pharynx and left there for several seconds while the remainder of the bolus continues to be chewed (Hiiemae & Palmer, 1999; Palmer, Rudin, Lara, & Crompton, 1992—see Figure 12–9). Although this can also happen with liquids (Linden, Tippett, Johnston, Siebens, & French, 1989), it is much less common, except in cases where a combined liquid-and-solid bolus is chewed and swallowed (Saitoh et al., 2007), such as with normal mealtime eating (Dua et al., 1997). For example, imagine milk without cookies or cookies without milk. Ridiculous.

Substances can be characterized on a viscosity continuum, ranging from substances as thin as water to substances as thick as pudding. Such differences in viscosity have been shown to influence swallowing. That is, higher viscosity (thicker) liquids tend to take longer to swallow than lower viscosity (thinner) liquids (Chi-Fishman & Sonies, 2002), as a result of longer oral and pharyngeal phase events and longer upper esophageal sphincter opening durations (Dantas et al., 1990). The swallowing of higher viscosity substances is also associated with larger tongue forces than the swallowing of lower viscosity substances (Miller & Watkin, 1996). As might be predicted, it is more difficult to maintain a cohesive (single) bolus when swallowing thinner liquids as compared to thicker liquids. As a result, laryngeal penetration (where part of the bolus moves into the laryngeal vestibule, but remains above the vocal folds—Robbins et al., 1992) is more common when swallowing thin liquids than when swallowing thicker substances (Daggett, Logemann, Rademaker, & Pauloski, 2006).

It is also relevant to mention that swallowing occurs regularly throughout the day and night without the introduction of an external substance. These are called nonbolus swallows, dry swallows, or saliva swallows and they constitute the swallowing of saliva. These swallows are sometimes stimulated by pooling of saliva in the pharynx and can be initiated in the absence of oral preparatory and oral transport phases (Logemann, 1998).

Volume

It seems intuitive that the volume (size) of the bolus might affect the swallow and most studies indicate that, in fact, it does (Chi-Fishman & Sonies, 2002; Cook et al., 1989; Kahrilas & Logemann, 1993; Logemann et al., 2000; Logemann, Pauloski, Rademaker, & Kahrilas, 2002; Perlman, Palmer, McCullough, & VanDaele, 1999; Perlman, Schultz, VanDaele, 1993; Tasko, Kent, & Westbury, 2002). When swallowing a larger bolus compared to swallowing a smaller bolus, tongue movements are generally larger and faster, hyoid bone movements begin earlier and are larger, pharyngeal wall movements and laryngeal movements are more extensive, and the upper esophageal sphincter opens earlier and stays open longer (Kahrilas & Logemann, 1993). This means that events related to tongue propulsion of the bolus, closing of the velopharynx, protection of the pulmonary airways, and opening of the upper esophageal sphincter are conditioned by bolus volume in ways that are more sustained and more vigorous for larger boluses than smaller boluses. Whether or not apnea is longer during the swallowing of larger (versus smaller) boluses has yet to be convincingly determined (Martin-Harris, 2006).

Despite the success of the adjustments made to accommodate a larger bolus, there tends to be a greater frequency of laryngeal penetration as bolus size increases, at least for liquid boluses. Specifically, part of the bolus penetrates the laryngeal vestibule more than twice as often when swallowing a 10-ml bolus than when swallowing a 1-ml bolus (Daggett et al., 2006). Nevertheless, when laryngeal penetration occurs in healthy individuals, the substance is almost always pushed away from the larynx and transported to the esophagus without being aspirated (going below the vocal folds).

Taste and Temperature

Taste and temperature contribute enormously to the enjoyment of the eating and drinking experience. Imagine, for a moment, eating a hot fudge sundae and how much of the pleasurable eating experience is derived from the special combination of vanilla and chocolate flavors and hot and cold temperatures.

Tastes include sweet, salty, sour, bitter, and other tastes (such as umami, meaning meaty or savory). Substances of different tastes (but of the same consistency and volume) may influence certain features of swallowing. For example, substances with taste (sweet, salty, sour), when compared to tasteless substances, are generally associated with higher peak

Gutsy Stuff

Taste receptors in the tongue get all the press and all the credit for making things taste sweet. Put a little sugar or artificial sweetener in your mouth and the taste receptors in your tongue will come to attention and tell your brain about it. But the taste of sweetness is not just limited to your mouth. Receptors that sense sugar and artificial sweetener have also been found in the gut (Margolskee et al., 2007). These gut receptors taste glucose in the same way that taste cells in your tongue signal sweetness to the brain. They've been found to influence the secretion of insulin and hormones that regulate blood sugar level and influence appetite. Those are two very important responsibilities. This is all very gutsy stuff and is touted by its discoverers as possibly leading to new treatment options for obesity and diabetes. Let's hope they're right.

station is shown in Figure 12–13 (also see the lower part of Figure 3–48 in Chapter 3 which shows nasal insertion of a flexible endoscope).

The examination usually includes a preliminary viewing of the velopharyngeal region, pharyngeal walls, back part of the tongue, epiglottis, aryepiglottic folds, epiglottic valleculae, pyriform sinuses, laryngeal vestibule, ventricular folds, vocal folds, and the inlet to the esophagus. Abnormalities in structure or color are noted and are used to help interpret abnormal swallow behaviors. Swallowing is evaluated in much the same way as for a videofluroscopic examination, by using food and liquid of different consistencies and volumes (the major difference being that no barium is required). Descriptions provided by the speech-language pathologist might include the presence/absence of substance remaining in the epiglottic valleculae or pyriform sinuses following the pharyngeal transport phase of swallowing, whether or not substance invaded the laryngeal vestibule (laryngeal penetration), and whether or not there is evidence that substance traveled below the vocal folds (aspiration).

Endoscopy offers certain advantages over other approaches to evaluating swallowing. To begin, the equipment is easily portable so that the examination can be done at bedside in a hospital, there is no exposure to x-rays and no need to use barium products, and it is possible to see structural and color abnormalities. In addition, the procedure can often be performed by a speech-language pathologist without the direct oversight of a physician or the aid of other health care professionals. Finally, the speech-language pathologist can observe the client eat an entire meal at the client's usual pace.

The major disadvantage of an endoscopic approach is that, during the pharyngeal transport phase of the swallow, there is a moment when the endoscopic view is blocked as the tongue and pharynx approximate. Also, there are some clients who cannot tolerate the procedure, including those with hyperkinetic movement disorders, bleeding disorders, or certain cardiac conditions. Furthermore, it is sometimes difficult to detect aspiration with endoscopy. Nevertheless, one way to improve such detection is to infuse the swallowed substance with

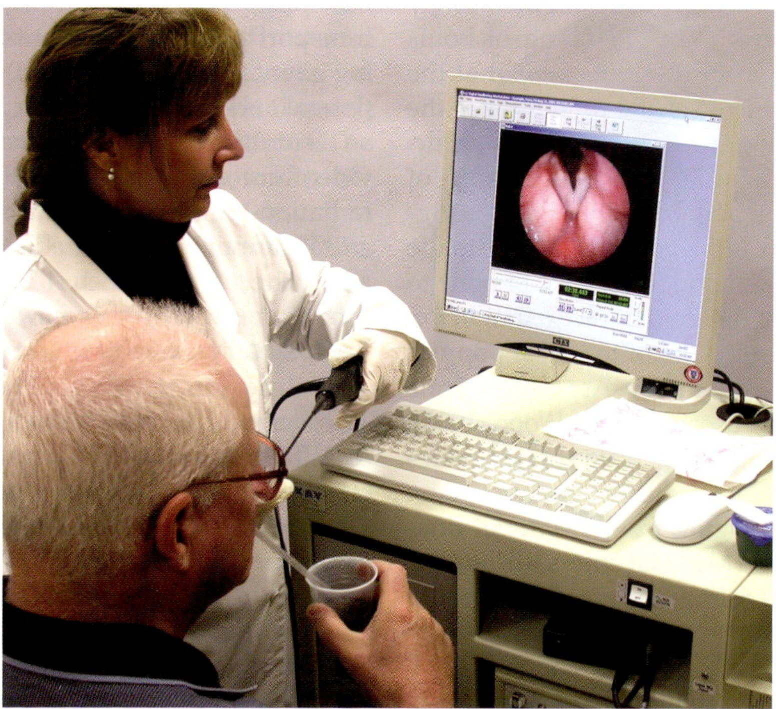

Figure 12–13. Fiberoptic endoscope used for evaluation of swallowing. Image provided courtesy of KayPENTAX, Lincoln Park, NJ. Reproduced with permission.

green or blue dye. In this way, the endoscope can be directed into the laryngeal vestibule immediately following the swallow to look for any green or blue substance that may have been deposited near or below the vocal folds.

Ultrasonography

Another way to visualize swallowing events is with ultrasonography. The use of ultrasonography as it applies to the measurement of speech production is discussed in Chapter 5, and similar procedures can be applied to the measurement of swallowing. Briefly, ultrasonography requires the use of a transducer that generates and receives a high-frequency signal (sound waves). The transducer is pressed against the skin (usually on the undersurface of the mandible) and the signal is transmitted through the tissue toward the airway. When the signal encounters air, it reflects back. The receiver senses the returning sound waves and the resultant signal is processed to provide an image of the outline of the proximal border of the airway.

Ultrasonography is applied to the measurement of swallowing much less frequently than are videofluoroscopy and flexible endoscopy. Nevertheless, it can offer some valuable information especially in relation to the behavior of the tongue (Stone & Shawker, 1986), lateral pharyngeal walls (Miller & Watkin, 1997), and other structures by way of images obtained in sagittal, frontal, and transverse planes. It may also be a useful biofeedback tool in the management of oral preparatory phase behavior (Shawker & Sonies, 1985). Its major limitation is that aspiration cannot be detected.

Manometry

Manometry refers to the measurement of pressure. In the context of swallowing, two types of manometric measurement approaches are of interest. One allows for measurement of pressure in the pharyngeal and upper esophageal sphincter regions and one allows inferences to be made regarding the temporal relationship between swallowing events and breathing events.

Technological advances have made manometric measurements of pharyngeal and upper esophageal sphincter events more accurate and have, therefore, made valuable additions to understanding swallowing events, especially those related to disordered swallow (Hila et al., 2001). A modern manometric device comprises a small-diameter catheter containing miniature pressure transducers, with perhaps two or more positioned in the pharynx and one positioned within the upper esophageal sphincter (or all of them positioned in the esophagus). The output signals can provide information about the magnitude of the pressures generated during the pharyngeal propulsive wave, the squeezing pressures exerted within the upper esophageal sphincter, and the magnitude of relaxation (pressure drop) of the upper esophageal sphincter during the passage of the bolus. Concurrent videofluoroscopic imaging can be used with manometry for more accurate interpretation of the pressure signals (Hila et al., 2001; Logemann, 1998). Although manometric measurements can be used to assess pharyngeal function, they are most often used to evaluate esophageal function. This form of manometry is conducted under the direction of a gastroenterologist (see section below on Clinical Professionals and Swallowing Disorders) and is typically accompanied by simultaneous videofluoroscopic imaging of the esophagus (barium swallow study).

A different type of pressure measurement can be used to determine the relationship between swallowing and breathing. This is nasal air pressure that is sensed near the nares using a small, double-barreled catheter connected to a pressure transducer. During nasal breathing, this pressure is below atmospheric for inspiration and above atmospheric for expiration. When nasal pressure is recorded simultaneously with videofluoroscopic imaging, it is possible to infer the temporal relationships among certain swallowing events and inspiration, expiration, and apnea (Martin-Harris et al., 2005a; Perlman, He, Barkmeier, & Van Leer, 2005).

SWALLOWING DISORDERS

Another word for swallowing disorder is dysphagia (pronounced dis-FAY-juh). Dysphagia comes in many forms and can have many different causes. Occasionally it can have a functional cause (no

The term swallowing is ingrained as a synonym for deglutition, and is used as such in this chapter, although swallowing technically involves only part of the deglutition process.

Many of the important anatomical and physiological components of the speech production apparatus, discussed in Chapters 2, 3, 4, and 5 of this text, are also important anatomical and physiological components of the swallowing apparatus.

The esophagus is a muscular tube that extends from the lower border of the pharynx to the stomach and is bounded at its two ends by high-pressure valves (the upper esophageal sphincter and the lower esophageal sphincter) that govern the passage of food and liquid into and out of the structure.

The stomach is a liter-sized sac whose upper end connects to the esophagus through the lower esophageal sphincter and whose lower end connects to the small intestine through the pyloric sphincter.

The forces of swallowing are greater and the movements of swallowing are generally slower than those associated with speech production.

Passive forces of swallowing come from the natural recoil of structures, surface tension between structures in apposition, gravity, and aeromechanical factors, whereas active forces result from the activation of breathing, laryngeal, velopharyngeal-nasal, and pharyngeal-oral muscles in various combinations.

Different pressure gradients are critical to the swallowing process and are influenced by pressures existing within the oral cavity, the upper esophageal sphincter, the esophagus, the lower esophageal sphincter, and the stomach.

The forces and movements associated with the act of swallowing can be categorized in four phases that include an oral preparatory phase, oral transport phase, pharyngeal transport phase, and esophageal transport phase.

The oral preparatory phase involves taking food or liquid in through the oral vestibule and manipulating it within the oral cavity to prepare the bolus (lump of food or liquid volume) for passage.

The oral transport phase involves movement of the bolus (or a part of it) through the oral cavity toward the pharynx by rearward propulsion.

The pharyngeal transport phase is usually "triggered" when the bolus passes the anterior faucial pillars, and results from a combination of compressive actions that force the bolus downward toward the esophagus.

The esophageal transport phase pushes the bolus through the esophagus toward the stomach by a series of peristaltic waves of muscular contraction and relaxation that progress down the muscular tube and which are followed by secondary waves that clear the esophagus.

Swallowing usually occurs during expiration and is associated with a brief apneic interval (cessation of breathing).

The neural control of swallowing is vested in the brainstem and in other higher brain centers that oversee automatic and voluntary aspects of the different phases of swallowing.

Characteristics of the bolus can influence the swallowing pattern, including bolus consistency, bolus volume, the taste evoked by the bolus, and bolus temperature.

The mode of swallowing has an impact on the swallowing process, with differences observed for single swallows versus sequential swallows, cued swallows versus spontaneous swallows, and with dependencies on how the food or liquid is presented.

Details of the swallowing pattern may change with changes in body position, including when swallowing occurs during the breathing cycle, the timing of certain swallowing events, and the magnitudes of certain pressures.

The development of swallowing is rapid and complex and moves through different sucking and chewing patterns toward adult-like eating and drinking behaviors, and carries with it important developmental processes related to social and emotional development.

Age influences swallowing in that the overall duration of the swallow increases in older individuals and the spatial and temporal coordination among certain structures of the swallowing apparatus undergo modification.

Sex of the individual makes little difference to the nature of swallowing.

Several methods are used to measure swallowing events, including videofluoroscopy (which uses x-rays to image all phases of swallowing), endoscopy (which uses a flexible endoscope to image the pharyngeal, laryngeal, and esophageal regions), ultrasonography (which uses ultrasound to image the structures of swallowing), and manometry (which uses pressure transducers to sense pressure change in the pharynx and/or esophagus, or air pressure change at the nares).

A swallowing disorder (also called dysphagia) may be characterized as oropharyngeal dysphagia or esophageal dysphagia and may have no apparent physical cause or, more commonly, has structural, neurogenic, or systemic causes.

Some of the more important clinical professionals who work with individuals with swallowing disorders include speech-language pathologists, radiologists, gastroenterologists, otolaryngologists, dietitians, and occupational therapists.

Scenario

There was no cure. No way to slow it down. There was nothing but nature and the ticking of time. Her referral to a speech-language pathologist had given her helpful strategies for drinking and eating more safely. Crackers, steak, and her beloved honey-roasted cashews gave way to pudding, oatmeal, and thick soups. She concentrated on taking small bites and on tucking her chin when she swallowed. She maintained her weight for a period of time, but her swallowing problem worsened. She choked often and came to dislike eating altogether, a combination that led to weight loss at a dangerous rate. Re-evaluation by the speech-language pathologist revealed that she was aspirating frequently. The medical option of choice was a feeding tube. She resisted but with the urging of her family she agreed to have a tube inserted into her stomach through which nutrition and hydration could be delivered safely. She was allowed to drink water as long as it was pure and her mouth was clean.

As time went by, breathing became the focus of her existence. She felt starved for air and would tend to exhaust herself to satisfy her air hunger. Eventually she could no longer breathe on her own and was placed on a positive-pressure ventilator by her pulmonologist. The ventilator evoked mixed feelings. She had sadness at the thought of being "on life support," but relief at no longer struggling to breathe. By this time, all attempts to maintain her residual speech were abandoned and she had transitioned to a "talking computer" that enabled her to carry on conversations with her family and the few friends who were comfortable enough with her condition to visit her. Nothing else was as important as this connection to the people she loved.

She left one quiet morning with a nurse sleeping at her side. She had been saying goodbyes in various forms for months. The time she chose was sometime between 4:00 and 5:00 AM, that mystical span when so many choose to steal away. The air was still and the lake was as smooth as glass.

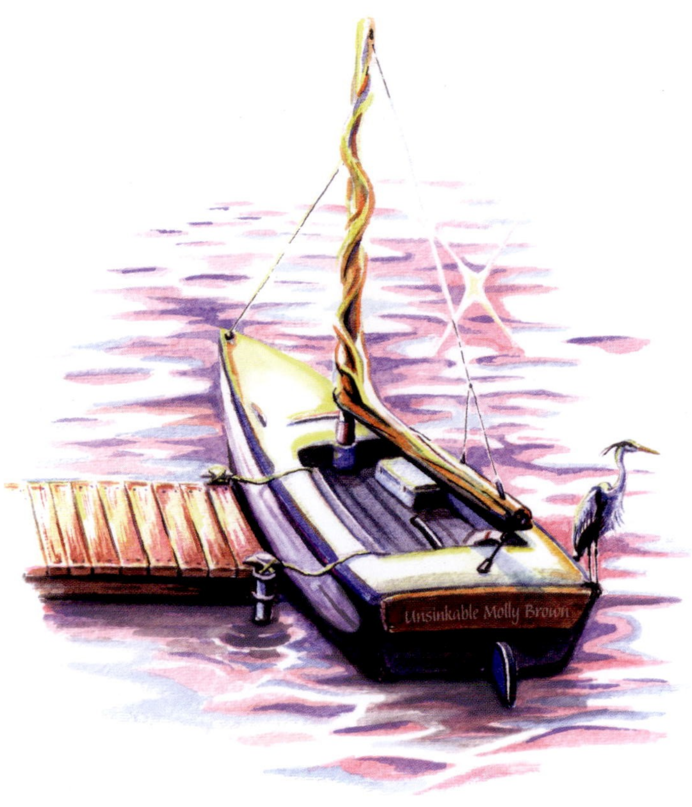

REFERENCES

Arvedson, J., & Brodsky, L. (2002). *Pediatric swallowing and feeding: Assessment and management* (2nd ed.). Clifton Park, NY: Thompson Learning (Singular Publishing Group).

Barkmeier, J., Bielamowicz, S., Takeda, N., & Ludlow, C. (2002). Laryngeal activity during upright vs. supine swallowing. *Journal of Applied Physiology, 93*, 740–745.

Barofsky, I., & Fontaine, K. (1998). Do psychogenic dysphagia patients have an eating disorder? *Dysphagia, 13*, 24–27.

Bisch, E., Logemann, J., Rademaker, A., Kahrilas, P., & Lazarus, C. (1994). Pharyngeal effects of bolus volume, viscosity, and temperature in patients with dysphagia resulting from neurologic impairment and in normal subjects. *Journal of Speech and Hearing Research, 37*, 1041–1059.

Bosma, J. (1986). Development of feeding. *Clinical Nutrition, 5*, 210–218.

Castell, J., Dalton, C., & Castell, D. (1990). Effects of body position and bolus consistency on the manometric parameters and coordination of the upper esophageal sphincter and pharynx. *Dysphagia, 5*, 179–186.

Chi-Fishman, G., & Sonies, B. (2000). Motor strategy in rapid sequential swallowing: New insights. *Journal of Speech, Language, and Hearing Research, 43*, 1481–1492.

Chi-Fishman, G., & Sonies, B. (2002). Effects of systematic bolus viscosity and volume changes on hyoid movement kinematics. *Dysphagia, 17*, 278–287.

Chi-Fishman, G., Stone, M., & McCall, G. (1998). Lingual action in normal sequential swallowing. *Journal of Speech, Language, and Hearing Research, 41*, 771–785.

Cook, I., Dodds, W., Dantas, R., Kern, M., Massey, B., Shaker, R., & Hogan, W.. (1989). Timing of videofluoroscopic, manometric events, and bolus transit during the oral and pharyngeal phases of swallowing. *Dysphagia, 4*, 8–15.

Cook, I., Weltman, M., Wallace, K., Shaw, D., McKay, E., Smart, R., & Butler, S.. (1994). Influence of aging on oral-pharyngeal bolus transit and clearance during swallowing: Scintigraphic study. *American Journal of Physiology, 266*, G972–G977.

Corbin-Lewis, K., Liss, J., & Sciortino, K. (2005). *Clinical anatomy and physiology of the swallow mechanism*. Clifton Park, NY: Thomson Delmar Learning.

Daggett, A., Logemann, J., Rademaker, A., & Pauloski, B. (2006). Laryngeal penetration during deglutition in normal subjects of various ages. *Dysphagia, 21*, 270–274.

Daniels, S., Corey, D., Hadskey, L., Legendre, C., Priestly, D., Rosenbek, J., & Foundas, A.. (2004). Mechanism of sequential swallowing during straw drinking in healthy young and older adults. *Journal of Speech, Language, and Hearing Research*, *47*, 33–45.

Daniels, S., & Foundas, A. (2001). Swallowing physiology of sequential straw drinking. *Dysphagia*, *16*, 176–182.

Daniels, S., Schroeder, M., DeGeorge, P., Corey, D., & Rosenbek, J. (2007). Effects of verbal cue on bolus flow during swallowing. *American Journal of Speech-Language Pathology*, *16*, 140–147.

Dantas, R., Kern, M., Massey, B., Dodds, W., Kahrilas, P., Brasseur, J., Cook, I., & Lang, I. (1990). Effect of swallowed bolus variables on oral and pharyngeal phases of swallowing. *American Journal of Physiology*, *258*, G675–G681.

Dejaeger, E., Pelemans, W., Ponette, E., & VanTrappen, G. (1994). Effect of body position on deglutition. *Digestive Diseases and Sciences*, *39*, 762–765.

Ding, R., Logemann, J., Larson, C., & Rademaker, A. (2003). The effects of taste and consistency on swallow physiology in younger and older healthy individuals: A surface electromyographic study. *Journal of Speech, Language, and Hearing Research*, *46*, 977–989.

Dodds, W., Hogan, W., Reid, D., Stewart, E., & Arndorfer, R. (1973). A comparison between primary esophageal peristalsis following wet and dry swallows. *Journal of Applied Physiology*, *35*, 851–857.

Dodds, W., Taylor, A., Stewart, E., Kern, M., Logemann, J., & Cook, I. (1989). Tipper and dipper types of oral swallows. *American Journal of Roentgenology*, *153*, 1197–1199.

Dua, K., Ren, J., Bardan, E., Xie, P., & Shaker, R. (1997). Coordination of deglutitive glottal function and pharyngeal bolus transit during normal eating. *Gastroenterology*, *112*, 73–83.

Ekberg, O., & Sigurjonsson, S. (1982). Movement of epiglottis during deglutition: A cineradiographic study. *Gastrointestinal Radiology*, *7*, 101–107.

Fink, B., & Demarest, R. (1978). *Laryngeal biomechanics*. Cambridge, MA: Harvard University Press.

Fink, B., Martin, R., & Rohrmann, C. (1979). Biomechanics of the human epiglottis. *Acta Otolaryngologica*, *87*, 554–559.

Goyal, R., & Cobb, B. (1981). Motility of the pharynx, esophagus, and esophageal sphincters. In L. Johnson (Ed.), *Physiology of the gastrointestinal tract* (pp. 359–390). New York: Raven Press.

Green, J., Moore, C., Ruark, J., Rodda, P., Morvee, W., & VanWitzenburg, M. (1997). Development of chewing in children from 12 to 48 months: Longitudinal study of EMG patterns. *Journal of Neurophysiology*, *77*, 2704–2716.

Hiiemae, K., & Palmer, J. (1999). Food transport and bolus formation during complete feeding sequences on foods of different initial consistency. *Dysphagia*, *14*, 31–42.

Hila, A., Castell, J., & Castell, D. (2001). Pharyngeal and upper esophageal sphincter manometry in the evaluation of dysphagia. *Journal of Clinical Gastroenterology*, *33*, 355–361.

Hirst, L., Ford, G., Gibson, G., & Wilson, J. (2002). Swallow-induced alterations in breathing in normal older people. *Dysphagia*, *17*, 152–161.

Humbert, I., & Robbins, J. (2007). Normal swallowing and functional magnetic resonance imaging: A systematic review. *Dysphagia*, *22*, 266–275.

Humphrey, T. (1970). Reflex activity in the oral and facial area of the human fetus. In J. Bosma (Ed.), *Second symposium on oral sensation and perception* (pp. 195–233). Springfield, IL: Charles C. Thomas.

Ingervall, B., & Lantz, B. (1973). Significance of gravity on the passage of bolus through the human pharynx. *Archives of Oral Biology*, *18*, 351–356.

Jean, A. (2001). Brain stem control of swallowing: Neuronal network and cellular mechanisms. *Physiological Reviews*, *81*, 929–969.

Johnson, F., Shaw, D., Gabb, M., Dent, J., & Cook, I. (1995). Influence of gravity and body position on normal oropharyngeal swallowing. *American Journal of Physiology*, *269*, G653–G658.

Kahrilas, P., & Logemann, J. (1993). Volume accommodation during swallowing. *Dysphagia*, *8*, 259–265.

Klaun, M., & Perlman, A. (1999). Temporal and durational patterns associating respiration and swallowing. *Dysphagia*, *14*, 131–138.

Koenig, J., Davies, A., & Thach, B. (1990). Coordination of breathing, sucking, and swallowing during bottle feedings in human infants. *Journal of Applied Physiology*, *69*, 1623–1629.

Langmore, S., Schatz, K., & Olson, N. (1988). Fiberoptic endoscopic evaluation of swallowing safety: A new procedure. *Dysphagia*, *2*, 216–219.

Leonard, R., & McKenzie, S. (2006). Hyoid-bolus transit latencies in normal swallow. *Dysphagia*, *21*, 183–190.

Leonard, R., & McKenzie, S. (2008). Dynamic swallow studies: Measurement techniques. In R. Leonard & K. Kendall (Eds.), *Dysphagia assessment and treatment planning: A team approach* (2nd ed., pp. 265–294). San Diego, CA: Plural.

Leow, L., Huckabee, M., Sharma, S., & Tooley, T. (2007). The influence of taste on swallowing apnea, oral preparation time, and duration and amplitude of submental muscle contraction. *Chemical Senses*, *32*, 119–128.

Lever, T., Cox, K., Holbert, D., Shahrier, M., Hough, M., & Kelley-Salamon, K. (2007). The effect of effortful swallow on the normal adult esophagus. *Dysphagia*, *22*, 312–325.

Linden, M., Hogosta, S., & Norlander, T. (2007). Monitoring of pharyngeal and upper esophageal sphincter activity with an arterial dilation balloon catheter. *Dysphagia, 22,* 81–88.

Linden, P., Tippett, D., Johnston, J., Siebens, A., & French, J. (1989). Bolus position at swallow onset in normal adults: Preliminary observations. *Dysphagia, 4,* 146–150.

Logemann, J. (1998). *Evaluation and treatment of swallowing disorders* (2nd ed.). Austin, TX: Pro-Ed.

Logemann, J., Boshes, B., Blonsky, E., & Fisher, H. (1977). Speech and swallowing evaluation in the differential diagnosis of neurologic disease. *Neurologia, Neurocirugia, and Psiquiatria, 18*(2–3 Suppl.), 71–78.

Logemann, J., Kahrilas, P., Kobara, M., & Vakil, N. (1989). The benefit of head rotation on pharyngo-esophageal dysphagia. *Archives of Physical Medicine and Rehabilitation, 70,* 767–771.

Logemann, J., Pauloski, B., Rademaker, A., Colangelo, L., Kahrilas, P., & Smith, C. (2000). Temporal and biomechanical characteristics of oropharyngeal swallow in younger and older men. *Journal of Speech, Language, and Hearing Research, 43,* 1264–1274.

Logemann, J., Pauloski, B., Rademaker, A., & Kahrilas, P. (2002). Oropharyngeal swallow in younger and older women: Videofluoroscopic analysis. *Journal of Speech, Language, and Hearing Research, 45,* 434–445.

Margolskee, R., Dyer, J., Kokrashvili, Z., Salmon, K., Ilegems, E., Daly, K., Ninomiya Y., Mosinger, B., & Shirazi-Beechey, S. (2007). T1R3 and gustducin in gut sense sugars to regulate expression of Na+-glucose cotransporter 1. *Proceedings of the National Academy of Sciences, 104,* 15075–15080.

Martin, B., Logemann, J., Shaker, R., & Dodds, W. (1994). Coordination between respiration and swallowing: Respiratory phase relationships and temporal integration. *Journal of Applied Physiology, 76,* 714–723.

Martin, R., & Sessle, B. (1993). The role of the cerebral cortex in swallowing. *Dysphagia, 8,* 195–202.

Martin-Harris, B. (May 16, 2006). Coordination of respiration and swallowing. *GI Motility Online.*

Martin-Harris, B., Brodsky, M., Michel, Y., Ford, C., Walters, B., & Heffner, J. (2005a). Breathing and swallowing dynamics across the adult lifespan. *Archives of Otolaryngology-Head and Neck Surgery, 131,* 762–770.

Martin-Harris, B., Brodsky, M., Price, C., Michel, Y., & Walters, B. (2003). Temporal coordination of pharyngeal and laryngeal dynamics with breathing during swallowing: Single liquid swallows. *Journal of Applied Physiology, 94,* 1735–1743.

Martin-Harris, B., Michel, Y., & Castell, D. (2005b). Physiologic model of oropharyngeal swallowing revisited. *Otolaryngology-Head and Neck Surgery, 133,* 234–240.

McFarland, D., & Lund, J. (1995). Modification of mastication and respiration during swallowing in the adult human. *Journal of Neurophysiology, 74,* 1509–1517.

McFarland, D., Lund, J., & Gagner, M. (1994). Effects of posture on the coordination of respiration and swallowing. *Journal of Neurophysiology, 72,* 2431–2437.

Mendell, D., & Logemann, J. (2007). Temporal sequence of swallow events during the oropharyngeal swallow. *Journal of Speech, Language, and Hearing Research, 50,* 1256–1271.

Meyer, G., Gerhardt, D., & Castell, D. (1981). Human esophageal response to rapid swallowing: Muscle refractory period or neural inhibition? *American Journal of Physiology, 241,* G129–G136.

Miller, J., & Watkin, K. (1996). The influence of bolus volume and viscosity on anterior lingual force during the oral stage of swallowing. *Dysphagia, 11,* 117–124.

Miller, J., & Watkin, K. (1997). Lateral pharyngeal wall motion during swallowing using real time ultrasound. *Dysphagia, 12,* 125–132.

Miyaoka, Y., Haishima, K., Takagi, M., Haishima, H., Asari, J., & Yamada, Y. (2006). Influences of thermal and gustatory characteristics on sensory and motor aspects of swallowing. *Dysphagia, 21,* 38–48.

Nishino, T., Yonezawa, T., & Honda, Y. (1985). Effects of swallowing on the pattern of continuous respiration in human adults. *American Review of Respiratory Disease, 132,* 1219–1222.

Palmer, J. (1998). Bolus aggregation in the oropharynx does not depend on gravity. *Archives of Physical Medicine and Rehabilitation, 79,* 691–696.

Palmer, J., & Hiiemae, K. (2003). Eating and breathing: Interactions between respiration and feeding on solid food. *Dysphagia, 18,* 169–178.

Palmer, P., McCullouch, T., Jaffe, D., & Neel, A. (2005). Effects of a sour bolus on the intramuscular electromyographic (EMG) activity of muscles in the submental region. *Dysphagia, 20,* 210–217.

Palmer, J., Rudin, N., Lara, G., & Crompton, A. (1992). Coordination of mastication and swallowing. *Dysphagia, 7,* 187–200.

Pelletier, C., & Dhanaraj, G. (2006). The effect of taste and palatability on lingual swallowing pressure. *Dysphagia, 21,* 121–128.

Perlman, A., Ettema, S., & Barkmeier, J. (2000). Respiratory and acoustic signals associated with bolus passage during swallowing. *Dysphagia, 15,* 89–94.

Perlman, A., He, X., Barkmeier, J., & Van Leer, E. (2005). Bolus location associated with videofluoroscopic and respirodeglutometric events. *Journal of Speech, Language, and Hearing Research, 48,* 21–33.

Perlman, A., Palmer, P., McCullough, T., & VanDaele, D. (1999). Electromyographic activity from human laryngeal, pharyngeal, and submental muscles during swallowing. *Journal of Applied Physiology, 86,* 1663–1669.

Perlman, A., Schultz, J., & VanDaele, D. (1993). Effects of age, gender, bolus volume, and bolus viscosity on oropharyngeal pressure during swallowing. *Journal of Applied Physiology*, *75*, 33–37.

Pitcher, J., Crandall, M., & Goodrich, S. (2008). Pediatric clinical feeding assessment. In R. Leonard & K. Kendall (Eds.), *Dysphagia assessment and treatment planning: A team approach* (2nd ed., pp. 117–136). San Diego, CA: Plural.

Preiksaitis, H., Mayrand, S., Robins, K., & Diamant, N. (1992). Coordination of respiration and swallowing: Effect of bolus volume in normal adults. *American Journal of Physiology*, *263*, R624–R630.

Preiksaitis, H., & Mills, C. (1996). Coordination of respiration and swallowing: Effects of bolus consistency and presentation in normal adults. *Journal of Applied Physiology*, *81*, 1707–1714.

Ramsey, G., Watson, J., Gramiak, R., & Weinberg, S. (1955). Cinefluorographic analysis of the mechanism of swallowing. *Radiology*, *64*, 498–518.

Ravich, W., Wilson, R., Jones, B., & Donner, M. (1989). Psychogenic dysphagia and globus: Reevaluation of 23 patients. *Dysphagia*, *4*, 35–38.

Robbins, J., Hamilton, J., Lof, G., & Kempster, G. (1992). Oropharyngeal swallowing in normal adults of different ages. *Gastroenterology*, *103*, 823–829.

Rosenbek, J., Robbins, J., Roecker, E., Coyle, J., & Wood, J. (1996) A penetration-aspiration scale. *Dysphagia*, *11*, 93–98.

Saitoh, E., Shibata, S., Matsuo, K., Baba, M., Fujii, W., & Palmer, J. (2007). Chewing and food consistency: Effects on bolus transport and swallow initiation. *Dysphagia*, *22*, 100–107.

Sears, V., Castell, J., & Castell, D. (1990). Comparison of effects of upright versus supine body position and liquid versus solid bolus on esophageal pressures in normal humans. *Digestive Diseases and Sciences*, *35*, 857–864.

Selley, W., Flack, F., Ellis, R., & Brooks, W. (1989). Respiratory patterns associated with swallowing: Part I. The normal adult pattern and changes with age. *Age and Ageing*, *18*, 168–172.

Shapiro, J., Franko, D., & Gagne, A. (1997). Phagophobia: A form of psychogenic dysphagia. A new entity. *Annals of Otolaryngology, Rhinology, and Laryngology*, *106*, 286–290.

Shawker, T., & Sonies, B. (1985). Ultrasound biofeedback for speech training. *Investigative Radiology*, *20*, 90–93.

Smith, J., Wolkove, N., Colacone, A., & Kreisman, H. (1989). Coordination of eating, drinking, and breathing in adults. *Chest*, *96*, 578–582.

Sonies, B., Parent, L., Morrish, K., & Baum, B. (1988). Durational aspects of the oral-pharyngeal phase of swallow in normal adults. *Dysphagia*, *3*, 1–10.

Steele, C., & Huckabee, M. (2007). The influence of orolingual pressure on the timing of pharyngeal pressure events. *Dysphagia*, *22*, 30–36.

Stone, M., & Shawker, T. (1986). An ultrasound examination of tongue movement during swallowing. *Dysphagia*, *1*, 78–83.

Tasko, S., Kent, R., & Westbury, J. (2002). Variability in tongue movement kinematics during normal liquid swallow. *Dysphagia*, *17*, 126–138.

Tracy, J., Logemann, J., Kahrilas, P., Jacob, P., Kobara, M., & Krugler, C. (1989). Preliminary observations on the effects of age on oropharyngeal deglutition. *Dysphagia*, *4*, 90–94.

VanDaele, D., Perlman, A., & Casell, M. (1995). Intrinsic fibre architecture attachments of the human epiglottis and their contributions to the mechanism of deglutition. *Journal of Anatomy*, *186*, 1–15.

Wilson, S., Thach, B., Brouillette, R., & Abu-Osba, Y. (1981). Coordination of breathing and swallowing in human infants. *Journal of Applied Physiology*, *50*, 851–858.

Witcombe, B., & Meyer, D. (2006). Sword swallowing and its side effects. *British Medical Journal*, *333*, 1285–1287.

Name Index

Subject Index

A

B

C

D

E

F

G

H

I

K

L

M

N

O

P

Q

R

S

T

U

W

X

Y

Z